Nursing Diagnosis
Application to Clinical Practice

D1399754

Nursing Diagnosis
Application to Clinical Practice

Third Edition

Lynda Juall Carpenito, R.N., M.S.N.
Nursing Consultant, Mickleton, New Jersey

with 35 additional contributors

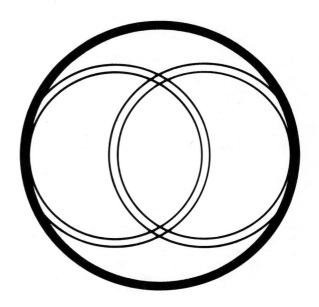

J. B. Lippincott Company
Philadelphia

Grand Rapids   New York   St. Louis   San Francisco
London   Sydney   Tokyo

Acquisitions Editor: Nancy Mullins
Coordinating Editorial Assistant: Ellen Campbell
Project Editor: Lorraine D. Smith
Manuscript Editors: Gail Turner and Dorothy Wright
Indexer: Ellen Murray
Design/Production Coordinator: Kathryn Rule
Compositor: Circle Graphics
Printer/Binder: R. R. Donnelley & Sons Company
Cover Printer: Phoenix Color Corp

Library of Congress Cataloging-in-Publication Data

Carpenito, Lynda Juall.
  Nursing diagnosis.

  Includes bibliographies and index.
  1. Diagnosis.   2. Nursing.   I. Title. [DNLM:
1. Nursing Assessment—outlines.   2. Patient Care
Planning—outlines. WY 18 C294n]
RI48.C37 1989   616.07'5'024613   89-8292
ISBN 0-397-54764-1

Any procedure or practice described in this book should
be applied by the health-care practitioner under
appropriate supervision in accordance with professional
standards of care used with regard to the unique
circumstances that apply in each practice situation. Care
has been taken to confirm the accuracy of information
presented and to describe generally accepted practices.
However, the author, editors, and publisher cannot
accept any responsibility for errors or omissions or for
consequences from application of the information in this
book and make no warranty, express or implied, with
respect to the contents of the book.

Every effort has been made to ensure that drug
selections and dosages are in accordance with current
recommendations and practice. Because of ongoing
research, changes in government regulations, and the
constant flow of information on drug therapy, reactions,
and interactions, the reader is cautioned to check the
package insert for each drug for indications, dosages,
warnings, and precautions, particularly if the drug is new
or infrequently used.

To Richard, my husband
Through bright and dark you are there, thank you again.

It was such a pretty day we decided
    to take a walk,
And we had not gone ten steps
    before I knew
That you and I are long past the point
    of no return.

Hand in hand we go.
Still close, still loving,
Still looking and overlooking
The flaws we hide from others.

Side by side we move,
Sometimes closer, sometimes farther apart.
Because of ways we read and talk,
Agree and disagree.

Step by step we advance
Against the cynics
Those all-knowing unknowings who
    honestly think
Marriage is dead.

—Lois Wyse, "I Still Love You"

Contributors

Rosalinda Alfaro, R.N., M.S.N., Lecturer, Immaculata College, Immaculata, Pennsylvania, Per Diem Staff Nurse, Intensive Care Unit, Paoli Memorial Hospital, Paoli, Pennsylvania

(Potential Altered Respiratory Function; Ineffective Airway Clearance; Ineffective Breathing Patterns; Activity Intolerance related to insufficient oxygenation secondary to impaired gas exchange; Diversional Activity Deficit; Impaired Verbal Communication; Fluid Volume Deficit; Fluid Volume Excess; Potential Altered Temperature Regulation; Altered Temperature Regulation, and Hyperthermia/Hypothermia)

Virginia Arcangelo, R.N., M.S.N., Nursing Consultant, Marlton, New Jersey

(Sexual Dysfunction)

Cynthia Balin, R.N., M.S.N., Director of Clinical Services, Kissimmee Memorial Hospital, Kissimmee, Florida

(Altered Nutrition: Less Than Body Requirements; Altered Nutrition: More Than Body Requirements; Powerlessness; and Impaired Swallowing)

Eleanor A. Bell, B.S., C.N.A., Director of Nursing, Bryn Mawr Rehabilitation Hospital, Malvern, Pennsylvania

(Self-Care Deficit)

Michelle Bockrath, R.N., M.S.N., Instructor, College of Nursing, University of Pennsylvania, Philadelphia, Pennsylvania

(Sleep Pattern Disturbance and sections of Sensory–Perceptual Alterations, First Edition)

Christine Cannon, R.N., M.S.N., Coordinator of Patient Education, Wilmington Medical Center, Wilmington, Delaware

(Altered Health Maintenance [selected sections, First Edition])

Nancy Conrad, R.N., M.S.N., Assistant Professor, Department of Nursing, Rutgers University, Camden, New Jersey

(Fear)

Janet Derrington, R.N., M.S.N., Psychiatric Clinical Specialist, Wilmington Medical Center, Wilmington, Delaware

(Selected sections of Potential for Violence, First Edition)

Linda Goldberg, R.N., M.A., Instructor, St. Joseph's School of Nursing, Reading, Pennsylvania

(Grieving, First Edition)

Judy A. Hartmann, Director of Nursing, Kansas Rehabilitation Hospital, Topeka, Kansas

(Altered Patterns of Urinary Elimination; Unilateral Neglect; Activity Intolerance [selected sections]; and Impaired Adjustment [selected sections])

Sandra Jansen, R.N., A.C.C.E., A.S.P.O., Certified Childbirth Educator, AASECT Sex Educator, Los Angeles, California

(Ineffective Breast-feeding and Altered Patterns of Sexuality related to changes in body function or image during and after pregnancy)

Elizabeth Keech, R.N., M.S.N., Instructor, College of Nursing, Villanova University, Villanova, Pennsylvania

(Selected sections of Altered Parenting, First Edition)

Margaret Kendrick, R.N., M.S.N., Assistant Professor, College of Nursing, Villanova University, Villanova, Pennsylvania

(Selected sections of Fluid Volume Deficit; Fluid Volume Excess; and Potential for Injury, First Edition)

Susan Kitchell, R.N., M.S., Pediatric Clinical Nurse Specialist, San Francisco, California

(Selected sections of Parental Role Conflict related to Hospitalized Child)

Deborah Lekan–Rutledge, M.S.N., R.N.C., Nursing Consultant

(High-Risk Elderly Assessment and High-Risk Elderly Principles and Rationale)

Carol Lillis, R.N., M.S.N., Instructor, Delaware County Community College, Media, Pennsylvania

(Altered Bowel Elimination, First Edition)

Jo Ann Maklebust, M.S.N., R.N., C.S., Case Manager, Surgical Patient Services, Harper Hospital, Detroit Medical Center, Detroit, Michigan

(Altered Tissue Integrity; Potential Altered Health Maintenance related to lack of knowledge of ostomy care; Impaired Skin Integrity; and Pruritus)

Bonnie McDonald Wakefield, R.N., M.A., Quality Assurance/Research, Nursing Service, VA Medical Center, Iowa City, Iowa

(Selected sections of Altered Health Maintenance, Second Edition)

Glenda S. McGaha, Ph.D., R.N., Department of Nursing, Southeast Missouri State University, Cape Girardeau, Missouri

(Altered Growth and Development)

Janet Hoffman Mennies, R.N.C., M.S.N., Adult Nurse Practitioner

(Noncompliance; Ineffective Individual Coping; Altered Health Maintenance; Selected sections of Altered Family Processes; and Health-Seeking Behavior)

Kathe H. Morris, R.N., M.S.N., Assistant Professor, College of Nursing, Villanova University, Villanova, Pennsylvania

(Rape Trauma Syndrome)

Nursing Diagnosis Discussion Group, Nancy A. Eppich, Chairwoman, Rainbow Babies and Children Hospital, University Hospitals of Cleveland, Cleveland, Ohio

(Parental Role Conflict)

Catherine Oblaczynski, R.N., M.S.N., Associate Professor, College of Nursing, Villanova University, Villanova, Pennsylvania

(Selected sections of Altered Thought Processes, First Edition)

Patricia O'Brien O'Riordan, R.N., M.S.N., Director, E. I. du Pont Division, Wilmington Medical Center, Wilmington, Delaware

(Impaired Physical Mobility, First Edition)

Mary M. Owen, R.N., B.S.N., P.H.N., Nurse Epidemiologist, Martin Luther Hospital Medical Center, Anaheim, California

(Potential for Infection and Potential for Infection Transmission)

Deborah Soholt, R.N., B.S.N., Head Nurse, Urology, St. Luke's Midland Regional Medical Center, Aberdeen, South Dakota

Mary Sieggreen, M.S.N., R.N., C.S., Case Manager, Surgical Patient Services, Harper Hospital, Detroit Medical Center, Detroit, Michigan

(Altered Peripheral Tissue Perfusion and Potential for Injury related to Effects Secondary to Orthostatic Hypotension)

Anna Mae Spaniolo, R.N., B.S.N., M.S.N., Nurse Educator, Bronson Methodist Hospital School of Nursing, Kalamazoo, Michigan

(Potential for Injury related to Maturational Age)

Katsuko Tanaka, R.N., M.S., C.S., Staff Nurse, Alcohol and Drug Dependent Treatment Program, Seattle Veterans Administration Medical Center, Seattle, Washington

(Post-Trauma Response)

Laura A. Terrill, R.N., M.S.N., Director of Nursing Education, Wilmington Medical Center, Wilmington, Delaware

(Disturbance in Self-Concept and Social Isolation)

Carol Van Antwerp, R.N., M.S., Nurse Educator, Bronson Methodist Hospital School of Nursing, Kalamazoo, Michigan

(Potential for Injury related to Maturational Age)

Mary Mishler Vogel, R.N., M.S.N., Instructor, Helene Fuld School of Nursing, Camden, New Jersey

(Selected sections of Altered Patterns of Urinary Elimination, First Edition)

Julie Waterhouse, R.N., M.S., Instructor, College of Nursing, University of Delaware, Newark, Delaware

(Spiritual Distress)

Janet R. Weber, R.N., M.S.N., Instructor, Southeast Missouri State University, Cape Girardeau, Missouri

(Hopelessness)

Anne E. Willard, R.N., M.S.N., Associate Professor, Cumberland County College, Vineland, New Jersey

(Anxiety; Potential for Violence; Ineffective Family Coping; Altered Thought Processes; Potential for Self-Harm; Impaired Social Interactions; Self-Esteem Disturbance; Defensive Coping; and Ineffective Denial)

Consultants

Philip N. Barkins, R.P.T., Private Practice, Dover, Delaware

Carol Bechtold, R.N., M.S.N., Assistant Administrator/Education, Department of Nursing, The Hospital Center at Orange, Orange, New Jersey

Benjamin M. Evans, R.N., O.N.P., M.S.C., Nurse Consultant and Counselor, Evansville, Indiana

Ann Feins, R.D., Assistant Professor, Saint Anselm College, Manchester, New Hampshire

Jean W. Fitzgerald, R.N., E.T., Enterostomal Therapist, Wilmington Medical Center, Wilmington, Delaware

Annette D. Friday, R.N., Head Nurse, Neonatal Intensive Care Unit, Wilmington Medical Center, Wilmington, Delaware

Margaret M. Hirst, R.N., M.S.N., Clinical Specialist in Oncology, Wilmington Medical Center, Wilmington, Delaware

Jacqueline W. Levett, R.N., M.S.N., Pediatric Clinical Specialist, Wilmington Medical Center, Wilmington, Delaware

Susan Ross, R.N., M.S., Assistant Professor, American International College, Springfield, Massachusetts

Rebecca Rush, M.Ed., Cognitive Therapist, The Center at Plaza Medical, Camden, New Jersey

Linda H. Snow, R.N., M.S., Assistant Professor, American International College, Springfield, Massachusetts

Fe Ayalin Tamparong, R.N., M.A., Director of Education, AMI Circle City Hospital, Corona, California

Carl K. Wyckoff III, D.D.S., Private practice, Wenonah, New Jersey

Preface

The practice of nursing often interfaces with the practices of the other health care providers.* Sometimes the nurse sees the client problems that require referral for treatment and ignores or fails to detect the problems that she can treat independently. *Nursing Diagnosis: Application to Clinical Practice* focuses on the diagnosis and treatment of client situations that the nurse can and should treat, legally and independently. It provides a condensed, organized outline of clinical nursing practice designed to communicate creative clinical nursing. It is not meant to replace textbooks of nursing, but rather to provide nurses in a variety of settings with the information they need without requiring a time-consuming review of the literature.

From assessment criteria to specific interventions, the book focuses on nursing. It will assist students in transferring their theoretical knowledge to clinical practice; it can also be used by experienced nurses to recall past learning and to intervene in those clinical situations that previously went ignored or unrecognized.

The author believes that nursing needs a classification system to organize its functions and define its scope. Use of such a classification system would expedite research activities and facilitate communication between nurses, consumers, and other health care providers. After all, medicine took over 100 years to develop its taxonomy. Our work, at the national level, was only begun in 1973 and is still in an early stage. It is hoped that the reader will be stimulated to participate at the local, regional, or national level in the utilization and development of these diagnostic categories.

Since the first edition was published, the use of nursing diagnosis has increased markedly throughout the United States and Canada. Practicing nurses vary in experience with nursing diagnosis from just beginning to full practice integration for over six years. With such a variance in use, questions posed from the neophyte, such as

- What does the label really mean?
- What kinds of assessment questions will yield nursing diagnoses?
- How do I tailor a diagnostic category for a specific individual?
- How should I intervene after I formulate the diagnostic statement?
- How do I care-plan with nursing diagnoses?

differ dramatically from the questions from experts as

- Can medical diagnoses be included in a nursing diagnosis statement?
- What is the difference between potential and possible nursing diagnoses?
- What kind of problem statement should I write to describe a person at risk for hemorrhage?
- What kind of nursing diagnosis should I use to describe a healthy person?

This third edition seeks to continue to answer these questions.

Section I begins with a chapter on the historic etiology of nursing diagnosis and the work of the North American Nursing Diagnosis Association (NANDA). The concepts of

*The model of interlocking circles on the cover depicts this relationship. The common area represents those activities on which all professionals collaborate; the rest denotes the dimensions for which each professional prescribes definitive interventions to prevent or treat.

classification and taxonomic issues are explored. The third edition discusses the review process of NANDA and describes the evolving taxonomy of NANDA's Human Response Patterns.

Chapter 2 presents the Bifocal Clinical Nursing Model, which differentiates nursing diagnoses from other problems that nurses treat. This edition further describes the Bifocal Clinical Nursing Model by the relationships of interventions and outcome criteria to nursing diagnoses and collaborative problems. The components of the diagnostic statement are explained, as are actual, potential, and possible nursing diagnoses.

Chapter 3 focuses on the assessment and diagnosis components of the nursing process with clinical application. This edition expands on the differentiation between a focus assessment and a data base assessment.

Chapter 4 describes the process of care planning and care planning systems. Techniques are presented for evolving diagnoses from the assessment data and for writing diagnostic statements and goals. This edition illustrates a defer component for an admission data base and includes an example of a nursing admission data base with discharge planning incorporated. Examples of outcome criteria from the literature are critiqued. Guidelines are presented to provide assistance in writing measurable goals with a time frame for achievement. Nursing interventions are discussed in the context of independent versus delegated. The types of evaluations are discussed and examples presented. The third edition expands the description of care planning systems, including standards of care and standardized care plans. Examples of standards for collaborative problems and nursing diagnoses are included. The concept of addendum care plans is introduced.

Section I concludes with two case studies which allow reader participation.

Section II is a compilation of the nursing diagnostic categories accepted by the North American Nursing Diagnosis Association and additional clinically useful categories.

The third edition has 101 diagnostic categories (95 NANDA approved with 6 added by the author). In addition to the new diagnostic categories, sections have been added on substance abuse, end-of-life decisions, perioperative teaching for children, socio/cultural implications of rape, remotivation therapy, prevention of AIDS transmission, dysfunctional grieving, body image, chemotherapy and dehydration in the elderly. A list of collaborative problems is presented in Appendix XI. Each diagnostic category is explained by the following components:

- Definition
- Defining characteristics
- Etiological, contributing, risk factors
- Focus assessment criteria
- Principles and rationale for nursing care

Author's notes have been included for each diagnostic category. The author's notes serve to assist the student and nurse by clarifying the category and by differentiating it from other similar categories.

Each diagnostic category is followed by one or more specific nursing diagnoses that relate to familiar clinical situations. These specific diagnoses are defined by subjective and objective assessment data. Outcome criteria for the diagnosis are provided with the related interventions, which represent activities in the independent domain of nursing derived from the physical and applied sciences, pharmacology, nutrition, mental health, and nursing research.

This book is intended to assist nurses in addressing all the human needs of individuals, with the expectation that—as more "nursing" is added to nursing—the profession, the nurse person, and, most importantly, the client will reap the rewards.

For no other reason than to avoid awkward and redundant reading, the author has chosen to use *she* and *her* when referring to the nurse and *he, his,* and *him* when referring to the client.

The author invites comments or suggestions from readers. Correspondence can be directed to the publisher or to the author's address: 66 East Rattling Run Road, Mickleton, NJ 08056.

Lynda Juall Carpenito,R.N., M.S.N.

Acknowledgments

A sincere thank you to all my good friends who continue to sustain our friendships, despite my schedule. I wish to thank my typist and friend Maria Manel for more than her typing. I am grateful for the ongoing professional support from J. B. Lippincott, the editorial guidance of editor-in-chief, Nancy Mullins, senior editor, Diana Intenzo, Ellen Campbell, and the creativity of the marketing department.

Since the first edition, hundreds of nurse colleagues have shared their experiences with nursing diagnoses and have challenged me to grow, learn, and change. I am grateful for their challenges. Also, thank you to those departments of nursing that have shared their success stories after integration of the Bifocal Clinical Nursing Model.

At last, I would like to thank Laura Terrill for her moral and professional support, the group in Detroit (JoAnn Maklebust, Mary Sieggreen, Linda Mondoux) for our late night talks, Rosalinda Alfaro, who recognized the need for the book and sought to make it a reality, and lastly, a very special person, my son, Olen Juall Carpenito, who too often is expected to understand the commitments of his Mom and to put his wishes on hold. I still owe you several games of monopoly.

Contents

V
Maternal Data Base Assessment Guide

VI
Noninvasive Pain Relief Techniques

VII
Guidelines for Problem-Solving and Crisis Intervention

VIII
Guidelines for Preparing Diagnostic Categories

IX
Guidelines for Play Therapy

X
Stress Management Techniques

XI
Collaborative Problems

Section I

The Nursing Process

Introduction

Nursing is primarily assisting individuals (sick or well) with those activities contributing to health or its recovery (or to a peaceful death) that they perform unaided when they have the necessary strength, will, or knowledge; nursing also helps individuals carry out prescribed therapy and to be independent of assistance as soon as possible.*

Individuals are open systems who continually interact with the environment, creating individual interaction patterns. These patterns are dynamic and interact with life processes (physiological, psychological, sociocultural, developmental, and spiritual) to influence the individual's behavior and health. A person becomes a client not only when an actual or potential alteration in this interaction pattern compromises his health but also when the person desires assistance to achieve a higher level of health.

Nursing diagnosis describes health states or disrupted interaction patterns with which the nurse can assist the client. The nurse provides the primary assistance to clients with these responses, just as the physician provides primary assistance for medical pathology. Nursing diagnoses focus on the human response as opposed to the cellular response.

Health is the state of wellness as defined by the client; it is no longer defined as whether or not a biological disease is present. Health is a dynamic, ever-changing state influenced by past and present interaction patterns. The individual is an expert on himself and is responsible for seeking or refusing health care.

The use of the term *client* in place of the term *patient* to identify the health care consumer suggests an autonomous person who has freedom of choice in seeking and selecting assistance. The client is no longer a passive recipient of services but an active participant who assumes responsibility for his choices and also for the consequences of those choices. *Family* is used to describe any person or persons who serve as support systems to the client. *Group* is used to describe support systems as well as communities such as senior citizen centers. Societal health needs have changed in the last decade; so must the nurse's view of the consumers of health care (individual, family, community).†

Nursing diagnosis provides nurses with an opportunity to pinpoint the health alterations of individuals in a concise and systematic manner while also describing the individual's unique situation.

---

* Henderson V, Nite G: Principles and Practice of Nursing, 5th ed, p 14. New York, Macmillan, 1960.

† Carpenito LJ, Duespohl TA: A Guide to Effective Clinical Instruction, 2nd ed, pp 3, 4. Rockville, MD, Aspen Systems Corp, 1985.

1

Nursing Diagnosis: The Beginning

Nursing diagnosis provides a useful mechanism for structuring nursing knowledge in an attempt to define the unique role and domain of nursing. The quest to define nursing and its functions began with the writings of Nightingale. In her words, the purpose of nursing is "to put the patient in the best condition for nature to act upon him." In the early 20th century, attempts to differentiate nursing from medicine stemmed from the need to define each of these disciplines for legislative and educational purposes. V. Henderson in 1955 and F. Abdellah in 1960 proposed organizing nursing curriculums according to nursing problems or patient needs, rather than medical diagnoses.

The trend to focus nursing education on the principal functions of nursing rather than on medicine continues today with the development of nursing models. During the late 1960s and '70s, nurses sought to organize nursing knowledge and practice through the construction of theoretical or conceptual frameworks. Examples of such frameworks are Roy's adaptation model, Johnson's behavioral system model, Orem's self-care concept of nursing, Rogers's life process theory, and Newman's health systems model. The work of these theorists can help distinguish nursing phenomena within the broad field of health care.

Criticism of most theories and frameworks usually arises from difficulty in applying them to clinical practice. In a critique of theory development in nursing, Kritek (p. 34) submits that most nursing theories "describe how nursing should be, not how it is in reality." She notes that the use of poorly defined or confusing terms by theorists only serves to limit professional application of these theories. Kritek advocates beginning with a theory that is operational in nature, one that describes "what we see and what we do," rather than with one that appears sophisticated but is obscure.

Nursing diagnosis can provide a solution to the quest of nursing because it serves to:

- Define nursing in its present state
- Classify the domain of nursing
- Differentiate nursing from medicine
- Identify nursing knowledge for students

The Concept of Nursing Diagnosis

The word *diagnosis* evokes many responses in nurses—some positive, some negative. Because nurses have historically linked the word diagnosis exclusively with medicine, some may tend to overlook the fact that teachers diagnose teaming disabilities, hair-dressers diagnose hair problems, and mechanics diagnose automotive disorders. In addition, many nurses were taught to avoid making definitive statements when documenting and were advised to use terms such as "seems to be" or "appears to be." This socialization process rewarded nurses *for* not diagnosing.

By dictionary definition, diagnosis is the careful, critical study of something in order to determine its nature. The question is not *whether* nurses can diagnose but *what* nurses can diagnose.

In 1953 the term *nursing diagnosis* was introduced by V. Fry to describe a step necessary in developing a nursing care plan. For the next 20 years, references to nursing diagnosis appeared only sporadically in the literature. However, from 1973 (when the first meeting of the National Group for the Classification of Nursing Diagnosis was held) to the present, attention in the literature has increased tenfold, and various definitions of nursing diagnosis have appeared, four of which follow. These definitions describe nursing diagnosis as problems, responses, evaluation, or judgment.

Definitions of Nursing Diagnosis

- An independent nursing function; an evaluation of a client's personal responses to his human experiences throughout the life cycle, be they developmental or accidental crises, illness, hardships, or other stresses (Bircher)
- Actual or potential health problems that nurses, by virtue of their education and experience, are able and licensed to treat (Gordon)
- Responses to actual or potential health problems that nurses, by virtue of their education and experience, are able, licensed, and legally responsible and accountable to treat (Moritz)
- A clinical judgment about an individual, family, or community that is derived through a deliberate, systematic process of data collection and analysis. It provides the basis for prescriptions for definitive therapy for which the nurse is accountable (Shoemaker)

In 1973, the American Nurses' Association (ANA) published the Standards of Practice; they were followed in 1980 by the ANA Social Policy Statement, which defined nursing as follows:

Nursing is the diagnosis and treatment of human response to actual or potential health problems.

Most state nurse practice acts describe nursing in accordance with the ANA definition.

Nursing Diagnosis: Process or Outcome?

A review of the literature reveals that, over time, the term *nursing diagnosis* has been used in three contexts:

- As the second step of the nursing process
- As a list of diagnostic labels or titles
- As a two-part or three-part statement

1. *As the second step of the nursing process.* In the second step of the nursing process, the data collected during the assessment of the client's health status is analyzed, and problems are identified. Some of the conclusions resulting from data analysis will lead to nursing diagnoses, but others will not. It is important to recognize that the outcome of this process can include problems that are primarily treated by nurses and problems that require treatment by several disciplines. For example, while assessing a particular client, the nurse may record observations that

point to the medical problems of seizures, hypoglycemia, and hypertension, as well as the nursing diagnosis of potential for injury. Using the term *nursing diagnosis* to designate the second step of the nursing process can be confusing and may have the undesirable effect of leading nurses to try to state all conclusions or problems as nursing diagnoses.

2. *As a list of diagnostic labels or titles.* After the first conference on nursing diagnosis in 1973, the term nursing diagnosis was applied to specific labels describing health states that nurses could legally diagnose and treat. The purpose of establishing these labels was to define and classify the scope of nursing. These labels are concise descriptors of a cluster of signs and symptoms like anxiety or altered family processes, or risk factors such as Potential for Infection.

3. *As a two-part or three-part statement.* Nurses use the term nursing diagnosis to describe a two-part or three-part statement about an individual's, a family's, or a group's response to a situation or a health problem.

Thus, it has become necessary to indicate clearly whether the term nursing diagnosis is being used in the context of problem identification (critical thinking), a classification system of diagnostic labels such as that developed by the North American Nursing Diagnosis Association (NANDA), or an individualized statement.

In order to avoid misuse and confusion, the author recommends using the following terms:

- For the second step of the nursing process: *diagnosis.*
- For the list of diagnostic labels or titles: *diagnostic categories.*
- For the two-part or three-part statement: *nursing diagnosis.*

Nursing diagnosis is a statement describing one specific type of problem or situation that nurses identify. It should not be used to label all the problems nurses can ascertain, since such usage will not emphasize the unique role of the nurse. For the purpose of clarity, the use of the term in this book will be restricted to describing the two-part or three-part statement. Thus, nursing diagnosis is defined as follows:

A nursing diagnosis is a statement that describes the human response (health state or actual/potential altered interaction pattern) of an individual or group which the nurse can legally identify and for which the nurse can order the definitive interventions to maintain the health state or to reduce, eliminate, or prevent alterations.

The North American Nursing Diagnosis Association

When the first conference on nursing diagnosis was held in 1973, its purpose was to identify nursing functions and to establish a classification system suitable for computerization. From this conference developed the National Group for the Classification of Nursing Diagnosis. This group is composed of nurses from all regions of the United States and Canada, representing all elements of the profession: practice, education, and research. From 1973 to the present, the National Group has met eight times and formulated a list of diagnostic categories. These diagnostic categories are listed in the first column of Table 1-1.

(*Text continues on page 8*)

Table 1-1. **Diagnostic Categories**

Accepted Diagnoses from the North American Nursing Diagnosis Assn.	Year Accepted	An Amended List of Nursing Diagnoses*
Activity Intolerance	1982	
Adjustment, Impaired	1986	
Airway Clearance, Ineffective	1980	*Listed under* Altered Respiratory Function
Anxiety	1973	
Aspiration, Potential for	1988	
Body Image Disturbance	1973	
Body Temperature, Potential Altered	1986	
Bowel Elimination, Altered	1975	
Constipation	1975	
Colonic Constipation	1988	
Perceived Constipation	1988	
Diarrhea	1975	
Incontinence	1975	Combined with Diarrhea
Breastfeeding, Ineffective	1988	
Breathing Patterns, Ineffective	1980	*Listed under* Altered Respiratory Function
Cardiac Output, Decreased	1975	
Comfort, Altered: Pain	1978	Acute pain
Chronic Pain	1986	
Communication, Impaired Verbal	1973	
Coping, Ineffective Individual	1978	
Coping, Ineffective Family: Compromised	1980	
Coping, Ineffective Family: Disabling	1980	
Coping, Family: Potential for Growth	1980	*Listed under* Altered Health Maintenance
Decisional Conflict	1988	
Defensive Coping	1988	
Denial, Ineffective	1988	
Disuse Syndrome, Potential for	1988	
Diversional Activity Deficit	1980	
Dysreflexia	1988	
Family Processes, Altered	1982	
Fatigue	1988	
Fear (specify)	1980	
Fluid Volume Deficit, Actual	1978 ⎫	*Combined* as Fluid Volume Deficit
Fluid Volume Deficit, Potential	1978 ⎭	
Fluid Volume Excess	1982	
Gas Exchange, Impaired	1980	*Listed under* Altered Respiratory Function
Grieving, Anticipatory	1980	*Combined as* Grieving (specify)
Grieving, Dysfunctional	1980	
Growth & Development, Altered	1986	
Health Maintenance, Altered	1982	
Health-Seeking Behaviors (specify)	1988	
Home Maintenance Management, Impaired	1980	
Hopelessness	1986	
Hyperthermia	1986	
Hypothermia	1988R	

(continued)

Table 1-1.   **Diagnostic Categories** (Continued)

Accepted Diagnoses from the North American Nursing Diagnosis Assn.	Year Accepted	An Amended List of Nursing Diagnoses*
Incontinence, Functional	1986	
Incontinence, Reflex	1986	
Incontinence, Stress	1986	Listed under Altered Patterns of Urinary Elimination
Incontinence, Total	1986	
Incontinence, Urge	1986	
Infection, Potential for	1986	
Injury, Potential for (specify)	1978	
Poisoning	1980	
Suffocation	1980	
Trauma	1980	
Knowledge Deficit (specify)	1980	
Mobility, Impaired Physical	1973	
Noncompliance (specify)	1973, 1980	
Nutrition, Altered Less Than Body Requirements	1975	Combined as Nutrition, Altered More Than Body Requirements
Nutrition, Altered More Than Body Requirements	1975	
Nutrition, Altered Potential for More Than Body Requirements	1980	
Oral Mucous Membrane, Altered	1982	
Parental Role Conflict	1988	
Parenting, Altered: Actual	1978	Combined as Parenting, Altered
Parenting, Altered: Potential	1978	
Personal Identity Disturbance	1978	
Post-Trauma Response	1986	
Powerlessness	1982	
Rape Trauma Syndrome	1980	
Role Performance, Altered	1978	
Feeding Self-Care Deficit		
Bathing/Hygiene Self-Care Deficit		
Dressing/Grooming Self-Care Deficit		
Toileting Self-Care Deficit		
Self-Concept Disturbance	1980	
Self-Esteem Disturbance	1988R	
Self-Esteem, Chronic Low	1988	
Self-Esteem, Situational Low	1988	
Sensory–Perceptual, Altered	1978, 1980	
Visual		
Auditory		
Kinesthetic		
Gustatory		
Tactile		
Olfactory		
Sexual Dysfunction	1980	
Sexuality Patterns, Altered	1986	
Skin Integrity, Impaired Actual	1975	Combined as Skin Integrity, Impaired
Skin Integrity, Impaired Potential	1975	
Sleep Pattern Disturbance	1980	
Social Interaction, Impaired	1986	

(continued)

Table 1-1. **Diagnostic Categories** (Continued)

Accepted Diagnoses from the North American Nursing Diagnosis Assn.	Year Accepted	An Amended List of Nursing Diagnoses*
Social Isolation	1982	
Spiritual Distress	1978	
Swallowing, Impaired	1986	
Thermoregulation, Ineffective	1986	
Thought Processes, Altered	1973	
Tissue Integrity, Impaired	1986	

Tissue Perfusion, Altered (specify type)
  Cerebral
  Cardiopulmonary
  Renal
  Gastrointestinal
  Peripheral
	1980	

Unilateral Neglect	1986	
Urinary Elimination, Altered Patterns of	1973	
Urinary Retention	1986	
Violence, Potential for	1980	

*Where no category is given, the title is unchanged.
Note: R next to date indicates a revision.

At its first meeting in 1973, the National Group also appointed a task force to:

1. Gather information and disseminate it through the Clearinghouse for Nursing Diagnosis.†
2. Encourage educational activities at regional and state levels to promote the implementation of nursing diagnoses. These activities include conferences to organize nurses to identify additional diagnostic labels and workshops to teach nurses about nursing diagnoses.
3. Promote and organize activities to continue the development, classification, and scientific testing of nursing diagnosis. These activities include planning national conferences, identifying criteria for accepting diagnoses, surveying current research activities, and exploring varied methods for classification.

A proposal from the task force for a more formal organization was approved at the fifth national conference, and the group was renamed the North American Nursing Diagnosis Association. NANDA has elected officers, a board of directors, and standing committees.

Breu et al describe assimilation of scientific advances like nursing diagnosis into practice as, usually, a three-step process. Initially the research question is formulated and the research conducted. Next, the research findings are disseminated at scientific meetings and in journals. The third step is the incorporation of the relevant findings into clinical practice. This process is usually linear with little feedback (Breu).

The North American Nursing Diagnosis Association has taken a different approach to the scientific assimilation of nursing diagnosis into practice. It involves three concurrent activities: consensus development, research, and infiltration occurring in an open

†The Clearinghouse collects material on nursing diagnosis, publishes a newsletter, and coordinates the national conference. The address is: North American Nursing Diagnosis Assn. 3525 Caroline Street, St. Louis, MO 63104.

NANDA Organization
President
Vice-President
Secretary
Treasurer
Board of Directors (7)
Committees
    Program
    Nominating
    Publications
    Membership/Public Relations
    Taxonomic
    Diagnostic Review
    Regional Affairs

system (Breu). As diagnostic categories are being identified, clinical research using selected designs (Gordon, Sweeney, Fehring) test and refine assumptions.

Clinicians utilize the diagnostic categories accepted by NANDA for clinical testing and submit revisions to NANDA. Integration of nursing diagnosis into nursing curricula and literature serves to further disseminate the work of NANDA. Figure 1-1 contrasts the traditional versus NANDA's method to incorporate scientific advances into practice.

In December 1986, an advisory panel on Classification for Nursing Practice of the American Nursing Association met with liaisons from NANDA. Their purpose was to formally submit a nursing system to the World Health Organization for possible inclusion

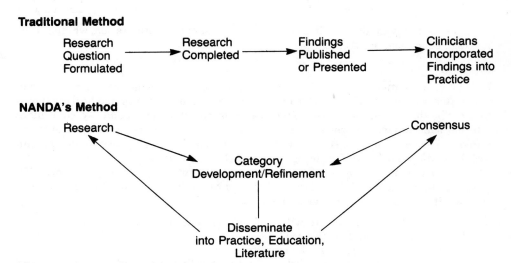

Fig. 1-1 Traditional method versus NANDA's method of incorporating scientific advances into practice.

in the tenth revision of the International Code of Diseases. The document that was submitted represented a compilation of the work of NANDA, the Omaha Classification System, and the Psychiatric–Mental Health Council of the ANA. In August 1987, as the result of collaborative work of the ANA and NANDA, a replacement document was sent to the WHO. This document represents the classification system of NANDA. Also, at this time the American Nursing Association officially sanctioned the North American Nursing Diagnosis Association as the organization to govern the development of a classification system of nursing diagnoses. The Councils of the ANA have been advised to submit proposed diagnostic categories to NANDA. This timely and significant action by the American Nurses Association will facilitate a uniform classification system for the nursing profession.

Why a Taxonomy?

Why does nursing need a classification system, or taxonomy? While perceived reasons will vary according to the individual nurse's focus, nursing in general needs a classification system to describe and develop a sound scientific foundation in order to fulfill one of the criteria for professional status. The requisites commonly demanded of an occupational group seeking to claim professional status are listed by Styles as follows:

An extensive university education
A unique body of knowledge
An orientation of service to others
A professional society
Autonomy and self-regulation

A classification system for nursing will define the body of knowledge for which nursing will be held accountable. The relationship of nursing diagnosis to accountability and autonomy can be expressed as follows:

Nursing Diagnosis ⟶ Clearer identification ⟶ Greater accountability ⟶ Greater
of the body of nursing   professional
knowledge   autonomy

A single taxonomy would benefit all nurses regardless of their orientation, whether it be practice, education, or research.

Practice

Using a classification system to identify nursing's domain provides nurses with a common frame of reference. Historically, nurses have been educated to use medical diagnoses to describe the nursing focus. Since medical terminology provides an easy, convenient solution, some nurses have resisted other, more nursing-oriented terminology. Clinicians would rather use terms like congestive heart failure, asthma, and placenta previa, than social isolation, impaired skin integrity, and self-care deficits.

The need for a common, consistent language for a profession was identified over 200 years ago by medicine. If physicians had elected to use just any word to describe their clinical situations, as nursing does, then:

- How could they communicate with each other? With nurses?
- How would research be organized?
- How would new practitioners be educated?
- How could quality assurance be achieved if the diagnoses could not be retrieved systematically?

For example, prior to the formal labeling Acquired Immunodeficiency Sy⁻
it was difficult or perhaps impossible to define or study the disease
records would have a variety of diagnoses or causes of death such a
hemorrhage, or Kaposi's sarcoma that were listed to describe the indiv...

A unified system of terminology will establish a common denominator that .
direct nurses to assess selected data and identify a potential or an actual client problem.
Nurses can then refer to the list of terms to assist them in describing the problem.
Consistent terminology makes oral and written communication easier and more efficient.
In addition, identifying definitive nursing functions will increase the nurse's accountability in assessing the patient, determining the diagnosis, and providing the treatment
called for by the diagnosis. Knowledge of the unique responsibilities of nursing will in
turn stimulate nurses to acquire new knowledge and skills to use as they intervene to
solve these problems.

From the viewpoint of health care delivery, a classification of nursing diagnoses
would establish a system suitable for computerization. With the potential for computer
use, nursing diagnosis would:

- Provide nurses with a system for retrieving client records using nursing, not medical,
  diagnoses
- Provide an opportunity for nurses to develop or be included in a computerized health
  care information system that would collect, analyze, and synthesize nursing data for
  practice, literature, and research
- Provide a mechanism for the reimbursement of nursing activities related to nursing
  diagnoses, not medical diagnoses

Clarifying nursing for nurses, employers, the public, and third-party payers can only
serve to strengthen and enrich the profession.

Research

A taxonomy of nursing diagnosis would provide a framework for clinical investigation
with the potential for growth in research and knowledge. Each diagnostic category—its
defining characteristics as well as the related nursing interventions should be developed
and tested through research.

In 1987, McLane reviewed computer listings, literature indexes, and the Proceedings
from the NANDA Conferences to locate research that contributed to the measurement
and validation of diagnostic concepts. Approximately 62 studies were identified. Recommendations for further studies include the need to focus on replication, reliability, and
validity of the instrument, use of case studies, and standardization of diagnostic concepts.

Publishers of nursing texts are encouraging authors to use the NANDA approved
diagnostic categories in their work. As the generation of nurses who were educated with
nursing diagnoses begin to publish, one can expect to see this terminology used exclusively.

Nursing diagnosis, because of its clear clinical implications, seems to stimulate
clinical nurses to investigate. Research on diagnostic categories has been stimulated by
the research models of Fehring, Gordon, and Sweeney. These models serve to measure the
degree of reliability and validity of a category. Since 1980, the published research on
nursing diagnosis has increased appreciably, as has the multitude of unpublished studies
conducted in health care agencies in the United States and Canada. This serves as
evidence that the development and refinement of nursing diagnostic categories have
taken on ownership by many and not just by a choice group.

ı education, nursing diagnosis will enable educators and students to focus on nursing phenomena rather than on medical phenomena. It challenges students to think critically, rather than simply to assume that because a client has a particular medical diagnosis, certain nursing actions are the only ones warranted.

In order to practice nursing, students of nursing need to learn content from the natural, physical, and behavioral sciences, the humanities, and nursing research. Often, nursing diagnosis is used as the vehicle to teach this content. This is an inaccurate use of nursing diagnosis.

Nursing diagnostic categories are not intended to encompass all the theoretical knowledge a nurse needs for practice. Impaired gas exchange should not replace the term pneumonia, nor should Sensory-Perceptual Alteration replace retinal detachment. The student should be taught pathophysiology, treatment, therapies, diagnostic studies, and so forth, and then the human response to these situations. Most of these situations can contribute to several nursing diagnoses rather than just one.

Students will be able to explore and appreciate the complexity and rigor of nursing as it relates to nursing diagnosis. The use of nursing diagnoses permits the nurse to go beyond the medical model and identify those problems that may or may not be related to the medical diagnoses. By relinquishing the practice of medicine to physicians, nurses can assume more completely their unique role as health care providers.

The steps that have been taken toward the development of a nursing taxonomy have been small, but at least they have been taken. The future movement on taxonomic development is linked, says Gebbie, "with the movement toward professional and scientific maturity, and each feeds on the other" (p. 12).

The Classification Process

Classification systems for other professionals (such as physicians, biologists, and pharmacists) developed over hundreds of years; nurses have only just begun. It is a slow and difficult process. Since nursing cannot stop and wait until the classification is complete, practice must continue while the classification evolves.

Two research methods can be used to identify and validate nursing diagnosis nomenclature, the inductive and the deductive. The inductive approach moves from specific observations to generalizations; it is a generalization based on observed relationships. The nurse's observations and additional support cited from related literature serve as a basis for a tentative explanation of the relationship. A prediction can then be derived to test the association. The deductive approach, on the other hand, begins with generalizations and moves toward specific observations.

Previously, NANDA used the inductive method to generate nursing diagnoses. Nurses with various clinical and educational experience collaborated to identify and describe health problems that nurses diagnose and treat. These nurses recalled from their experiences and from the related literature those clinical phenomena that describe varied states of health. Defining characteristics were identified to describe these states. It was expected that this approach would initially yield fairly general diagnostic categories that could be used by most nurses.

The process for generating and accepting diagnostic categories changed in 1984 when NANDA established a Diagnostic Review Committee (DRC) to create a review process for the approval of new diagnoses. The review process begins when a nurse or a group of nurses submits a new diagnosis according to the guidelines for submission (see Appendix VIII). Figure 1-2 outlines the diagnosis review cycle. In 1986, several new diagnostic categories were approved. A more concise style of wording was used for some of the new

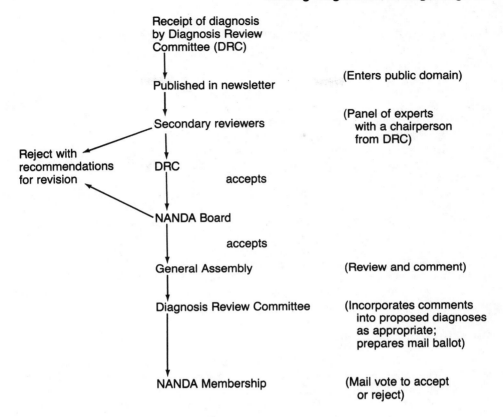

Receipt of diagnosis
by Diagnosis Review
Committee (DRC)

Published in newsletter   (Enters public domain)

Secondary reviewers   (Panel of experts
                                      with a chairperson
                                      from DRC)

Reject with
recommendations   DRC
for revision   accepts

NANDA Board

                  accepts

General Assembly   (Review and comment)

Diagnosis Review Committee   (Incorporates comments
                                      into proposed diagnoses
                                      as appropriate;
                                      prepares mail ballot)

NANDA Membership   (Mail vote to accept
                                      or reject)

Fig. 1-2 The diagnosis review cycle.

categories (for example, Altered Sexuality Patterns instead of Alterations in Sexuality Patterns).

The 1988 review cycle reviewed 61 categories; 39 were rejected, 17 were accepted, and five were placed on hold. Two categories were revisions (Self Esteem Disturbance and Hypothermia). Several diagnostic categories represented more specification of previously accepted categories, such as Colonic Constipation and Perceived Constipation under Altered Bowel Elimination, and Chronic Low Self-Esteem and Situational Low Self-Esteem under Self-Esteem Disturbance.

At the review sessions at the General Assembly in March 1988, much discussion focused on the present review process and suggestions for improvement. Of particular concern were the changes made to diagnoses after submission and in response to the General Assembly Review.

The rigor in the development of the 16 diagnostic categories (one of the 17 originally accepted had later been rejected) that were accepted was evident. Nine of the categories had validation studies prior to submission. Conference participants suggested that proposed diagnostic categories be returned to the submitter with the review and comments for their revision. Perhaps submitters whose work is accepted by the reviewers and the DRC can present their work formally at the NANDA Conference. This process would provide the submitter with additional dialogue with interested nurses. The diagnosis could then be reexamined again for revisions if indicated for final DRC review.

Nurses using NANDA's diagnostic categories will note variations in the level of conceptualization. Some nurses have criticized the list for being too broad or too restrictive, and certain diagnoses as being too medical, too abstract, or too unfamiliar. Some nurses are philosophically opposed to the use of such diagnoses as *Noncompliance* or *Knowledge Deficit*.

Disagreement with particular items in any classification system can be expected. However, the individual has always had the prerogative of simply not using those items. For example, in medicine a physician may disagree with the diagnosis *schizophrenia* and will refrain from using it in his practice. This physician does not reject the entire medical classification system, only one diagnosis. And systems change. When the medical classification system was still evolving, dropsy was listed as an accepted diagnosis; years later, it was removed.

If nursing is to become a full profession, it needs to develop and accept one classification system for those functions and responsibilities that are solely those of the nurse. Individual practitioners who are uncomfortable with the list should use only those labels that have meaning for them and develop diagnoses to describe the other clinical responses they treat. The use of the list by these nurses will help to refine and expand it. New proposed diagnostic categories can then be submitted to NANDA for consideration. (Guidelines for preparing diagnostic categories appear in Appendix VIII.) The task of developing additional diagnostic categories should be the responsibility of nurses from all practice and educational settings.

Classification Systems

The classification efforts that began in 1973 produced categories that are listed alphabetically. The alphabet, although well known to all, does not provide a theoretical basis for the work of classification. In 1976, Sister Callista Roy proposed convening a group of nurse theorists to assist with developing a framework for the classification system. This framework would provide (Roy):

- Rules for eligibility for acceptance into the system
- The place the label will hold in the system
- Rules for the set of labels and subsets

The work of the initial theorist group and subsequently of the taxonomic committee of NANDA has produced the beginnings of a conceptual framework for the diagnostic classification system. This framework is named NANDA Nursing Diagnosis Taxonomy I; the taxonomy is composed of nine patterns of human response:

- Exchanging
- Communicating
- Relating
- Valuing
- Choosing
- Moving
- Perceiving
- Knowing
- Feeling

Each pattern that is too abstract for clinical use is followed by two or more levels of abstraction that are more concrete and clinically useful. The second level could become the category structure for assessment, while the third and below levels would serve as the diagnostic label for the individual or group (Kritek, 1986). The diagnostic categories at level five are more clinically specific than those at level four. Ineffective Individual Coping still remains a useful category but does require very specific etiological or contributing factors in order to determine nursing prescriptions for treatment. Figure

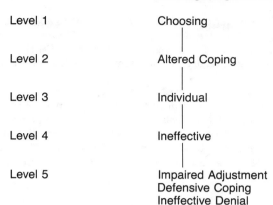

Level 1	Choosing
Level 2	Altered Coping
Level 3	Individual
Level 4	Ineffective
Level 5	Impaired Adjustment
	Defensive Coping
	Ineffective Denial

Fig. 1-3 Diagram showing one set of multiple levels of abstraction associated with the human response pattern of choosing.

1-3 illustrates the levels of abstraction related to one of the human response patterns—choosing.

For further discussion of the diagnostic classification system and for material on the concept of the unitary person, the reader is referred to the proceedings of the fifth and sixth NANDA conferences.

Diagnostic Category Components

Each diagnostic category has four components: the title (label); the definition; the defining characteristics; and the etiological, contributing, and risk factors.

Title
The title, or label, offers a concise description of the state (actual, potential) of the individual's health. Qualifying terms such as *altered, impaired, deficit,* and *ineffective* reflect a change in health status but do not label the degree of change. These terms are used in place of more subjective qualifying words such as maladaptive, poor, and inappropriate.

Definition
The definition expresses a clear, precise meaning of the category and differentiates this category from all others.

Defining Characteristics
Defining characteristics are the clinical criteria that validate the presence of a diagnostic category. Clinical criteria can be either a sign or a symptom (or a cluster of signs and symptoms), or risk factors that are expressed or observed in the person or group with the response. They can be both subjective and objective. Previously, all defining characteristics were listed together without regard for rank. It was often difficult to determine which signs and symptoms were critical for validation of the actual diagnosis. In 1986, NANDA began to separate signs and symptoms into two categories—major and minor. Major signs and symptoms are those that must be present in order to validate a particular diagnosis. The minor category includes signs and symptoms that appear to be present in many but not all individuals to whom the diagnosis could be applied.

In 1988, NANDA further defined major as "present in 80%–100% of the persons or groups with the diagnosis" and minor as "present in 50–79% of persons or groups with the diagnosis." Through the use of research designs such as Fehring's diagnostic content validity (DCV) scores, the category can be researched to differentiate between major and minor.

All the categories accepted by NANDA are approved for clinical testing, but many have not been clinically tested. This author uses the consensus of experts to differentiate between major and minor. The consensus method is more valid if major is defined as "must be present (100%)." Thus, when clinical validation studies identify the major as between 80% and 100%, this author will reflect the major as 80%–100% instead of 100%. In this edition, the following categories use 80%–100%, not 100%, as the criterion for major:

Hypothermia
Colonic Constipation
Perceived Constipation
Fatigue
Decisional Conflict
Situational Low Self-Esteem
Chronic Low Self-Esteem
Self-Esteem Disturbance
Defensive Coping

Etiological, Contributing, and Risk Factors (Related To's)

The etiological and contributing factors are those clinical and personal situations that can change health status or influence problem development. These are often the "related to's" of the nursing diagnosis statement.

The factors listed under each category are those that are frequently seen, but they do not represent a complete list. The nature of human variability and uniqueness prohibits a complete listing. Situations can be pathophysiological (biological or psychological), treatment-related, situational (environmental, personal), or maturational.

Etiological, Contributing, and Risk Factors
Pathophysiological (biological or psychological)
    Diabetes mellitus
    Anorexia nervosa
Treatment-related
    Medications
    Diagnostic studies
    Surgery
    Treatments
Situational
    Environmental
        Community
        Institution
    Personal
        Life experiences
        Roles
Maturational
    Age-related

To illustrate the components of a diagnostic category, let us take the nursing diagnosis *Powerlessness* and list its components.

Powerlessness

Definition

Powerlessness: The state in which an individual perceives a lack of personal control over certain events or situations.

Defining Characteristics
1. Major (must be present)
   Expresses dissatisfaction over inability to control situation (*e.g.*, illness, prognosis, care, recovery rate)
2. Minor (may be present)
   Refuses or is reluctant to participate in decision-making

Apathy	Uneasiness
Aggressive behavior	Resignation
Violent behavior	Acting-out behavior
Anxiety	Depression

Etiological, Contributing, Risk Factors
1. Pathophysiological
   Any disease process, acute or chronic, can cause or contribute to powerlessness. Some common sources are:
   Inability to communicate (CVA, Guillain-Barré syndrome, intubation)
   Inability to perform activities of daily living (CVA, cervical trauma, myocardial infarction, pain)
   Inability to fulfill role responsibilities (surgery, trauma, arthritis)
   Progressive debilitating disease (multiple sclerosis, terminal cancer)
2. Situational (Personal, Environmental)
   Lack of knowledge
   Personal characteristics that value control highly (*e.g.*, internal locus of control)
   Altered personal territory
   Social isolation
   Lack of explanations from caregivers
   Lack of client participation in making decisions
   Social displacement
   Relocation
   Insufficient finances
   Sexual harassment
3. Treatment-related
   Hospital or institutional limitations
   Some control relinquished to others
   No privacy
4. Maturational
   Adolescent: Dependence on peer group, independence from family
   Young adult: Marriage, pregnancy, parenthood
   Adult: Adolescent children, physical signs of aging, career pressures
   Elderly: Sensory deficits, motor deficits, losses (money, significant others)

Even with defining characteristics and etiological factors for each diagnostic category, nurses continue to have difficulty in using nursing diagnoses, as is illustrated by the questions cited in the Preface:

• What does the label really mean?

- What kinds of assessment questions will yield nursing diagnoses?
- How do I tailor a diagnostic category for a specific individual?
- How should I intervene after I formulate the diagnostic statement?
- How do I develop a care plan with nursing diagnoses?

To assist the nurse in using nursing diagnoses, Section II of this book, Manual of Nursing Diagnoses, has been designed so that each diagnostic category is described in terms of

- Definition
- Etiological, contributing, and risk factors
- Defining characteristics
- Focus assessment criteria (subjective and objective)
- Principles and rationale for nursing care

Each diagnostic category is further described in terms of one or more specific nursing diagnoses within the category. For example, take the diagnostic category *Impaired Tissue Integrity*. A specific diagnosis under this category would be *Impaired Skin Integrity*.

Each specific diagnosis is explained in terms of

- Assessment data (subjective and objective)
- Outcome criteria
- Clinical nursing interventions

Thus, Section II provides an explanation of each diagnostic category, along with related interventions that will assist the nurse in applying nursing diagnoses in clinical practice.

Functional Health Patterns

Gordon has developed a system for organizing a nursing assessment based on function, in order to direct the nurse in collecting data to determine an individual's or group's health status and functioning. After data collection is complete, the nurse and client can determine positive functioning, altered functioning, or at-risk status for altered functioning. Altered functioning is defined as functioning that is perceived as a negative change or as undesirable by the client (individual, group). The functional health patterns are

1. Health perception–health management pattern
2. Nutritional–metabolic pattern
3. Elimination pattern
4. Activity–exercise pattern
5. Sleep–rest pattern
6. Cognitive–perceptual pattern
7. Self-perception pattern
8. Role–relationship pattern
9. Sexuality–reproductive pattern
10. Coping–stress tolerance pattern
11. Value–belief pattern

The current diagnostic categories are grouped under functional health patterns in Table 1-2.

This standardization of assessment data should not interfere with the nurse's theoretical or philosophical beliefs. It simply directs the nurse to the data that should be collected, not to the approach that should be used in interpreting the data or determining

Table 1-2. **Nursing Diagnostic Categories Grouped Under Functional Health Patterns***

1. Health Perception–Health Management
† Breastfeeding, Ineffective
Growth & Development, Altered
Health Maintenance, Altered
† Health-Seeking Behaviors
Noncompliance
Potential for Injury
Potential for Suffocation
Potential for Poisoning
Potential for Trauma

2. Nutritional–Metabolic
Body Temperature, Potential Altered
Hypothermia
Hyperthermia
Thermoregulation, Ineffective
Fluid Volume Deficit
Fluid Volume Excess
Infection, Potential for
‡ Infection Transmission, Potential for
Nutrition, Altered: Less than Body Requirements
Nutrition, Altered: More than Body Requirements
Nutrition, Altered: Potential for More than Body Requirements
Swallowing, Impaired
Tissue Integrity, Impaired
Oral Mucous Membrane, Altered
Skin Integrity, Impaired

3. Elimination
‡ Bowel Elimination, Altered
Constipation
† Colonic Constipation
† Perceived Constipation
Diarrhea
Bowel Incontinence
Urinary Elimination, Altered Patterns of
Urinary Retention
Total Incontinence
Functional Incontinence
Reflex Incontinence
Urge Incontinence
Stress Incontinence
‡ Maturational Enuresis

4. Activity–Exercise
Activity Intolerance
Cardiac Output, Decreased
† Disuse Syndrome, Potential for
Diversional Activity Deficit
Home Maintenance Management, Impaired
Mobility, Impaired Physical
‡ Respiratory Function, Potential Altered
Ineffective Airway Clearance
Ineffective Breathing Patterns
Impaired Gas Exchange
(Specify) Self-Care Deficit (Total‡, Feeding, Bathing/Hygiene, Dressing/Grooming, Toileting)
Tissue Perfusion, Altered (Specify type: Cerebral, Cardiopulmonary, Renal, Gastrointestinal, Peripheral)

(continued)

Table 1-2.   **Nursing Diagnostic Categories Grouped Under Functional Health Patterns*** *(Continued)*

5. Sleep–Rest
   Sleep Pattern Disturbance

6. Cognitive–Perceptual
   ‡ Comfort, Altered
       Pain
       ‡ Acute Pain
       Chronic Pain
   ‡ Pruritis
   ‡ Nausea/Vomiting
   † Decisional Conflict
   † Dysreflexia
     Knowledge Deficit (specify)
   † Potential for Aspiration
     Sensory–Perceptual Alteration: (Specify: visual, Auditory, Kinesthetic, Gustatory, Tactile, Olfactory)
     Thought Processes, Altered
     Unilateral Neglect

7. Self-Perception
     Anxiety
   † Fatigue
     Fear
     Hopelessness
     Powerlessness
   ‡ Self-Concept Disturbance
       Body Image Disturbance
       Personal Identity Disturbance
     † Self-Esteem Disturbance
       † Chronic Low Self-Esteem
       † Situational Low Self-Esteem

8. Role–Relationship
   ‡ Communication, Impaired
       Communication, Impaired Verbal
     Family Processes, Altered
   ‡ Grieving
       Grieving, Anticipatory
       Grieving, Dysfunctional
     Parenting, Altered:
   † Parenting Role Conflict
     Role Performance, Altered
     Social Interaction, Impaired
     Social Isolation

9. Sexuality–Reproductive
     Sexual Dysfunction
     Sexuality Patterns, Altered

10. Coping–Stress Tolerance
     Adjustment, Impaired
     Coping, Ineffective Individual
       †Defensive Coping
       †Ineffective Denial
     Coping: Disabling, Ineffective Family
     Coping: Compromised, Ineffective Family
     Coping, Family: Potential for Growth

(continued)

Table 1-2. **Nursing Diagnostic Categories Grouped Under Functional Health Patterns*** *(Continued)*

Post-Trauma Response
  Rape Trauma Syndrome
‡ Self-Harm, Potential for:
  Violence, Potential for:

11. Value–Belief
  Spiritual Distress

*The Functional Health Patterns were identified by M. Gordon in *Nursing Diagnosis: Process and Application* (New York, McGraw-Hill, 1982) with minor changes by the author.
  †These categories were accepted by the North American Nursing Diagnosis Association in 1988.
  ‡These diagnostic categories are not currently on the NANDA list but have been included for clarity and usefulness.

the interventions. Thus, the nurse who subscribes to Roy's adaptation framework, Orem's self-care model, or Rogers's life process model can use the functional health pattern framework developed by Gordon (p. 81) to gather baseline data. From that point, she can continue with her individual philosophy or framework after collecting the initial data.

The data base assessment guide presented in Appendix I is organized according to functional health patterns. It is designed to assist the nurse in gathering initial data. Should questions arise concerning a pattern, the nurse is instructed to gather more data about the diagnostic category by using the assessment criteria under the category. This additional data is based on a focus assessment, a procedure that will be discussed in Chapters 2 and 3.

Wellness and Nursing Diagnosis

Since 1973, many nurses have been concerned because the NANDA list primarily represents alterations (Popkess-Vawter, Gleit). Many nurses practice with clients who are healthy. Examples may include new parents and school children, as well as clients of college health services and well-baby clinics. Nurses also help individuals with illnesses to pursue optimal health. Examples may include stress management, exercise programs, or nutritional counseling.

Using the functional health pattern format to guide data collection, the nurse and client can determine positive functioning, altered functioning, or at-risk status for altered functioning. Table 1-3 illustrates statements that describe strengths for each of the eleven functional health patterns. These statements are also incorporated into the case study application in Chapter 4. When the nurse and client conclude that there is positive functioning in a functional health pattern, this conclusion is an assessment conclusion but by itself is not necessarily a nursing diagnosis. The nurse utilizes this data to help the client reach a higher level of functioning or uses the identified strengths in planning interventions for altered functioning or at-risk for altered functioning.

For example, after assessing the role–relationship pattern with a client, the conclusion is positive functioning. If this client has recently received a diagnosis of cancer of the breast, the nurse can use the client's strength to assist her in dealing with the diagnosis. Another example would be a young couple who recently became parents. They report positive functioning in the role–relationship pattern. The nurse could use this informa-

Table 1-3.   **Positive Functioning Assessment Statements Grouped Under the Functional Health Patterns**

Functional Pattern	Positive Functioning Assessment Statements
1. Health perception–health management pattern	1. Positive health perception Effective health management
2. Nutritional–metabolic pattern	2. Effective nutritional–metabolic pattern
3. Elimination pattern	3. Effective elimination pattern
4. Activity–exercise pattern	4. Effective activity–exercise pattern
5. Sleep–rest pattern	5. Effective sleep–rest pattern
6. Cognitive–perceptual pattern	6. Positive cognitive–perceptual pattern
7. Self-perception pattern	7. Positive self-perception pattern
8. Role–relationship pattern	8. Positive role–relationship pattern
9. Sexuality–reproductive pattern	9. Positive sexuality–reproductive pattern
10. Coping–stress tolerance pattern	10. Effective coping–stress tolerance pattern
11. Value–belief pattern	11. Positive value–belief pattern

tion and the addition of a new baby to the family unit to assist the family to maintain effective role–relationship. The diagnosis

Health-Seeking Behaviors Related to Adjustment to Parenting Role

could be used to describe the situation for which the nurse would teach specific interventions to deal with stressors of new parenthood.

Labeling both of these clients—the woman with the new diagnosis of cancer and the new parents—with the nursing diagnoses

Positive Role–Relationship Pattern
or
Positive Role–Relationship Functioning

will provide diagnoses that the nurse can assist the individual to maintain. What may prove problematic is the daily use of this type of diagnosis with individuals who are acutely ill. Hospitalized clients have approximately 22 nursing diagnoses (Kiley). The nurse, weighing resource allocations (staffing, length of stay), determines the priority set of nursing diagnoses and collaborative problems that can be managed responsibly during the client's length of stay. The nurse providing care to an acutely ill individual can identify strengths and draw on these strengths to assist the individual with problems related to other functional health patterns.

One could incorporate positive functioning assessment statements under each functional health pattern on the admission assessment tool. Figure 1-4 illustrates an example under the Sleep–Rest Pattern.

Some nurses use potential nursing diagnoses to describe situations in which individuals need specific assistance to prevent the occurrence of a problem. This is sometimes useful, but caution is advised.

Theoretically, all new parents are at risk for *Altered Parenting*. Since parenting skills are considered part of the health maintenance–promotion model, it may be more advisable to use

Health-Seeking Behaviors: Effective Parenting Skills

to describe the need of most new parents for information.

Sleep/Rest Pattern

Habits: 8 hrs/night ___   <8 hrs   _X_ >8 hrs ___ AM nap ___ PM nap

Feel rested after sleep _X_ Yes ___ No

Problems: _X_ None ___ Early waking ___ Insomnia ___ Nightmares

☒ Effective Sleep/Rest Pattern

Fig. 1-4 Positive functioning statements related to sleep/rest pattern.

However, when the new parent is an adolescent, additional factors may be involved that place her at risk for *Altered Parenting*. In this situation, *Potential Altered Parenting* related to conflict between adolescent and parental roles may more appropriately describe the situation.

It is true that the health maintenance diagnostic category is very broad. Nurses should be directed to use their clinical knowledge and clinical studies to identify more specific descriptive labels for designating health promotion topics under the broad abstract category Health-Seeking Behaviors.

Summary

Nursing diagnoses provide a method for describing a client's health status in a clear and concise way in order to enhance communication and recognition. Difficulty in formulating diagnostic statements can be greatly reduced if the nurse uses the list of nursing diagnoses from NANDA for the majority of diagnostic statements. Those states that cannot be described by the current list of labels can be stated using guidelines presented in Appendix VIII. Nurses are encouraged to submit new diagnostic labels to NANDA.

The use of nursing diagnoses can stimulate nurses to explore interaction patterns that were previously ignored or unknown and to address all the human needs of individuals, with the expectation that the nurse and, most important, the client will reap the benefits.

References

Bircher A: On the development and classification of nursing diagnoses. Nurs Forum 14:10–29,1975

Breu C, Dracup K, Walden J: Integration of nursing diagnoses in the critical care literature. Heart Lung 16:605–616, 1987

Fehring RJ: Validating diagnostic labels: Standardized methodology. In Hurley M (ed): Classification of Nursing Diagnoses: Proceedings of the Sixth Conference, pp 183–190. St. Louis, CV Mosby, 1986.

Fry VS: The creative approach to nursing. Am J Nurs 53:301–302, 1953

Gebbie K: Toward the theory development for nursing diagnoses classification. In Kim MJ, Moritz DA (eds): Classification of Nursing Diagnoses, p 12. New York, McGraw-Hill, 1982

Gleit C, Tatro S: Nursing diagnoses for healthy individuals. Nurs Health Care 2:456–457, 1981

Gordon M: Historical perspective: The National Group for classification of nursing diagnoses. In Kim MJ, Moritz DA (eds): Classification of Nursing Diagnoses, p 3. New York, McGraw-Hill, 1982

Gordon M, Sweeney MA: Methodological problems and issues in identifying and standardizing nursing diagnoses. Adv Nurs Sci 2:1–15, 1979

Kiley ML: Nursing complexity of two groups of surgical ICU patients. Presented at the Nursing Diagnosis in Critical Care Conference, Milwaukee, Wisconsin, March 1987

Kritek PB: The generation and the classification of nursing diagnoses: Toward a theory of nursing. Image 10(2):33–40, 1978

Kritek P: Development of a taxonomic structure for nursing diagnosis. In Hurley M (ed): Classification of Nursing Diagnosis: Proceedings of the Sixth Conference, pp 23–38. St Louis, CV Mosby, 1986

McLane A: Measurement and validation of diagnostic concepts: A decade of progress. Heart Lung 16:616–624, 1987

Popkess-Vawter S: Strength-oriented nursing diagnoses. In Kim MJ, McFarland G, McLane A (eds): Classification of Nursing Diagnosis, pp 443–440. St Louis, CV Mosby, 1984

Roy C: Framework for classification systems development: Progress and issues. In Kim MJ, McFarland G, McLane A (eds): Classification of Nursing Diagnoses, pp 26–46. St Louis, CV Mosby, 1984

Shoemaker JK: Essential features of a nursing diagnosis. In Kim MJ, McFarland G, McLane A (eds): Classification of Nursing Diagnosis, p 109. St Louis, CV Mosby, 1984

Styles MM: On Nursing: Toward a New Endowment, pp 53–54. St Louis, CV Mosby, 198

2

Differentiating Nursing Diagnoses From Other Client Problems

The Dimensions of Nursing

References to nursing diagnosis in the literature have increased tenfold since the first meeting of the National Group for the Classification of Nursing Diagnosis in 1973 (renamed North American Nursing Diagnosis Association in 1982). Nationwide, health care facilities are beginning to implement nursing diagnosis in response to accreditation pressures, or the need to computerize records, or because the nursing department subscribes to its importance for the profession. These priorities are passed on to practicing nurses, who are now expected to implement nursing diagnosis in their practice and documentation. Because of the complexity of nursing practice, this requirement is not easily met. A clear understanding of the dimensions of nursing is needed to distinguish nursing diagnoses from other client problems.

The theoretical knowledge of nursing is derived from the natural, physical, and behavioral sciences, the humanities, and nursing research. Preparation for clinical practice adds another dimension of knowledge. Nursing curricula are designed to teach students, in the classroom and in clinical settings, about a number of situations encountered in practice. These situations can be organized into four categories: pathophysiological (both biological and psychological), treatment-related, situational (personal, environmental), and maturational. The following are examples of each category:

Pathophysiological
    Pneumonia
    Dependent personality disorder
    Hepatitis
Treatment-related
    Antibiotics
    Dialysis
    Foley catheterization
Personal
    Loss of job
    Relocation
    Lack of regular exercise
Environmental
    Admission to nursing home
    Lack of handrail on stairs
    Toxic waste dump
Maturational
    Aging
    Peer pressure
    Parenthood

Recognizing Nursing Diagnoses

It is essential for the nurse to be knowledgeable about these practice situations and equally important to understand how they are related to nursing diagnosis. In the quest to integrate nursing diagnosis into practice, nurses have often found it convenient to present these situations as nursing diagnoses simply by renaming them. In this way, pneumonia is often called *Impaired Gas Exchange*. However, such an approach is not accurate.

The nurse diagnoses the client's response to a given situation, not the situation itself. In treating the client, the nurse is addressing his response to a situation.

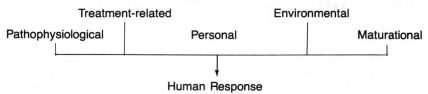

The practice focus for clinical nursing is at the human response level, not above it.

The concept of nursing diagnosis acquired a more clearcut and workable definition in 1973, when human response was designated as the area to which nursing diagnosis should be applied. Since that time, it has been assumed by some that nursing practice consists solely of those aspects of care that can be expressed as nursing diagnoses. NANDA has no official statement regarding the other situations nurses treat. This view has had some unfortunate effects, notably the response of attempting to attach a nursing diagnosis label to every facet of nursing practice. For example, nurses have been directed to use nursing diagnoses exclusively to document their care on care plans and progress notes. Such endeavors have led inevitably to individual frustration and universal misuse of the diagnostic categories. Questions that face the nurse are (Carpenito, 1987):

1. Can nursing diagnoses result in independent and delegated interventions?
2. Should the nurse write a client goal that medicine is legally responsible to accomplish?
3. How can nursing interventions for joint diagnoses be recorded on care plans?
4. What diagnostic label should be used to describe such conditions as shock or disseminated intravascular coagulation?

In addition, the attempt to label all situations in which nurses intervene with nursing diagnostic categories has created a number of serious clinical dilemmas. Several of these have been identified and described as follows (Carpenito, 1985).

Using Nursing Diagnoses without Validation. The nurse is encouraged to change data "to fit the label." This situation results when, even though the data collected do not include the signs and symptoms (defining characteristics) of a particular diagnostic category, the nurse is pressured to describe the data with a nursing diagnostic label. In this circumstance, the label is used without validation. Not only is this practice unscientific, but it can also lead to erroneous and injurious misdiagnosing. For example, labeling all NPO clients with the diagnosis

Altered Nutrition: Less Than Body Requirements

is inaccurate.

Renaming Medical Diagnoses. Since nurses have had and continue to have a responsibility to monitor the responses of patients with medical diagnoses to treatment, a specific vocabulary is needed to describe these situations. Restricting nurses to the use of nursing diagnoses in documenting their practice has contributed to the renaming of medical diagnoses with nursing diagnosis terminology. Perhaps *Impaired Gas Exchange* and *Decreased Cardiac Output* may be said to represent the renaming of medical diagnoses. This activity has serious implications. If nursing diagnosis as a classification system is intended to describe the domain of professional nursing for the purposes of accountability and autonomy, how will nursing be served if medical diagnoses (renamed) are included? Many state nurse practice acts now identify the legal responsibility of professional nurses as the diagnosis and treatment of human responses (as described in nursing diagnoses). Placing situations that represent medical diagnoses within nursing's classification system may prove legally hazardous.

Omitting Problem Situations in Documentation. Recently the documentation systems used by nurses have been changed to require that care plans and standards of care include only nursing diagnoses. This requirement encourages nurses to omit from their documentation situations not described by the list of diagnostic categories. These omissions can seriously jeopardize nursing's present effort to justify and clarify the need for professional nurses in all health care settings.

In addition to the serious problems just discussed, other difficulties exist. Some nurses reject the NANDA classification system because they object to using *Altered Cerebral Tissue Perfusion* as a new term for increased intracranial pressure. Do nurses need a new word for hemorrhage or ICP in order to communicate nursing's unique contribution to treatment?

Recognizing Collaborative Problems

The practice of nursing often involves a collaborative relationship with other members of the health team. Figure 2-1 illustrates this relationship. In a collaborative relationship, functions and activities sometimes overlap. When this occurs, experience has shown that classification problems can arise. Some basic questions may be asked:

- Should nursing diagnosis represent the exclusive focus of nursing?
- Should the areas of collaboration be renamed and designated as nursing diagnoses?
- If the collaborative areas are not identified as nursing diagnoses, is their importance to nursing diminished?

Bifocal Clinical Nursing Model

In 1983, a model for practice was designed that directed nurses to describe their areas of concern with nursing diagnoses and clinical problems (Carpenito, 1983). As this model

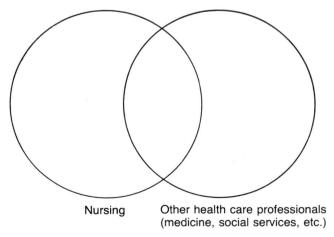

Nursing   Other health care professionals
(medicine, social services, etc.)

Fig. 2-1 Collaborative relationships between nursing and other health care professions.

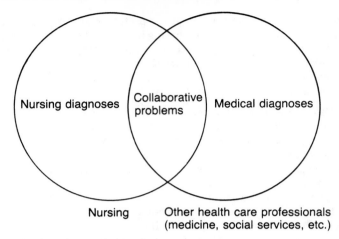

Fig. 2-1A Schematic of the Bifocal Clinical Practice Model.

evolved, clinical problems (both medical and nursing) were incorporated into one category and renamed collaborative problems (Carpenito, 1984). This bifocal model for nursing identifies two clinical situations in which nurses intervene—nursing diagnoses and collaborative problems. The collaborative relationship between nursing and medicine is illustrated in Figure 2-1A.

Human responses are involved in both nursing diagnoses *and* collaborative problems. Figure 2-2 represents the bifocal model. Nursing diagnosis is defined as follows:

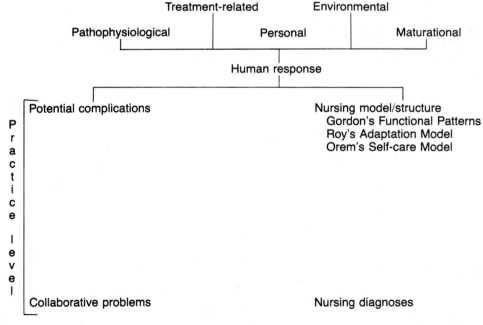

Fig. 2-2 Bifocal clinical nursing model. (© 1985, Lynda Juall Carpenito)

> Nursing diagnosis is a statement that describes the human response (health state or actual/potential altered interaction pattern) of an individual or group that the nurse can legally identify and for which the nurse can order definitive interventions to maintain the health state or to reduce, eliminate, or prevent alterations.

For nursing diagnoses, nurses prescribe interventions that are definitive for prevention and treatment. Collaborative problems are defined as follows:

> Collaborative problems are the physiological complications that have resulted or may result from pathophysiological, treatment-related, and other situations. Nurses monitor to detect their onset/status and collaborate with medicine for definitive co-treatment.

Examples:

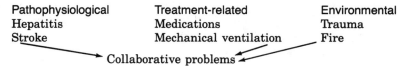

Pathophysiological	Treatment-related	Environmental
Hepatitis	Medications	Trauma
Stroke	Mechanical ventilation	Fire

Collaborative problems

For collaborative problems, nurses prescribe and implement monitoring interventions that are in the domain of nursing. Some of the interventions indicated for collaborative problems are also indicated for nursing diagnoses.

In 1987, Carpenito wrote that the relationship of diagnosis to interventions is a critical element when nursing diagnosis is defined. In many definitions of nursing diagnosis there is a focus on the relationship of selected interventions to the diagnosis. A certain type of intervention appears to distinguish a nursing diagnosis from a medical diagnosis or other problems that nurses treat. Bulechek and McCloskey wrote in 1985 that "a nursing intervention is an autonomous action based on scientific rationale that is executed to benefit the client in a predicted way related to the nursing diagnosis and goal." Nursing interventions can be categorized into two types: independent and delegated (Maryland). Independent are nurse-prescribed, while delegated are physician-prescribed. Both types of interventions require judgment. For whether it is an independent or delegated intervention, legally, the nurse must determine if it is appropriate to initiate.

The nurse makes independent decisions regarding both collaborative problems and nursing diagnoses. The decisions differ in that, for nursing diagnoses, the nurse prescribes most of the definitive treatment for the situation; for collaborative problems, the nurse primarily monitors the patient's condition to detect onset or status of physiologic complications to prevent a worsened condition or death. When a nurse diagnoses a collaborative problem, the nurse confers with the physician regarding treatment. When a nurse makes a nursing diagnosis, this collaboration is usually not warranted.

The nature of collaborative problems is that they are present or at risk of being present whenever the pathology or the treatment is present. For example, all postoperative abdominal surgery clients will be at risk for hemorrhage, hypoxia, and so on. Expert nursing knowledge will be required to determine who is at risk and to identify these individuals at an early stage in order to prevent morbidity and mortality.

The nature of nursing diagnoses is that they sometimes can be predicted or expected with a high degree of certainty but often require repeated assessments for validation. Because of the variability and uniqueness of individuals, nursing diagnoses are often more complex than collaborative problems, *but they are not more important.*

A single format for labeling collaborative problems is needed in order to provide consistency for documentation and computer coding. The following is recommended as a logical way of labeling collaborative problems:

Potential Complication: (specify)

Examples:
Potential Complication: Cardiac
Potential Complication: Sepsis
Potential Complication: Hypoglycemia

Refer to Appendix XI for the list of Collaborative Problems.

If the nurse is monitoring for a cluster or group of potential complications, this situation can be recorded as follows:

Potential Complication of Chemotherapy:
Necrosis/phlebitis at IV site
Thrombocytopenia
Anemia
Leukopenia
Peripheral nerve toxicity
Anaphylaxis
Pulmonary fibrosis
Central nervous system toxicity

Figure 2-3 outlines the nursing diagnoses that may be identified and the collaborative problems that are present in a client with pneumonia. For a complete listing of collaborative problems grouped under medical diagnoses and treatment, refer to the reference under Figure 2-3.

Some physiologic complications, such as pressure ulcers and infection from invasive lines, are problems that nurses can prevent. Prevention is different from detection. Nurses do not prevent hemorrhage or paralytic ileus but, instead, can detect their presence early to prevent greater severity of illness or even death. Physicians cannot treat collaborative problems without nursing's knowledge, vigilance, and judgment. For collaborative problems, nurses institute orders in addition to monitoring, such as ordering position changes, patient teaching, or specific protocols.

Figure 2-4 is a diagram designed to assist the nurse in differentiating a collaborative problem from a nursing diagnosis. As nursing's body of knowledge evolves, some of the collaborative problems of today may be nursing diagnoses tomorrow. Nurses are cautioned not to try to make a collaborative problem a nursing diagnosis simply because the latter is perceived as having greater value.

PNEUMONIA

Collaborative Problems
Potential Complications: Septic shock
Respiratory insufficiency   Paralytic ileus

Nursing Diagnoses
Activity Intolerance related to compromised respiratory function
Potential Altered Oral Mucous Membrane related to mouth breathing and frequent expectorations
Potential Fluid Volume Deficit related to increased insensible fluid loss secondary to fever and hyperventilation
Potential Altered Nutrition: Less than Body Requirements, related to anorexia, dyspnea, and abdominal distention secondary to air swallowing
Ineffective Airway Clearance related to pain, tracheobronchial secretions, and exudate
Potential for Infection Transmission related to communicable nature of the disease
Potential Altered Body Temperature related to body's response to infectious process
Altered Comfort related to hyperthermia, malaise, and pulmonary pathology
Potential Impaired Skin Integrity related to prescribed bed rest

Fig. 2-3 Collaborative problems and nursing diagnoses grouped under the medical diagnosis *pneumonia*. (Carpenito LJ: Handbook of Nursing Diagnosis, 2nd ed. Philadelphia, JB Lippincott, 1987)

Differentiating Nursing Diagnoses From Other Client Problems

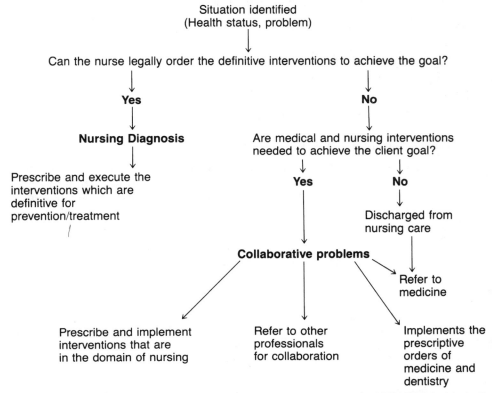

Fig. 2-4 Differentiation of nursing diagnoses from collaborative problems. (© 1988, 1985, Lynda Juall Carpenito)

- Collaborative problems are not more important than nursing diagnoses.
- Nursing diagnoses are not more important than collaborative problems.
- Priorities for the client will be determined by conditions, the nurse, and the client.

Using the criteria questions from Figure 2-4, the nurse can differentiate collaborative problems from nursing diagnoses, as is illustrated in the following case study vignettes.

Case Study 1

Mr. Smith is a 35-year-old male admitted for a possible concussion after a car accident, with a physician's order for

- Clear liquid diet
- Neurological assessment q 1 hour

On admission the nurse records

- Is oriented and alert
- Pupils at 6 mm, equal and reactive to light
- B.P. 120/72, pulse 84, resp 20, temp 99° F

Two hours later the nurse records

- Vomiting
- Restlessness
- Pupils at 6 mm, equal, with a sluggish response to light
- B.P. 140/60, pulse 65, resp 12, temp 99° F

Problem: Possible increased intracranial pressure.

Now apply the criteria questions to Case Study 1.

Q. Can the nurse legally order the definitive interventions to achieve the client goal (which would be a reversal of the increasing intracranial pressure)?
A. No, nurses do not definitively treat or prevent increased intracranial pressure. They collaborate with the physician for definitive treatment.
Q. Are medical and nursing interventions needed for goal achievement?
A.

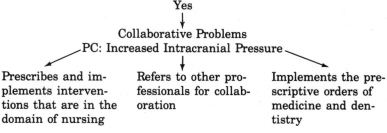

In this situation, the nurse would monitor to detect ICP or increasing levels of intracranial pressure. The nurse also prescribes interventions that reduce ICP, but these interventions are not considered definitive. This problem is the joint responsibility of medicine and nursing.

Case Study 2

Mr. Green is a 45-year-old male with a cholecystectomy incision (10 days postop). The incision is not healing, and there is continual purulent drainage. The nursing care consists of

- Inspecting and cleansing the incision and the surrounding area q 8 hours
- Applying Stomahesive and drainage pouch to contain drainage and protect skin
- Promoting optimal nutrition and hydration to enhance healing

Problem: Adjacent skin at risk for erosion.

Now apply the criteria questions to Case Study 2.

Q. Can the nurse legally order the definitive interventions to achieve the goals (which would be continued intact surrounding tissue)?

↓

A. Yes, nurses do prescribe the interventions that will prevent skin erosion from occurring as a result of wound drainage.

↓

Nursing Diagnosis

↓

Potential Impaired Skin Integrity related to draining purulent wound

In this situation the nurse would prescribe the interventions to preserve adjacent skin area. No collaboration with medicine is warranted.

Nursing diagnoses and collaborative problems have different implications for expected outcomes. Bulechek and McCloskey define goals as "guideposts to the selection of nursing interventions and criteria in the evaluation of nursing interventions." These authors continue by saying that "readily identifiable and logical links should exist between the diagnoses and the plan of care, and the activities prescribed should assist or enable the patient to meet the identified expected outcome." Alfaro wrote that client outcomes are "statements describing a measurable behavior of client/family which denote a favorable status (changed or maintained) after nursing care has been delivered." Thus, outcome criteria and interventions may be critical to differentiating nursing diagnoses from collaborative problems that nurses treat.

For example, if the following diagnosis is formulated:

Potential Fluid Volume Deficit Related to Loss of Fluid During Surgery and Possible Hemorrhage Postop

the following client outcome may be written:
The client will demonstrate continued fluid balance, as evidenced by

- Absence of bleeding
- B/P and pulse within normal limits

Client goals are used to determine the success or appropriateness of the nursing care plan. If the goals are not achieved or progress to achievement is not evident, then the nurse must:

- Reevaluate the appropriateness of the goal and/or
- Revise the plan

In the above example, if the client shows evidence of bleeding, is it appropriate for the nurse to change the goals? What changes in the nursing care plan would the nurse make to stop the bleeding?

Neither action is appropriate. The nurse would confer with the physician for delegated orders to treat the bleeding.

When the nurse writes client outcomes that require delegated medical orders for goal achievement, the situation is not a nursing dignosis but a collaborative problem.

Potential Fluid Volume Deficit Related to Loss of Fluid During Surgery and Possible Hemorrhage Postop would be better described as

Potential Complication: Hemorrhage

Client outcomes are not necessary for collaborative problems because they do not serve as indicators for evaluating nursing care. If client outcomes are written for collaborative problems, it should be clear that they are achieved by nursing-prescribed (independent) and medical-prescribed (delegated) interventions. Figure 2-5 illustrates these relationships. Figure 2-6 illustrates the difference between interventions for nursing diagnoses and for collaborative problems. Chapter 4 describes the documentation of nursing diagnoses and collaborative problems.

Since each individual is unique, it is difficult to develop exclusive criteria that will always differentiate nursing diagnoses from other client problems. Ultimately, the decision to use or not to use the diagnostic label will rest with the individual nurse until more refined defining characteristics for each category are developed and tested.

Learning to formulate nursing diagnoses is a skill that requires knowledge and practice. The nurse needs to familiarize herself with the diagnostic categories and their components. Certain ones such as *Altered Bowel Elimination* and *Altered Nutrition* are familiar to most nurses and thus will be easier to use. Section II provides specific information on each category to increase a working knowledge of the various diagnoses.

Actual, Potential, and Possible Nursing Diagnoses

The terms *actual, potential,* and *possible* describe the present state of the diagnosis. Each diagnostic category has a label, definition and defining characteristics. Defining charac-

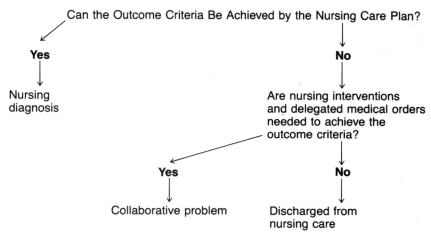

Fig. 2-5   Relationship of goals to nursing diagnoses and collaborative problems.

	Nursing Diagnoses	*Collaborative Problems*
Definitive treatment	Prescribed by nurse	Prescribed by nursing and medicine
Primary focus of nursing interventions	Reduce, eliminate, prevent, promote	Monitor to detect
Type of goal	Client or outcome criteria	Not needed unless jointly made by nursing and medicine

Fig. 2-6 Compare and contrast nursing diagnoses and collaborative problems.

teristics, as discussed in Chapter 1, are the clinical criteria that represent the presence of the diagnosis. For actual nursing diagnoses, these are major signs and symptoms, while for potential nursing diagnoses, defining characteristics are the risk factors that are present.

Actual

The use of a nursing diagnosis without the word *possible* or *potential* means that the state has been clinically validated by identifiable major defining characteristics. An example of an actual nursing diagnosis is:

Activity Intolerance Related to Insufficient Oxygenation for Activities of Daily Living

Defining Characteristics
Dyspnea on exertion
Failure of pulse to return to a resting state of 74 three minutes after activity

Potential

A potential nursing diagnosis describes an altered state that may occur if certain nursing interventions are not ordered and implemented. Defining characteristics are present as risk factors (as related to's). For example:

Potential Altered Respiratory Function Related to Postop Immobility and Postanesthesia State

The use of the term *potential* with a nursing diagnosis can also describe a state in which health promotion activities are needed, as illustrated with:

Potential Altered Nutrition: Less Than Body Requirements, Related to Adolescent Eating Patterns and Lack of Knowledge Regarding Diet During Pregnancy

The Following Assessment Data Supported the Related To's:
Primigravida, 17 years old
Diet history
    Breakfast: none
    Lunch: sandwich, soda
    Dinner: meat, vegetable, potato, soda
    Snacks: potato chips, candy bars

Thus, the validation to support an actual diagnosis is signs and symptoms, while the validation to support a potential diagnosis is risk factors.

For example:
Impaired Skin Integrity related to
   immobility secondary to pain
   as manifested by *2 cm erythematous sacral*
   lesion

Validation
(defining
   characteristics)

Potential Impaired Skin Integrity related
   to *immobility secondary to pain*

Possible

It is unfortunate that many nurses have recently been socialized to avoid appearing tentative. In scientific decision-making, a tentative approach is not a sign of weakness or indecision but an essential part of the process. One must reserve judgment until the necessary information has been gathered and analyzed in order to arrive at a sound scientific conclusion. Physicians demonstrate tentativeness with the statement *rule-out (R/O)*. Nurses should also adopt a tentative attitude until data collection and evaluation have been completed and they are able to confirm or rule out. The word *possible* is used in nursing diagnoses to describe problems that may be present but that require additional data to be confirmed or ruled out. *Possible* serves to alert nurses to the need for additional data. Usually, defining characteristics have not been identified, but factors that have led the nurse to suspect the diagnosis are present.

Possible Self-Concept Disturbance Related to Recent Loss of Role Responsibilities Secondary to Exacerbation of MS

When a nurse records a possible nursing diagnosis, other nurses are now alerted to assess for more data to support or refute the tentative diagnosis. After additional data collection, the nurse may:

- Confirm the presence of major signs and symptoms, thus labeling the diagnosis, or
- Confirm the presence of potential risk factors, or
- Rule out the presence of a diagnosis (actual or potential) at this time

---

Summary: Three Types of Nursing Diagnoses

Actual: problem is present
Potential: problem may occur
Possible: problem may be present

A decision tree to be used in differentiating actual, potential, and possible nursing diagnoses is shown in Figure 2-7.

Associated Interventions

The interventions for each type of nursing diagnosis—actual, potential, and possible—have a different focus.

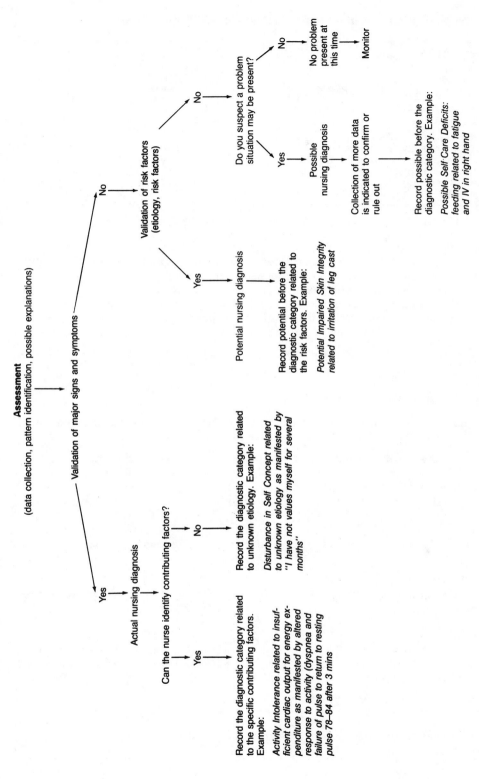

Fig. 2-7 Decision tree for differentiating actual, potential, and possible nursing diagnoses. (© Lynda Juall Carpenito)

Nursing Diagnosis	Interventions
Activity Intolerance related to insufficient oxygenation for A.D.L.	1. Provide for rest periods before activities 2. Monitor response to activity
Potential Altered Respiratory Function related to postop immobility, post anesthesia	1. Instruct to cough and deep breaths q 1–2 hours 2. Monitor respiratory status 3. Ambulate evening of surgery
Possible Sexual Dysfunction related to effects of abdominal perineal surgical resection (3 months prior) on the ability to have or sustain an erection	1. Assess if sexual function has changed since surgery

Fig. 2-8   Interventions corresponding to the three types of nursing diagnoses.

1. For an actual nursing diagnosis, the nurse prescribes interventions to reduce or eliminate. If the diagnosis is a healthy response, the nurse prescribes promotion activities. The nurse also monitors status/response.
2. For a potential nursing diagnosis, the nurse prescribes interventions to prevent by reducing risk factors and also monitors the status and onset.
3. For a possible nursing diagnosis, the nurse prescribes additional data collection to rule out or confirm an actual or potential nursing diagnosis.

Figure 2-8 illustrates the relationship of interventions to the three types of nursing diagnosis.

The Diagnostic Statement

The diagnostic statement is a statement that describes the health status of an individual or group and the factors that have contributed to the status.

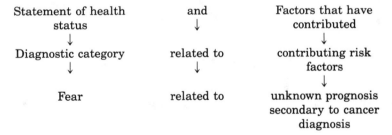

The diagnostic statement or the nursing diagnosis should have either two or three parts.

Two-Part Statement

Potential and possible nursing diagnoses are two-part statements. The validation for a potential nursing diagnosis is the presence of risk factors. The risk factors are the second part of the statement.

> Potential Nursing Diagnosis   related to   risk factors

Example:

Potential Altered Oral Mucous Membrane Related to Prolonged NPO State

Possible nursing diagnoses are suspected because of the presence of certain data. This data is insufficient for the nurse to make a conclusion. The nurse or other nurses will assess for more data in order to rule out or confirm the existence of an actual or a potential diagnosis.

Possible Nursing Diagnosis   related to   factors that led you to suspect the
                                                diagnosis

Three-Part Statement

Actual nursing diagnoses consist of three parts.

Diagnostic label + contributing factors + signs and symptoms

Example:

Grieving Related to Recent Loss of Job, as Manifested by Statements of Anger at Co-workers and Sadness about Loss of Routine

The presence of signs and symptoms (defining characteristics) provides the clinical validation needed to confirm an actual diagnosis.

Statements of potential or possible diagnoses do not have a third part because in those situations signs and symptoms do not exist.

Documentation of Signs and Symptoms

The third part of an actual nursing diagnosis can be documented with one of four methods: the P.E.S. format, the nursing care plan, the S.O.A.P.I.E. format, and focus charting.

1. P.E.S. format. Gordon identified the following format for recording the signs and symptoms of an actual diagnosis: problem, etiology, and symptom (P.E.S.).

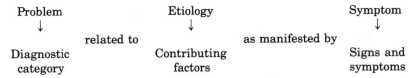

Problem		Etiology		Symptom
↓		↓		↓
	related to		as manifested by	
Diagnostic		Contributing		Signs and
category		factors		symptoms

    This format cannot be used for potential or possible diagnoses because signs and symptoms are not present in those instances.

2. Nursing Care Plan. Although the literature has encouraged nurses to formulate concise nursing diagnoses, it is inappropriate for nurses to try to shorten statements simply for the purpose of conciseness. Specific contributing or risk factors will assist the nurse in planning individualized care. If the P.E.S. format creates too long a statement, the nurse can choose to document the supporting signs and symptoms under the diagnostic label, as in Figure 2-9.

Date	Diagnosis	Plan
9/23	Fear related to possible negative effects secondary to scheduled myelogram	1. Allow her to share her concerns about the procedure. Correct all misconceptions.
		2. Explain in detail: Pretest preparation Procedure
	Signs and symptoms:	Sensations Positions during test Medications
	Stated "I am afraid something terrible will happen."	Post-test procedures Position restrictions Fluid replacement
	"My neighbor had a myelogram and suffered with a headache for a month afterward."	Assessments (vital signs, motor and sensory function) 3. Explain that water-soluble contrast agents now used are less likely to produce headaches because they are reabsorbed more readily.

Fig. 2-9 Diagnostic label with supporting defining characteristics.

3. S.O.A.P.I.E. format. The S.O.A.P.I.E. format of documentation is a systematic method for recording some events. The acronym refers to the following elements:

    S = Subjective data
    O = Objective data
    A = Analysis or diagnosis
    P = Plan
    I = Implementation
    E = Evaluation

The following is an example of the S.O.A.P.I.E. format for a newly validated nursing diagnosis:

    S = "I am afraid something terrible will happen."

        "My neighbor had a myelogram and suffered with a headache for a month afterward."

    O = N/A

    A = Fear related to possible negative effects secondary to scheduled myelogram

    P = Refer to care plan

If the nurse uses the S.O.A.P.I.E. format, the initial recording of the diagnosis will reflect the signs and symptoms. It is then unnecessary for the nurse to use the P.E.S. method.

4. Focus Charting. Lampe developed focus charting to provide a concise systematic method for recording client status and/or response. Focus charting uses the acronym DAR to record data. The following is an example of focus charting used to record a newly validated nursing diagnosis.

Focus: Fear related to possible negative effects secondary to scheduled myelogram

    Data = Stated, "I am afraid something terrible will happen."

        "My neighbor had a myelogram and suffered with a headache for a month afterward."

    Action = Initiate care plan

    Response = N/A

Directions for Care

The literature has specified that the nurse will direct interventions toward reducing or eliminating etiological or contributing factors (Bulechek, Gordon). Specifically, if the nurse cannot treat the contributing factors, then the nursing diagnosis is considered incorrect. This is problematic.

As the diagnostic categories evolve into more specific labels, the nurse may encounter nursing diagnoses with contributing factors that are not treatable by nursing. Example:

Potential for Infection Related to Compromised Immune System

The nurse does not prescribe for compromised immune system, but the nurse can prevent infection in some of these individuals. Forcing the nurse to rewrite the contributing factors to reflect direction for treatment as

Potential for Infection Related to Susceptibility to Environmental Contagions Secondary to Compromised Immune System

may not be necessary except for beginning students of nursing.

In some instances, the categories direct the interventions, and the etiological or contributing factors are not involved.

Examples of such categories are:

- Impaired swallowing
- Functional incontinence
- Potential for infection

Figure 2-9 illustrates this relationship.

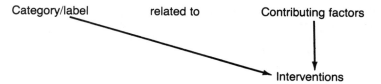

Fig. 2-10 Deriving interventions from the nursing diagnosis. (The author wishes to acknowledge the authors of this diagram as clinical nurse specialists at Harper Division of Detroit Medical Center.)

The nurse should be able to prescribe the definitive therapy for the diagnostic category.

> Q. Can the nurse prescribe the definitive interventions to achieve a client goal for the following nursing diagnosis?

Sensory Perceptual Alteration: Visual Related to Progressive Loss of Vision

> A. No. The nurse should rewrite the diagnosis or reevaluate; perhaps the category is incorrect and would be better stated as:

Fear Related to Progressive Loss of Vision

However, as Figure 2-10 illustrates, sometimes the interventions are derived from the category, not from the contributing factors.

"Related to"

The use of the words *related to* reflects a relationship between the first and the second parts of the statement. It is important that the nurse not link the statements with words implying liability, because such a relationship can result in legal or professional difficulty. Examples of such errors are:

- Impairment of Skin Integrity: Pressure sores related to infrequent turning
- Potential for Injury related to the mother's frequently leaving the children at home unsupervised

On the other hand, using the diagnostic label by itself without a *related to* etiological or contributing factor would result in a vaguely stated problem that is not specific enough to direct individualized interventions.

The more specific the second part of the statement, the more specialized the interventions can be. The linking of the diagnostic category with contributing factors also assists the nurse in validating the category. For example, the diagnostic category *Noncompliance* when stated by itself usually conveys the negative implication that the client is not cooperating. When the nurse relates the noncompliance to a factor, this diagnosis can transmit a very different message. For example:

- Noncompliance: related to the negative side-effects of the drug (reduced libido, fatigue), as manifested by "I stopped my B/P medicine."
- Noncompliance related to inability to understand the need for weekly blood pressure measurements, as manifested by "I don't keep my appointments if I am busy."

If the defining characteristics of a diagnostic category are present, but the etiological and contributing factors are unknown, the statement can be written as:

- Fear related to unknown etiology, as manifested by rapid speech, pacing, and "I am worried."

The use of the term *unknown etiology* alerts the nurse and other members of the nursing staff to assess for contributing factors at the same time as they are intervening for the present manifestation.

A diagnostic category that may represent an exception to the need to use the phrase *related to* is Rape Trauma Syndrome.

As more specific diagnostic categories evolve, it may be unnecessary for the nurse to write *related to's*. Thus, the nursing diagnoses of tomorrow may be single-part statements such as

Functional Incontinence

Unilateral Neglect

Errors in Diagnostic Statements

The nursing diagnostic statement will reflect either some alteration in the individual's health state related to factors that have contributed or could contribute to its development, or a healthy state that may be threatened or achieved. Like any other new skill, the writing of diagnostic statements takes practice and probably will not be completely without error. Remember to refer to the criteria questions previously presented to help differentiate a nursing diagnosis from a collaborative problem. You may formulate your own diagnostic category if one of the current categories does not accurately describe the problem. This diagnostic label should be shared with nurse colleagues to clinically validate it. After validation (research), submit the category to NANDA.

In an attempt to increase the accuracy and usefulness of the statement (and also to reduce the nurse's frustration), some common errors of diagnostic statements should be avoided.

Common Statement Errors

Nursing diagnoses are *not*

- Medical diagnoses—*e.g.*, diabetes mellitus
- Medical pathology—*e.g.*, decrease in cerebral tissue oxygenation
- Treatments or equipment—*e.g.*, hyperalimentation, Levin tube
- Diagnostic studies—*e.g.*, cardiac catheterization

The nurse, however, may assess for the response of the individual to the situations just mentioned and may validate a nursing diagnosis as

Potential Altered Health Maintenance Related to Lack of Knowledge of Relationship of Activity to Insulin and Diet Requirements in Diabetes Mellitus

Nursing diagnostic statements should *not* be written in terms of

- Cues—*e.g.*, crying, hemoglobin level
- Inferences—*e.g.*, dyspnea
- Goals—*e.g.*, should perform own colostomy care
- Client needs—*e.g.*, needs to walk every shift; needs to express fears
- Nursing needs—*e.g.*, change dressing; check blood pressure

Avoid legally inadvisable or judgmental statements, such as:

- Fear related to frequent beatings by her husband
- Ineffective Family Coping related to mother-in-law's continual harassment of daughter-in-law

- Potential Altered Parenting related to low IQ of mother
- Noncompliance related to failure to return for follow-up visits

A nursing diagnosis should not be related to a medical diagnosis. For example:

Disturbance in Self-Concept Related to Multiple Sclerosis or Anxiety Related to Myocardial Infarction

If the use of a medical diagnosis adds clarity to the diagnosis, it can be linked to the statement with a *secondary to* (2°), as follows:

Self-Concept Disturbance Related to Recent Losses of Role Responsibilities Secondary to Multiple Sclerosis, as Manifested by, "My Mother Comes Every Day to Run My House," "I Can No Longer be the Woman in Charge of My House."

Summary

Nurses diagnose and treat human responses to situations. Situations can be pathophysiological, treatment-related, environmental, personal, and maturational.

Human responses in which nurses intervene can be expressed as nursing diagnoses or collaborative problems. Both require expert nursing interventions, but with different focuses. Interventions for nursing diagnoses are definitive for prevention or treatment. Most interventions are independent nursing prescriptions. Interventions for collaborative problems primarily involve monitoring to detect and are interdependent with medicine. The bifocal model that differentiates nursing diagnoses from collaborative problems provides nurses with a clearer definition of the two dimensions of nursing practice.

References

Bulechek G, McCloskey J: Nursing Interventions: Treatments for Nursing Diagnoses. Philadelphia, WB Saunders, 1985

Carpenito LJ: Nursing Diagnosis: Application to Clinical Practice, pp 15–18. Philadelphia, JB Lippincott, 1983

Carpenito LJ: Is the problem a nursing diagnosis? Am J Nurs 84:1418–1419, 1984

Carpenito LJ: Impact of nursing diagnosis on practice and outcomes. Heart Lung 16(6):595–600, 1987

Gordon M: Nursing Diagnosis: Process and Application. New York, McGraw-Hill, 1982

Lampe S: Focus Charting. Creative Nursing Management Inc, 4950 Dupont Ave South, Minneapolis, MN 55409

Maryland Nurse Practice Act, July 1986, p 4

3

Deriving Nursing Diagnoses: Assessment and Diagnosis

Nursing diagnosis cannot be taken out of the context of the nursing process. To do so would result in a misuse of the concept and would lead to premature labeling or stereotyping. This, in turn, would interfere with accurate and careful observations and result in inappropriate nursing interventions.

Each client is an autonomous and precious person who interacts in a unique manner with his environment and must be assessed within the context of his uniqueness. Because nursing diagnoses are derived from these assessments and because people are continually interacting with their environment, the nurse must apply the process in a continuous round of assessment, diagnosing, planning, implementing, and evaluating.

Figure 3-1 illustrates the cyclic relationship of each step of the nursing process to the other steps and to the whole. Each step is dependent upon the accuracy of the step preceding it. Assessment and evaluation are related to diagnosis, planning, and implementation. For example, when the nurse is implementing the plan, she or he also assesses for other problems or needs and evaluates the person's response to the interventions.

The Nursing Process

After a client has entered the health care setting (home, office, clinic, hospital), the nurse uses systematic observational and problem-solving techniques to identify his functional status: Is it positive, or altered, or is the client at risk for altered functioning? The nurse and client collaborate on appropriate interventions and on the evaluation of the effectiveness of these interventions. The nursing process describes this method, for through its five components—assessment, diagnosis, planning, intervention, and evaluation—it sets the practice of nursing in motion.

The professional acknowledgment that the nursing process is pivotal to nursing is made evident by the fact that it is included in the definition of nursing in most nurse practice acts and in the conceptual framework of most curriculums. Despite this emphasis, many nurses fail to apply the process systematically in their practice. The expertise and efficiency of nursing interventions depend on the accurate utilization of the nursing process. A nurse who is expert in this problem-solving technique can intervene in a skillful and successful manner with clients in a variety of settings.

The depth and breadth of the knowledge of the individual nurse will directly influence the suitability and relevance of the care given. Students with a limited knowledge base can learn the nursing process by focusing initially on a selected area. As they gain more knowledge and experience, they can then increase their process skills. Experienced nurses can enhance their process skills by identifying areas that were previously avoided or misunderstood.

Assessment

Assessment, the first phase of the nursing process, is the deliberate and systematic collection of data to determine a client's current health status and to evaluate his present and past coping patterns. Data are obtained by five methods:

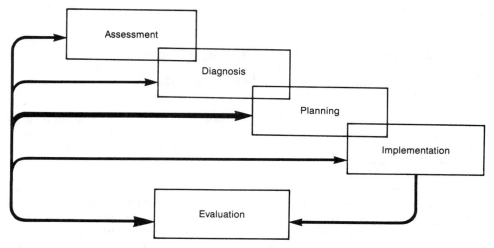

Fig. 3-1   Relationships between the steps of the nursing process. (Alfaro R: Application of Nursing Process: A Step-by-Step Guide. Philadelphia, JB Lippincott, 1986)

- Interview
- Physical examination
- Observation
- Review of records and diagnostic reports
- Collaboration with colleagues

The purpose of collecting data is to identify the client's

- Present and past health status
- Present and past coping patterns (strengths and limitations)
- Response to present alterations
- Response to therapy (nursing, medical)
- Risk for potential problems

Nurses collect data to determine nursing activities and to assist other professionals (pharmacists, nutritionists, social workers, physicians) in determining their activities. It is therefore important that health care professionals freely exchange data about their clients in order to increase the quality and the validity of health care. For example, a nurse assesses the signs of orthostatic hypotension in a client. The problem is referred to the physician to investigate the cause and determine the treatment. The nurse plans nursing activities to help the client reduce those factors that contribute to the vertigo and also to prevent injury.

Unfortunately, many nurses primarily gather physiological data for other professionals to use and ignore the other life processes, those which involve psychological, sociocultural, developmental, and spiritual considerations. From a holistic view, an understanding of the interaction patterns in all five areas is needed to identify the individual's strengths and limitations and help him achieve an optimal level of health. Ignoring any of the life processes can result in frustration and failure for all concerned.

Like the other components of the nursing process, the assessment process is dynamic and ongoing. During every nurse–client interaction, the nurse is continually processing data. The types of data gathered depend on the nurse's knowledge base, experience, and philosophy.

Data Collection Formats

Data collection usually consists of two formats, the nursing data-base interview and the focus assessment, each of which can be used either alone or in conjunction with the other.

Historically, the assessment forms used by nurses were organized under a body-system format. Information collected under a body-system model is useful to nursing, but it is incomplete because it does not include data on the areas of sleep, activity, spirituality, and so on. In an attempt to focus data collection on concerns that are more relevant to nursing, the body-system model was discarded and replaced by a nursing model. Unfortunately, the nursing model alone failed to provide the nurse with complete data about physiological functioning.

As was discussed in Chapter 2, nurses encounter, diagnose, and treat two types of human responses—those that can be described by nursing diagnoses and those that represent collaborative problems. Each type requires a different assessment focus.

Data-Base or Admission Interview

The data-base interview involves the collection of a predetermined set of facts during the initial contact with the client. The interviewer should gather data in all five life processes to determine patterns, strengths, and alterations. The assessment criteria in the data-base interview should be clear and concise in order to provide the nurse with a tool for gathering data in a systematic and efficient manner. This interview should not duplicate data gathered by other professionals; the focus should clearly be a nursing focus. Appendix I represents a sample nursing data-base interview designed for nurses in an adult acute care setting. It can be modified if either the setting or the client requires additional data. (Appendixes II, III, IV, and V are data bases for mental health settings, pediatric clients, high-risk elderly clients, and maternal clients.) Refer to Chapter 4 for characteristics of an efficient data collection tool.

Focus Assessment

Focus assessment is the acquisition of selected or specific data as determined by the nurse and the client or family or by the condition of the client. A focus assessment can take a few minutes or a longer period of time. The nurse who assesses the condition of a new postoperative client (vital signs, incision, hydration, comfort) is performing a focus assessment.

A focus assessment can also be carried out during the initial interview if the data collected suggest a possible problem area that needs to be validated or ruled out. For example, during the data base interview, the nurse suspects that certain data may represent a nursing diagnosis. The nurse considers a possible or tentative diagnosis. The nurse then collects additional data (focus assessment) to confirm or rule out the tentative diagnosis. This process can be depicted as:

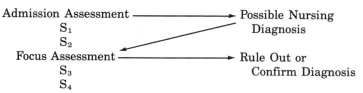

In Section II, each diagnostic category is described in terms of focus assessment criteria to identify specific data that may need to be collected to confirm or rule out the diagnosis. These focus assessment criteria can be used in conjunction with the data-base interview or in an isolated situation requiring additional information. Focus assessments can yield collaborative problems (*e.g.*, postoperative hypovolemia) or nursing diagnoses (*e.g.*, anxiety).

The Assessment Process

In order to perform an accurate assessment, the nurse must have the ability to

- Communicate effectively
- Observe systematically
- Perform a nursing physical assessment
- Differentiate between cues and inferences
- Identify interaction patterns
- Validate impressions

Communicating Effectively

All nurse–client interactions are based on communication. The term *therapeutic communication* is used to describe techniques that provide an opportunity for the client or family to share views and feelings openly. The technique incorporates verbal and nonverbal skills, as well as empathy and a sense of caring. Verbal techniques include asking closed- and open-ended questions, exploring the answers, and summarizing the content for the client. Nonverbal techniques include active listening, the use of silence, touch, and eye contact. Active listening, which is most vital in data collection, is also the most difficult skill to learn. Few people listen objectively; most tend to concentrate on their own forthcoming responses rather than on what the other person is saying. The elements of active listening are

- Channeling attention to the sender and staying quiet within oneself
- Reducing or eliminating barriers
- Maintaining eye contact
- "Squaring off" eye-to-eye, shoulder-to-shoulder (positioning one's body in alignment with the other person's body)
- Avoiding interruptions

Barriers to active listening are always present, and the professional nurse must take the appropriate measures to eliminate them or their influence on an interaction. Figure 3-2 illustrates the barriers to active listening.

Learning effective communication skills requires knowledge of self and of communication and learning theory, as well as continuous practice. Above all, it calls for the determination to retain sensitivity, which is often lost as one develops more advanced communication skills (Ramackers).

Observing Systematically

The ability to observe systematically is dependent on the nurse's knowledge base. With increased knowledge about human interaction, the nurse will look for specific data. Knowing what contributes to or causes a particular problem enables the nurse to explore these areas with the client. If the nurse does not know what a problem looks like, she will be unable to recognize and diagnose it. For example, if the nurse does not know the signs and symptoms of *Self-concept Disturbance*, she may overlook the presence of this response. Systematic observations can be enhanced when written guidelines are used. Such guidelines are invaluable because they identify the specific types of data that need to be collected. Once one becomes familiar with the guidelines, one can gather the data without referring to a written guide.

1. Internal
   - The person's views are different from the nurse's perceptions.
   - The person's dialect or accent is different.
   - The person's appearance is different or distracting.
   - The person is in pain or is anxious.
   - The person is telling the nurse something that he or she does not want to hear.
   - The nurse feels a dislike toward the person.
   - The nurse is thinking of something else.
   - The nurse is planning the next statement.
   - The nurse is anxious or apprehensive.
2. External
   - Noise from equipment, speakers, television, radio, etc.
   - Lack of privacy
   - Physical hindrances such as desks, equipment, space, etc.
   - Verbal remarks such as clichés, trite comments, or interruptions

Fig. 3-2 Barriers to active listening. (Carpenito LJ, Duespohl TA: A Guide to Effective Clinical Instruction, 2nd ed. Rockville, MD, Aspen Systems Co, 1986)

For each diagnostic category listed in Section II, a focus assessment is presented to direct the nurse in gathering data in order to confirm or rule out the nursing diagnosis. Each specific nursing diagnosis has its assessment signs and symptoms to further assist in diagnosing.

Performing a Nursing Physical Assessment

Physical assessment is the collection of objective data concerning the client's physical status. The techniques used include inspection, palpation, percussion, and auscultation. Physical assessment incorporates the examination of an individual from head to toe with a focus on the body systems.

To determine the purpose of the physical exam from a nursing perspective, we must ask the following question: What can a staff nurse do with the data acquired from performing a data-base physical assessment? If the answer is only to report the findings to the physician, perhaps the nurse should leave that portion of the examination to the physician. The important thing is to stress the assessment skills that are crucial for the nurse generalist. For example, the nurse needs to be able to assess signs of increased intracranial pressure but not necessarily to perform an entire neurological exam. However, this does not mean that advanced skills should not be learned by nurses who routinely screen, case-find, and treat selected problems.

Table 3-1 lists those areas of physical diagnosis in which nurses should be proficient. The examination of these areas by the nurse can yield valuable data from which nursing care can be planned. Physical diagnosis as determined by nurses should be clearly "nursing" in focus. The diagnosis of pathophysiology should be left to the physician. The individual nurse must decide how important it is to her own practice to learn to palpate livers, auscultate murmurs, or use an ophthalmoscope. By examining her philosophy and definition of nursing, the nurse should seek to develop expertise in those areas that will enhance her nursing practice.

Differentiating Between Cues and Inferences

In order to recognize and validate information accurately, the nurse must acquire a method of identifying that information. Little and Carnevali have identified such a process as cue identification and inferencing.

A *cue* is information that one acquires through the use of the five senses (taste, touch,

Table 3-1.   **Physical Assessment by Nurse Generalists**

Physical System	Criteria
Sensory-Perceptual	Mental status Vision and appearance of eyes Hearing Touch Taste and smell
Skin	Condition (color, turgor, character) Lesions Edema Hair distribution Breast
Respiratory	Rate, character Breath sounds Cough

Cardiovascular	Pulses (rate, quality, rhythm)
	   Apical Radial
	   Carotid Dorsalis pedis
	   Brachial Posterior tibial
	   Femoral
	Blood pressure
	Circulation (mucous membranes, nail beds)

Neurological	Pupillary reactions Orientation Level of consciousness Grasp strength
Gastrointestinal	Mouth, gums, teeth, and tongue (color and condition) Gag reflex Bowel sounds Presence of distention, impaction, hemorrhoids (external)
Genitourinary	Presence of retention Discharge (vaginal, urethral) Uterine response (pregnancy, postpartum) External genitalia
Musculoskeletal	Muscle tone, strength Gait, stability Range of motion

smell, hearing, and sight). Primary sources of cues are the subjective statements of the client and the objective facts observed by the nurse. Secondary sources are family, other health care providers, and diagnostic studies. An *inference* is the nurse's judgment or interpretation of these cues. Inferences are always subjective and are influenced by the knowledge base, values, and experiences of the nurse. For example:

Cue	*Corresponding Inference*
Hgb 9.1	Abnormal
Crying	Possible fear, sadness
5 ft 1 in, 220 lb	Obesity

Differentiating between inferences and cues is important. Although an inference is a subjective judgment, nurses will frequently report it as a fact or fail to gather sufficient cues to confirm it or rule it out. Inferences made with fewer or no supporting cues can result in inappropriate and sometimes dangerous care, especially when invalid inferences are passed on to other members of the health team.

Diagnosis

Diagnosis, the second component of the nursing process, incorporates the intellectual activities that focus on identifying patterns, validating the findings, and evolving a conclusion. As was mentioned in Chapter 1, the term *nursing diagnosis* is used frequently in place of the term *problem identification* as a step in the nursing process, as specified in the ANA standards of practice. This author will use diagnosis to represent the second component of the nursing process.

Nurses make judgments regarding a variety of assessment data. Some of these judgments are nursing diagnoses, some are not. When a nurse concludes that a certain EKG pattern is abnormal, the nurse has made a diagnosis. When the nurse labels certain tonic–clonic movements a seizure, the nurse has made a diagnosis. In both of these situations the nurse had diagnosed, but neither one is a nursing diagnosis. Both of these situations require nursing and medical interventions for successful outcomes to be achieved. The reader is referred to Chapter 2 for an in-depth discussion of nursing diagnoses versus the other problems nurses treat.

Identifying Alternatives

Diagnosis involves complex thinking about the data gathered from the client, family, records, and other health care providers. This thinking, combined with relevant information stored in the nurse's memory, is used to generate possible explanations for the data. These intellectual (cognitive) activities are difficult to teach and learn; many nurses who acquire expertise in assessment often flounder when asked to synthesize the data and identify a pattern. Aspinall and Tanner (1981) found that nurses take various approaches to problem identification, ranging from systematic testing of several possible explanations to the quick generation of one explanation. However, if the nurse does not take an approach that considers more than one explanation, the validity and effectiveness of the plan of care are jeopardized. According to Aspinall and Tanner, potential problems that can result when alternative explanations are not considered and tested include

- Overvaluing the probability of one explanation
- Failing to include the accurate diagnosis in the initial hypothesis
- Failing to consider all the data because of the narrow focus
- Reaching an incorrect diagnosis because of speed, bias, or assumptions based on experience

To assist in identifying alternative explanations and in confirming or ruling out alternatives, the nurse should supplement her own memory-stored information by consulting references on the subject or by talking with other members of the health team. Unfortunately, nurses do not always utilize the most valuable resource available to them—other nurses.

Nursing staff conferences on client care are a nonthreatening and productive method for helping staff members identify alternative solutions to problems and interventions. After the background of the problem has been shared with the group, the members are asked to think of possible explanations for the data. These explanations are then written on a blackboard, after which the group considers what data are needed to confirm or rule out each possibility. Explanations that have been ruled out are crossed off. The nurse caring for the client will then proceed to confirm or rule out the remaining explanations while caring for the client.

As the nurse gains more knowledge and experience, she will need less time to think of alternative explanations. However, this step should never be eliminated. Identifying alternatives is also important when determining interventions, in order to avoid failure, stereotyping, and monotony.

Identifying Nursing Diagnoses

After collecting the necessary data, the nurse then clusters or organizes the information according to various areas of functioning and determines the client's *pattern of functioning* in each area (positive functioning, altered functioning, or at-risk-for-altered functioning). The following questions may be applied to each area of functioning (listed below) to assist the nurse in formulating a conclusion about the data collected for that category.*

- Is there a problem (actual), or is there a high risk for developing a problem (potential) in this area of functioning, or
- Do the data collected lead one to suspect a problem (possible) in this area?

    1. Health perception–health management
        Health management?
        Compliance?
        Injuries?
    2. Nutritional–metabolic
        Nutrition?
        Fluid intake?
        Peripheral edema?
        Infection?
        Oral cavity health?
    3. Elimination
        Bowel elimination?
        Incontinence?
    4. Activity–exercise
        Activities of daily living?
        Leisure activities?
        Home care?
        Respiratory function?
    5. Sleep–rest
        Sleep?
    6. Cognitive–perceptual
        Decisions?
        Comfort?
        Knowledge?
        Sensory input?
    7. Self-perception
        Anxiety/fear?
        Control?
        Self-concept?

* Copyright 1985, Lynda Juall Carpenito

8. Role–relationship
   Communication?
   Family?
   Loss?
   Parenting?
   Socialization?
   Violence?
9. Sexuality–reproductive
   Sexuality?
10. Coping–stress tolerance
    Coping?
11. Value–belief
    Spirituality?

Identifying Collaborative Problems

Is a physiological complication present, or is there a *high* risk for one developing because of a disease, treatment, diagnostic study, or medication that you want to monitor?

- Cardiac
- Circulatory
- Respiratory
- Renal
- Neurological
- Muscular
- Skeletal
- Endocrine
- Gastrointestinal

Assessment Conclusions

After the data have been gathered and examined and alternative explanations tested and ruled out, the nurse will reach one of the following three conclusions:

1. No problem evident at this time; health promotion activities indicated
2. Collaborative problem
3. Actual, potential, possible nursing diagnosis

Figure 3-3 is a schematic diagram of the diagnosing phase.

Conclusion 1

No problem evident at this time
Health promotion activities indicated

If at the time of the assessment, no problem is identified, but certain teaching needs are indicated to maintain the present level of wellness or to promote a higher level of wellness, conclusion 1 is reached. The nurse, along with the client, then determines the complexity of the health promotion activities needed. If the teaching can be accomplished at the initial session without the need for the follow-up meetings, the situation remains a 1. Thus, the session would probably conclude with the nurse specifying those indicators that suggest the need for future contact. This situation could occur in acute settings when a nurse has a specialized role that allows her to act as a consultant. Examples include enterostomal therapists, operating room nurses performing preoperative visits, clinical specialists, and nurses in private practice.

Assessment

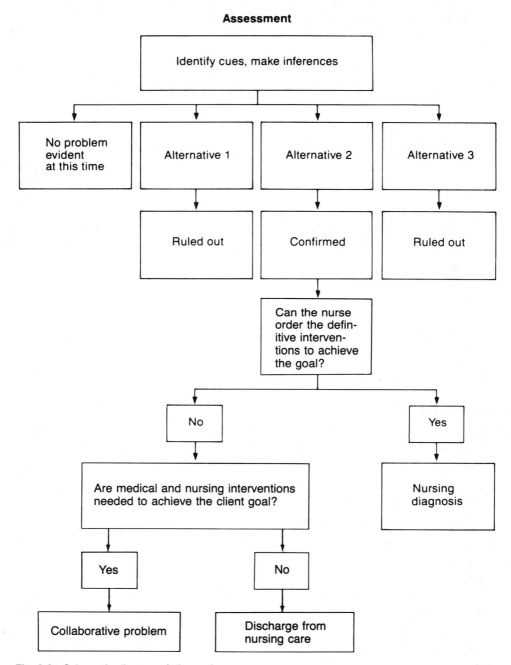

Fig. 3-3   Schematic diagram of diagnosing.

A client is admitted for surgery for a cataract removal. Since the client has a colostomy, the enterostomal therapist visits him to assess his present status. After discussing his stomal care and his postoperative expectations, the nurse concludes that follow-up visits for teaching are not indicated. The nurse instructs him to call her if needed during his hospitalization.

If the health promotion activities cannot be accomplished in one session, the nurse would then use the nursing diagnosis *Health-Seeking Behaviors* and develop a teaching plan for future sessions. Other nursing diagnoses are also appropriate to describe interventions that promote health, as illustrated in the following example:

Mrs. Green is a 32-year-old woman who recently gave birth to her first child. She works for a large publishing company as an editor and has taken a 9-month leave of absence because of the baby. During a routine examination of her newborn in the pediatrician's office, Mrs. Green expresses concern to the nurse that she is bored and feels useless. She indicates that she has recently gained 10 pounds, is sleeping about 12 hours out of 24, and has frequent arguments with her husband. The nurse validates with Mrs. Green that these problems have developed since the birth of the baby. Since the health of the family unit is influenced by the interaction patterns of its members, the nurse identifies potential problems in the areas of parenting and coping. In analyzing the data, the nurse selects the nursing diagnosis *Self-Concept Disturbance* to describe Mrs. Green's problem (see Section II). In order to complete the diagnosis and determine the appropriate interventions, the nurse needs to identify the contributing factors and incorporate them into the diagnosis. In the case of Mrs. Green, the complete diagnosis would appear as:

Self-Concept Disturbance Related to Change in Life-style from That of an Editor to the Mother Role as Manifested by Negative Statements Regarding Self and Activities

Having made the diagnosis, the nurse can assist Mrs. Green to identify activities that will increase her productivity and improve her self-concept. Follow-up phone calls or visits should be used to evaluate progress and to reassess the situation.

Conclusions 2 and 3

Conclusion 2 involves a collaborative problem, whereas Conclusion 3 is an actual, potential, or possible nursing diagnosis. These situations were discussed and differentiated in Chapter 2.

Case Study Application

A clinical situation often encountered by nurses, the confused elderly client, exemplifies the dangers of incomplete assessments and impulsive problem-solving. Many nurses dismiss confusion in the elderly as an outcome of aging and fail to treat it as a signal. Before labeling a client as "Altered Thought Processes Related to Aging Associated With Atherosclerosis," the nurse should assess for other explanations. The assessment criteria in Figure 3-4 represent factors to be assessed when considering the history of the confusion and possible contributing factors.

The following case study illustrates two methods of problem-solving.

Mrs. D is an 86-year-old woman admitted to a medical unit because she had a blood sugar of 260. Mrs. D has intermittent periods of confusion, especially at night. In an attempt to control her outbursts (she kept screaming that she was "being held prisoner"), the nurses requested and received an order for a hypnotic at night, a sedative PRN, and a jacket restraint. Mrs. D became more agitated and confused.

History of the Confusion	
At home and in agency	Sudden or gradual
Onset and duration	Continuous or intermittent
Acute or chronic	Time of day or night
History of the Individual	
Life-style	Interests
(past and present)	Support system
Work history	Coping patterns
Presence of Physiological Contributing Factors	
Respiratory status (blood gases)	Nutritional status (weight, hydration)
Renal status (output, BUN, creatinine)	Circulatory status (pulses, skin)
Endocrine status (glucose)	Medication (overdose or side-effect)
Fluid and electrolyte balance (Na, K,	
specific gravity)	
Presence of Situational Contributing Factors	
Fear of unknown, loss	Philosophy of family and health care
Actual loss of control, income, significant	providers
others, routine, familiar objects or sur-	Attitude toward aging
roundings (house, pets)	Beliefs about confusion
Sensory overload or deprivation	Tone, speed, volume of speech
	Content of communication

Fig. 3-4 Focus assessment criteria for confusion.

Nursing Diagnosis: Altered Thought Processes Related to Hypoxic Effects of Cerebral Arteriosclerosis (Aging Process)

After noticing that Mrs. D was usually not confused when her granddaughter or daughter was present, the nurse initiated an assessment of Mrs. D's confusion by acquiring data from Mrs. D and her granddaughter, as follows:

History of Individual

The confusion began the first night of admission. Mrs. D lives alone and is very independent. She has had a history of forgetting some facts but has not had episodes of confusion. She has strong family ties and communicates with her daughter daily via visit or phone.

Physiological Contributing Factors

In reviewing the possible physiological factors that could contribute to confusion in Mrs. D, the nurse identified hyperglycemia and possible side-effects of hypnotic medications and sedatives.

Situational Contributing Factors

The sudden hospitalization caused Mrs. D to lose control over her activities: her normal routine, her familiar surroundings, her significant others. All these losses contributed to her fear. Since most of the nursing staff had never known Mrs. D before her apparent confusion, their communications with her were loud and rapid, occurring primarily while they helped her with her activities of daily living (eating, ambulating, hygiene). In contrast, her family talked slowly and quietly with her about her grandchildren and about their activities. She listened carefully and responded appropriately to them. As a result, the nursing diagnosis had to be revised.

Revised Nursing Diagnosis: Altered Thought Processes Related to Unfamiliar Surroundings and Inability to Differentiate Increased Incoming Stimuli

The nurse collaborated with the physician concerning the medications ordered, and both the sedative and the hypnotic were discontinued. Blood glucose levels were ordered at bedtime and at 6:00 A.M. to assess the need for insulin twice a day.

A care plan was formulated with the interventions designed to:

1. Reduce unfamiliar incoming stimuli by slowly explaining procedures and activities
2. Institute reality orientation by introducing familiar objects from home, photographs, music
3. Encourage staff to talk to client about her interests: cooking, crocheting, her grandchildren

As is illustrated in this case study, the deliberate search for alternative explanations for data is important to prevent problems that can be injurious to clients and frustrating to nurses.

Summary

Data is systematically collected in the assessment phase by means of collaborative observation, examination, interviewing, and record review. Strengths and limitations of the individual and the family are considered, as are the client's patterns and perceptions. Validation of the data is sought from the client, family, nursing colleagues, other professionals, client records, and reference material.

The quality and validity of the cues and inferences are dependent on the knowledge base, experiences, and values of the nurse.

After considering several alternative explanations for the data, the nurse concludes the problem-identification phase with one of the following outcomes:

- No problem at this time
- Health promotion activities indicated
- Collaborative problem
- Actual, potential, possible nursing diagnosis

References

Alfaro R: Application of Nursing Process: A Step-by-Step Guide. Philadelphia, JB Lippincott, 1986

Aspinall MJ, Tanner C: Decision-making for Patient Care, pp 7–12. New York, Appleton-Century-Crofts, 1981

Gordon M: Nursing diagnoses and the diagnostic process. Am J Nurs 76:1298–1300, 1976

Little D, Carnevali D: Nursing Care Planning. Philadelphia, JB Lippincott, 1976

Ramackers MJ: Communication blocks revisited. Am J Nurs 79:1079–1081, 1979

Smith VN, Bass T: Communication for Health Professionals. Philadelphia, JB Lippincott, 1979

4

Application to Care Planning

In order to become a full profession, nursing must identify its unique focus and demonstrate accountability in terms of that focus. The classification system of nursing diagnoses is a mechanism for identifying the domain of nursing, and care planning is the mechanism for demonstrating accountability. Care plans serve to communicate to the nursing staff the specific problems of the client and the prescribed interventions for directing and evaluating the care given. In order to prepare a care plan, the nurse must deliberately and systematically engage in problem-solving.

Care Plans

Care plans have two professional purposes—administrative and clinical. The administrative purposes of care plans are:

- To define the nursing focus for the client or group
- To differentiate the accountability of the nurse from that of other members of the health team
- To provide the criteria for reviewing and evaluating care (quality assurance)
- To provide the criteria for patient classification

The care plan serves the following clinical purposes:

- Provides a blueprint to direct charting
- Communicates to the nursing staff
  what to teach
  what to observe
  what to implement
- Provides outcome criteria for reviewing and evaluating care
- Directs specific interventions for the individual, family, and other nursing staff members to implement

In order to direct and evaluate nursing care, the care plan should include the following:

- Diagnostic Statement
  Collaborative problems
  Nursing diagnoses
- Outcome criteria (client goals)
- Nursing orders or interventions
- Evaluation (status of plan)

Some institutions require that the nursing care plan include only nursing diagnoses and not collaborative problems. However, since nurses treat clients with other problems in addition to those designated by nursing diagnoses, this restriction creates a dilemma. Where is the nurse to record the planned interventions for collaborative problems? Faced with this situation, nurses have tended to respond by rewording all problems as nursing diagnoses, a practice that further confuses the issue and dilutes the effectiveness of nursing as a whole.

Nurses need a system for recording the nursing actions that address problems not covered by nursing diagnoses. Since nurses often find it difficult to separate the collaborative from the independent dimension of nursing, it would be best to use a system that provides a way to designate and include both collaborative problems and nursing diagnoses. Complex collaborative problems and nursing diagnoses could be recorded with the related interventions on the care plans, while routine problems could be addressed on the standard of care. This type of documentation will be explained later in this chapter.

Assessment and Diagnosis

The assessment component of the nursing process is addressed in the admission data base and in the care plan. The admission data base is gathered during the nursing interview conducted at the time of initial contact with the client. A preprinted form directs the nurse to gather data in order to assess the client for present or potential alterations in health. This form should be organized in a manner that permits efficient data collection and provides space for elaboration when needed.

The assessment component is also addressed on the care plan in the intervention column, which directs the nurse to monitor or assess for a problem. For example:

Diagnosis

Potential Complication:
Cardiogenic shock (post M.I.)

Interventions

Monitor
  Urinary perfusion <30 ml/hr
  Level of consciousness, skin (temp., color)
  Blood pressure (systolic <80 mm)
  Cardiac pattern

Identifying Interaction Patterns

Many questions arise as the nurse gathers initial data with the data-base assessment.

1. What is the person's usual pattern?
2. What represents an altered pattern?
3. Does the person's usual pattern present a risk of contributing to an altered functional pattern?
4. Is the person at risk for a physiological complication due to disease, injuries, treatments, or diagnostic studies?
5. What health promotion teaching is indicated?
6. When should the nurse defer the collection of data?

What is the Person's Usual Pattern? What Represents an Altered Pattern?

During the assessment, the nurse elicits data that reflect the past and present functional patterns of the person. The nurse must be careful not to diagnose patterns with isolated data. Isolated data may be important in the content of the usual pattern, but the usual pattern must be determined before analysis can take place. The following is an example of this error.

Mrs. F is a 33-year-old woman. In response to a 24-hour recall of her diet, she reports:

Breakfast: coffee (1 cup)
Morning break: coffee (1 cup)
Lunch: yogurt
Afternoon break: pound cake (1 slice)
Dinner: pizza, salad, coffee (2 cups)

The inference drawn from this data could be: Inadequate intake of basic four food groups. The nurse should ask Mrs. F, "Is this your usual daily intake?" Mrs. F's response will help the nurse determine the reason for the diet: *e.g.*, financial factors, lack of knowledge of nutrition, unusual circumstances.

If the nurse determines a diagnosis of possible altered nutrition related to inadequate consumption of the four basic food groups, she then looks to other assessment data to validate the existence of the altered state: *e.g.*, skin, bowel elimination, weight/height ratio.

If the nurse is uncertain of what data are needed to confirm the nursing diagnosis, she can refer to the specific diagnostic category in Section II for the focus assessment criteria and the defining characteristics.

Does the Person's Usual Pattern Present a Risk of Contributing to an Altered Functional Pattern?

In the case of Mrs. F, if the diet recall presented is her usual state, the nurse can infer that this diet is nutritionally deficient and with additional questions can elicit contributing factors. When the nurse diagnoses the state of risk she utilizes the diagnosis of:

> **Potential Altered Health Maintenance Related to Lack of Knowledge of Implications of Inadequate Diet and Daily Nutritional Requirements, and the Inconvenience of Preparing Meals for One Person**

Is the Person at Risk for a Physiological Complication due to Disease, Injuries, Treatments, or Diagnostic Studies?

Prior to the assessment, the nurse may receive information about the person's medical diagnosis and treatment. During the assessment, the nurse will acquire data regarding medical history and treatment. With this information the nurse can predict physiological complications for which the individual is at risk and for which the nurse must monitor.

For example, a person admitted for elective surgery who also has diabetes mellitus will be monitored for blood sugar fluctuations under the collaborative problem of *Potential Complication: hypo/hyperglycemia*. (See Chapter 2 for a complete discussion of collaborative problems.)

What Health Promotion Teaching Is Indicated?

The expanding focus of nursing on health promotion and wellness is an attempt to balance the previous focus, which centered on illness. It must be appreciated, however, that in some situations in acute care settings the priority for the client and the nurse is the resolution of the compromised function. As length of stay is reduced and severity of illness increases, it will become more difficult for nurses in acute care settings to focus on health promotion. Rather than discard health promotion as an option, nurses in acute care settings can use some nontraditional teaching strategies to foster wellness. The following are some examples:

- Printed take-home material
- Audiovisual material (lending library)
- Classes (community-based)

In order to determine the type and amount of teaching indicated, the nurse assesses the individual's knowledge of the following factors that contribute to the promotion and maintenance of health.

- Knowledge of disease and preventive behavior
- Appropriate screening practices for age and risk

- Optimal nutrition and weight control
- Regular exercise program
- Constructive stress management
- Supportive social networks

For specific directions for assessment and interventions, please refer to *Altered Health Maintenance and Health-Seeking Behaviors* in Section II.

When Should the Nurse Defer the Collection of Data?

A printed data-assessment form should be viewed as a guide for the nurse, not a mandate. All data-base forms should have a provision for allowing the nurse to defer the collection of selected data. Before requesting information from a client, the nurse should ask herself, What am I going to do with the data? If certain information is useless or irrelevant for a particular client, then its collection is a waste of time and often distressing to clients. Asking a terminally ill man how much he smokes or drinks, for example, is inexcusable, unless the nurse has a specific goal. If a client will be NPO for an unlimited period of time, it is probably unnecessary for the nurse to collect data on nutritional patterns. The assessment will be indicated when the person resumes a diet.

If the client is extremely stressed, the nurse should collect only necessary data and defer the collection of functional patterns to another time or day. A stressed person may not be the best source of data because his memory is often clouded.

The admission interview form can be structured to allow for deferring the collection of data. The following codes illustrate the defer options:

1 = N/A, not applicable: applies to sections that are not suitable

2 = Unable to acquire: applies to items or sections that need to be assessed but cannot be addressed at this time. For example, a confused patient may be unable to provide the needed information.

3 = Not a priority: applies to items or sections that are not appropriate to assess at this time

4 = Other: applies to items or sections that are not assessed for reasons other than 2 or 3. For example, the admission interview may be discontinued in order to transport the patient for emergency surgery. This option requires an explanatory note in the chart.

If desired, the admission assessment form can be marked to indicate selected items that must always be assessed, unless, of course, the situation is an Option 2—unable to acquire. Figure 4-1 is an example of an admission assessment form. It contains several characteristics that facilitate its use for the defer options and has a format that allows for checking options rather than writing them. Some data collection is not facilitated by checking choices, such as support system, emotional status, sexual concerns, etc.

Planning Conferences

Client care conferences are an excellent way to help nurses with planning care. These conferences can be held daily and should be restricted to 15 to 20 minutes. If you are initiating conferences, it is sometimes advantageous to begin with weekly sessions and move gradually to daily or three-times-a-week sessions. Planning conferences should not be restricted to the day shift. They should also be conducted on evening and night shifts. The client or clients discussed can be those who are new admissions, those who have complex problems or conflicts with the staff, or those who are difficult to diagnose from a nursing diagnosis standpoint. The conference time provides nurses with an opportunity

(*Text continues on page 65*)

**NURSING ADMISSION
DATA BASE**

Date _____ Arrival Time _____ Contact Person _____ Phone _____
ADMITTED FROM: ____ Home alone   ____ Home with relative   ____ Long-term care
                ____ Homeless   ____ Home with _____   facility
                ____ ER   ____   (Specify)   ____ Other _____
MODE OF ARRIVAL: ____ Wheelchair   ____ Ambulance   ____ Stretcher
REASON FOR HOSPITALIZATION: _____
_____

LAST HOSPITAL ADMISSION: Date _____ Reason _____
_____

PAST MEDICAL HISTORY: _____
_____

MEDICATION (Prescription/Over-the-Counter)	DOSAGE	LAST DOSE	FREQUENCY

HEALTH MAINTENANCE–PRESCRIPTION PATTERN
USE OF:
Tobacco: ____ None ____ Quit (date) ____ Pipe ____ Cigar ____ <1 pk/day
             ____ 1–2 pks/day ____ >2 pks/day Pks/year history _____
Alcohol: ____ None ____ Type/amount ____ /day ____ /wk ____ /month
Other Drugs: ____ No ____ Yes Type _____ Use _____
Allergies (drugs, food, tape, dyes): _____ Reaction _____
_____

ACTIVITY/EXERCISE PATTERN
SELF-CARE ABILITY:
  0 = Independent   1 = Assistive device   2 = Assistance from others
  3 = Assistance from person and equipment   4 = Dependent/Unable

	0	1	2	3	4
Eating/Drinking					
Bathing					
Dressing/Grooming					
Toileting					
Bed Mobility					
Transferring					
Ambulating					
Stair Climbing					
Shopping					
Cooking					
Home Maintenance					

ASSISTIVE DEVICES: ____ None ____ Crutches ____ Bedside commode ____ Walker
                   ____ Cane ____ Splint/Brace ____ Wheelchair ____ Other ____

CODE: (1) Non-applicable (2) Unable to acquire
      (3) Not a priority at this time (4) Other (specify in notes)

Side One

Fig. 4-1. Sample admission data base.

NUTRITION/METABOLIC PATTERN
Special Diet/Supplements _____
Previous Dietary Instruction: ___ Yes ___ No
Appetite: ___ Normal ___ Increased ___ Decreased ___ Decreased taste sensation
___ Nausea ___ Vomiting ___ Stomatitis
Weight Fluctuations Last 6 Months: ___ None _____ lbs. Gained/Lost
Swallowing Difficulty (Dysphagia): ___ None ___ Solids ___ Liquids
Dentures: ___ Upper (_ Partial _ Full) ___ Lower (_ Partial _ Full)
With Patient ___ Yes ___ No
History of Skin/Healing Problems: ___ None ___ Abnormal Healing ___ Rash
___ Dryness ___ Excess Perspiration

ELIMINATION PATTERN
Bowel Habits: ___ # BMs/day ___ Date of last BM ___ Within normal limits
___ Constipation ___ Diarrhea ___ Incontinence
___ Ostomy: Type ___ Appliance ___ Self-care ___ Yes ___ No
Bladder Habits: ___ WNL ___ Frequency ___ Dysuria ___ Nocturia ___ Urgency
___ Hematuria ___ Retention
Incontinency: ___ No ___ Yes ___ Total ___ Daytime ___ Nighttime
___ Occasional ___ Difficulty delaying voiding
___ Difficulty reaching toilet
Assistive Devices: ___ Intermittent catheterization
___ Indwelling catheter ___ External catheter
___ Incontinent briefs ___ Penile implant type _____

SLEEP/REST PATTERN
Habits: ___ hrs/night ___ AM nap ___ PM nap
Feel rested after sleep ___ Yes ___ No
Problems: ___ None ___ Early waking ___ Insomnia ___ Nightmares

COGNITIVE–CONCEPTUAL PATTERN
Hearing: ___ WNL ___ Impaired (_ Right _ Left) ___ Deaf (_ Right _ Left)
___ Hearing Aid ___ Tinnitus
Vision: ___ WNL ___ Eyeglasses ___ Contact lens
___ Impaired ___ Right ___ Left
___ Blind ___ Right ___ Left
___ Cataract ___ Right ___ Left
___ Glaucoma
___ Prosthetis ___ Right ___ Left
Vertigo: ___ Yes ___ No
Discomfort/Pain: ___ None ___ Acute ___ Chronic ___ Description _____
_____

Pain Management: _____

COPING STRESS TOLERANCE/SELF-PERCEPTION/SELF-CONCEPT PATTERN
Major concerns regarding hospitalization or illness (financial, self-care): _____
_____
Major loss/change in past year: ___ No ___ Yes _____
_____

CODE: (1) Non-applicable (2) Unable to acquire
(3) Not a priority at this time (4) Other (specify in notes)

Side Two

Fig. 4-1. (continued)

SEXUALITY/REPRODUCTIVE PATTERN

LMP: _____

Menstrual Problems: ____ Yes ____ No _____

Last Pap Smear: _____

Monthly Self-Breast/Testicular Exam: ____ Yes ____ No

Sexual Concerns R/T Illness: _____

ROLE-RELATIONSHIP PATTERN

Occupation: _____

Employment Status: ____ Employed ____ Short-term disability
____ Long-term disability ____ Unemployed

Support System: ____ Spouse ____ Neighbors/Friends ____ None
____ Family in same residence ____ Family in separate residence
____ Other _____

Family concerns regarding hospitalization: _____

VALUE-BELIEF PATTERN

Religion: ____ Roman Catholic ____ Protestant ____ Jewish ____ Other

Religious Restrictions: ____ No ____ Yes (Specify) _____

Request Chaplain Visitation at This Time: ____ Yes ____ No

PHYSICAL ASSESSMENT (Objective)

1. **CLINICAL DATA**

   Age _____ Height _____ Weight _____ (Actual/Approximate)

   Temperature _____

   Pulse: ____ Strong ____ Weak ____ Regular ____ Irregular

   Blood Pressure: Right Arm ____ Left Arm ____ Sitting ____ Lying ____

2. **RESPIRATORY/CIRCULATORY**

   Rate _____

   Quality: ____ WNL ____ Shallow ____ Rapid ____ Labored ____ Other _____

   Cough: ____ No ____ Yes/Describe _____

   Auscultation:

   Upper rt lobes ____ WNL ____ Decreased ____ Absent ____ Abnormal sounds ____

   Upper lt lobes ____ WNL ____ Decreased ____ Absent ____ Abnormal sounds ____

   Lower rt lobes ____ WNL ____ Decreased ____ Absent ____ Abnormal sounds ____

   Lower lt lobes ____ WNL ____ Decreased ____ Absent ____ Abnormal sounds ____

   Right Pedal Pulse: ____ Strong ____ Weak ____ Absent

   Left Pedal Pulse: ____ Strong ____ Weak ____ Absent

3. **METABOLIC-INTEGUMENTARY**

   SKIN:

   Color: ____ WNL ____ Pale ____ Cyanotic ____ Ashen ____ Jaundice ____ Other ____

   Temperature: ____ WNL ____ Warm ____ Cool

   Turgor: ____ WNL ____ Poor

   Edema: ____ No ____ Yes/Description/location _____

   Lesions: ____ None ____ Yes/Description/location _____

   Bruises: ____ None ____ Yes/Description/location _____

   Reddened: ____ No ____ Yes/Description/location _____

   Pruritus: ____ No ____ Yes/Description/location _____

   Tubes: Specify _____

   MOUTH:

   Gums: ____ WNL ____ White plaque ____ Lesions ____ Other _____

   Teeth: ____ WNL ____ Other _____

   ABDOMEN:

   Bowel Sounds: ____ Present ____ Absent

Side Three

Fig. 4-1. (continued)

4. NEURO/SENSORY
Mental Status: ____ Alert ____ Receptive aphasia ____ Poor historian
____ Oriented ____ Confused ____ Combative ____ Unresponsive
Speech: ____ Normal ____ Slurred ____ Garbled ____ Expressive aphasia
Spoken language_____ Interpreter _____
Pupils: ____ Equal ____ Unequal

Left: • • • • • ● ● ● ●

Right: • • • • ● ● ● ● ●

Reactive to light:
Left: ____ Yes ____ No/Specify _____
Right: ____ Yes ____ No/Specify _____

Eyes: ____ Clear ____ Draining ____ Reddened ____ Other _____

5. MUSCULAR–SKELETAL
Range of Motion: ____ Full ____ Other _____
Balance and Gait: ____ Steady ____ Unsteady
Hand Grasps: ____ Equal ____ Strong ____ Weakness/Paralysis (__ Right __ Left)
Leg Muscles: ____ Equal ____ Strong ____ Weakness/Paralysis (__ Right __ Left)

DISCHARGE PLANNING
Lives: Alone ____ With _____ No known residence _____
Intended Destination Post Discharge: ____ Home ____ Undetermined ____ Other _____
Previous Utilization of Community Resources:
____ Home care/Hospice ____ Adult day care ____ Church groups ____ Other _____
____ Meals on Wheels ____ Homemaker/Home health aide ____ Community support group
Post-discharge Transportation:
____ Car ____ Ambulance ____ Bus/Taxi
____ Unable to determine at this time
Anticipated Financial Assistance Post-discharge?: ____ No ____ Yes _____
Anticipated Problems with Self-care Post-discharge?: ____ No ____ Yes _____
Assistive Devices Needed Post-discharge?: ____ No ____ Yes _____
Referrals: (record date)
Discharge Coordinator _____ Home Health _____
Social Service _____ V.N.A. _____
Other Comments: _____
_____

SIGNATURE/TITLE _____ DATE _____

Side Four

Fig. 4-1. (continued)

to share assessment data, feelings, problems, and knowledge (theory and practice). It can provide nurses who are reluctant to care-plan with an opportunity for collaboration.

Planning conferences should include all levels of nursing staff. Other members of the health team (therapists, social workers) may attend when appropriate. It is not appropriate for other health care professionals to coordinate or conduct these conferences. The planning of nursing care such as discharge planning should be coordinated by the professional nurse. Other disciplines can be consulted as indicated.

When conferences are being initiated, their success can be influenced positively if the following guidelines are considered:

- Manage the conference time judiciously by starting and ending on time
- Include all levels of nursing personnel and encourage their participation when appropriate
- Have personnel rotate covering unit during conferences
- Discourage interruptions
- Select an experienced group leader for beginning sessions

- Introduce inexperienced group leaders only after the conferences are firmly established

The Process of Care Planning

After the actual or potential problems have been identified, the nursing activities to monitor, prevent, reduce, or eliminate the problems need to be formulated. Thus, the planning phase of the nursing process is activated. Care plans represent the planning of care, not the delivery of care. The planning phase has three components:

1. Establishing priorities of care
2. Designating expected outcome criteria (client goals)
3. Prescribing the nursing care plan through the nursing orders

Priorities of Care

Priorities of care are established to identify which nursing interventions will be provided when an individual has multiple problems or alterations. The setting of priorities does not mean numbering problems in priority. It is a method by which the nurse and the client select which problems will be addressed on the care plan. Theoretically, some clients could have as many as 20 nursing diagnoses on a care plan, a number that would render its use almost impossible. Often, priorities are identified without collaboration when a well-intentioned nurse believes she knows what the client's most important problem is, as in the following example:

> Mrs. Gaul, a 44-year-old single parent, is admitted to the hospital because of hyperglycemia and a blood glucose level of 265. Mrs. Gaul has been an insulin dependent diabetic for 19 years. The nurse, on reading the admitting diagnosis, asks Mrs. Gaul, "Have you been following your diet?" Her reply is "No." The nurse orders a consultation with the dietician, who spends 40 minutes with Mrs. Gaul explaining the therapeutic diet. The nurses continue to reinforce the importance of adhering to the diet. After three days Mrs. Gaul shares with a nurse the discipline problems she has been having with her 15-year-old daughter. She relates that she becomes so frustrated she eats and eats.

The nurse, at the time of admission, should have assessed for the reasons why Mrs. Gaul had not been adhering to her diet, instead of inferring that she lacked knowledge about it (knowledge deficit). Questions concerning recent changes in life-style and added stressors would have supported a more accurate diagnosis:

Noncompliance Related to Indiscriminate Eating When Faced with Discipline Problems with Daughter, as Manifested by Reports of Lack of Adherence to Diabetic Diet

If the nurse had sought validation for the initial lack-of-knowledge diagnosis, valuable time and money would have not been spent on diet teaching. Any nurse can recall countless medical and nursing problems that were misdiagnosed or prioritized erroneously.

Process Criteria vs. Outcome Criteria

Goals for nursing interventions are written to direct care, to identify desired outcomes, and to measure the effectiveness of the interventions. Goals can be process criteria goals or outcome criteria goals. Goals are sometimes also called objectives, expected outcome, or outcomes.

Process Criteria

Process criteria—also called *nursing goals*—direct the nurse toward the prevention or alleviation of the altered state of wellness. Process criteria can focus on three major areas to assist the client to:

- Use his resources more effectively to facilitate an optimal level of coping
- Seek other resources to facilitate an optimal level of coping
- Modify his activities of daily living and usual life-style when resources are diminished or inadequate

These goals serve to indicate what the nurse should seek to accomplish with a client.

Process goals or nursing goals are not written on care plans in practice. Students can be requested to write nursing goals in order to help them plan care. Faculty members need to evaluate whether teaching students to write both nursing goals and patient goals only serves to confuse the students.

Most often, the interventions associated with nursing goals are repetitive:

Nursing Goal	*Interventions*
The individual will be monitored for signs and symptoms of hemorrhage	Monitor for signs and symptoms of hemorrhage
	• Vital signs
	• Intake and output
	• HCT and Hgb

Nursing or process goals are unnecessary for care planning. If one finds a nursing goal more realistic to write than a client goal, perhaps the problem is that the situation is a collaborative problem, not a nursing diagnosis. A more complete discussion of goals for collaborative problems is found in the Outcome Criteria section in this chapter.

Outcome Criteria

Bulechek and McCloskey define goals as "guideposts to the selection of nursing interventions and criteria in the evaluation of nursing interventions." These authors continue by saying that "readily identifiable and logical links should exist between the diagnoses and the plan of care, and the activities prescribed should assist or enable the patient to meet the identified expected outcome." Alfaro wrote that client outcomes are "statements describing a measurable behavior of client/family which denote a favorable status (changed or maintained) after nursing care has been delivered."

Thus, client goals are the criteria to measure the effectiveness of the plan. Outcome criteria for nursing diagnoses should represent favorable statuses that can be achieved or maintained through nursing-prescribed interventions (independent). Thus, outcome criteria may be critical in differentiating nursing diagnoses from collaborative problems. As discussed in Chapter 2, client goals related to nursing diagnoses should be the criteria used to determine the success or failure of nursing actions on the nursing care plan.

In several care plan books, the authors frequently present patient or client outcomes with nursing diagnoses that may prove problematic. Figure 4-2 represents selected examples. Examine the goals outlined in Figure 4-2. Picture caring for a client with one or more of the goals in Figure 4-2. For example, the client has outcome criteria such as:

- Will not experience cardiac dysrhythmias
- Vital signs within normal limits for patient

If this man experiences premature ventricular contractions (PVCs) or a decrease in pulse or blood pressure, how will the nurse respond?

- ABG's are within patient's normal limits (p. 26)
- Blood sugar/electrolytes are within acceptable limits (p. 243)
- Blood loss from mediastinal or pleural tubes is within acceptable limits (p. 23)
  (From Moorhouse, Geissler, Doenges)

- Will not develop paralytic ileus (p. 23)
- Will not experience cardiac dysrhythmias (p. 253)
- Will not experience uremia (p. 420)
  (From Ulrich, Canale, Wendell)

- Blood pressure will not increase more than 30 mm Hg systolic or 15 mm Hg diastolic (p. 112)
- The causative organism will respond to treatment (p. 116)
- Will progress through labor and delivery without incident of severe fluid deficit, hemorrhage and/or shock (p. 124) (From Aukamp)

- Cardiac rhythm and rate are stable and within normal limits for patient (p. 252)
- No signs and symptoms of hypothermia (p. 251) (Kim, McFarland, McLane)

Fig. 4-2 Literature examples of client goals.

- What nursing orders will be added or deleted to correct the problem?
- Should the nurse change the goal because it was not achievable?

Neither of these responses is correct. The nurse will respond to the above situation by either initiating delegated orders from medicine (protocols, standing orders) or contacting the physician for delegated orders. Changing nursing orders will not correct the situation.

Client Goals or Outcomes for nursing diagnoses should be of such a nature that if they are not achieved, or if progress to achievement is not evident, the nurse must reevaluate the attainability of the goal and/or revise the nursing care plan.

Thus, outcome criteria, or *client goals*, are the maintenance of or change to a favorable status of the client after nursing care. Outcome criteria or client goals can represent resolution of a problem or evidence of progress toward resolution of a problem. Because the length of stay in acute care settings is reduced, it is unrealistic to view most problems as resolved at discharge. For example, for the nursing diagnosis

Impaired Tissue Integrity Related to Immobility, as Manifested by 6 cm Ulcer Below Dermis

the goal would be: will demonstrate evidence of granulation tissue rather than evidence of a healed ulcer. Outcome criteria are utilized to:

- Direct interventions to achieve the desired changes or maintenance
- Measure the effectiveness and validity of the interventions

Outcome criteria can be formulated to direct and measure positive and negative outcomes. Goals found on care plans are outcome criteria, or client goals. These goals are written in terms of what the client is expected to do, not the nurse.

Positive outcome criteria seek to direct interventions to provide the client with:

1. An improvement in health status by increasing comfort (physiological, psychological, social, spiritual) and coping abilities
   - Example: The client will discuss relationship between activity and carbohydrate requirements and walk unassisted to end of hall four times a day.

2. Maintenance of present optimal level of health
   - Example: The client will relate the signs, symptoms, and associated interventions for angina.
3. Optimal levels of coping with significant others
   - Example: The client will relate an intent to discuss with her husband her concern about returning to work.
4. Optimal adaptation to deterioration of health status
   - Example: The client will visually scan the environment while walking, to prevent injury.
5. Optimal adaptation to terminal illness
   - Example: The client will consume protein and high-calorie supplements (800 ml/day) to compensate for periods of anorexia and nausea.
6. Collaboration and satisfaction with health care providers
   - Example: The client will ask questions concerning the care of his colostomy.

Negative outcome criteria seek to direct interventions to prevent negative alterations in the client, such as:

1. Complications
   - Example: The client will not develop the complications of imposed bed rest.
2. Disabilities
   - Example: The client will elevate left arm on pillow and exercise fingers on sponge ball to reduce edema.
3. Unwarranted death
   - Example: The infant will be attached to an apnea monitor at night.

Components of Outcome Criteria. The essential characteristics of outcome criteria are as follows. Outcome criteria should:

- Be long-term or short-term
- Have measurable verbs
- Be specific in content and time
- Be attainable

Client goals can be *long-term* or *short-term goals*. They may be defined as follows:

- Long-term: An objective that is expected to be achieved over a longer period of time, usually over weeks or months.
- Short-term: An objective that is expected to be achieved in a short period of time, usually in less than a week (Alfaro, p. 93).

Sometimes short-term goals are objectives for care.

Previously, when hospital stays were frequently longer than a week, it was appropriate to formulate short-term and long-term goals. With current schedules, this is no longer necessary for many hospitalized clients.

Long-term goals are appropriate for individuals in long-term care facilities, rehabilitation units, mental health units, community nursing settings, and ambulatory services.

The following represents a long-term goal with the associated short-term goals for an individual at home (Scherman, p. 118).

Long-term: The individual will perform activities of daily living independently in eight weeks.
Short-term: The individual will:

1. Feed self after 3 RN visits
2. Dress self after 6–8 RN visits
3. Toilet self after 5–6 RN/PT visits
4. Ambulate with a cane after 6–10 RN/PT visits

Measurable verbs are verbs that describe the exact behavior of the client/family that you expect will occur when the goal has been met. The action/behavior must be such that the nurse can validate it by seeing or hearing.

The other senses—touch, taste, and smell—can also be used to measure goal achievement, but their use is infrequent.

If the verb used does not describe a result that can be seen or heard, as in:

The individual *will experience* less anxiety,

the nurse can change the verb to a behaviorally measurable one, as in:

The individual *reports* less anxiety.

Examples of verbs that are *not* measurable by sight or sound are:

Accepts	Appreciates
Knows	Understands

Examples of verbs that are measurable are:

States	Has an increase in
Performs	Has an absence of
Identifies	Specifies
Has a decrease in	Administers

Measurement of goal achievement can be made easier in the following ways:

1. By using the phrase *as evidenced by* to introduce measurable evidence of a reduction in signs and symptoms, as in:

    The individual will experience less anxiety, as evidenced by a reduction in signs and symptoms of racing, rapid pulse >90.

    and in:

    The individual will demonstrate tolerance to activity, as evidenced by a return to resting pulse 76, 3 min. postactivity.

2. By adding the expression *within normal limits* (W.N.L.), as in:

    The individual will demonstrate healing W.N.L., as evidenced by absence of redness, purulent discharge, or edema.

The outcome criteria should describe the *specific response* planned. Three elements add to the specificity of a goal: content, modifiers, and achievement time.

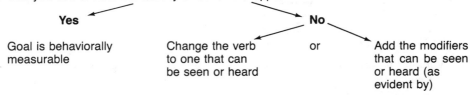

Fig. 4-3 Steps to formulate behaviorally measurable goals.

The *content* area indicates what the individual is to do, experience, or learn (usually a verb), such as drink, walk, cough, or learn.

Associated with the verb are *modifiers*, which add the specifics or individual preferences to the goal. Modifiers are usually adjectives or adverbs; they explain what, where, when, and how. For example: drink (what and when), walk (where and when), learn (what), and cough (how and when).

The *time for achievement* of a goal can be added to the goal using one of three options:

By discharge
Will relate an intent to discuss with wife by discharge fears regarding diagnosis
Continued
Will demonstrate continued intact skin
By date
Will walk ½ of hallway with assistance by Friday A.M.

Often, the nurse has limited data when initial care plans are formulated. Thus, the goals and interventions may lack specificity. As the nurse interacts with the client, more data will be collected. The longer the nurse–client interactions, the more specific the plan would be.

The outcome criteria for each nursing diagnosis in Section II are stated in measurable terms but must be made specific to each client by adding modifiers. These outcome criteria serve to guide the nurse in the areas that need to be observed and measured. The following is an example of an outcome criterion for the diagnosis *Pain* that has been rewritten to reflect the goal for a particular client on a rehabilitation unit.

Outcome Criterion	*Individualized Outcome Criteria*
The client will report a reduction in pain and improve mobility by discharge	The client will 1. Complete his bath without assistance 2. Relate a reduction of pain and request less medication (<250 mg/24 hr) 3. Remain out of bed from 11 A.M. to 2 P.M. and 5 P.M. to 9 P.M.

The nurse must ask herself, How will I measure that the client is experiencing less pain and has increased mobility? For this particular client, the goals stated above will serve as measurements. As this client's mobility increases, the nurse may have to revise the goals to reflect the client's changing status.

Goals for Possible Nursing Diagnoses and Collaborative Problems. Many students and nurses have been instructed to write only client goals (outcome criteria) for the problem statements on the care plan. Since outcome criteria refer to the expected change in the client's status after he has received nursing care, it is inappropriate for the nurse to formulate outcome criteria for collaborative problems and for possible nursing diagnoses.

The following examples illustrate this problem:

Possible Feeding Self-Care Deficit related to I.V. in right hand	The individual will feed self.
Potential Complication: hemorrhage	The individual will not bleed.

As one can easily see, both of these goals are problematic. How can a client goal be written for a possible nursing diagnosis if it is not known whether or not the individual has a problem?

For the collaborative problem *Potential Complication: hemorrhage*, the nurse does not prevent bleeding but detects the early signs of bleeding to prevent morbidity. Thus, client goals or outcome criteria are not appropriate for possible nursing diagnoses or collaborative problems. This author recommends that goals for these two situations be omitted because they are not needed. Another alternative is to write nursing goals or process criteria for these two situations, as follows:

Possible Feeding Self-Care Deficit related to I.V. in right hand	The individual will be assessed for his ability to feed himself.
Potential Complication: hemorrhage	The individual will be monitored for changes in vital signs and urinary output.

Nurses are often confused about the difference between a nursing goal and a client goal. To reduce confusion, it is advisable not to write nursing goals on care plans. Write client goals for actual and potential nursing diagnoses, and omit goals for collaborative problems and possible nursing diagnoses.

Nursing Interventions

As previously discussed in Chapter 2, there are two types of nursing intervention, nurse-prescribed (independent) and physician-prescribed (delegated). Independent interventions are those prescriptions formulated by nurses for themselves or other nursing staff to implement. Delegated interventions are prescriptions formulated by physicians for nursing staff to implement.

Both types of interventions require independent nursing judgment, because legally the nurse must determine whether it is appropriate to initiate the action (independent or delegated).

Examples of each are:

Independent	*Delegated*
Increase fluid intake to 1500 ml/day	Initiate oxygen therapy by nasal cannula
Perform passive range of motion exercises to left shoulder, elbow, wrists, fingers	Administer analgesic
	Irrigate wound

When independent *and* delegated interventions are needed to treat a situation and to accomplish the outcome, the problem is a collaborative problem. Figure 4-4 illustrates the independent and delegated interventions indicated to treat the collaborative problem

PC: Increased Intracranial Pressure

The reader should review the interventions in Section II for nursing diagnoses. They represent independent actions for goal achievement.

After the nursing diagnoses and the outcome criteria have been stated, the nurse focuses on prescribing the care required to prevent, reduce, or eliminate the alteration or to promote health. After the collaborative problem has been identified, the nurse prescribes actions that monitor the onset or status of the complication and prevent morbidity and mortality. The specific directions for nursing care are called *nursing orders*. Nursing orders are composed of the following: (Carnevali)

- Date
- Directive verb
- What, when, how often, how long, where
- Signature

The objective of the nursing order is to direct individualized care to a client. Nursing

STANDARD OF CARE

Potential Complication: Increased Intracranial Pressure

I   1. Monitor for signs and symptoms of increased intracranial pressure
- Pulse changes: Slowing rate to 60 or below; Increasing rate to 100 or above
- Respiratory irregularities: Slowing rate with lengthening periods of apnea
- Rising blood pressure or widening pulse pressure with moderately elevated temperature
- Temperature rising
- Level of responsiveness: Variable change from baseline (alert, lethargic, comatose)
- Pupillary changes (size, equality, reaction to light, movements)
- Eye movements (doll's eyes, nystagmus)
- Vomiting
- Headache: Constant, increasing in intensity; aggravated by movement/standing
- Subtle changes: Restlessness, forced breathing, purposeless movements and mental cloudiness
- Paresthesia, paralysis

I   2. Avoid:
- Carotid massage
- Prone position
- Neck flexion
- Extreme neck rotation
- Valsalva maneuver
- Isometric exercises
- Digital stimulation (anal)

I   3. Maintain a position with slight head elevation
I   4. Avoid rapidly changing positions
I   5. Maintain a quiet, calm environment (soft lighting)
I   6. Plan activities to reduce number of interruptions
I   7. Intake and output; use infusion pump to ensure accuracy
Del   8. Consult for stool softeners
Del   9. Maintain fluid restrictions as ordered (may be restricted to 1000 ml/day for a few days)
Del   10. Administer fluids at an even rate as prescribed
Del   11. Administer medications (osmotic diuretics, *e.g.,* mannitol and corticosteroids, *e.g.,* dexamethasone, methylprednisolone if administered)

(Del = Delegated; I = Independent)

Fig. 4-4

orders differ from nursing actions, which are broad interventions that can apply to any number of individuals sharing a similar problem. Examples of nursing actions are:

- Increase fluid intake
- Ambulate client
- Reassure client
- Monitor for dysrhythmias

In order to translate the nursing action into a nursing order, the nurse must have data from the client to answer the following: what, when, how often, how long, and where?

The following example illustrates the translation of a nursing action to a nursing order.

Nursing Action	Nursing Order

Increase fluid intake	Increase fluids to at least 2500 ml/24 hr
	  1000 ml 7–3
	  700 ml 3–11
	  100 ml 11–7
	Likes orange and apple juice
	Dislikes carbonated beverages
	Do not count coffee or tea in the 2500 ml

This nursing order reflects the need to hydrate an individual with tenacious secretions, considers preferences, and indicates that coffee and tea are permitted, although not as part of the measured increase, since they act as diuretics.

The nursing interventions outlined in Section II for each nursing diagnosis are guidelines for the nurse. The nurse rewrites these interventions considering the components of a nursing order: What, when, how often, how long, and where? The example below illustrates the rewriting of a nursing intervention from Section II as a nursing order.

Nursing Diagnosis: Sleep Pattern Disturbance Related to Decreased Daytime Activity Level

Nursing Action	Individualized Nursing Order
Promote a well-scheduled daytime program of activity	Assist to dining room for each meal Have another resident accompany him on a daily afternoon walk around grounds

As with outcome criteria, the nurse must have specific knowledge of an individual in order to write nursing orders. Student nurses can write care plans for clients they are yet to meet based on information from their instructors, but it must be specified that they are writing guidelines for care, not nursing orders. After caring for the client, the student can revise the plan with specific orders.

As a nurse increases her knowledge about a client, she may need to revise the nursing orders to reflect changes or to make them more specific. The following example illustrates a nursing order that underwent such revisions.

Nursing Diagnosis: Fear Related to Uncertain Future

Initial order (Day 1)	Provide opportunities to ventilate concerns
Order Day 2	Encourage client to share her concerns Explore with husband his concerns for the future
Order Day 4	Reinforce necessity for preserving present function (refer to problem *Impaired Physical Mobility*) Discuss a plan for increasing self-care activities Assess the communication pattern between husband and wife Provide the husband with a time to talk outside wife's room

Implementation

The implementation component of the nursing process involves applying the skills needed to implement the nursing order. The skills and knowledge necessary for the implementation of nursing care usually focus on:

- Performing the activity for the client or assisting the client.
- Performing nursing assessments to identify new problems and determine the status of existing problems.

- Performing patient teaching to help clients gain new knowledge concerning their own health or the management of a disorder.
- Counseling clients to make decisions about their own health care.
- Consulting with and referring to other health care professionals to obtain appropriate direction.
- Performing specific treatment actions to remove, reduce, or resolve health problems.
- Assisting clients to perform activities themselves.
- Assisting clients to identify risks or problems and to explore options available. (Alfaro)

As discussed in Chapter 2, the major focus of interventions differs for actual, potential, and possible nursing diagnoses and collaborative problems.

1. For *actual nursing diagnoses*, the interventions will seek to:
   - Reduce or eliminate contributing factors and
   - Prevent the occurrence of the diagnostic category
   - Monitor status
2. For *potential nursing diagnoses*, the interventions will seek to:
   - Reduce or eliminate risk factors and/or
   - Prevent the occurrence of the diagnostic category
   - Monitor for onset
3. For *possible nursing diagnoses*, the interventions will seek to:
   - Collect additional data to rule out or confirm the diagnosis
4. For *collaborative problems*, interventions will seek to:
   - Monitor to detect onset/status and collaborate with other members of the health team for treatment

Not only must the nurse possess these skills, but she must also assess, teach, and evaluate them in the nursing personnel she manages. Often, the nurse is responsible for planning the care but not for its actual implementation. This requires that the nurse also possess the management skills of delegation, assertion, evaluation, and knowledge of change and motivational theory. The nurse should consult the appropriate literature on these topics.

Evaluation

Evaluation in relation to the nursing process and care planning has three different operations or purposes: evaluation of the quality of the written care plan, evaluation of the client's progress, and evaluation of the status/currency of the care plan.

Evaluation of the Quality of the Written Care Plan

This evaluation is performed by the individual nurse who wrote the care plan or by another nurse for peer review or audit. Figure 4-5 represents questions that the nurse can use to evaluate the completeness and quality of the plan.

Evaluation of the Client's Progress

This type of evaluation enables the nurse and client to determine how well the nursing care plan has worked. It consists of three distinct but related activities:

- Establishing outcome criteria to observe and measure
- Assessing the present response for evidence
- Recording the present response to the established outcome criteria

Nursing Diagnosis	Goals	Interventions
Is the statement clearly stated?	Is the goal a client goal or a nursing goal?	Are the nursing orders clear (what, when, how often, how long, and where)?
Is the terminology correct?	Is the goal realistic and attainable?	Do the nursing orders reflect creativity (thinking, unusual references)?
Is there a two-part statement?	Is it measurable? (Can the nurse validate it by seeing or hearing?)	
Does the second part of the statement reflect the specific factors that have contributed or may contribute to the development of the nursing diagnosis?	Are the verbs measurable (states, demonstrates) or not measurable (knows, understands, experiences)?	
Is there documentation of validation (signs and symptoms) for actual diagnosis?	Has the content been clearly specified (how much, when, where)?	
Does the nursing diagnosis statement reflect a situation in which a nurse can order the primary interventions in order to achieve the goal?	Can a time for achievement be realistically identified?	
Does the nurse need additional client contact to individualize the diagnostic statement?	*Does the nurse need additional client contact to individualize the goals?*	*Does the nurse need additional client contact to individualize the interventions?*

Fig. 4-5 Evaluation of care plan components. (© 1985, Lynda Juall Carpenito)

Establishing Criteria to Observe and Measure

The goals that have been established with the client are the criteria that will be measured.

Will walk unassisted ½ the length of the hall by 6/5.

Assessing the Present Response for Evidence

In this step, the nurse observes the client's response to interventions.

How far did the client walk?
Was assistance needed?

Recording the Present Response

In this step, the nurse compares the client's response after the intervention with the established outcome criteria. The recording of the client's response can be on flow charts or progress notes (narrative, S.O.A.P.I.E., Focus).

- Flow charts can be used to record clinical data such as vital signs, skin condition, presence or absence of side effects, and wound assessments.
- Progress notes should be used to record specific responses that are not appropriate for flow charts, such as response to counseling, response of family to client, or unusual responses.

Evaluation of the Status and Currency of the Care Plan

This type of evaluation relies on the conclusions derived from the evaluation of the client's progress. After examining the client's response, the nurse will ask the following questions:

1. *Nursing diagnosis*
   - Does the diagnosis still exist?
   - Does the potential diagnosis still exist?
   - Has the possible diagnosis been confirmed or ruled out?
   - Does a new diagnosis need to be added?
2. *Goals*
   - Have they been resolved?
   - Do they reflect the present focus of care?
   - Can more specific modifiers be added?
3. *Interventions*
   - Are they acceptable to the client?
   - Are they specific to the client?
   - Do they provide clear instructions for the nursing staff?

In reviewing the problem and interventions, the nurse will record one of the following decisions in the evaluation column at the time prescribed for evaluation.

Continue: The diagnosis is still present, and the goals and interventions are appropriate.

Revised: The diagnosis is still present, but the goals or nursing orders require revision. The revisions are then recorded.

Ruled out/confirmed: A possible diagnosis has been confirmed or ruled out by additional data collection. Goals and nursing orders are written.

Resolved: A diagnosis has been resolved, and that portion of the care plan is discontinued.

Reinstate: A diagnosis that had been resolved returns.

An evaluation like that above is appropriate only when the nurse-client relationship will be long-term (over weeks or months), as in long-term-care facilities and rehabilitation units. Care plans representing short-term nurse–client relationships should have a status column instead of an evaluation column to reflect diagnoses that have been resolved, discontinued, or ruled out. The nurse can then indicate which sections of the plan are no longer active. An example of a status column is presented later in this chapter.

Students who care for clients for only a short time (less than two weeks) usually incorporate this evaluation into the evaluation of the client's response. Both are then recorded on the care plan in the evaluation section. It is, however, important that students recognize that practicing nurses record client response on the flow record or nursing note, not on the care plan.

Minor revisions can be made daily on a care plan by the nurse caring for or directing the care of the client. A yellow felt-tip marker (Hi-Liter) is an excellent pen with which to revise a plan, marking out those areas that are no longer being used. Because it is still possible to read through the yellow marking, the nurse can always refer to what was planned previously. In addition, the marking will not interfere with photocopying. (Documentation examples of evaluation are presented later in this chapter.)

Evaluation of nursing care is a process to measure the client's progress or lack of progress toward the goal. The problem list is examined for its current relevancy, and the prescribed interventions are assessed for their appropriateness and acceptance by the client.

Care Planning Systems

Care planning systems can consist of:

Kardex care plans (not permanent record)
Standard of care
Standardized care plan
Care plan (addendum)

A care planning system can consist of a Kardex care plan or a care plan with or without standardization.

Standards of Care

Standards of care are detailed guidelines to direct the nurse to intervene in a selected situation.

Standards of care can direct care for an individual/family:

- With a selected medical diagnosis
    e.g., myocardial infarction
       fractured hip
- In a selected situation
    e.g., normal neonate
       postpartum
- Undergoing a treatment or diagnostic study
    e.g., hemodialysis
       anticoagulant therapy
       arteriogram
- With a selected Nursing Diagnostic Category
    e.g., Potential for Self-Harm
       Potential Impaired Skin Integrity
- With a collaborative problem
    e.g., Potential Complication: dysrhythmia
       Potential Complication: hyper/hypoglycemia

Standards of care do not direct nurses to provide medical interventions but offer an efficient method for retrieving generic (general) nursing interventions. Standards of care are not permanent chart records but are permanent hospital records. Standards of care identify a set of problems (actual, potential) that usually occur in a selected situation. The set of problems and/or health states can be called a diagnostic cluster. Diagnostic clusters may prove to be useful for measuring nursing intensity and reimbursement for selected situations (Diagnosis-Related Groups, etc.). Figure 4-6 represents a diagnostic cluster for clients undergoing a total hip replacement. The reader can refer to Carpenito, LJ: *Handbook of Nursing Diagnoses*, Section II, for diagnostic clusters in a variety of settings (medical, surgical, maternal, child, mental health).

The nursing staff would be held accountable for intervening in these diagnoses or problems with individuals experiencing this surgery. Of course, additional diagnoses and/or interventions can also be added. Nursing, however, should be cautioned that it may be unrealistic and legally inadvisable for nurses to place on care plans diagnoses that cannot be addressed because of priorities and length of stay. Due to the multifarious nature of nursing knowledge and the complex nature of individuals and personal situations, nurses cannot address the numerous diagnoses that exist with each encounter (hospitalization, home visit, office visit). Therefore, it is necessary for the nurse to analyze each client situation and determine with the client which diagnoses and problems will be addressed. Referrals can be made for assistance in areas that require interventions but are not a priority at this time.

Since it would not be clinically useful to include *all* actual or potential problems in

Preoperative
Anxiety r/t impending surgery and lack of knowledge of pre-postoperative routines

Postoperative
Collaborative Problems
   PC: Fat emboli
   PC: Hematoma formation
   PC: Sepsis
   PC: Dislocation of joint
   PC: Stress fractures
   PC: Neurovascular alterations
   PC: Synovial herniation
   PC: Thromboemboli formation
   PC: Compartmental syndrome

Nursing Diagnoses
Potential for injury r/t altered gait and use of assistive devices
Impaired physical mobility r/t pain, stiffness, fatigue, restrictive equipment and prescribed
   activity restrictions
Potential impaired skin integrity r/t pressure and immobility secondary to pain and
   restrictions
Potential altered health maintenance r/t lack of knowledge of:
   Activity restrictions
   Use of assistive devices
   Signs of complications
   Follow-up care

Fig. 4-6 Example of a diagnostic cluster for an individual experiencing total hip replacement surgery.

the standard, only those that are serious and/or are priority are addressed. Standards of care should represent "responsible care" that can be provided to clients, not "impossible care." These documents should represent the care that nurses are responsible to provide.

When formulating standards of care, nurses must consider the length of stay and the acuity related to the client population. Nurses cannot address all the problems clients have. Problems that will not be addressed should be referred to both the client and family for interventions postdischarge. Referrals to community agencies may be indicated for assistance after discharge, *e.g.*, weight loss program, smoking cessation program, counseling.

Addendum care plans (ACP) are the interventions that are to be given in addition to the usual standard of care. These additional interventions may be added to a preprinted standardized care plan, or they can be written on a blank care plan form. The initial care of most hospitalized clients can be given responsibly using standards of care. With additional nurse–client interactions, specified data may warrant addendum additions to the standard plan.

For example, a standard of care for a post-total hip replacement surgery client could contain two preoperative diagnoses and seven postoperative diagnoses, some of which are nursing diagnoses and others collaborative problems. For each nursing diagnosis there are outcome criteria, nursing orders, and interventions that are usually required. However, the nurse is not required or encouraged to copy or write routine interventions on a care plan; instead, she should document the delivery of the care and the client's response as outlined on the standard on a flow record and/or a progress note. Figure 4-7 is an example of typical standard of care content.

8. Potential Complications:
   neurovascular deficits
   joint dislocation

8a. Neurovascular check q 4 hr. Report any inability to dorsiflex foot.
   b. Quad setting exercises 10 × q 1 hr while awake! Knee flexion exercises 10 × q 1 hr while awake!
   c. Out of bed, to sit on elevated chair with 1 or 2 pillows. Sit with operative foot always in front of opposite foot; keep knees apart. Toe touch to partial weight bearing or may bear weight as tolerated. Operative hip flexion *no more than 75°.*
   d. Ambulate with walker, with supervision tid.
   e. Ambulate with crutches tid.
   f. BRP. Use elevated toilet seat.
   g. Use knee exerciser q 1 hr.

Fig. 4-7 Section of a standard of care showing collaborative problems for an individual who has had total hip replacement surgery.

Standardized Care Plans

Standardized care plans are similar to standards of care but differ in that they:

- Are permanent chart records
- Contain additions or deletions from standard of care
- Can provide for individualization of goals and interventions

Figure 4-8 is a section of a standardized care plan with areas for individualization.

It is not always necessary to convert the standard of care to a standardized care plan. The detailed standard of care provides specific directions for nurses who are inexperienced or unfamiliar with the particular problem. In this situation, the less detailed document (standardized care plan) would not be useful because the nurse would need either the detailed standard of care or none. Experienced nurses may not need any reference in order to deliver the care.

9. Potential Colonic Constipation related to decreased peristalsis secondary to immobility, anesthesia effects, and pain medication

9a. Explain the causes of constipation.
   b. Assess bowel sounds (presence, quality).
   c. Urge client to increase fluid intake. Include prune juice prn. Specify amounts
   _____ 7–3
   _____ 3–11
   _____ 11–7
   Specify likes _____
   Specify dislikes _____
   d. Discuss the need to include foods with high fiber content in diet (*e.g.,* fruit, bran).
   Specify likes _____

Fig. 4-8 Standardized care plan for an individual who has experienced total hip replacement surgery (postoperative phase).

How, then, would the nurse communicate that a particular problem existed if it was not written on a care plan? Each client would have a problem list that would represent the nursing diagnoses and collaborative problems that are a priority for this client/ family. The problem list would indicate where directions for care could be found—on a standardized form (standard of care, standardized care plan) and/or client care plan. Figure 4-9 is an example of a nursing problem list.

For example, nursing interventions for the collaborative problem—*Potential Complication: neurovascular deficits*—can be found on a standard of care. Since frequency of monitoring may differ from client to client, the nurse can use the Kardex (disposable) to indicate how often monitoring should be done and can record the data acquired on flow charts or progress notes. The nurse should not have to create a care plan on this problem just to communicate frequency.

Certainly, like any concept or system, standardized forms have both advantages and disadvantages. The advantages are:

- Eliminates the need to write routine nursing interventions
- Teaches new employees or transferred personnel the standard of care
- Directs nursing staff to selected documentation requirements
- Provides the criteria for the quality assurance program
- Allows the nurse to spend more time on delivering care than on documenting care

The disadvantages are:

- May take the place of a needed individualized intervention
- May encourage nurses to focus on predictable problems instead of additional ones

Many nurses experienced the above disadvantages when standardized care plans were introduced into their clinical setting.

When these problems were experienced, the solution was to eliminate standardized care plans. When they were eliminated, care plan audits revealed that the nurses were writing what previously was contained on the standard of care, *e.g.*, turn q2h or administer pain relief medication.

Nurses have also been socialized to view standardization as mediocre nursing—unprofessional. Standards of care or standardized care plans should represent responsible nursing care that is predicted to be needed in certain situations. Nurses should view these predictions as scientific. When problems arise with the use of standardized forms, the solution is not to change the forms but to address the nurse's misuse of the forms.

In order to minimize the disadvantages of standardized care plans, certain strategies can be implemented. Standardized care plans should be formulated only for certain

NURSING PROBLEM LIST

Nursing Diagnosis/ Collaborative Problem	Status	Standard of Care	ACP (Addendum Care Plan)
1. Potential Complications:			
Neurovascular deficit	A	✓	
Joint dislocation	A	✓	
2. Potential Constipation	A		✓

Code: A = Active   R = Resolved   RO = Ruled-out

Fig. 4-9 Example of a nursing problem list, including priority nursing diagnosis and collaborative problems, the status of each, and the location of directions for care.

client problems that direct a set of common nursing interventions, for example, for a postfemoral arteriogram or total hip replacement (pre- and postoperatively).

Interposed in standardized care plans should be spaces where the nurse can add specific points to the nursing interventions. This will help avoid the problem of the staff's ignoring the printed care plans. For example, next to the intervention for increased fluid intake, space is allocated for the amount taken within a certain time span.

Increase fluid intake to: _____ per 24 hours
                        _____ ml 7 A.M.–3 P.M.   Likes _____
                        _____ ml 3 P.M.–11 P.M.   Dislikes _____
                        _____ ml 11 P.M.–7 A.M.

In addition, the nurse who initiates the plan will cross out all sections that do not apply to her particular client. Requiring that the nurse individualize parts of the standardized care plan will reduce the chances of misusing it.

However, with clinical use, in time it may prove unnecessary to require additions to all standardized care plans. The staff may find it more efficient to use the Kardex to communicate minor variations, *e.g.*, frequency, quantities. Other interventions not appropriate for a Kardex can be entered on an addendum care plan to indicate that additional interventions have been added to a standardized plan. This will prevent the experienced nurse from having to read through known standardized interventions to find addendum interventions.

The documentation of implementation does not take place on a care plan but requires a separate form. Several formats are available—flow chart, graphic chart, or nursing progress notes—depending on the types of data being recorded.

Flow charts are excellent formats for recording treatments, activities of daily living, selected teaching, and observations. Figure 4-10 is an example of a flow chart.

Flow charts should not be used to record interactions in the spiritual, cultural, social, and psychological domains. These responses are recorded in the progress notes, as are explanations and counseling given to clients and families and unusual or unexpected situations (*e.g.*, injuries, clinical emergencies).

If the nurses are recording the same data over and over in the progress notes, it may be possible to adapt a flow sheet to accommodate these data more efficiently.

Case Study Applications

The following two case studies and related documentation illustrate care planning for the individuals discussed. Functional health patterns are used in organizing the assessment and the analysis of the data.

Case Study 1

Mrs. Gates, a 42-year-old woman, is admitted with metastatic carcinoma of the breast (recently diagnosed).

Medical History

Mrs. Gates went to see her medical doctor because of a lump she discovered under her left arm. After a biopsy confirmed a diagnosis of metastatic carcinoma of the breast, Mrs. Gates was admitted for further diagnostic studies. A mammogram revealed a lesion in the left breast. Mrs. Gates is scheduled for a left lower quadrant resection of the breast and node dissection on Thursday (three days away).

Medical Plan

Present
    Schedule for surgery on Thursday 9/20

Harper-Grace Hospitals
☐ Harper Hospital Division (48201)
☐ Grace Hospital Division (48235)

NURSING SHIFT ASSESSMENT

DATE

INITIAL ASSESSMENT	2300–0700	0700–1500	1500–2300
2. NUTRITION/ METABOLIC PATTERN	Skin: ☐ NP OTHER _____	Skin: ☐ NP OTHER _____	Skin: ☐ NP OTHER _____
3. RESPIRATION/ CIRCULATION PATTERN	Breath Sounds: ☐Normal ☐Abnormal ☐NA Cough: ☐YES ☐NO ☐Productive ☐Non-productive Pulse: ☐Regular ☐Irregular Calf Tenderness: ☐+☐−☐NA Peripheral Pulses: ☐NA☐+☐− Edema: ☐+☐−☐NA	Breath Sounds: ☐Normal ☐Abnormal ☐NA Cough: ☐YES ☐NO ☐Productive ☐Non-productive Pulse: ☐Regular ☐Irregular Calf Tenderness: ☐+☐−☐NA Peripheral Pulses: ☐NA☐+☐− Edema: ☐+☐−☐NA	Breath Sounds: ☐Normal ☐Abnormal ☐NA Cough: ☐YES ☐NO ☐Productive ☐Non-productive Pulse: ☐Regular ☐Irregular Calf Tenderness: ☐+☐−☐NA Peripheral Pulses: ☐NA☐+☐− Edema: ☐+☐−☐NA
4. ELIMINATION PATTERN	☐Nausea ☐Vomiting ☐Diarrhea ☐NP Abdomen: ☐Distended ☐Non-Distended Bowel Sounds: ☐+☐−☐NA	☐Nausea ☐Vomiting ☐Diarrhea ☐NP Abdomen: ☐Distended ☐Non-Distended Bowel Sounds: ☐+☐−☐NA	☐Nausea ☐Vomiting ☐Diarrhea ☐NP Abdomen: ☐Distended ☐Non-Distended Bowel Sounds: ☐+☐−☐NA
5. ACTIVITY/EXERCISE PATTERN	ROM: ☐Full ☐Impaired ☐NA	ROM: ☐Full ☐Impaired ☐NA	ROM: ☐Full ☐Impaired ☐NA
7. COGNITIVE/ PERCEPTUAL PATTERN	LOC: ☐Person ☐Place ☐Time Follows Commands: ☐+☐− Thought Process: ☐Logical ☐Illogical Mood: ☐Sad ☐Angry ☐Calm ☐Withdrawn ☐Other Discomfort: ☐+☐− Type: _____ Location: _____	LOC: ☐Person ☐Place ☐Time Follows Commands: ☐+☐− Thought Process: ☐Logical ☐Illogical Mood: ☐Sad ☐Angry ☐Calm ☐Withdrawn ☐Other Discomfort: ☐+☐− Type: _____ Location: _____	LOC: ☐Person ☐Place ☐Time Follows Commands: ☐+☐− Thought Process: ☐Logical ☐Illogical Mood: ☐Sad ☐Angry ☐Calm ☐Withdrawn ☐Other Discomfort: ☐+☐− Type: _____ Location: _____
ONGOING ASSESSMENT			
1. HEALTH PERCEPTION/ HEALTH MANAGEMENT PATTERN	Safety: Siderails x _____ ☐Restraints ☐Equipment ☐Special Precautions	Safety: Siderails x _____ ☐Restraints ☐Equipment ☐Special Precautions	Safety: Siderails x _____ ☐Restraints ☐Equipment ☐Special Precautions
2. NUTRITION/ METABOLIC PATTERN	Snacks _____ Food Taken: ☐Full ☐Partial ☐Refused ☐NPO ☐No Food Taken	Diet _____ Breakfast: ☐Full ☐Partial ☐Refused ☐NPO Lunch: ☐Full ☐Partial ☐Refused ☐NPO	Diet _____ Dinner: ☐Full ☐Partial ☐Refused ☐NPO
4. ELIMINATION PATTERN	Void: x _____ ☐Incontinent x _____ ☐Constipated ☐Diarrhea ☐Incontinent of stool x _____ Devices _____	Void: x _____ ☐Incontinent x _____ ☐Constipated ☐Diarrhea ☐Incontinent of stool x _____ Devices _____	Void: x _____ ☐Incontinent x _____ ☐Constipated ☐Diarrhea ☐Incontinent of stool x _____ Devices _____
5. ACTIVITY/EXERCISE PATTERN	Hygiene: ☐Complete ☐Partial ☐Self-Care ☐NA Ambulated x _____ Chair x _____ Bedrest ☐ Positioned x _____	Hygiene: ☐Complete ☐Partial ☐Self-Care ☐NA Ambulated x _____ Chair x _____ Bedrest ☐ Positioned x _____	Hygiene: ☐Complete ☐Partial ☐Self-Care ☐NA Ambulated x _____ Chair x _____ Bedrest ☐ Positioned x _____
6. SLEEP/REST PATTERN	☐Restless ☐Sleeping ☐NA	☐Restless ☐Sleeping ☐NA	☐Restless ☐Sleeping ☐NA
7. COGNITIVE/PERCEPTUAL PATTERN	Patient Teaching: Knowledge Deficit ☐+☐−☐NA Discomfort ☐+☐− Type: _____ Location: _____ Relieved ☐+☐− Method _____	Patient Teaching: Knowledge Deficit ☐+☐−☐NA Discomfort ☐+☐− Type: _____ Location: _____ Relieved ☐+☐− Method _____	Patient Teaching: Knowledge Deficit ☐+☐−☐NA Discomfort ☐+☐− Type: _____ Location: _____ Relieved ☐+☐− Method _____
10. ROLE/RELATIONSHIP PATTERN	Visitors ☐YES ☐NO Communication Patterns ☐Effective ☐Ineffective	Visitors ☐YES ☐NO Communication Patterns ☐Effective ☐Ineffective	Visitors ☐YES ☐NO Communication Patterns ☐Effective ☐Ineffective
SIGNATURE & TITLE			

Asterisks (*) on this sheet indicate further notations on the Nursing Progress Notes (Including any changes in health status).

FORM 300955 (REV. 4/86)

CODE: LOC = LEVEL OF CONSCIOUSNESS + = POSITIVE
ROM = RANGE OF MOTION − = NEGATIVE
NA = NOT APPLICABLE x = TIMES
NP = NO PROBLEM

(continued)

Fig. 4-10 Sample flow chart. (Courtesy of the Detroit Medical Center, Detroit, Michigan)

NURSING PROCEDURES/TREATMENTS

_____
DATE

TREATMENTS *See Nurses Notes for Patient Teaching and Special Problems	2300-0700 (Time & Initial)	0700-1500 (Time & Initial)	1500-2300 (Time & Initial)
SPECIMENS			

INITIALS	TIME	SPECIAL PROCEDURES	DEPARTMENT	MODE OF TRANSPORTATION

INITIALS	SIGNATURE	INITIALS	SIGNATURE	INITIALS	SIGNATURE

Fig. 4-10 (_continued_)

Schedule bone scan, liver scan, chest x-ray
Complete blood count and urinalysis
SMA 24 blood studies
ECG
Future
Dr. Drong discussed with Mrs. Gates that approximately three weeks after surgery he will begin a course of chemotherapy to last eight months, followed by radiation.

Admission Data Base	*Assessment Conclusions:* • *Positive Functioning* • *Collaborative Problems* • *Nursing Diagnoses (actual, potential, possible)*

Health History

Past unusual childhood diseases
Appendectomy at age 21
Menarche at age 13 with a 28-day cycle

Health Perception/Health Management Pattern	
Does not smoke Drinks 1 glass of wine with dinner Does not exercise regularly States she "just signed up for an exercise dance class but will have to cancel now"	Altered Health Maintenance related to insufficient exercise

Nutritional–Metabolic Pattern	
(24-hour diet recall) Breakfast: 2 eggs, 1 slice toast, orange juice, coffee Lunch: Yogurt or cottage cheese with fruit, water Dinner: Meat, potatoes, vegetable, salad, water, 1 glass wine Other: 2–3 cups coffee, 1–2 pieces fruit, 1 serving ice cream/cake, cookies Water: 2 glasses/day	Effective nutritional pattern

Elimination Pattern	
Chronic constipation, which she treats with over-the-counter laxatives Bowel movement q 3–4 days	Colonic Constipation related to possible inadequate water intake, insufficient exercise as manifested by reports of BM q 3–4 days

Admission Data Base	*Assessment Conclusions:*

Activity–Exercise Pattern	
Works full-time as a librarian Spends most of her free time sewing, gardening, and activities with husband (plays, day trips)	Refer to Health Perception Pattern

Sleep–Rest Pattern	
Sleeps 7–8 hours a night Retires at 11 P.M., awakens at 6 A.M. Falls asleep easily	Effective sleep–rest pattern

Cognitive–Perceptual Pattern	
Master's degree	Effective cognitive–perceptual pattern

Self-Perception Pattern

States she "hoped that their relationship would not change after the surgery."	Potential Self-Concept Disturbance related to change in appearance 2° surgery

Role–Relationship Pattern

Married 22 years	Positive role–relationship pattern
Relies on husband for daily support	
Married sister with 2 children (ages 12 and 14) lives 20 minutes away; they talk q.o.d. (every other day) on telephone and usually have Saturday or Sunday dinner together	

Sexuality–Reproductive Pattern

No children: "I never got pregnant, so we both accepted it as God's will."	Positive sexuality pattern
States that both she and her husband are very happy and satisfied with their sex life	
Engages in intercourse approximately 5 times/month	

Coping–Stress Management Pattern

Is worried what her husband will do without her at home (*e.g.,* meals)	Fear related to cancer diagnosis, uncertainty about treatments and future
Expressed concern about getting sick with chemotherapy	
Related that her cousin, who had chemotherapy for leukemia, vomited all the time and lost all her hair but has been doing well for 5 years now	Potential Impaired Home Maintenance Management related to uncertainty about husband's ability to manage household

Value–Belief Pattern

Is active in her church (Lutheran)	Positive value–belief pattern
Teaches Sunday school each week	

Present Medical Status

Left lower quadrant resection of left breast and node dissection surgery 9/20	Postoperative Potential Complications: hemorrage paralytic ileus

Figure 4-11 is the nursing problem list for Mrs. Gates one day after surgery. It contains the priority nursing diagnoses and collaborative problems for this client, with the status of each, and also indicates where directions for care are recorded.

The two diagnoses, *Colonic Constipation* and *Fear*, have both standardized and addendum interventions, as indicated by a check in each column (Standard, ACP). The diagnosis *Potential Self-Concept Disturbance* has interventions that are represented exclusively on the addendum care plan.

Case Study 2

While wrestling with her 15-year-old brother, 11-year-old JS sustained a fracture of her left tibia. She was admitted to the pediatric floor and placed in Buck's extension traction with a boot.

Medical Plan

Continuous traction for 5 weeks
Diazepam (Valium) 2 mg P.O. q 8 hr
Meperidine (Demerol) 50 mg P.O. q 4 hr
Regular diet

NURSING PROBLEM LIST

Nursing Diagnosis/ Collaborative Problem	Status	Standard of Care	ACP (Addendum Care Plan)
1. Standard Postoperative Plan	A 9/20	✓	
2. Pot. Fluid Volume Excess: left arm related to effects of mastectomy and dependent positions	A 9/20	✓	
3. Colonic constipation related to possible inadequate water intake, insufficient exercise as manifested by reports of bowel movements q 3–4 days	A 9/20	✓	✓
4. Potential Self-Concept Disturbance related to fears that change in appearance will influence relations with spouse	A 9/21		✓
5. Fear related to cancer diagnosis, uncertainty about treatments and future as manifested by expressions of concern about chemotherapy and its success	A 9/21	✓	✓
6. Potential Altered Health Maintenance related to lack of knowledge of arm exercises, self-breast exams, hazards to affected arm, community services	A 9/20	✓	

Code: A = Active   R = Resolved   RO = Ruled-out

Fig. 4-11   Nursing problem list for Mrs. Gates 1 day postoperatively, showing priority nursing diagnoses and collaborative care problems, the status of each, and indicating where directions for care are recorded.

Medical Diagnosis

Pathological fracture due to a benign cyst
Plan to discharge in 5 weeks in body cast; duration of body cast approximately 10 weeks

Medical History

Systems review unremarkable
1–2 episodes of upper respiratory infection each winter

Health Maintenance—Health Perception Pattern

Up-to-date with immunizations
Dental checkup q 6 months

Nutritional–Metabolic Pattern

Reports a usual daily intake of:
Breakfast: Pancakes or cereal, orange juice
Lunch: Sandwich, hot dog or pizza, ice cream, milk

Dinner: Meat, potatoes, vegetables (carrots, peas, corn only)
Snacks: Cookies, popcorn
Water: 4 glasses

Elimination Pattern

Reports a soft, formed BM qd

Activity–Exercise Pattern

Reports:
She is well liked in school
Enjoys sports (soccer)
Likes to cook
Likes school (excels in math and science, has to work at her reading skills)
States she is bored in the hospital

Sleep–Rest Pattern

Retires at 9:00 P.M. on weekdays
Awakes at 7:00 A.M.
Bedtime ritual: Bath, oral hygiene, reads a short story

Cognitive–Perceptual Pattern

Three days postadmission:
JS experiences intermittent leg spasms that were visible the first two days. She
continues to complain of spasms that are no longer visible. She responds to the
spasms by screaming.
JS is placed in private room at the end of the hall, and the door is kept closed to muffle
her screams.
JS's mother arrives at 10:30 A.M. and remains until 6:30 P.M. Her husband arrives at
6:30 P.M. and stays until 8:30 or 9:00 P.M.
JS spends her day watching TV, conversing with her mother, and experiencing
spasms. Her contact with the nursing staff is limited to hygiene needs and
medications.
JS complains that her pain meds are often late, and then her spasms are "really bad."

Self-perception Pattern

Reports she is well liked in school
Expects to be "as good as before, after the fracture heals."

Role–Relationship Pattern

Has a 15-year-old brother
Mother is a former librarian
Father is a pharmacist who teaches at the local university
Reports her family has a good time together

Sexuality–Reproductive Pattern

Reports she learned about sexuality, pregnancy and menses "from her mom and dad
before the health teacher had a class"

Coping–Stress Management Pattern

Says when she is sad, she talks to her mother, father, or brother depending on the
reason

Value–Belief Pattern
>   Attends Catholic church every Sunday
>   Believes in God and prays for assistance and to say, "Thank you"

You are a part-time nurse caring for JS today.
  I. Examine the preceding data. For each of the following functional patterns, are there
     data to support:
>   positive functioning?
>   altered functioning?
>   at high risk for altered functioning?*

    A. Health Perception–Health Management Pattern
>   Health management?
>   Compliance?
>   Injuries?

    B. Nutritional–Metabolic Pattern
>   Nutrition?
>   Fluid intake?
>   Peripheral edema?
>   Infection?
>   Oral cavity health?

    C. Elimination Pattern
>   Bowel elimination?
>   Incontinence?

    D. Activity–Exercise Pattern
>   Activities of daily living?
>   Leisure activities?
>   Home care?
>   Respiratory function?

    E. Sleep–Rest Pattern
>   Sleep?

    F. Cognitive–Perceptual Pattern
>   Comfort?
>   Knowledge?
>   Sensory input?

    G. Self–Perception Pattern
>   Anxiety/fear?
>   Control?
>   Self-concept?

    H. Role–Relationship Pattern
>   Communication?
>   Family?
>   Loss?
>   Parenting?
>   Socialization?
>   Violence?

    I. Sexuality–Reproductive Pattern
>   Knowledge of?
>   Sexuality?

* Copyright 1985, Lynda Juall Carpenito

    J. Coping–Stress Tolerance Pattern
       Coping?
    K. Value–Belief Pattern
       Spirituality?

II. Is there a physiological complication present, or is there a *high* risk for one developing because of a disease, treatment, diagnostic study, or medication? That you want to monitor for?

    Cardiac
    Circulatory
    Respiratory
    Renal
    Neurological
    Muscular
    Skeletal
    Endocrine
    Gastrointestinal

III. After you have determined which functional patterns are altered or at risk for altered functioning, review the list of nursing diagnostic categories under that pattern and select the appropriate diagnosis.*

    A. If you select an actual diagnosis
       Do you have signs and symptoms to support its presence? (refer to Section II of Manual of Diagnostic Categories under the selected diagnosis)
          Write the actual diagnosis in three parts:
             (1) category (2) related to contributing factors (3) as manifested by signs and symptoms
    B. If you select a potential diagnosis
       Do you have risk factors present?
       Write the potential diagnosis in two parts:
          (1) category (2) related to risk factors
    C. Check each nursing diagnosis with the following review question*:
       1. Is the statement clearly stated?
       2. Is the terminology correct?
       3. Is there a two-part statement?
       4. Does the second part of the statement reflect the specific factors that have contributed or may contribute to the development of the nursing diagnosis?
       5. Is there documentation of validation (signs and symptoms) for actual diagnoses?
       6. Does the nursing diagnosis statement reflect a situation for which a nurse can order the primary interventions to treat or prevent? (If medical orders are needed for outcome achievement, refer to IV.)
       7. *Do you need additional client contact to individualize the diagnostic statement?*

IV. After you have identified which physiological complications should be monitored for, list them as:
    Potential Complications: (list here)

V. A. Write short-term outcome (client goals) for each actual and potential nursing diagnosis. (Remember that collaborative problems do not have client goals; place a dash (—) in the goal column for collaborative problems.)
    B. Check each goal with the following review questions*:

1. Is the goal a client goal or a nursing goal?
2. Is the goal realistic and attainable?
3. Is it measurable? (Can the nurse validate it by seeing or hearing?)
4. Are the verbs measurable (states, demonstrates) or not measurable (knows, understands, experiences)?
5. Has the content been clearly specified (how much, when, where)?
6. Can a time for achievement be realistically identified?
7. *Do you need additional client contact to individualize the goals?*

VI. A. Write interventions for both the nursing diagnoses and the collaborative problems.

    B. Check each intervention with the following review questions*:

1. Are the nursing orders clear (what, when, how often, how long, and where)?
2. Do the nursing orders reflect creativity (thinking, unusual references)?
3. *Do you need additional client contact to individualize the interventions?*

Now review the following care plan (Fig. 4-12), which represents the priority problems for JS. This care plan illustrates a format different from the problem list in Figure 4-11.

(Text continues on page 96)

---

* Copyright 1985, Lynda Juall Carpenito; used with permission

Adult Patient Care Plan

Activities of Daily Living

Complete dependence   ☐ Ind–Independent (No assistance needed)

Mobility:
Ability to turn self   ☐ Ind. ☒ Assistance needed _____
Ability to sit   ☐ Ind. ☒ Assistance needed _____   Number of People _____
☐ Wheelchair   ☐ Crutches   ☐ Cane   ☐ Walker   ☐ Braces   ☐ Prosthesis   Gait: ☐ Stable   ☐ Unstable
Bathing: ☐ Ind. ☒ Assistance needed
☐ Shower   ☐ Sink ☐ Bathtub ☒ Bed bath–(partial) self, complete
Dressing: ☐ Ind. ☒ Assistance needed _____ *with pants*
Toileting: ☐ Ind. ☒ Assistance needed _____   ☐ Bathroom   ☐ Commode   ☐ Bed pan
Eating: ☒ Ind. ☐ Assistance needed _____
     Ability to: Swallow liquids ☒ Yes ☐ No   Chew ☒ Yes ☐ No
              Swallow solids ☒ Yes ☐ No   Feed self ☒ Yes ☐ No

Date	Diagnosis	Goals The individual will:		Diagnosis	Goals The individual will:
5/1	1. acute pain related to ineffective relief of muscle spasms	1. Report less pain 2. Practice selected distraction techniques during pain episodes	5/1	Potential complication: Impaired circulation	N/A
5/1	2. Potential impaired skin integrity related to: – Imposed bedrest – Traction equipment	1. Be free from skin complications of immobility	5/2	Diversional activity deficit related to: Imposed bedrest, isolation	1. Occupy his time with activities other than TV viewing
5/1	3. Potential Colonic Constipation related to: Dietary patterns (low fiber) Embarrassment	1. Have a daily bowel movement 2. Consume daily (at least): 3 fruit exchanges 6 vegetables 10 glasses of water	5/4	Potential impaired home maintenance management related to discharge with body cast to home for 10 weeks	1. Parents will ask questions concerning home care 2. Demonstrate care of daughter's cast and other needs

Reviewed with client, family _____ _____ _____
                            (date)   (date)   (date)

Initials/Signature

1.	7.	13.	19.
2.	8.	14.	20.
3.	9.	15.	21.
4.	10.	16.	22.
5.	11.	17.	23.
6.	12.	18.	24.

Fig. 4-12 Care plan for Case Study 2. (Courtesy of the Wilmington Medical Center, Wilmington, Delaware)

Date	Diagnosis		Plan	Ints.	Status
5/1	1. Acute Pain related to ineffective relief of muscle spasms as manifested by frequent reports of inadequate relief	nDx	1. Teach her rhythmic abdominal breathing to practice during muscle spasms 2. Coach her to practice breathing during episodes of spasms 3. Administer pain medications on time 4. Encourage her to use her radio with earphones during episodes of spasms, and to increase the volume as pain increases		
5/1	2. Potential impaired skin integrity related to: Imposed bedrest Traction equipment	nDx	1. Inspect back and heels at bath time, rinse soap off well. 2. Massage skin over bony prominences 3. Protect heel under traction boot with a clear skin barrier dressing. Do not remove unless skin alterations are seen through dressing		
5/1	3. Potential colonic constipation related to: Dietary patterns (low fiber) Imposed bedrest Embarrassment	nDx	1. Teach the relationship of activity, diet, and bowel elimination 2. Teach her to contract abdominal muscles several times a day 3. Have her keep a record of her daily intake of: Vegetables (low starch), fruits, bran, nuts, fluids, juices		

Initials/Signature

1.	7.	13.	19.
2.	8.	14.	20.
3.	9.	15.	21.
4.	10.	16.	22.
5.	11.	17.	23.
6.	12.	18.	24.

Fig. 4-12 (continued)

Date	Diagnosis		Plan	Ints.	Status
			4. Teach her to avoid: Bakery products Foods high in starch (corn, white bread, noodles, rice)		
			5. Request parents to bring in nutritious snacks (carrots, celery, apples) to keep on unit		
			6. Give her a bedpan after lunch: — Tell her no one will interrupt her — Give her a room deodorizer to use — Put the TV or radio on to make noise.		
5/1	4. Potential Complications: skeletal misalignment Impaired circulation	CP	1. Assess limb (toes, skin around traction, popliteal pulse) for temperature, color, tingling, loss of sensation. Rid and hs 2. Remind her to wiggle toes at least 10 times each hour 3. Assure that: — Weights hang free — Ropes are away from bed — Ropes and pulleys are in straight alignment — Traction is never interrupted — She is in good alignment and has not slipped down in bed		

Initials/Signature			
1.	7.	13.	19.
2.	8.	14.	20.
3.	9.	15.	21.
4.	10.	16.	22.
5.	11.	17.	23.
6.	12.	18.	24.

Fig. 4-12 (continued)

Date	Diagnosis		Plan	Ints.	Status
5/2	5. Diversional activity deficit related to: imposed bedrest / isolation as manifested by statements of boredom	NDx	1. Consult with recreational therapist for appropriate activities		
			2. Encourage other children on floor to visit and play cards with her		
			3. Encourage her to read stories to small children on unit in her room		
			4. Arrange for tutoring with school district		
			5. Try to stimulate her to do something other than watching TV, e.g. Hook rug, electronic games		
			6. Allow her opportunities to share her feelings of loneliness		
5/4	6. Potential impaired home maintenance management related to discharge with body cast to home for 10 weeks (approximate discharge date 6/10)	NDx	1. Allow parents to share their concern about care of daughter after discharge		
			2. Assure them that they will have an opportunity to care for daughter under supervision in hospital		
			3. Discuss and teach each of the following when indicated: Cast care / Hygienic measures / Nutrition (& calcium restr.) / Elimination / Diversional activities / Tutoring / Relief periods for parents from care		

Initials/Signature					
1.	7.	13.	19.		
2.	8.	14.	20.		
3.	9.	15.	21.		
4.	10.	16.	22.		
5.	11.	17.	23.		
6.	12.	18.	24.		

Fig. 4-12 (continued)

References/Bibliography

Alfaro R: Application of Nursing Process: A Step by Step Guide. Philadelphia, JB Lippincott, 1986
Carnevali DL: Nursing Care Planning: Diagnosis and Management, 3rd ed, p 222. Philadelphia, JB Lippincott, 1983
Scherman S: Community Health Nursing Care Plans. New York, John Wiley & Sons, 1985

General (Nursing Process, Research)

Aspinall MJ, Tanner C: Decision-Making for Patient Care, Applying the Nursing Process. New York, Appleton-Century-Crofts, 1981
Carnevali D, Mitchell PH et al: Diagnostic Reasoning in Nursing. Philadelphia, JB Lippincott, 1984
Carnevali D: Nursing Care Planning: Diagnosis and Management. Philadelphia, JB Lippincott, 1983
Carpenito LJ, Duespohl TA: The nursing process. In A Guide to Effective Clinical Instruction, 2nd ed. Rockville, MD, Aspen Systems Corp, 1985
Dickoff J, James P: A theory of theories: A position paper. Nurs Res 17:200–201, 1968
Diers D: Research in Nursing Practice, pp 44–52. Philadelphia, JB Lippincott, 1979
Ellis R: Characteristics of significant theories. Nurs Res 17:217–222, 1968
Fry VS: The creative approach to nursing. Am J Nurs 53:301–302, 1953
Griffith J, Christensen P: Nursing Process: Application of Theories, Frameworks, and Models, 2nd ed. St Louis, CV Mosby, 1986
Harris RB: A strong vote for the nursing process. Am J Nurs 81:1999–2001, 1981
McLane A: Measurement and validation of diagnostic concepts: A decade of progress. Heart Lung 16:616–624, 1987
Polit D, Hungler B: Nursing Research: Principles and Methods, 3rd ed. Philadelphia, JB Lippincott, 1987
Woodtli A: Validation of defining characteristics: Retrospective design. Neurosci Nurs 20(2):81–83, 1988

Assessment

Bellack JP, Bamford PA: Nursing Assessment: A Multidimensional Approach. Monterey, CA, Wadsworth Health Sciences Division, 1984
Block GJ, Nolan JW: Health Assessment for Professional Nursing: A Developmental Approach, 2nd ed. New York, Appleton-Century-Crofts, 1986
Communicating with patients. Am J Nurs 79:1074–1085, 1979
Dossey B: Perfecting your skill for systematic patient assessments. Nursing 9:42–45, 1979
Eggland ET: How to take a meaningful nursing history. Nursing 7(7):22–30, 1977
Mahoney EA, Verdisco L: How to Collect and Record a Health History. Philadelphia, JB Lippincott, 1982
Miakowski C, Nielson B: A cancer nursing assessment tool. Oncol Nurs Forum 12(6):37–42, 1985

Diagnosis

Books

Carpenito LJ: Handbook of Nursing Diagnoses, 2nd ed, Philadelphia, JB Lippincott, 1987
Gebbie K: Summary of the Second National Conference Classification of Nursing Diagnoses. St Louis, The Clearinghouse, St Louis University, 1976
Gordon M: Nursing Diagnosis: Process and Application. St Louis, McGraw-Hill, 1982
Hurley ME (ed): Classification of Nursing Diagnoses: Proceedings of the Sixth Conference. St Louis, CV Mosby, 1986
Kim MJ, Moritz D: Classification of Nursing Diagnosis/Proceedings of the Third and Fourth National Conferences. New York, McGraw-Hill, 1982
Kim MJ, McFarland G, McLane H: Classification of Nursing Diagnoses: Proceedings of the Fifth Conference. St Louis, CV Mosby, 1984

McLane A (ed): Classification of Nursing Diagnoses: Proceedings of the Seventh National Conference. St Louis, CV Mosby, 1987

Soares C: Nursing and medical diagnoses: A comparison of variant and essential features. In Chaska N (ed): The Nursing Profession: Views Through the Mist. New York, McGraw-Hill, 1978

Periodicals

Alberts ME: Nursing diagnosis (editorial). J Iowa Med Soc 73:275–276, 1983

Aspinall M: Nursing diagnoses—The weak link. Nurs Outlook 24:433–437, 1976

Aspinall MJ: Use of decision tree to improve accuracy of diagnosis. Nurs Res 28:182–185, 1979

Bircher A: On the development and classification of diagnoses. Nurs Forum 14:10–29, 1975

Bruce J: Implementation of nursing diagnosis: A nursing administrator's perspective. Nurs Clin North Am 14:509–515, 1979

Carpenito LJ: Is the problem a nursing diagnosis? Am J Nurs 84:1418–1419, 1984

Carpenito LJ: Actual, potential, or possible? Am J Nurs 85:458, 1985

Carpenito LJ: Diagnosing nutritional problems. Am J Nurs 85:584, 1985

Carpenito LJ: Nursing diagnosis: Selected dilemmas in practice. Occup Health Nurs 33: 397–400, 1985

Carpenito LJ: Nursing diagnosis in critical care: Impact on practice and outcomes. Heart Lung 16(6):595–600, 1987

Fadden TC et al: Nursing diagnosis: A matter of form, Am J Nurs 84:470–472, 1984

Field L: The implementation of nursing diagnosis in clinical practice. Nurs Clin North Am 14:497–508, 1979

Gebbie K, Lavin M: Classifying nursing diagnoses. Am J Nurs 74:250–253, 1974

Gleit C, Tatro S: Nursing diagnoses for healthy individuals. Nurs Health Care 2:456–457, 1981

Gordon M: Nursing diagnoses and the diagnostic process. Am J Nurs 76:1298–1300, 1976

Herberth L, Gosnell D: Nursing diagnosis for oncology nursing practice. Cancer Nurs 10(1):41–51, 1987

Kritek P: Nursing diagnosis in perspective: Response to a Critique. Image 17:3–8, 1985

Lyons J, Hester N: Research Generated Nursing Diagnoses for Healthy School-Age Children. Issues in Comprehensive Pediatric Nursing 10:149–159, 1987

McKay RP: What is the relationship between development and utilization of a taxonomy and nursing theory. Nurs Res 26:222–224, 1977

Nursing diagnosis. Top Clin Nurs 5:1–96, 1984

Nursing diagnosis. Nurs Clin North Am 20(4):1985

Nursing diagnosis. AORN J 40(8), 1984

Nursing diagnosis. Occup Health Nurs 33, 1985

Nursing diagnoses: Implementation. Nurs Clin North Am 22(4):879–1099, 1987

Peplau HE: In defense of nursing diagnosis (letter to editor). Nurs Outlook 32:240, 1984

Popkess SA: Diagnosing your patient's strengths. Nursing 11:34–37, 1981

Price MR: Nursing diagnosis: Making a concept come alive. Am J Nurs 80:668–671, 1980

Roy C: A diagnostic classification system for nursing. Nurs Outlook 23:90–94, 1975

Shamansky SL, Yanni CR: In opposition to nursing diagnosis: A minority opinion. Image 15:47–50, 1983

Care Planning

Aukamp V: Nursing Care Plans for Childbearing Family. Norwalk, CT, Appleton-Century-Crofts, 1984

Bailey JT, Claus KE: Decision-making in Nursing. St Louis, CV Mosby, 1975

Beck J: Standards as a guide for nursing care plans. Oncol Nurs Forum 7(4):28–30, 1980

Bulechek G, McCloskey J: Nursing Interventions: Treatments for Nursing Diagnoses. Philadelphia, WB Saunders, 1985

McCloskey JC: Nurse's orders: The next professional breakthrough. RN 43(2):99–100, 1980

McFarland G, Wasli E: Nursing Diagnoses and Process in Psychiatric Mental Health Nursing. Philadelphia, JB Lippincott, 1986

McNally J, Stair J, Somerville E (eds): Guidelines for Cancer Nursing Practice. Orlando, FL, Grune & Stratton, 1985

Randolph D, Bernau K: Dealing with resistance in the nursing care conference. Am J Nurs 77:1955–1958, 1977

Roeder MA: Patient care plans and the evaluation of the nursing process. Supervisor Nurse 11(1):57–58, 1980

Ulrich S, Canale S, Wendell S: Nursing Care Planning Guides: A Nursing Diagnosis Approach. Philadelphia, WB Saunders, 1986

Evaluation

Barba M, Bennett B, Shaw WJ: The evaluation of patient care through use of ANA's standards of nursing practice. Supervisor Nurse 9(1):42–54, 1978

Block D: Evaluation of nursing care in terms of process and outcome: Issues in research and quality assurance. Nurs Res 24:256–263, 1975

Block D: Criteria, standards, norms—crucial terms in quality assurance. J Nurs Adm 7(9):20–30, 1977

Brown K, Dunn K, et al: Nursing diagnosis and process evaluation: Implications for continuing education. Journal of Continuing Education in Nursing 18(5):172–178, 1987

Chow RK: Assuring the quality of care: A personal perspective—from tailoring to outcome measurement. Nurs Leadersh 1(3):11–22, 1978

Hover J, Zimmer MJ: Nursing quality assurance: The Wisconsin system. Nurs Outlook 26: 242–248, 1978

Hushower G, Gamberg D, Smith N: The nursing process in discharge planning. Supervisor Nurse 9(9):55–58, 1978

Mayers MG, Norby RB, Watson AB: Quality Assurance for Patient Care: Nursing Perspectives. New York, Appleton-Century-Crofts, 1976

Phaneuf MC: The Nursing Audit: Self-Regulation in Nursing Practice. New York, Appleton-Century-Crofts, 1976

Spotts ST: A nursing diagnosis taxonomy for quality assurance and reimbursement. P Nurse 36:5, 1981

Warren J: Accountability and nursing diagnosis. J Nurs Adm 13:34–37, 1983

Section II

Manual of Nursing Diagnoses

Introduction

The Manual of Nursing Diagnoses consists of 98 diagnostic categories. Each category is described with the following:
- Definition
- Etiological, contributing, and risk factors, organized according to pathophysiological, treatment-related, situational, and maturational factors that may contribute to or cause the altered state
- Defining characteristics, signs and symptoms, or risk factors of the diagnosis
- Focus assessment criteria, subjective and objective, which serve to guide the nurse to specific data collection in order to help confirm or rule out the diagnosis
- Outcome criteria—statements that describe a favorable status after nursing care has been delivered
- Principles and rationale for nursing care—statements that serve to explain the diagnosis or the rationale for assessing and intervening

Each diagnostic group is then further explained by one or more specific nursing diagnoses. These specific diagnoses were selected because of their frequency in nursing and do not in any respect represent exclusive categories. For example, *Potential for Injury* has four specific contributing factors:

Related to sensory/motor deficits

Related to lack of awareness of environmental hazards

Related to maturational age of hospitalized child

Related to vertigo secondary to orthostatic hypotension

But the nurse can utilize this diagnostic category to describe other client situations; for example:

Potential for Injury Related to Unstable Gait Secondary to Total Hip Replacement

Some diagnostic categories are listed with no specific "related to's"; for example: *Anxiety, Fear, Hopelessness, Potential for Self-Harm*. Instead, each of these categories has one group of interventions that focuses on the treatment associated with the diagnostic category, regardless of the etiological and contributing factors.

Each specific nursing diagnosis is further explained with:
1. Assessment data—the subjective and objective signs and symptoms of the specific diagnosis
2. Outcome criteria—the goals for clients with the diagnosis
3. Interventions, which specifically direct the nurse to:
   - The assessment of causative and contributing factors
   - The reduction or elimination of the factors
   - The promotion of selected activities
   - Health teaching
   - Referrals

Each diagnostic category concludes with a bibliography containing books and periodicals in which the nurse can obtain more information about the diagnosis. Pertinent literature and organizations for the consumer are also cited when appropriate. Several of the diagnostic categories represent broad categories under which more specific categories fall. As the taxonomic work of NANDA continues, more specific categories will evolve, making the broader categories no longer clinically useful. For example, the addition of the seven new categories (six NANDA-approved) related to incontinence:

Functional Incontinence
Reflex Incontinence
Stress Incontinence
Total Incontinence
Urge Incontinence
Urinary Retention
Maturational Enuresis

makes *Altered Patterns of Urinary Elimination* too broad for clinical use.

The diagnostic categories are organized alphabetically by the major category. When more specific categories are present under the broad category, they appear under the broad category but not in alphabetical order. The following are the broad categories with the more specific categories listed under them:

Body Temperature, Altered
    Hypothermia
    Hyperthermia
Bowel Elimination, Altered
    Constipation
    Colonic Constipation
    Perceived Constipation
    Diarrhea
    Bowel Incontinence
Comfort, Altered
    Acute Pain
    Chronic Pain
    Pruritus
    Nausea/Vomiting
Communication, Impaired
    Communication, Impaired Verbal
Coping, Ineffective Individual
    Defensive Coping
    Ineffective Denial
Grieving
    Grieving, Anticipatory
    Grieving, Dysfunctional
Health Maintenance
    Health Maintenance, Altered
Infection, Potential for
    Infection Transmission, Potential for
Nutrition, Altered: Less than Body Requirements
    Swallowing, Impaired
Parenting, Altered
    Parental Role, Altered
Post Trauma Response Syndrome
    Rape Trauma Syndrome
Respiratory Function, Potential Altered
    Ineffective Airway Clearance
    Ineffective Breathing Patterns
    Impaired Gas Exchange

Self-Concept Disturbance
   Body Image Disturbance
   Personal Identity Disturbance
   Self-Esteem Disturbance
      Chronic Low Self-Esteem
      Situational Low Self-Esteem
Sexuality Patterns, Altered
   Sexual Dysfunction
Tissue Integrity, Impaired
   Skin Integrity, Impaired
   Oral Mucous Membrane, Altered
Urinary Elimination, Altered Patterns of
   Maturational Enuresis
   Functional Incontinence
   Reflex Incontinence
   Stress Incontinence
   Total Incontinence
   Urge Incontinence
   Urge Retention

Readers of this manual are encouraged to become familiar with all of the diagnostic categories in order to incorporate them into their nursing practice. Until you become familiar with the diagnostic categories and their defining characteristics, the following guidelines are suggested:

1. Collect data, both subjective and objective, from client, family, other health care professionals, and records.
2. Examine the data described above. For each of the following functional patterns, are there data to support
      positive functioning?
      altered functioning?
      at high risk for altered functioning?*
   • Health perception–health management pattern
      Health management?
      Compliance?
      Injuries?
   • Nutritional–metabolic pattern
      Nutrition?
      Fluid intake?
      Peripheral edema?
      Infection?
      Oral cavity health?
   • Elimination pattern
      Bowel elimination?
      Incontinence?
   • Activity–exercise pattern
      Activities of daily living?
      Leisure activities?
      Home care?
      Respiratory function?

* Copyright 1985, Lynda Juall Carpenito

- Sleep–rest pattern
    Sleep?
- Cognitive–perceptual pattern
    Decisions?
    Comfort?
    Knowledge?
    Sensory input?
- Self-perception pattern
    Anxiety/fear?
    Self-concept?
- Role–relationship pattern
    Communication?
    Family?
    Loss?
    Parenting?
    Socialization?
    Violence?
- Sexuality–reproductive pattern
    Knowledge of?
    Sexuality?
- Coping–stress tolerance pattern
    Coping?
- Value–belief pattern
    Spirituality?

3. Is a physiological complication present, or is there a *high* risk of one developing because of a disease, treatment, diagnostic study, or medication that you want to monitor for? (collaborative problem)
    Cardiac
    Circulatory
    Respiratory
    Renal
    Neurological
    Muscular
    Skeletal
    Endocrine
    Gastrointestinal

4. After you have selected which physiological complications or collaborative problems are indicated to be monitored for, list them as:
    Potential Complication: (list here)

5. Write the collaborative problem on the care plan and add the appropriate interventions that direct nurses to monitor for the problems and intervene accordingly. (Refer to Chapter 2 for a discussion of collaborative problems.)

6. After you have selected which functional patterns are altered or present a risk for altered functioning, review the list of nursing diagnostic categories under that pattern and select the appropriate diagnosis (see pages 19–21).

7. If you select an actual diagnosis,
    Do you have signs and symptoms to support its presence? (Refer to Section II, Manual of Diagnostic Categories, under the selected diagnosis.)
    Write the actual diagnosis in three parts:
        category related to contributing factors, as evidenced by signs and symptoms

8. If you select a potential diagnosis,
   Are risk factors present?
   Write the potential diagnosis in two parts:
   category related to risk factors
9. If you need assistance in writing the nursing diagnosis, refer to Chapters 2 and 4 for guidelines.
10. If you suspect a problem but have insufficient data, refer to the focus assessment data under the category and gather the additional data to confirm or rule out the diagnosis. If this additional data collection needs to be done at a later time or by other nurses, label the diagnosis *possible.* . . on the care plan. (Refer to Chapter 2 for a discussion of possible nursing diagnoses.)
11. For the nursing diagnoses that you have validated, refer to that category and review the outcome criteria. Rewrite the outcome criteria adding the individualized criteria for the specific client. (Refer to Chapter 4 for specific guidelines.)
12. Review the interventions under the category and select those that are appropriate. Rewrite the interventions, adding individualization when needed. Add other interventions as indicated.

Activity Intolerance

Related to **(Specify)**

Related to **Insufficient Oxygenation 2° Decreased Cardiac Output**

Related to **Insufficient Oxygenation 2° Chronic Impaired Gas Exchange**

Definition

Activity intolerance: The state in which the individual experiences an inability, physiologically and psychologically, to endure or tolerate an increase in activity.

Defining Characteristics

Major (must be present)

Altered response to activity (*e.g.*)

Respiratory
- Dyspnea
- Shortness of breath

Pulse
- Weak pulse
- Decrease in rate
- Excessive increase in rate

Blood pressure
- Failure to increase with activity
- Increase in diastolic 15 mm Hg
- Decrease

Weakness

Fatigue

Excessive increase in rate

Decrease in rate

Failure to return to resting after 3 minutes

Rhythm change

Minor (may be present)

Pallor or cyanosis

Confusion

Vertigo

Etiological, Contributing, Risk Factors

Any factor that compromises oxygen transport can cause activity intolerance. Some common factors are listed below.

Pathophysiological

Alterations in the oxygen transport system

Cardiac
- Congestive heart failure
- Dysrhythmias

Angina

Myocardial infarction

Respiratory
- Chronic obstructive pulmonary disease

Circulatory
  Anemia
  Peripheral arterial disease
Acute infection
  Viral infection
  Mononucleosis
  Hepatitis
Chronic infection
  Endocarditis
  Tuberculosis
Endocrine or metabolic disorders
  Diabetes mellitus
  Hypothyroidism
  Pituitary disorders
  Addison's disease
Chronic diseases
  Renal   **Musculoskeletal**
  Hepatic   **Neurological**
  Inflammatory
Nutritional disorders
  Obesity   **Malnourishment**
  Inadequate diet
Hypovolemia
Electrolyte imbalance
Malignancies

Treatment-related
  Surgery
  Diagnostic studies
  Treatment schedule/treatments (frequency)
  Prolonged bed rest
  Medications
    Antihypertensives
    Minor tranquilizers
    Hypnotics
    Antidepressants
    Antihistamines

Situational (personal, environmental)
  Depression
  Lack of motivation
  Sedentary life-style
  Extreme stress
  Crisis—personal or developmental, career, family, financial
  Stressors (*e.g;.*)
    Impaired language function
    Impaired sensory function
    Impaired motor function
    Pain
  Fatigue, caused by (*e.g.*)
    Sensory overload

Sensory deprivation
Interrupted sleep
Equipment that requires strength (walkers, crutches, braces)
Stress

Maturational

Elderly (sensory/motor deficits)

Focus Assessment Criteria

Subjective Data

Does person complain of

Weakness?	Fatigue?
Dyspnea?	Lack of sleep?

Difficulty performing activities of daily living?

Objective Data

1. Assess for the presence of factors that increase fatigue (subjective or objective)
   Situational
   Personal
   Lack of incentive   Age
   History of ineffective coping   Lack of support system
   Environmental
   Social isolation   Sensory deprivation
   Sensory overload
   Insufficient rest/sleep periods
   Disease-related
   Cardiopulmonary disorders
   Musculoskeletal disorders
   Neurological disorders
   Fluid and electrolyte imbalances
   Nutritional deficiencies
   Chronic diseases
   Pain
   Treatment-related
   Bed rest/immobility
   Medications
   Treatment schedule
   Diet
   Surgery
   Diagnostic studies
   Caregivers' expectations
   Assistance equipment (*e.g.*)
   Crutches
   Braces
   Walkers
2. Assess for effects of fatigue on activity level
   Assess persons' ability to:
   Turn in bed
   Assume sitting position
   Maintain alignment

Table II-1.   **Physiological Response to Activity (Expected and Abnormal)**

	Pulse	Blood Pressure	Respiration
Resting			
Normal	60–90	<140/90	<20
Abnormal	>100	>140/90	>20
Immediately After Activity			
Normal	↑ Rate ↑ Strength	↑ Systolic	↑ Rate ↑ Depth
Abnormal	↓ Rate ↓ Strength Irregular rhythm	Decrease or no change in systolic	Excessive ↑ ↓ Rate
3 Minutes After			
Normal	Within 6 beats of resting pulse		
Abnormal	>7 beats of resting pulse or complaints of confusion, incoordination, dyspnea, pallor		

       Ambulate

       Perform self-care activities

3. Assess response to activity
   - Take resting vital signs (see Table II-1)

     Pulse (rate, rhythm, quality)

     Blood pressure

     Respirations (rate, depth)
   - Have person perform the activity
   - Take vital signs immediately after the activity
   - Have person rest for 3 minutes; take vital signs again
   - Assess for presence of

       Pallor   Confusion

       Cyanosis   Disequilibrium

Principles and Rationale for Nursing Care

General

1. Endurance is the ability to withstand the mental and physical work required to accomplish a task.
2. An individual's endurance will directly influence his progress in rehabilitation.
3. The ability to maintain a given level of performance is dependent on strength, coordination, reaction time, alertness, and motivation.
4. Fatigue is the perception of tiredness, lack of energy, and an inability to continue. Fatigue is a person's total response to physiologic, psychological, and situational factors.
5. Fatigue can result from loss of endurance, lack of motivation, pathophysiology, treatments, diagnostic studies, and medications.
6. Any stressor (personal, environmental, disease-related, or treatment-related) can reduce a person's tolerance for activity (see Etiological and Contributing Factors).
7. Any factor that compromises cardiopulmonary, vascular, neurological, or musculoskeletal function will reduce tolerance to activity.
8. The response of the person to activity can be evaluated by pulse rate, blood pressure, and respirations (see Table II-1).
9. The daily schedule of the person must be coordinated by the nurse in order to reduce periods of excess energy expenditure.

Table II-2. **Effects of Chronic Hypoxia**

Thought Processes	Confusion and lethargy Mood swings, anxiety, depression Sleep disturbances Headache
Respiratory System	Tachypnea, bradypnea, arrhythmic breathing Abnormal flow rates (increased inspiratory/expiratory [I/E] ratio) Pursed-lip breathing Use of accessory muscles (neck, shoulders, abdomen) Gasping before speech effort Inability to speak or cry Orthopnea (assumption of 3-point position) Cough, shortness of breath, exercise intolerance Increased sputum production Inability to move secretions Mouth breathing Abnormal breath sounds (rales, rhonchi) Decreased breath sounds Fremitus
Circulatory System	Neck vein distention Edema, decreased cardiac output, enlarged heart Cyanosis Chest pain
Gastrointestinal System	Decreased bowel sounds Constipation Anorexia, nausea, vomiting
Genitourinary System	Decreased kidney function Decreased urinary output Decreased libido
Skeletal System	Hypertrophy of accessory breathing muscles (neck and shoulders) Atrophy or weakness of extremity muscles Barrel chest, horizontal sloping of ribs Cachexia (malnutrition) Skeletal muscle pain or weakness

Chronic Diseases of the Lung (Asthma, Bronchitis, Emphysema, COPD)

1. The normal range of arterial blood gases for a person with chronic lung disease may be much different from the range of the normal individual because of body adaptation to chronically high CO_2 levels. (*Baseline* normals are of utmost importance.)
2. Sustained moderate breathlessness from supervised exercise improves accessory muscle strength and respiratory function.
3. In normal individuals, the work of breathing is very limited. In people with obstructive lung disease, however, the work of breathing may be increased 5 to 10 times above normal. Under such conditions, the amount of oxygen consumed *just for breathing activities* may be a large fraction of total oxygen consumption.
4. Consciously controlled breathing techniques can improve alveolar gas exchange and prevent air entrapment in the lungs, thus causing each breath to be more efficient.
    Pursed-lip breathing causes expiratory resistance, which helps air passages to stay open longer, allows for more movement of air, and prevents air entrapment within the lungs.
    Diaphragmatic breathing is accomplished by lifting the walls of the abdomen up and out, which causes decreased pressure within the abdomen and easier downward movement of the diaphragm.

5. People who suffer from chronic lung disease experience permanent effects on every body system due to chronic hypoxemia Table II-2).

Cardiac Output

1. All living cells require oxygen. The degree of oxygenation of cells is dependent on the functions of the heart, lungs, and circulatory systems in the presence of adequate atmospheric oxygen.

2. Cardiac output is the amount of blood (liters) that is pumped by the heart per minute and is calculated by:

$$\text{heart rate} \times \text{stroke volume} = \text{cardiac output}$$

Units can be beats/min; ml/min; liters/min.

3. Stroke volume is the amount of blood ejected with each contraction of the heart.

4. Cardiac output increases with an increase in filling of the ventricles, up to a certain point. When "overfilling" of the ventricles occurs, as in congestive heart failure (CHF), myocardial fibers are overstretched and lose some of their contractility, thus ultimately reducing cardiac output.

5. Cardiac output is affected by the heart rate, the amount of ventricular filling during diastole, the contractility of the myocardial fibers, and the degree of peripheral resistance.

6. Decreased cardiac output affects the body systems. Decreased cardiac output results in early compensatory mechanisms of selected vasoconstriction (which serve to provide oxygen to the vital organs by shunting blood from the abdominal organs and peripheral areas [arms, legs, skin] to the brain and heart). The results of this shunting are cold clammy skin and reduced urine output.

   The heart responds by increasing its rate (tachycardia), as does the respiratory system (tachypnea), in an attempt to increase the amount of circulating oxygen.

   If cardiac output continues to decline, hypoxia of brain tissue will produce restlessness, then coma, and the heart will indicate ischemia with angina and dysrhythmias.

   Sustained tissue hypoxia results in anaerobic metabolism, producing metabolic acidosis and eventual death if not corrected.

7. Exercise and physical activity increase cardiac output, heart rate, and blood pressure. Regular exercise, leading to physical fitness, makes the heart more efficient so that stroke volume increases and heart rate is not greatly altered with exercise. Warning signs that the heart is not able to meet demands placed on it by exercise include chest pain, dyspnea, dizziness, and pulse and blood pressure alterations that do not return to normal resting rates 3 minutes after the activity has ceased.

8. The heart is required to work harder following the ingestion of larger meals, as opposed to smaller meals. Intake of large amounts of fluid increases blood volume and, in turn, blood pressure, especially when sodium intake is high.

9. The two main sources of pain in low cardiac output states are (a) ischemia resulting from diminished oxygenation and (b) venous congestion and engorgement caused by the backup of blood that enters the heart.

10. The effects of reduced cardiac output are:

    Physical symptoms (pain, fatigue, edema, weight loss)

    Altered life-style (occupational, social, sexual, financial, role responsibilities)

    Altered self-concept

11. Required reduction in the level of personal activity may result in role identification conflict and, in the case of married couples, may disrupt the division of labor among the partners.

Nutritional

1. Dietary management of persons with decreased cardiac output varies with the amount of decompensation present. Restrictions may be placed on calories (weight reduction), sodium (edema reduction), fluids (edema reduction), and fat (lipid reduction).
2. Individuals on sodium-restricted diets must be monitored for hyponatremia resulting from sodium restrictions in the presence of renal insufficiency. Hypokalemia (potassium loss) can result from the loss of potassium with certain diuretics.
3. The four levels of sodium restriction diets are severe (250 mg daily), strict (500 mg daily), moderate (1000 mg daily), and mild (2000–3000 mg daily).
4. Food restrictions occur at each level (these restrictions do not apply to persons also on low-fat diets).

	Severe	*Strict*	*Moderate*	*Mild*
Milk	Low-sodium 2 cups	2 cups	2 cups	2 cups
Low-salt meat/eggs	Meat 4 oz Eggs 3 wk	6 oz daily	Moderation	Moderation
Fruits	2–3	2–3	2–3	2–3
Bread (slices)	4 salt-free	4 salt-free	2	4
Vegetables	Low-sodium	Low-sodium	Moderate use of high-sodium types	No restrictions; limit canned vegetables
Table salt	None	None	None	¼ tsp

5. A high intake of sodium causes increased retention of water.

   Foods with high sodium content include salted snacks, bacon, cheddar cheese, pickles, soy sauce, processed luncheon meats, MSG (monosodium glutamate), canned vegetables, catsup, mustard; also, some over-the-counter drugs such as bicarbonate of soda, antacids, cough suppressants, and many oral hygiene products.

   Foods with moderate sodium content include eggs, milk, hamburger, canned corn, and canned tomato juice.

   Foods with low sodium content include fruits, chicken, liver, fresh vegetables, unsalted bread, and unsalted crackers.
6. Foods with a high potassium content include bananas, dates, raisins, oranges, puffed wheat cereal, potatoes, liver, Pepsi, and Gatorade.

Activity Intolerance
Related to (Specify)

Assessment
See preceding Defining Characteristics

Outcome Criteria

The person will
- Identify factors that reduce his activity tolerance
- Progress to (specify the highest level of mobility possible)
- Exhibit a decrease in hypoxic signs of increased activity (pulse, blood pressure, respirations)

Interventions

The following interventions apply to most individuals with activity intolerance, regardless of the etiology.

A. Assess for causative and contributing factors

Disorders of oxygen transport system (see Activity Intolerance Related to Insufficent Oxygen Transport)

Nutritional deficiencies (see Alterations in Nutrition: Less Than Body Requirements)

Fluid and electrolyte imbalances (see Fluid Volume Deficit and Fluid Volume Excess)

Insufficient sleep or rest

Pain

Prolonged immobility

Treatment-related considerations
  Medication
  Diagnostic studies
  Staff expectations
  Surgery
Personal factors
  Lack of incentive
  Depression

B. Reduce or eliminate contributing factors if possible

1. Inadequate rest or sleep periods

   Plan rest periods according to the person's daily schedule (rest periods may occur between activities)

   Encourage person to rest during the first hour following meals (rest can take the form of napping, sitting and watching TV, or sitting with legs elevated)

   Assess nocturnal sleep (refer to Sleep Pattern Disturbance for additional information)

2. Pain

   Evaluate pain and the present treatment regimen (refer to *Altered Comfort: Pain* for specific assessment criteria and interventions)

3. Treatment-related factors

   a. Medications

      Assess for side-effects of medication

      Reduce side-effects, if possible (*e.g.*, for diuretic-induced hypokalemia, teach person to increase dietary potassium—oranges, tomatoes, bananas, dried fruit; for antibiotic-induced diarrhea, teach person to consume yogurt two or three times a day)

b. Daily schedule
   Assess the person's present daily schedule
   Consider treatments, diagnostic studies, etc.
   Adjust schedule to reduce energy expenditure when possible (*e.g.*, cancel
   morning shower or bath when a diagnostic study is scheduled for the
   morning)
4. Lack of incentive
   Identify progress and encourage record keeping by patients in selected cases
   (*e.g.*, "Today you walked four feet farther and your pulse did not go as high as
   yesterday")
   Allow person to set activity schedule and functional activity goals (if his goal is
   too low, contract with him: *e.g.*, "If you walk halfway up the hall, I will play
   three games of cards with you")
   Plan a purpose for the ambulation, such as walking to the dayroom for a group
   activity or meal or walking to the hall to see a grandchild
   Promote a sincere "can do" attitude to provide a positive atmosphere to encourage
   increased activity; convey to the person the belief that he can improve his
   mobility status
   Explore possible incentives with the person and his family; consider what the
   person values (*e.g.*)
   Playing with grandchild
   Returning to work
   Performing a task, such as a craft
   For additional interventions, refer to *Ineffective Individual Coping Related to
   Depression*

C. Assess the individual's response to activity

Take resting pulse, blood pressure, and respirations
Consider rate, rhythm, and quality (if signs are abnormal—*e.g.*, pulse above 100—
   consult with physician about the advisability of increasing activity)
Have person perform the activity
Take vital signs immediately after activity; take pulse for 15 seconds and multiply by
   4 instead of for a full minute
Have person rest for 3 minutes; take vital signs again
Discontinue the activity if the individual responds to the activity with:
   Complaints of chest pain, dyspnea, vertigo, or confusion
   Decrease in pulse rate
   Failure of systolic rate to increase
   Decrease in systolic blood pressure
   Increase in diastolic rate 15 mm Hg
   Decrease in respiratory rate
Reduce the intensity, frequency, or duration of the activity if:
a. The pulse takes longer than 3–4 minutes to return within 6 beats of the resting
   pulse rate
b. The respiratory rate increase is excessive after the activity
c. Other signs of hypoxia are present, *e.g.*, confusion, vertigo
Prevent the complications of immobility (refer to *Potential for Disuse Syndrome*)

D. Progress the activity gradually

1. For a person who is or has been on prolonged bed rest, begin range of motion (ROM) at
   least b.i.d.

If the person is unable, the nurse should perform passive ROM

If the person is able, have him perform active ROM

Encourage isometric exercises

Progress to functional ROM after the person can perform active ROM

Monitor vital signs before and after exercise

Refer to *Impaired Physical Immobility* for additional interventions

2. Increase the person's tolerance for the activity by having him perform the activity more slowly, or for a shorter period of time with more rest pauses, or with more assistance.

(Strenuous activity may increase the pulse by 50 beats. Such a rate is still satisfactory, as long as it returns to the resting pulse within 3 minutes.)

Encourage the person to turn and lift himself actively unless contraindicated

Raise the bed to a high position so that the person can slide out of bed to a standing position rather than try to get up from a very low position

Provide support when the person begins to stand

If the person is unable to stand without buckling his knees, he is not ready for ambulation; have him practice standing in place with assistance

3. Promote optimal sitting balance and tolerance by increasing muscle strength

Gradually increase exercise tolerance by starting with 15 minutes for the first time out of bed

Have the person get out of bed 3 times a day, increasing the time out of bed by 15 minutes each day

Practice transfers, having the person do as much active movement as possible

4. Promote ambulation with or without assistance devices

Choose a gait that is safe for the individual (If his gait appears awkward but he has stability, allow him to continue; stay close by, giving clear coaching messages: *e.g.*, "Look straight ahead, not down")

Allow the person to gauge the rate of the ambulation

Prevent the person from falling (stand slightly behind him on his weaker side, one hand on his belt and one on his shoulder)

Encourage person to wear comfortable walking shoes (slippers do not support the feet properly)

E. Initiate health teaching or referrals as indicated

1. Teach the person safety precautions to prevent falls (see *Potential for Injury*)

2. Teach the person the proper use of walking aids (crutches, walkers, canes) and ensure the proper fit of such devices

3. Teach the person methods of preventing the complications of immobility

Encourage frequent turning and repositioning

Encourage exercises—range of motion, isometrics—provide bedside exercise equipment if needed

Encourage adequate fluid intake, 2–3 quarts per day

Encourage good dietary habits with adequate roughage

Encourage coughing and deep-breathing exercises (see *Potential for Disuse Syndrome*)

4. Consult with a physical therapist for assistance in increasing activity tolerance

Activity Intolerance
Related to Insufficient Oxygenation Secondary to Decreased Cardiac Output

Assessment

Subjective Data
The person reports:
Pain with activity
Dyspnea with activity
Fatigue after activity

Objective Data
Rapid pulse
Low blood pressure
Dysrhythmias

Outcome Criteria

The person will
- Identify factors that increase cardiac workload
- Describe adaptive techniques needed to perform activities of daily living
- Demonstrate cardiac tolerance to increased activity, as evidenced by stable pulse, respirations, and blood pressure

---

Interventions

The nursing interventions for this diagnostic category represent interventions for individuals with decreased cardiac output regardless of the etiological and contributing factors.

A. Assess for causative and contributing factors that increase cardiac workload
Activity
Stress
Smoking
Edema
Overweight/obesity

B. Reduce or eliminate causative factors if possible
1. Activity
   a. Plan nursing strategies to promote rest, incorporating them into the care plan
      - Organize care to minimize unnecessary disturbances
      - Provide scheduled periods for rest and sleep when no one is permitted to disturb patient (except in emergencies)
      - Acknowledge the importance of visitors but assist the family to meet the needs of the individual without compromising sleep/rest patterns

- Encourage increases in activity and ambulation to prevent a sudden increase in cardiac workload
- Minimize activity prior to planned periods that require exertion, such as treatments, ambulation, meals

b. Decrease fatigue at mealtime
- Encourage a light meal in the evening to promote a more comfortable night's rest
- Initially provide easily digestible and chewable foods
- Schedule meals to avoid interfering with other activities
- Offer food preferences, avoiding dislikes
- Consider sociocultural influences

c. Teach the person energy conservation methods for activities
- Take rest periods during activities, at intervals during the day, and 1 hour after meals
- Sit rather than stand when performing activities, unless this is not feasible
- When performing a task, rest every 3 minutes for 5 minutes to allow the heart to recover
- Stop an activity if fatigue or signs of cardiac hypoxia are present (*e.g.*, ↑ pulse, dyspnea, chest pain)

d. Instruct the person to avoid certain exercises
- Isometric exercises, *e.g.*, using arms to lift himself up, lifting objects (slide them instead)
- Valsalva maneuver, *e.g.*, bending from the waist, straining during a bowel movement

e. Monitor the person's response to increased activity in the hospital or teach him to monitor (see *Principles and Rationale for Nursing Care*)
- Take a resting pulse
- Take a pulse immediately after or during activity
- Take a pulse 3 minutes after
- Instruct him to report
  Rate decreases on activity
  Rates >110
  Irregular pulse
  Pulses that do not return to within six beats of resting pulse after 3 min
  Dyspnea
  Cyanosis
  Chest pain
  Palpitations

2. Stress
a. Assist the person to identify stressors (home, work, social)
b. Discuss his usual response to stressors (*e.g.*, anger, depression, avoidance, discussion)
c. Explain the effects of stress on the cardiovascular system (*e.g.*, increased heart rate, increased blood pressure, increased respirations)
d. Discuss various methods for stress reduction
- Deliberate problem-solving (see Appendix VII)
  What is the problem?
  Who/what is responsible for the problem?
  What are the options?
  What are the advantages of each option?
  What are the disadvantages and risks of each option?

- Relaxation techniques (see Appendix VI)
- Yoga, biofeedback
- Regular exercise (30 min at least 3 times a week)
  e. See *Ineffective Individual Coping* for additional assessment and intervention information
3. Smoking
   a. Discuss with the person the effects of smoking on his cardiovascular system (*e.g.*, vasoconstriction increases workload of the heart)
   b. Teach person when not to smoke: before an activity and after an activity
   c. Discuss methods that can help reduce the amount of cigarettes smoked
   d. See *Altered Health Maintenance Related to Tobacco Use.*
4. Edema
   a. Assess for the presence of edema in ankles and sacral area
   b. See *Fluid Volume Excess* for interventions for edema
5. Overweight/obesity
   a. Assess whether the person is overweight or obese by securing height and weight of person and comparing these findings with a standardized weight/height chart, or use anthropometric measurements (See *Altered Nutrition: More Than Body Requirements* for charts of weight for heights and anthropometric norms)
   b. If weight reduction is indicated and the person has validated an interest to lose weight, refer to *Altered Health Maintenance*

C. **Discuss with the person his perceived effects that his condition will have on role responsibilities (social, home, sexual), occupation, and finances**

D. **Provide the family with an opportunity to share their concerns**
- Assess their knowledge of the condition, treatment, and prognosis
- Encourage them to share their concerns about the future and about role responsibilities

E. **Initiate health teaching and referrals if indicated**
- Instruct the person to consult his physician and physiatrist for a long-term exercise program, or to contact the American Heart Association for names of cardiac rehabilitation programs
- Explain the diet restrictions to the person and his family (*e.g.*, give them written instructions, or refer them to pertinent literature on preparation of food for restricted diets)
- Explain the prescribed drug therapy (*e.g.*, diuretics, vasodilators, dosage, side-effects, administration, and storage)
- Refer to one or more selected nursing diagnoses, if indicated, for additional information
    Constipation
    Diversional Activity Deficit
    Sexual Dysfunction
    Altered Family Processes Related to Ill Family Member
    Grieving Related to a Perceived Loss

Activity Intolerance
Related to Insufficient Oxygenation Secondary to Chronic Impaired Gas Exchange

Assessment

Subjective Data
Because chronic tissue hypoxia affects all body systems, data are presented by systems.

Respiratory history

Lung disease (chronic)

Shortness of breath or dyspnea on exertion

Chronic cough

Orthopnea (sleeping with extra pillows)

Circulatory history

Chest pain aggravated by activity

Enlarged heart

Gastrointestinal history

Anorexia

Nausea and vomiting

Constipation

Mental history

Confusion or lethargy

Mood swings, anxiety, depression

Sleep disturbances

Headache

Skeletal history

Skeletal muscle pain aggravated by activity

Muscle weakness

Chronic fatigue

Genitourinary history

Decreased kidney function

Decreased libido or impotence

Objective Data
Respiratory

Tachypnea, bradypnea, arrhythmic breathing

Abnormal chest film

Abnormal flow rates; increased inspiratory/expiratory (I/E) ratio

Pursed-lip breathing

Abnormal blood gases ($\downarrow$ PO_2 $\uparrow$ CO_2)

Use of accessory muscles (neck, shoulders, abdomen)

Gasping before speech effort/inability to speak or cry

Orthopnea/assumption of 3-point position (sitting, leaning forward with one hand on each knee)

Cough

Increased sputum production and inability to remove secretions

Mouth breathing

Abnormal breath sounds (rales and rhonchi)

Decreased breath sounds

Fremitus

Circulatory

Neck vein distention

Edema

Cyanosis

Gastrointestinal
   Decreased bowel sounds
Genitourinary
   Decreased kidney function (↑ Creatinine, ↑ BUN)
   Decreased urinary output
Skeletal system
   Hypertrophy of accessory breathing muscles (neck and shoulder)
   Atrophy or weakness of extremity muscles
   Barrel chest/horizontal sloping ribs
   Cachexia (malnutrition)

Outcome Criteria

The person will
- Preserve pulmonary function by maintaining optimal activity level and preventing infection
- Demonstrate methods of effective coughing, breathing, and conserving energy
- Relate methods to relieve symptoms of pain, weakness, and dyspnea
- Relate how to prevent further pulmonary problems

Interventions

A. Assess causative or contributing factors

Inadequate pulmonary hygiene regimen
Maladaptive breathing techniques
Inadequate nutritional intake
Insufficient level of activity
Lack of knowledge
Smoking or inhaling other irritants or allergens

B. Eliminate or reduce causative factors

1. Inadequate pulmonary hygiene routine
   - Instruct person to practice controlled coughing four times a day, 1/2 hour before meals and at bedtime (allow 15–30 minutes' rest after coughing session and before meals)
   - Consider use of inhaled humidity and postural drainage, chest clapping before coughing session (assess for use of prescribed aerosol bronchodilators to dilate airways and thin secretions)
   - Explain the importance of adhering to daily coughing schedule for clearing the lungs (this is a lifetime commitment)
   - Teach the proper method of coughing
     a. Breathe deeply and slowly while sitting up as upright as possible
     b. Use diaphragmatic breathing
     c. Hold the breath for 3 to 5 seconds and then slowly exhale as much of this breath as possible through your mouth (lower rib cage and abdomen should sink down as you exhale)

    d. Take a second deep breath, hold, and cough forcefully from deep in the chest (not from the back of the mouth or throat); use two short forceful coughs

    e. Rest after session

2. Maladaptive breathing techniques

- Encourage conscious controlled breathing techniques during increased activity and times of emotional and physical stress (techniques include pursed-lip and diaphragmatic breathing)
- For pursed-lip breathing, the person should breathe in through his nose; then he should breathe out slowly through partially closed lips while counting to seven and making a "pu" sound (often this is learned naturally by person with progressive lung disease)
- For diaphragmatic breathing
  - a. The nurse should place her hands on the person's abdomen below the base of the ribs and keep them there while he inhales
  - b. To inhale, the person should relax his shoulders, breathe in through his nose, and push his stomach outward against the nurse's hands, holding his breath for 1 to 2 seconds to keep the alveoli open
  - c. To exhale, the person should breathe out slowly through his mouth while the nurse applies slight pressure at the base of the ribs
  - d. This breathing technique should be practiced several times with the nurse; then the person should place his own hands at the base of the ribs and practice on his own
  - e. Once the person has learned, he should practice this exercise a few times each hour

3. Inadequate nutritional intake

- Suggest that person brush teeth and use mouthwash before meals (and especially after coughing session, because there is frequently an associated bad taste in the mouth, causing a decreased appetite and a decrease in tasting ability)
- Encourage smaller, more frequent meals (large portions require more oxygen/energy to digest and also limit the downward movements of the diaphragm during inspiration)
- Choose foods that are easy to chew and swallow (food that must be chewed extensively will require more work, causing fatigue); assist in food preparation (*e.g.,* cutting meat) if person is extremely fatigued
- Avoid gas-producing foods or liquids
- Discourage talking while eating; encourage thorough chewing and slow eating
- Encourage drinking 2 to 3 quarts of liquid a day (minimum) if sodium and fluids are unrestricted (consult with physician for desired daily fluid intake)
- Assure satisfactory bowel elimination

4. Insufficient level of activity

- Encourage gradual increase in daily activity to prevent "pulmonary crippling"
- Encourage person to use adaptive breathing techniques to decrease the work of breathing
- Discuss physical barriers at home and at work (*e.g.,* number of stairs) and ways of alternating expenditure of energy with rest pauses (place a chair in bathroom near sink to rest during daily hygiene)
- Encourage verbalization of feelings about disease and limitations and discuss methods of coping with daily stressors (see *Ineffective Individual Coping*)
- Encourage socialization with others and methods of reducing depression (taking a walk, visiting with a friend)
- Give calm, consistent emotional support in time of increased respiratory distress, in hopes of reducing oxygen demands

- Support person by suggesting that he follow your breathing pattern and by demonstrating pursed-lip and diaphragmatic breathing

5. Lack of knowledge
   - Assess person's understanding of the prescribed therapeutic regimen; proceed with health teaching, using simple, clear instructions and including family members*
   - Explain that the person with chronic pulmonary disease is susceptible to infection and must detect symptoms early and consult with physician for treatment (frequently, early antibiotic therapy is necessary)
   - Discuss the need for annual immunizations (against flu, bacteria)
   - Instruct person to wear warm dry clothing; avoid crowds, heavy smoke, fumes, and irritants; avoid exertion in cold, hot, or humid weather; and balance work, rest, and recreation to conserve energy
   - Teach person to observe his sputum, note changes in color, amount, and odor, and seek professional advice if sputum changes
   - Emphasize importance of maintaining a good wholesome diet (high calorie, high vitamin C, high protein, and 2 to 3 quarts of liquid a day, unless on fluid restriction)
   - Specifically assess
     a. Knowledge and skill of adaptive breathing techniques
     b. Knowledge of medicines (when taken, why, how much, how often, and food and drug interactions)
     c. Knowledge of the care, cleansing, and use of inhalatory equipment
     d. Awareness of fire hazards (if on oxygen therapy, especially at home); explain need for home extinguisher

6. Smoking
   - Teach person to avoid factors that aggravate symptoms and advance disease (excessive allergens, pollution)
   - Discourage smoking
   - If person insists on smoking, discourage smoking immediately before meals or activity
   - See further interventions under *Altered Health Maintenance Related to Tobacco Use* if person wishes to reduce or stop smoking

C. Initiate health teaching and referrals as indicated

- Give clear written and verbal instructions; be specific
- Reassess knowledge of skills and rationale frequently; keep clear progress notes on strengths and weaknesses of person's knowledge
- Encourage person to keep a daily written log of his activities and symptoms and of measures that relieve symptoms
- Refer to community nurse for follow-up if needed
- Refer to organizations and pertinent literature for the person with lung disorders

References/Bibliography

General

Allen S: Step by step: Renew a patient's initiative. Nursing 11:56–57, 1981

Basmajian JV (ed): Therapeutic Exercise, 4th edition. London, Williams & Wilkins, 1984

---

* A person who is chronically hypoxic should always be taught in simple terms and assured of support by family and caretakers, because thought processes frequently become confused during periods of hypoxia.

Bouman HD: An exploratory analytical survey of therapeutic exercise. Am J Phys Med 46:26–31, 1967

Jacobs MM, Giels W: Signs and Symptoms in Nursing Interpretation and Management. Philadelphia, JB Lippincott, 1985

Licht S (ed): Therapeutic Exercise. Baltimore, Waverly Press, 1965

Louis MC, Pouse S: Aphasia and endurance: Consideration in assessment and care of the stroke patient. Nurs Clin North Am 15:265–292, 1980

Lunsford B: Clinical indicators of endurance. Phys Ther 58:704–790, 1978

Ziegler J: Physical reconditioning. Nursing 10:67–69, 1980

Cardiac

Adler J: Patient assessment: Pulses. Am J Nurs 79:115–132, 1979

Alexy BJ: Monitoring cardiovascular status with noninvasive techniques. Nurs Clin North Am 13:423–435, 1978

Arlin M: Controversies in nutrition: A brief review. Nurs Clin North Am 14:199–214, 1979

Cole C, Levin EM, Whitley JO et al: Brief sexual counseling during cardiac rehabilitation. Heart Lung 8:124–129, 1979

Coyle N: Analgesics at the bedside. Am J Nurs 79:1554–1557, 1979

Jordan J: Your fingers on the pulse: Evaluating what you feel. Nursing 10(11):33–39, 1980

Respiratory

See Bibliography for *Potential Altered Respiratory Function*.

Adjustment, Impaired

Related to **(Specify)**

Definition

Impaired adjustment: The state in which the individual is unwilling to modify his/her life-style/behavior in a manner consistent with a change in health status.

> **Author's Note:** The term *adjustment* describes an individual's psychosocial regulatory processes to establish equilibrium in a person–environment. This individual is having difficulty adapting to a health status change.

Defining Characteristics

Major (must be present)

Verbalization of nonacceptance of health status change or inadequate capacity to be involved in problem-solving or goal-setting.

Minor (may be present)

Lack of movement toward independence; extended period of shock, disbelief, or anger regarding health status change; lack of future-oriented thinking.

Etiological, Contributing, Risk Factors

Adjustment impairment can result from a variety of situations and health problems. Some common sources are listed below.

Pathophysiological

Spinal-cord injury
Paralysis
Loss of limb
Cerebrovascular accident (CVA)
Myocardial infarction
Progressive neurological diseases
Cancer
Chronic obstructive pulmonary disease (COPD)

Treatment-related

Dialysis

Situational (personal, environmental)

Inadequate support systems
Unavailable support systems
Impaired cognition
Depression
Loss (object, person, job)
Divorce

Maturational
>   Child/adolescent: chronic disease, disability
>   Adult: loss of ability to practice vocation, role reversal
>   Elderly: normal physiological aging changes

Focus Assessment Criteria

See *Ineffective Individual Coping*

Principles and Rationale for Nursing Care

1. Individuals have a concept of self that includes feelings about self, worth, attractiveness, lovability, and capabilities (Peretz). One's mental image of one's own body and person is assaulted after a physical injury. This injury or loss involves the grieving process.
2. The grieving process in response to a recent disability has been described as (Friedman-Campbell):
   a. Shock-denial
      - Denies injury or severity of the injury
      - Minimally allows self to think of loss to protect self
      - Intellectually accepts the loss, but denies it emotionally
   b. Developing awareness
      - Realizes the impact of the loss on self
      - Experiences acute somatic feelings of loss
      - Displaces anger
      - Is preoccupied with guilt and blaming
      - Mourns the loss and withdraws
      - Shuns change and clings to routines
   c. Managing loss of body function
      - Begins to deal with the impact of the loss on self
      - Frees self slowly from the bondage of the loss
      - Readjusts to changed environment
      - Invests in new relationships
3. Everyone has implicit or explicit goals. Through experience, patterns of successful behavior in achieving these individual goals are developed. The person then regularly uses this behavior to achieve goals.
4. Goals are established to maintain:
   >   Physical well-being
   >   Self-esteem
   >   Productive satisfying interactions with others
5. The behavior of individuals is such that:
   >   People act to meet needs and achieve goals
   >   Relatively stable patterns of behavior are developed
   >   Behavior is disrupted when both needs and goals are threatened
6. Coping attempts to remove the threats to meeting needs and achieving goals. Lazarus states that coping refers to efforts to master conditions of harm, threat, or challenge when a routine or automatic response is not available.
7. Successful coping with physical injury or loss (Hamburg)
   >   Reduces stress to manageable limits
   >   Maintains feelings of personal worth
   >   Restores relationships with significant others
   >   Seeks recovery of physical functions
   >   Initiates a situation that is a positive contribution

Initiates a situation (project, job, tasks) after maximum recovery that is viewed as socially acceptable and personally valued

Gains pleasure from mastery

8. A person who is ill or disabled continues to have needs and goals. Previous coping patterns, if effective, may assist the individual to achieve goals and meet needs.
9. Responses to illness, disability or treatments are influenced by:

Attitude toward event (punishment, weakness, challenge, etc.)

Developmental level or age

The extent of interference of the disability in goal-directed activity and the significance of the goal

10. Recognize that gender, level of intelligence, social and cultural background, value systems, and the cognitive and behavioral style of the person falling ill may importantly influence his/her coping style.
11. Crisis is defined by Miller and Iscoe as "the experiencing of an acute situation where one's repertoire of coping responses is inadequate in effecting a resolution of the stress." For an individual it usually represents a turning point in his/her life and a reorganization of some of the important aspects of his/her psychological structure.
12. An individual crisis can be described in four sequential stages: shock, defensive retreat, acknowledgment, and adaptation.
13. Optimal intervention can occur only when the defensive attempts have failed and the person has begun a self-examination of the current situation.
14. Adaptation is the process whereby an individual strives to achieve comfortable and effective functioning in the environment. Adaptation is not static; it is an ongoing process.

Impaired Adjustment
Related to (Specify)

Assessment

See Defining Characteristics

Outcome Criteria

The individual will:
- Identify the temporary and long-term demands of the situation
- Differentiate coping behavior that is effective versus ineffective

---

Interventions

1. Assess and identify the person's:

Premorbid life-style

Premorbid coping style

Amount and type of resources available

Extent of current disruption on life-style

Current level of stress
Current coping methods and their effectiveness
2. Identify factors that interfere with or delay effective adjustment:
   - Unmanageable level of stress (see *Anxiety*)
   - Inability to identify the problem or ineffective problem solving (see Appendix VII, Guidelines for Problem Solving and Crisis Interventions)
   - Lack of mastery of developmental tasks for age
   - History of patterns of ineffective coping and unresolved conflicts
   - Inadequate or unavailable resources
        Faith (see *Hopelessness*)
        Knowledge about illness/disability
        Money
        Support system
        Skills to manage illness/disability
3. Assess the family's or significant other's response to situation:
        Perception of the effects (long-term and short-term) of the illness or disability
        Past family dynamics
        Present family dynamics (verbal, nonverbal)
4. Assist the family and significant others to cope:
   - Explore with them their perception of how the situation will progress
   - Identify behaviors that facilitate adaptation
   - Stress the importance of trying to maintain usual roles and behavior
   - When appropriate, include the affected individual in family decision-making
   - Discuss the reality of everyday emotions: anger, guilt, jealousy; relate the hazards of denying these feelings
   - Discuss the hazards of trying to minimize the grief and trying to distract the grievers from grieving
5. Assess for the presence of denial as a coping mechanism:
   - Focus on present situation
   - Accept denial as an initial response
   - Give feedback about current reality: identify positive achievements regardless of how minor
6. Reduce stress if possible by manipulating the environment:
   - Establish an active constructive relationship with the individual and family by acknowledging the person's increased dependence and initiating a collaborative approach to care (Friedman-Campbell)
   - Reduce environmental noise, barriers
   - Remove distressing people, objects, or situations from person
   - Give permission to the person to express feelings, if desired. For example: "It must be very hard to have someone wash you."
   - Share your perception of injury
7. Identify dysfunctional coping mechanisms; *e.g.*, use of chemical substances, avoidance, morbid preoccupation with the disability.
8. When appropriate, begin health teaching (Friedman-Campbell):
   - Share your perceptions of the injury and the person's response to it
   - Explain the nature of the illness or injury
   - Discuss the anticipated changes in life-style
   - Teach health behaviors that need to be learned in order to adapt to a new life-style
9. Explore goals with individual and also with family:
        Career

Relationships

Recreation

Compare pre-morbid goals with post injury/illness goals.

10. Explore with individual his/her fears. Role-play fearful or stressful situations.

11. Initiate referrals as indicated.

    a. Identify resources available: community, financial, counseling, role models, self-help groups

    b. Refer individuals and family to appropriate self-help literature (see Literature for Consumer)

References/Bibliography

Beglinger JE: Coping tasks in critical care: Patient and families. Dimens Crit Care Nurs 2(2):80–89, 1983

Burgess AW, Baldwin BA: Crisis Intervention: Theory and Practice. Englewood Cliffs, NJ, Prentice-Hall, 1981

Cheney RJ: Emotional adaptation to disability. Rehab Nurs 9(5):36–37, 1984

Crate M: Nursing functions in adaptation to chronic illness. Am J Nurs 65:72–76, 1965

Fink SL: Crisis and motivation: A theoretical model. Arch Phys Med Rehab Nov. 592–597, 1967

Friedman-Campbell M, Hart CA: Theoretical strategies and nursing interventions to promote psychological adaptation to spinal cord injuries and disability. J Neurosurg Nurs 16(6):335–342, 1984

Gentry WD et al: Type A/B differences in coping with acute myocardial infarction: Further consideration (editorial). Heart Lung 13(3):212–214, 1983

Hamburg DA, Adams JE: A perspective on coping behavior. Arch Gen Psychiatry 17:1–20, 1953

Kiely WF: Coping with severe illness. Adv Psychosom Med 8:105–118, 1972

Lazarus RS, Monat A: Stress and Coping, An Anthology. New York, Columbia University Press, 1977

Martin N, Holt NB, Hicks D: Comprehensive Rehabilitation Nursing. New York, McGraw-Hill, 1981

Miller K, Iscoe I: The concept of crisis current status and mental health implications. Human Organizations 22:195–201, 1963

Miller P et al: Family health and psychosocial responses to cardiovascular diseases. Health Values 7(6):10–15, 1983

Peretz D: Reaction to loss. In Carr AC, Peretz D (eds): Loss and Grief Psychological Management in Medicine. New York. Columbia University Press, 1970

Oberst MT et al: Going home: Patient and spouse adjustment following cancer surgery. Top Clin Nurs 7(1):46–57, 1985

Ott CR et al: A controlled randomized study of early cardiac rehabilitation: The sickness impact profile as an assessment tool. Heart Lung 12(2):162–170, 1983

Resources for the Consumer

Literature

COPE: Living with Cancer (magazine), PO Box 54679, Boulder, CO 80322

Accent on Living (magazine), PO Box 700, Bloomington, IL 61702

Anxiety

Related to **(Specify)**

Related to **Lack of Knowledge of**
   Preoperative Routines
   Postoperative Exercises/Activities
   Postoperative Alterations/Sensations

Definition
Anxiety: A state in which the individual/group experiences feelings of uneasiness (apprehension) and activation of the autonomic nervous system in response to a vague, nonspecific threat.

Author's Note: Anxiety differs from fear in that the anxious person cannot identify the threat. With fear, the threat can be identified. Anxiety can be present without fear; however, anxiety is usually present with fear.

Defining Characteristics

Major (must be present)
Manifested by symptoms from each category—physiological, emotional, and cognitive, Symptoms vary according to the level of anxiety.

Physiological
Increased heart rate
Elevated blood pressure
Increased respiratory rate
Diaphoresis
Dilated pupils
Voice tremors/pitch changes
Trembling
Palpitations
Nausea and/or vomiting
Frequent urination
Diarrhea

Insomnia
Fatigue and weakness
Flushimg or pallor
Dry mouth
Body aches and pains (especially chest, back, neck
Restlessness
Faintness/dizziness
Paresthesias
Hot and cold flashes

Emotional
Person states that he has feelings of
Apprehension
Helplessness
Nervousness
Fear
Lack of self-confidence

Losing control
Tension or being "keyed up"
Inability to relax
Unreality
Anticipation of misfortune

Person exhibits

Irritability/impatience

Angry outbursts

Crying

Tendency to blame others

Startle reaction

Criticism of self and others

Withdrawal

Lack of initiative

Self-depreciation

Cognitive

Inability to concentrate

Lack of awareness of surroundings

Forgetfulness

Rumination

Orientation to past rather than to present or future

Blocking of thoughts (inability to remember)

Hyperattentiveness

Etiological, Contributing, Risk Factors

Pathophysiological

Any factor that interferes with the basic human needs for food, air, and comfort.

Situational (personal, environmental)

Actual or perceived threat to self-concept

Change in status and prestige

Lack of recognition from others

Failure (or success)

Loss of valued possessions

Ethical dilemmas

Actual or perceived loss of significant others

Death

Divorce

Cultural pressures

Moving

Temporary or permanent

separation

Actual or perceived threat to biological integrity

Dying

Assault

Invasive procedures

Disease

Actual or perceived change in environment

Hospitalization

Moving

Retirement

Safety Hazards

Environmental pollutants

Actual or perceived change in socioeconomic status

Unemployment

New job

Promotion

Transmission of another person's anxiety to the individual

Maturational (threat to developmental task)

Infant/child: Separation, mutilation, peer relationships, achievement

Adolescent: Sexual development, peer relationships, independence

Adult: Pregnancy, parenting, career development, effects of aging

Elderly: Sensory losses, motor losses, financial problems, retirement

Focus Assessment Criteria

Subjective Data

1. History of the individual from client and significant others

Life-style
 Interests   Strengths, limitations
 Work history   Previous level of functioning,
 Coping patterns (past, present)   handling stress
Support system
 Availability   Quality of support
History of medical problems/treatments
 Alcohol and drug abuse   Medications
Activities of daily living
 Ability to perform   Desire to perform

2. History of unusual sensations (*e.g.*, palpitations, tingling, dyspnea, dry mouth, nausea, diaphoresis)
 Precipitating factors   Routine time of occurrence
 Frequency   Description in individual's own
 Duration   words

3. Assess for feelings of
 Extreme sadness and worthlessness Harm from others
 Guilt for past actions   Mind being controlled by
 Apprehension   external agents
 Rejection or isolation   Being unable to cope
 Living in an unreal world   Falling apart
 Mistrust or suspiciousness of others Thoughts racing
 Manipulation by others   Being held prisoner

4. Orientation
 Person
  "What is your name?"
  "What is your occupation?"
  "Tell me about yourself"
 Time
  "What season is it?"
  "What month is it?"
 Place
  "Where are you?"
  "Where do you live?"

5. Usual coping behavior
 "How do you usually handle a particular situation (i.e., anger, disappointment, loss, rejection, etc.)?"
 "What did you usually do when you were faced with similar situations in the past?"
 "What happens when you do that?"
 (relevant coping mechanism)
 Assess for:
  Level of awareness of behavior
  Range of coping behavior
  Adaptive/maladaptive
  Secondary gains

Subjective and Objective Data

1. General appearance
 Facial expression (*e.g.*, sad, hostile, expressionless)
 Dress (*e.g.*, meticulous, disheveled, seductive, eccentric)

2. Behavior during interview
    Withdrawn   Cooperative
    Hostile   Quiet
    Apathetic

3. Communication pattern
    Content
        Appropriate   Sexually preoccupied
        Rambling   Delusions (of grandeur, persecution,
        Suspicious   reference, influence, control or
        Denial of problem   bodily sensations)
        Homicidal plans   Hallucinations (visual, auditory,
        Suicidal ideas   gustatory, olfactory, tactile)
    Flow of thought
        Appropriate   Jumps from one topic to another
        Blocking of ideas (unable to   Unable to come to conclusion, be
           finish idea)   decisive
        Circumstantial (unable to get   Difficulty concentrating
           to point)   States he is unable to follow what
        Ideas loosely connected   is being said
                                          Difficulty grasping circumstances or
                                          events

    Rate of speech
        Appropriate   Reduced
        Excessive   Pressured
    Nonverbal behavior
        Affect appropriate/inappropriate to verbal content
        Gestures, mannerisms, facial grimaces
        Posture

4. Interaction skills
    With a nurse
        Inappropriate   Shows dependency
        Relates well   Demanding/pleading
        Withdrawn/preoccupied with self   Hostile
    With significant others
        Relates with all family   Does not seek interaction
           members or with some   Does not have visitors
        Hostile toward one member/
           all members

5. Activities of daily living
    Emotionally capable of caring for self
    Physically capable of caring for self

6. Nutritional status
    Appetite   Weight (within normal limits, de-
    Eating patterns   creased, increased)

7. Sleep/rest pattern
    Recent change   Early wakefulness
    Sleeps too much/too little   Insomnia

8. Personal hygiene
    Cleanliness (body, hair, teeth)   Clothes (condition, appropriateness)
    Grooming (clothes, hair, makeup)

9. Motor activity
   Within normal limits
   Increased   Agitated
   Decreased   Repetitive
10. Present coping behavior
   "Acting-out" behaviors
      Derogating   Resentfulness
      Fighting   Motor restlessness
      Arguing   Pacing
      Intimidating   Physical exertion
      Ritualistic behavior
      Smoking, alcohol, drugs
      Manipulation of others to do tasks he is capable of
   Paralysis and retreating behaviors
      Withdrawal   Dissociation
      Depression   Ritualistic behavior
      Denial   Blocking
      Diverts attention
      Sleeping
      Avoids talking about self
      Minimizes signs and symptoms
   Somatizing
      Headache   Syncope
      Dyspnea
      Muscle tension
      Hives, eczema
      Anorexia
      Colitis
      Menstrual disturbance
   Constructive action
      Seeks support from others
      Ventilates
      Seeks information
      Uses positive thinking techniques
      Sets realistic goals
      Maintains social activities
      Plans rest periods

Principles and Rationale for Nursing Care

1. Anxiety is conceptually different from fear, in that fear has an identified stimulus. Anxiety is a feeling aroused by a vague, nonspecific threat.
2. Anxiety is communicated interpersonally.
3. Anxiety varies in intensity depending on the severity of the threat, as perceived by the person, and the success or failure of his efforts to cope with his feelings.
4. Coping behaviors used to manage anxiety occur at various levels of awareness and may be used simultaneously.
5. Individuals develop a range of coping behaviors; in some situations they are adaptive, in others, maladaptive.
6. The effectiveness of coping strategies depends on the individual and the situation, not on the behavior itself.

7. Patterns of coping with anxiety are
   a. Acting-out: converting anxiety into anger that is either overtly or covertly expressed
   b. Paralysis or retreating behaviors: withdrawing or being immobilized by own anxiety
   c. Somatizing: converting anxiety into physical symptoms
   d. Constructive action: using anxiety to learn and problem-solve (includes goal-setting, learning new skills, and seeking information)
8. Maladaptive coping mechanisms are characterized by inability to make choices, conflict, repetition and rigidity, alienation, and secondary gains. Refer to *Ineffective Individual Coping* for further information.
9. The term anxiety is used to refer to both a response to a particular situation—state anxiety—and the differences among people in interpreting situations as threatening—trait anxiety (Spielberger).
10. Persons with relatively high levels of trait anxiety tend to perceive greater danger in situations that threaten self-esteem than do persons with lower levels. These individuals respond with higher levels of state anxiety (Spielberger).
11. The effects of anxiety on a person's abilities are as follows:

   Mild
   > Perception and attention heightened; alert
   > Able to deal with problem situations
   > Can integrate past, present, and future experiences
   > Uses learning; can consensually validate; formulates meanings
   > Curious, repeats questions
   > Sleeplessness

   Moderate
   > Perception somewhat narrowed; selectively inattentive, but can direct attention
   > Slightly more difficult to concentrate; learning requires more effort
   > Views present experiences in terms of past
   > May fail to notice what is happening in a peripheral situation; will have some difficulty in adapting and analyzing
   > Voice/pitch changes
   > Increased respiratory and heart rates
   > Tremors, shakiness

   Severe
   > Perception greatly reduced; focuses on scattered details; cannot attend to more even when instructed to
   > Learning severely impaired; highly distractable, unable to concentrate
   > Views present experiences in terms of past; almost unable to understand current situation
   > Functions poorly; communication difficult to understand
   > Hyperventilation, tachycardia, headache, dizziness, nausea

   Panic
   > Perception distorted; focuses on blown-up detail; scattering may be increased
   > Learning cannot occur
   > Unable to integrate experiences; can focus only on present; unable to see or understand situation; lapses in recall of thoughts
   > Unable to function; usually increased motor activity and/or unpredictable responses to even minor stimuli; communication not understandable

Feelings of impending doom/unreality

Dyspnea	Dizziness/faintness
Palpitations	Trembling
Choking	Paresthesia
Hot/cold flashes	Sweating

12. The most common sign of anxiety in children and adolescents is increased motor activity. Signs of anxiety can be viewed developmentally and may be reflected in the following ways:

    Birth to 9 months: disruption in physiological functioning (*e.g.*, sleep disorders, colic)

    9 months to 4 years: major source is loss of significant others and loss of love; therefore, anxiety may be seen as anger when parents leave, somatic illnesses, motor restlessness, regressive behaviors (thumb sucking, head banging, rocking), regression in toilet training

    4 to 6 years: major source is fear of body damage; belief that his bad behavior causes bad things to happen (*e.g.*, illness); somatic complaints of headache, stomachache

    6 to 12 years: excessive verbalization, compulsive behavior (*e.g.*, repeating a task over and over)

    Adolescence: similar to 6 to 12 years plus types of negativistic behavior

13. Aggression is a response to a threat or frustration in which verbal and/or physical aggressive action offers relief to the anxiety experienced. Operationally, the steps are:
    a. The individual experiences a threat or frustration
    b. Anxiety is felt
    c. Feelings of insecurity and helplessness occur
    d. Increasing anxiety is decreased through verbal or physical aggression
14. Aggressive behavior may vary from irritation to rage and may be directed toward self, others, or objects.
15. Limits provide a sense of security. There is a need for predictability about self and environment.
16. Feelings of anger can be expressed either overtly or covertly. Examples of overt expression include hitting or fighting, nonverbal glaring, and verbal attack. Examples of covert expression of anger include somatizing, depression, and suicide.
17. Feelings of anxiety or anger may be unacceptable to the individual, and avoidance coping mechanisms may be used. Examples include denial, projection, and rationalization.
18. In managing inappropriate aggressive behavior, use the least amount of external control possible.
19. Individuals with severe or panic anxiety may be more agitated by attempts to communicate.
20. Anger is a response to frustration and anxiety.
21. Anger differs from hostility in that anger is usually short-lived and compatible in relationships. Hostility is a feeling of antagonism accompanied by a wish to hurt or humiliate others.
22. Children need opportunities and encouragement to express anger in a controlled, acceptable manner (*e.g.*, choosing not to play a particular game, choosing not to play with a particular person, slamming a door, or voicing anger). Unacceptable expressions of anger include throwing an object, hitting a person, and breaking an object.
23. Children who are not permitted to express their anger may develop hostility and perceive the world as unfriendly.

24. Hostility is usually the result of frustrated or unfulfilled needs or wishes (*e.g.*, unrealistic expectations of others, unrealistic expectations for self, low self-concept, and feelings of humiliation).
25. The hostile person may respond by repressing his hostility and withdrawing (depression), denying the hostility and overreacting with extreme compliance (politeness), or engaging in overt hostile behavior (verbal or nonverbal).

Anxiety
Related to (Specify)

Assessment
See Defining Characteristics

> **Outcome Criteria**
>
> The person will
> - Describe his own anxiety and coping patterns
> - Relate an increase in psychological and physiological comfort
> - Use effective coping mechanisms in managing anxiety, as evidenced by (specify)

Interventions
The nursing interventions for the diagnosis Anxiety apply to any individual with anxiety regardless of the etiological and contributing factors.

A. Assist the person to reduce his present level of anxiety
  1. Assess level of anxiety (See Principles and Rationale for Nursing Care for specific differentiation)

     Mild   Severe

     Moderate   Panic

  2. Provide reassurance and comfort
     - Stay with the person
     - Do not make demands or ask him to make decisions
     - Support present coping mechanisms (*e.g.*, allow client to walk, talk, cry); do not confront or argue with his defenses or rationalizations
     - Speak slowly and calmly
     - Be aware of your own concern and avoid reciprocal anxiety
     - Convey a sense of empathic understanding (*e.g.*, quiet presence, touch, allowing crying, talking, etc.)
     - Provide reassurance that a solution can be found
  3. Decrease sensory stimulation
     - Use short, simple sentences
     - Give concise directions

- Focus on the here and now
- Remove excess stimulation (*e.g.*, take person to quieter room); limit contact with others—patients or family—who are also anxious
- If person is hyperventilating, have him take slow, deep breaths and breathe with him
- Attempt to occupy person with a simple, repetitive task
- Consult physician for possible pharmacological therapy if indicated

B. **When anxiety is diminished enough for learning to take place, assist person in recognizing his anxiety in order to initiate learning or problem-solving**

- Request validation of your assessment of anxiety (*e.g.*, "Are you uncomfortable now?")
- If person can say yes, continue with the learning process; if he is not able to acknowledge anxiety, continue supportive measures until he is able (refer to A)
- When able to learn, determine usual coping mechanisms: "What do you usually do when you get upset?"
- Assess for unmet needs or expectations; encourage recall and description of what the person experienced immediately prior to feeling anxious
- Assist in reevaluation of the perceived threat by discussing the following:
  1. Were expectations realistic?
  2. Was it possible to meet his expectations?
  3. Where in the sequence of events was change possible?
- Encourage the person to recall and analyze similar instances of anxiety
- Explore what alternative behaviors might have been used if coping mechanisms were maladaptive
- Encourage the person to recall and analyze similar instances of anxiety

C. **Reduce or eliminate problematic coping mechanisms**

1. Depression, withdrawal (see *Ineffective Individual Coping*)
2. Violent behavior (see *Potential for Violence*)
3. Denial*
   - Develop an atmosphere of empathic understanding
   - Assist in lowering level of anxiety
   - Focus on present situation
   - Give feedback about current reality; identify positive achievements
   - Have person describe events in detail; focus on getting specifics of who, what, when, and where
4. Numerous physical complaints with no known organic base
   - Encourage expression of feelings
   - Give positive feedback when the person is symptom-free
   - Acknowledge that the symptoms must be burdensome
   - Encourage interest in external environment (*e.g.*, outside activity, volunteering, helping others)
   - Listen to the complaints
   - Evaluate the secondary gains the person receives and attempt to interrupt cycle; see the person on a regular basis, not simply in response to somatic complaints
   - Discuss with the person how others are reacting to him; attempt to have him identify his behavior when others react negatively (withdrawal? anger?)

---

* Denial serves a protective function and is not always maladaptive.

- Avoid "doing something" to each complaint; set limits when appropriate (*e.g.*, may refuse to call MD in response to a request for headache medication)
- When setting limits, provide an alternative outlet (*e.g.*, redirect to use relaxation technique) (see Appendix X, Stress Management Techniques)

5. Anger† (*e.g.*, demanding behavior, manipulation)

a. With adults
- Identify the presence of anger (*e.g.*, feelings of frustration, anxiety, helplessness, presence of irritability, verbal outbursts)
- Recognize your reactions to an individual's behavior; be aware of your own feelings in working with angry individuals
- If person can verbalize feelings, assist in identifying sources of frustration and anger
- Assist in making connections between feelings of frustration and subsequent behavior
- Have person analyze consequences of behavior
- Convey a sense of understanding of those things over which he has little control
- Set limits on manipulative or irrational demands
- State limits clearly; tell person exactly what is expected (*e.g.*, "I cannot allow you to scream [throw objects, etc.]")
- When stating an unacceptable behavior, give an alternative (*e.g.*, suggest a quiet room, physical exertion, a chance for one-to-one communication)
- State the consequences if limits are violated
- Develop behavior modification strategies; discuss with all personnel involved for consistency
- When discussing a limit with the person, avoid stating it in such a way that it is perceived as a challenge
- Give a brief explanation for the limit; if behavior continues, enforce the limit; encourage the person to express his feelings about the limit
- Structure experiences that the person can do successfully
- Provide positive feedback
- Interact with the person when he is not demanding or manipulative
- Discuss your feelings and the person's behavior with entire team; support each other and provide a consistent approach

b. With children
- Encourage the child to share his anger (*e.g.*, "How did you feel when you had your injection?" "How did you feel when Mary would not play with you?")
- Tell the child that being angry is okay (*e.g.*, "I sometimes get angry when I can't have what I want")
- Encourage and allow the child to express his anger in acceptable ways (*e.g.*, loud talking, hitting a play object, or running outside around the house)

D. Initiate health teaching and referrals as indicated

1. For patients identified as having chronic anxiety and maladaptive coping mechanisms, refer for ongoing psychiatric treatment.
2. Instruct patient in nontechnical, understandable terms regarding his illness and associated treatments. Repeat explanations, since anxiety may interfere with learning.

---

† Anger is a response to frustration and anxiety. Not all anger is problematic. It can be used for problem-solving.

3. Instruct patient in maintenance of physical well-being (*i.e.*, nutrition, exercise, elimination).
4. Instruct (or refer) person for assertiveness training.
5. Instruct person in use of relaxation techniques (see Appendix X)
6. Instruct person in constructive problem-solving (see Appendix VII)
7. Assist parents to respond constructively to age-related developmental needs (see Appendix IX)
8. Provide telephone numbers for emergency intervention
   - Hotlines
   - Psychiatric emergency room
   - On-call staff if available

Anxiety
Related to Lack of Knowledge of Preoperative Routines
Related to Lack of Knowledge of Postoperative Exercises/Activities
Related to Lack of Knowledge of Postoperative Alterations/Sensations

Assessment

Subjective Data
The person states that he
   Is anxious and fearful of unfamiliar situations
   Needs instruction

Objective Data
The person
   Exhibits anxious behavior, such as

Increased verbalization	Restlessness
Inability to concentrate and retain information	Sweating palms
	Tremulousness

   Behaves in a way that indicates a knowledge deficit, regarding
      Preparation for diagnostic study, examination, surgical procedure
      The need for diagnostic study, examination, surgical procedure, or treatment and follow-up medical supervision
      What is involved with the diagnostic study, examination, surgery, or treatment prescribed

---

Outcome Criteria

The individual will
- Verbalize, if asked what to expect (routines, environment)
- Demonstrate postoperative exercises, splinting, and respiratory regimen
- Relate less anxiety after teaching

Interventions

1. Before hospitalization, the person's physician should explain
   Nature of surgery needed
   Reason for and anticipated outcomes of surgery
   Risks involved
   Type of anesthesia
   Expectations regarding length of recovery and limitations imposed during the recovery period
2. Determine level of understanding of surgical procedure.
   Reinforce physician's explanation of surgical procedure. Notify physician if additional explanations are indicated.
3. Assess
   a. Past experiences related to surgery and positive or negative effect on client
   b. Nature of concerns, fears
   c. Factors affecting learning (refer to Etiological, Contributing, Risk Factors and Focus Assessment Criteria)
4. Document and communicate these data to others involved with care to meet the client's needs and ensure continuity of care.
5. Utilize efficient and effective teaching methods
   a. Give bedside instruction concerning specific type of surgery and sensations and appearances (presence of machines, tubes, etc.) that client and family may encounter postoperatively
   b. Provide instruction (bedside or group) on general information pertaining to the need for active participation, routines, environment, personnel, postoperative exercises
      - Give general information, pertaining to most people having surgery, in a group session for patients and families
      - Present information or reinforce learning with the use of written materials (booklets, posters for room on exercises, instruction sheets) or audiovisual aids (slides of surgical areas, personnel, films, videotapes)
      - Demonstrate and conduct practice session for postoperative exercises
      - Explain the rationale for routines, focusing on positive aspects. For example, "An enema may be ordered preoperatively, which will decrease your need to use the bedpan for a few days postoperatively"
      - Encourage participation by making person feel (without frightening him) that he will be susceptible to complications if he does not participate
      - Give feedback on progress, rewarding person frequently
6. Explain all procedures, the reasons for them, and their importance:
   a. Preoperative
      Enema   Preparation
      NPO   Laboratory work

  b. Postoperative
    Parenteral fluids
    Vital signs
    Dressings
    Nasogastric and other tubes
    Indwelling bladder catheter
    Pain and availability of medications
  c. Teach person, using return demonstration:
    To turn, cough, and breathe deep, depending on surgical procedure
    To support incision during coughing
    To deep breathe hourly postoperatively
    To exercise actively and how passive ROM exercises will be done
    To sit up, get up, and ambulate—sitting in a chair should be avoided
    Importance of progressive care
    Early ambulation
    Self-care, as soon as patient is able
7. For Children (Smallwood)
  a. Organize tours for children about 5–7 days before the surgery
  b. Group children with similar problems together
  c. Encourage the participation of parents and siblings to provide added security for the child
  d. Involve as many senses as possible. Explain how it feels and smells and whether or not it will hurt.
  e. Using a doll, demonstrate the OR garments, blood sample acquisition
  f. Using a volunteer child, demonstrate the taking of blood pressure, temperature, heart and respiration rate.
  g. Take children on OR cart to show them where their parents will be waiting while they're in surgery.
  h. Have an OR nurse (fully dressed) explain:
    • The reasons for OR attire
    • Anesthesia machine
    • Anesthesia as "hospital air" or "hospital sleep" to avoid confusion
    • Postanesthesia recovery room
    Explain/Demonstrate on doll or child:
    • Straps on OR table
    • Monitoring devices (EKG, pulse)
    • Anesthesia mask (on each child, or on parent if child is frightened)
    • Intravenous lines (inserted after induction; removed after child is eating and drinking)
  i. Increase the effectiveness of the teaching program and promote security
    • Use name tags so children can be addressed by name.
    • Involve children in discussion, *e.g.*, ask them the colors of objects; ask them to point to their nose.
    • Do not force any child to do anything.
    • If a child resists, have parent perform the activity and encourage child to help. Allow child to handle equipment.
    • Avoid calling anesthesia gas. It may be confused with gas in a car or gas used in euthanasia of animals.
    • Explain that anesthesia does not affect memories.
    • Allow children to take home masks, hats, and EKG buttons.
    • Encourage child to bring a favorite toy when returning for surgery.

j. If tours are not feasible or child cannot attend, consider using or developing a book for parents to use at home with child which they can receive from their surgeon's office, *e.g.*, *Your Operation Day*, by Margary Doroshow and Deborah London (1984).

8. Discuss purpose of recovery room with patient and family
     Visiting policies
     Type of care
     Length of stay, if applicable
     Possibility of placement in intensive care unit (ICU) if needed or indicated

9. Explain other hospital policies as indicated
     Visiting hours
     Number of visitors
     Location of waiting rooms
     How physician will contact them after operation

10. Evaluate
     a. Person's/family's ability to meet preset, mutually planned learning goals (behaviors)
     b. Need for further teaching and support

References/Bibliography

Refer also to Patient Teaching Bibliography in *Health Maintenance*

Brink R: How serious is the child's behavioral problem? Matern Child Nurs J 7:33–36, 1982

Bulechek G, McCloskey J: Nursing Interventions:Treatment for Nursing Diagnosis. Philadelphia, WB Saunders, 1985

Carlson C, Blackwell B: Behavioral Concepts and Nursing Interventions, pp 128–131. Philadelphia, JB Lippincott, 1978

Cohn L: Coping with anxiety: A step-by-step guide. *Nursing* 9(12):34–37, 1979

Decker N: Anxiety in the general hospital. In Fann W, Karacau I, Parkorny A et al (eds): Phenomenology and Treatment of Anxiety, pp 287–298. Jamaica, NY, Spectrum Publications, 1979

Doroshow M, London D: Surgery and Children, AORN J 47(3):696–700, 1988

Felton G: Preoperative teaching. In Bulechek G, McCloskey J (eds): Nursing Interventions: Treatments for Nursing Diagnoses. Philadelphia, WB Saunders, 1985

Holderly R, McNulty E: Feelings, feelings: How to make a rational response to emotional behavior, Nursing 10(3):39–43, 1979

Knowles R: Dealing with feelings: Managing anxiety. Am J Nurs 81:110–111, 1981

Knowles R: Handling anger: Responding vs. reacting, Am J Nurs 81:2196–2197, 1981

Lyon G: Limit setting as a therapeutic tool. In Backer B, Dubbert P, Eisenman E: Psychiatric/Mental Health Nursing: Contemporary Readings, pp 99–111. New York, Van Nostrand Reinhold, 1978

Melichar M: Using crisis theory to help parents cope with a child's temper tantrums. Matern Child Nurs J 5:181–185, 1980

Nissley B, Townes N: Guidelines for intervention in aggressive behavior. In Backer B, Dubbert P, Eisenman E: Psychiatric/Mental Health Nursing: Contemporary Readings, pp 174–180. New York, Van Nostrand Reinhold, 1978

Silver L: Recognition and treatment of anxiety in children and adolescents. In Fann W, Karacau I, Parkorny A et al (eds): Phenomenology and Treatment of Anxiety, pp 93–109. Jamaica, NY, Spectrum, 1979

Smallwood S: Preparing Children for Surgery. AORN J 47(1):177–182, 1988

Spielberger C, Sarason I (eds): Stress and Anxiety, vol I. Washington, DC, Hemisphere, 1975

Stewart A: Handling the aggressive patient. Perspect Psychiatr Care 16:5–6, 228–232, 1978

Stewart G, Sundeen S: Principles and Practice of Psychiatric Nursing, 2nd ed. St Louis, CV Mosby, 1983

Thomas M, Baker J, Estes N: Anger: A tool for self-awareness. Am J Nurs 70:2586–2590, 1970

Weisinger H: Dr. Weisinger's Anger Work-out Book. New York, Quill, 1985

Books and Articles

Becker H (ed): The Health Belief Model and Personal Health Behavior. Thorofare, NJ, Charles B Slack, 1974

Edel MK: Noncompliance: An appropriate nursing diagnosis? Nurs Outlook 33(4):183–185, 1985

Haynes R, Taylor D, Sackett D: Compliance in Health Care. Baltimore, Johns Hopkins Press, 1979

Kinnaird LS, Yoham MA, Kieval YM: Patient compliance in rehabilitative programs. Nurs Clin North Am 17(3):523–532, 1982

Komaroff L: The practitioner and the compliant patient. Am J Public Health 66(9):833–835, 1976

Marston MV: Compliance with medical regimes: A review of the literature. Nursing Res 19(4):312–323, 1970

Ryan P, Falco SM: A pilot study to validate the etiologies and defining characteristics of the nursing diagnosis of noncompliance. Nurs Clin North Am 20(4):685–695, 1985

Steckel SB: Predicting, measuring, implementing and following-up on patient compliance. Nurs Clin North Am 17(3):491–497, 1982

Scherwitz L, Leventhal H: Strategies for increasing patient compliance. Health Values 2(6)301–306, 1978

Thomson PS, Willis JC: Compliance changes in a black lung clinic. Nurs Clin North Am 17(3):513–521, 1982

Resources for the Consumer

Literature

Food–drug interactions: Can what you eat affect your medication? Elizabeth, NJ, Wakefern Food Corporation

Body Temperature, Potential Altered

Related to **(Specify)**

Hyperthermia

Related to **(Specify): Potential**

Hypothermia

Related to **(Specify): Potential**

Thermoregulation, Ineffective

Related to **Newborn Transition to Extrauterine Environment**

Definitions

Potential Altered Body Temperature: The state in which the individual is at risk of failing to maintain body temperature within normal range because of internal factors.

Hyperthermia: The state in which an individual has or is at risk of having a sustained elevation of body temperature of greater than 37.8° C (100° F) orally or 38.8° C (101° F) rectally because of external factors.

Hypothermia: The state in which the individual has or is at risk of having sustained reduction of body temperature to below 35° C (95° F) orally or 35.5° C (96° F) rectally because of external factors.

Ineffective Thermoregulation: The state in which an individual experiences or is at risk of experiencing an inability to effectively maintain normal body temperature in the presence of adverse or changing external factors.

Author's Note: These diagnostic categories represent two different thermal problems. *Potential Altered Body Temperature* describes an individual at risk for an abnormal body temperature because of disease and treatments, *e.g.,* infection, surgery. The nursing interventions would focus on comfort measures and maintaining hydration. *Hypothermia* and *Hyperthermia* are abnormal temperature states that are treatable by nursing interventions such as correcting the external causes, *e.g.,* inappropriate clothing, exposure to elements (heat, cold), dehydration. The nursing focus for *hypothermia* and *hyperthermia* is prevention or treatment of mild hypothermia and hyperthermia. I recommend that these diagnoses be termed *Potential Hyperthermia* and *Potential Hypothermia* to more appropriately describe the nursing role. *Severe Hypothermia* and *Hyperthermia* are life-threatening situations that require medical and nursing interventions for treatment. Such situations are collaborative problems and should be labeled *Potential Complication: Hypothermia or Hyperthermia.*

Body Temperature, Potential Altered

Related to **(Specify)**

Definition

Potential Altered Body Temperature: The state in which the individual is at risk of failing to maintain body temperature within normal range because of internal factors.

Defining Characteristics

Major (must be present)
     Presence of risk factors (See etiological, contributing, risk factors)

Etiological, Contributing, Risk Factors

Pathophysiological

Illness or trauma affecting temperature regulation:
     Coma/increased intracranial pressure
     Brain tumor/hypothalamic tumor/head trauma
     Cerebrovascular accident (CVA)
     Infection
     Integument (skin) injury
     Anemia
     Neurovascular disease/peripheral vascular disease
     Pheochromocytoma (tumor of the adrenal medulla)
     Altered metabolic rate

Treatment–related

     Medications (*e.g.*, vasodilators/vasoconstrictors)
     Sedation
     Parenteral fluid infusion/blood transfusion
     Dialysis
     Surgery

Maturational

     Extremes of age (*e.g.*, newborn, elderly)

Focus Assessment Criteria

Subjective Data

  1. Assess history of symptoms
          Onset?
          Associated symptoms.
               Pain (Specify: head/abdomen/dysuria/other)
               Nausea/vomiting/thirst
               Cough (productive/dry)

Sweats (night/day)
Rash (have client describe course)
Symptoms relieved by what?
2. Assess for presence of contributing or causative factors
Recent exposure to communicable disease without known immunity (*e.g.*, measles without vaccine or previous illness)
Recent overexposure to sun heat
Recent overactivity
Radiation/chemotherapy/immunosuppression
Medications
What? How often? When was last dose taken?
Effect on symptoms?
Home environment:
Adequate heating?
Adequate clothing (*e.g.*, socks, hat, gloves)?
Poverty?
Recent exposure to cold/dampness
Inactivity
3. Under medical treatment?
Medications:
Vasodilators/vasoconstrictors?
How often taken? Last dose taken when?
Effect on circulatory system?
4. Note if clothing is appropriate for environment
5. Assess past medical history
History of repeated infections
Pulmonary disease
Previous urinary tract infection
Inability to sweat

Objective Data

1. Vital signs
Elevated temperature?
Tachycardia?
Tachypnea?
Abnormal blood pressure?
2. Assess mental status
Alert/drowsy/confused/oriented/comatose
3. Assess skin and circulation
Intact?
Burned (specify degree and site)?
Injured (specify)?
Rash (specify type and site)?
Bites (specify site)?
Turgor: normal/dehydrated
Temperature/feel: hot/warm/cold/damp
Appearance: flushed/pale
Quality of peripheral pulses (radial, pedal)
4. Assess for possible signs of infection
Pain/redness/swelling (specify site)
Cloudy urine

Abnormal discharge or drainage

Foul odor (specify site)

5. Assess for signs of dehydration

Parched mouth/furrowed tongue/dry lips

Determine fluid intake and output

6. Analyze pertinent laboratory studies

White blood count: WNL/elevated/decreased (specify)

Hemoglobin and hematocrit: WNL/elevated/decreased (specify)

Serum electrolytes: WNL/abnormal (specify)

Principles and Rationale for Nursing Care

General

1. The nursing focus for this diagnosis is that of reducing the harmful effects of the altered body temperature (*e.g.*, maintaining hydration, nutrition, comfort).
2. Sustained altered body temperature must be referred to a physician so that collaborative treatment may be implemented (*e.g.*, medications).
3. All of the principles listed under hyperthermia and hypothermia can also apply to *Potential Altered Body Temperature.*
4. Rectal temperature reading is 1° higher than oral temperature reading.

Axillar temperature reading is 1° lower than oral temperature reading.

Hyperthermia

1. Adding clothes or blankets to a person inhibits the body's natural ability to reduce body temperature.
2. Perspiring is a sign of the human effort to reduce body temperature.
3. Increased metabolic rate increases body temperature, and vice versa (increase in body temperature causes an increased metabolic rate).
4. Shivering causes an increase in metabolic rate and body temperature.
5. Increased calories and fluids are required to maintain metabolic functions when fever is present.
6. Fever is a major sign of onset of infection, inflammation, and disease: treatment with aspirin or acetaminophen without medical consultation may mask important symptoms that should be noted.
7. Fever associated with immunosuppression, stiff neck, rashes, infection, mental confusion, prolonged vomiting, respiratory difficulty, or abdominal tenderness should be referred to the physician.
8. High fevers (102° F or above) in children predispose them to seizures or convulsions.
9. People with fevers often are subject to irritability, generalized aches, pains, and discomfort.
10. Blood is the cooling fluid of the body: low blood volume due to dehydration predisposes one to fever.
11. Seventy percent (70%) of all heatstroke victims are over 60 years of age. (Bafitis)

Hypothermia

1. Hypothermia reduces blood pressure and contributes to shock.
2. Vasodilatation promotes heat loss and predisposes one to hypothermia.
3. The elderly and the very young require more heat to maintain normal body temperature (room temperature should be 70°–74° F).
4. During the immediate postoperative period, patients are prone to hypothermia related to prolonged exposure to cold in the operating room and the infusion of large quantities of cool intravenous fluids.

5. People with known peripheral vascular disease should minimize exposure to cold because hypothermia causes the body to try to conserve heat by means of vaso-constriction (which creates an even greater vascular compromise).
6. The greatest amount of heat loss occurs by way of the head, feet, and hands.
7. Severe hypothermia can cause life-threatening cardiac arrhythmias and must be referred to a physician.
8. There is an increase in mortality in children (especially 0–4 years old) during the winter months. (Morris)
9. The elderly are compromised in their ability to produce heat because of decreased muscle bulk and a lower basal metabolic rate.
10. Immobility (*e.g.*, surgery) reduces muscle activity, thus producing less heat.

Body Temperature, Potential Altered
Related to (Specify)

Assessment

Subjective
The person reports a history of fevers

Objective
Presence of risk factors (see etiological, contributing, risk factors)

Outcome Criteria

The individual will
- Identify methods to prevent changes in temperature
- Maintain normal body temperature

Interventions
1. Maintain fluid balance by increasing fluid intake.
   - Remember to account for the increased fluid loss of perspiration.
   - See *Fluid Volume Deficit.*
2. Increase caloric intake.
   - Explain the need to increase caloric intake because of increased metabolic rate.
   - Have the patient maintain a written record of food intake/caloric intake.
   - Provide favorite high-calorie snacks
3. Provide for periods of uninterrupted rest.
   - Rest before and after activity (*e.g.*, meals)
4. Maintain good skin care and comfort.
   - Provide frequent sponge baths/cleansing baths.
   - Use alcohol rubs to refresh and cleanse.

- Provide frequent change of bedclothes (absorbent cotton is better than silk or nylon) and linens to minimize dampness.
- Use powder unless allergic.
- Provide for safety.
- Monitor mental status closely for confusion.
- Keep siderails up.
- Assist the person when ambulating.

5. Consult with physician
- To determine frequency of assessment of vital signs (monitor temperature, pulse, respirations, blood pressure).
- Regarding use of medication (*e.g.*, aspirin) or necessity for cultures, should early symptoms of hyperthermia become evident (*e.g.*, shaking, chills).

Hyperthermia

Related to **(Specify): Potential**

Definition

Hyperthermia: The state in which an individual has or is at risk of having a sustained elevation of body temperature of greater than 37.8° C (100° F) orally or 38.8° C (101° F) rectally due to external factors.

> **Author's Note:** These diagnostic categories represent two different thermal problems. *Potential Altered Body Temperature* describes an individual at risk for an abnormal body temperature because of disease and treatments, *e.g.*, infection, surgery. The nursing interventions would focus on comfort measures and maintaining hydration. *Hypothermia* and *Hyperthermia* are abnormal temperature states that are treatable by nursing interventions such as correcting the external causes, *e.g.*, inappropriate clothing, exposure to elements (heat, cold), dehydration. The nursing focus for *hypothermia* and *hyperthermia* is prevention or treatment of mild hypothermia and hyperthermia. I recommend that these diagnoses be termed *Potential Hyperthermia* and *Potential Hypothermia* to more appropriately describe the nursing role. *Severe Hypothermia* and *Hyperthermia* are life-threatening situations that require medical and nursing interventions for treatment. Such situations are collaborative problems and should be labeled *Potential Complication: Hypothermia or Hyperthermia.*

Defining Characteristics

Major (must be present)

Temperature greater than 37.8° C (100° F) orally or 38.8° C (101° F) rectally

Minor (may be present)

    Flushed skin
    Warm to touch
    Increased respiratory rate
    Tachycardia
    Shivering/goose pimples
    Dehydration
    Specific or generalized aches and pains (*e.g.*, headache)
    Malaise/fatigue/weakness
    Loss of appetite

Etiological, Contributing, Risk Factors

Situational (personal, environmental)

    Exposure to heat, sun
    Inappropriate clothing for climate

Poverty
Extremes of weight
Dehydration
Vigorous activity

Maturational
Extremes of age (*e.g.*, newborn, elderly)

Focus Assessment
See *Potential Altered Body Temperature.*

Principles and Rationale for Nursing Care
See *Potential Altered Body Temperature*

Potential Hyperthermia
Related to (Specify)

Assessment

Subjective Data
The person reports history of heat stroke

Objective Data
Presence of risk factors (see etiological, contributing, risk factors—*Potential Altered Body Temperature)*

Outcome Criteria

The person will
* Identify risk factors for hyperthermia
* Relate methods of preventing hyperthermia
* Maintain normal body temperature

Interventions

A. Assess for the presence of contributing risk factors

1. Dehydration
2. Environmental warmth/exercise

B. Remove or reduce contributing risk factors

1. For dehydration:
   * Monitor intake and output and provide favorite fluids to maintain a balance between intake and output.
   * Teach the person the importance of maintaining an adequate fluid intake (at

least 2000 ml a day unless contraindicated by heart or kidney disease) to prevent dehydration.
- See also, *Fluid Volume Deficit*

2. For environmental warmth/exercise:
- Assess whether clothing or bedcovers are too warm for the environment or planned activity.
- Remove excess clothing and/or blankets (remove hat, gloves, or socks, as appropriate) to promote heat loss.
- Provide air conditioning or fan, if appropriate.
- Teach the importance of increasing fluid intake during warm weather and exercise.

C. Initiate health teaching as indicated

- Explain the relationship of age as a risk for hyperthermia.
- Teach the early signs of hyperthermia or heat stroke:

Flushed skin	Headache
Fatigue	Loss of appetite

Hypothermia

Related to **(Specify): Potential**

Definition

Hypothermia: The state in which an individual has or is at risk of having a sustained reduction of body temperature of below 35° C (95° F) orally or 35.5° C (96° F) rectally because of external factors.

Defining Characteristics*

Major (80%–100%)

Reduction in body temperature below 35° C (95° F) orally or 35.5° C (96° F) rectally.
  Cool skin
  Pallor (moderate)
  Shivering (mild)

Minor (50%–79%)

  Mental confusion/drowsiness/restlessness
  Decreased pulse and respiration
  Cachexia/malnutrition

Etiological, Contributing, and Risk Factors

Situational (personal, environmental)

  Exposure to cold, rain, snow, wind
  Inappropriate clothing for climate
  Poverty (inability to pay for shelter or heat)
  Extremes of weight
  Consumption of alcohol
  Dehydration/malnutrition
  Operating suite

Maturational

Extremes of age (*e.g.*, newborn, elderly)

Focus Assessment

See *Potential Altered Body Temperature*

Principles and Rationale for Nursing Care

See *Potential Altered Body Temperature*

---

* Adapted from Carroll SM: Nursing diagnosis: Hypothermia. In Carroll-Johnson RM (ed): Classification of Nursing Diagnoses: Proceedings of the North American Nursing Diagnosis Association Eighth Conference, pp 425–428. Philadelphia, JB Lippincott, 1989

Potential Hypothermia
Related to (Specify)

Assessment

Subjective Data

The person reports:
"I get cold easily/I'm always cold."
"I can't afford to pay the heat."
"I don't have the right clothes to go out."
"I have poor circulation."
"My feet are always cold."

Objective Data

Presence of risk factors (see etiological, contributing, risk factors—*Potential Altered Body Temperature*)

Outcome Criteria

The person will
• Identify risk factors for hypothermia
• Relate methods of maintaining warmth/preventing heat loss
• Maintain body temperature within normal limits

Interventions

A. Assess for the presence of risk factors
1. Prolonged exposure to cold environment (either at home or outside)
2. Poverty/inability to pay for adequate heat/shelter
3. Extremes of age (*e.g.*, newborn, elderly)
4. Neurovascular/peripheral vascular disease
5. Malnutrition/cachexia
6. Perioperative experience

B. Reduce or eliminate causative or contributing factors if possible
1. For prolonged exposure to cold environment:
   • Assess room temperatures at home.
   • Teach the person to keep room temperatures at 70°–72° F or to layer clothing with sweaters.
   • Explain the importance of wearing a hat, gloves, and warm socks and shoes to prevent heat loss.
   • Encourage the person to limit going outside when temperatures are very cold.
   • Acquire an electric blanket, warm blankets, or down comforter for bed.

2. For poverty/inability to pay for heat:
   - Consult with social service to identify sources of financial assistance/warm clothing/blankets.
   - Teach the person the importance of preventing heat loss before body temperature is actually lowered.
   - Acquire warm socks, sweaters, gloves, and hats.
3. For extremes of age (newborn, elderly):
   - Maintain room temperature at 70°–74° F.
   - Have the client wear hat, gloves, and socks if necessary to prevent heat loss.
   - Explain to family members that newborns, infants, and the elderly are more susceptible to heat loss (see also *Ineffective Thermoregulation*).
4. For neurovascular/peripheral vascular disease:
   - Keep room temperature between 70°–74° F.
   - Assess for adequate circulation to extremities (*i.e.,* satisfactory peripheral pulses).
   - Have the person wear warm gloves and socks to reduce heat loss.
   - Teach the person to take a warm bath if he is feeling unable to get warm.
5. For children and elderly during intraoperative experience: (Burkle)
   - Increase ambient temperature of OR room prior to case.
   - Use a portable radiant heating lamp to provide additional heat during surgery.
   - Cover person with warm blankets when arriving in OR.
   - When possible, use a warming mattress.
   - During prepping and surgery, keep as much of body surface covered as possible.
   - Warm prep set, blood, fluids, anesthesia, irrigants.
   - Keep head covered well.
   - Continue heat-conserving interventions postoperatively.
6. Initiate health teaching if indicated.
   - Explain the relationship of age as a risk for hypothermia.
   - Teach the early signs of hypothermia:
     Cool skin
     Pallor, blanching, redness

Bibliography

Articles

Bafitis H, Sargent F: Human physiological adaptability through the life sequence. Gerontology 32(4):402–410, 1977

Barnes A, Bell J: Preventing shivering during hypothermia treatment. Nursing 14(9):56–57, 1984

Bindler RN, Howry RN: Nursing care of children with febrile seizures. Am J Nurs 78:270–273, 1978

Boyd Shurett PH, Coburn C: Heat and heat related illness. Am J Nurs 81:1298–1301, 1981

Burkle N: Inadvertent hypothermia. J Gerontol Nurs 14(6):26–29, 1988

Castle M, Watkins J: Fever: Understanding the sinister sign. Nursing 9(2):26–33,1979

Epstein Y et al: Fluid balance in hot climate: Sweating, water intake and prevention of dehydration. Pub Health Rev 13(1/2):115–137

Hayes K: Dealing with heat injuries. RN 47(7):41–44, 1984

Jones S: The use and misuse of hypothermia blankets. RN 47(3):55, 1984

Lavoy K: Dealing with hypothermia and frost bite. RN 47(1):53–56, 1985

Lepsky J: Saving the elderly from the killing cold. Nursing 14(2):42–43, 1984

Morris M: Tiredness and fatigue. In Norris C (ed): Concept Clarification in Nursing, pp 263–275. Rockville, MD, Aspen Systems Corp, 1982

Smith D: Don't let hypothermia fool you into making a fatal mistake. RN 4(6):48, 1983

Books

Bulechek G, McCloskey J: Nursing Interventions. Philadelphia, WB Saunders, 1985
Carnevali D, Patrick M: Nursing Management for the Elderly. Philadelphia, JB Lippincott, 1985
Carpenito L: Handbook of Nursing Diagnosis. Philadelphia, JB Lippincott, 1985
Jacobs M, Geels W: Signs and Symptoms in Nursing. Philadelphia, JB Lippincott, 1985
Patrick M, Woods et al: Medical Surgical Nursing. Philadelphia, JB Lippincott, 1985
Porth C: Pathophysiology. Philadelphia, JB Lippincott, 1985
Potter P, Perry A: Fundamentals of Nursing. St Louis, CV Mosby, 1985

Thermoregulation, Ineffective

Related to **Newborn Transition to Extrauterine Environment**

Definition

Ineffective Thermoregulation: The state in which an individual experiences or is at risk of experiencing an inability to effectively maintain normal body temperature in the presence of adverse or changing external factors.

> **Author's Note:** This diagnostic category is indicated when the nurse can maintain or assist an individual to maintain a body temperature within normal limits by manipulating external factors (*e.g.*, clothing) and environmental conditions. Individuals who are at high risk for this diagnosis are elderly persons and neonates. For individuals with temperature fluctuations due to disease, infections, or trauma, see *Potential Altered Body Temperature*.

Defining Characteristics

Major (must be present)

Temperature fluctuations related to limited metabolic compensatory regulation in response to environmental factors

Etiological, Contributing, Risk Factors

Situational (personal, environmental)

Fluctuating environmental temperatures
Cold or wet articles (clothes, cribs, equipment)
Inadequate heating system
Inadequate housing
Wet body surface
Inadequate clothing for weather (excessive, insufficient)

Maturational

Neonate
Large surface area relative to body mass
Limited ability to produce heat (metabolic)
Limited shivering ability
Increased basal metabolism
Premature
(Same as neonate but more severe)
Elderly
Decreased basal metabolism
Loss of adipose tissue (limbs)

Focus Assessment Criteria

Subjective

1. Tone/activity (neonate)
   Active
   Quiet
   Irritable
2. Cry (neonate)
   Vigorous
   High-pitched
   Weak
3. History of hypothermia or hyperthermia

Objective

1. Skin
   Color
   Nailbeds
   Integrity (cord, lacerations)
   Rashes
2. Temperature
   a. Environment (home, infant [ambient, radiant, Isolette])
   b. Body (adult, child [rectal, oral], newborn [axillary])
3. Vital signs
   a. Respiratory (rate, rhythm, presence of retractions, breath sounds)
   b. Heart rate

Principles and Rationale for Nursing Care

See *Potential Altered Body Temperature* for principles on hypothermia and hyperthermia.

General (adult)

1. Thermoregulation involves the balancing of heat production and heat loss.
2. Heat production is caused by increasing the metabolic rate by:
   a. Hypothalamic activity, which stimulates
      • Increased muscular activity (*e.g.*, shivering)
      • The release of thyroxine
      • Norepinephrine and sympathetic chemical thermogenesis
   b. Cellular response to produce heat
3. Heat loss is controlled by:
   • Insulator system (skin, subcutaneous tissues [fat])
   • Cellular response to conserve heat (vasoconstriction)
4. The elderly have compromised ability to respond to changes in environmental temperature because of:
   • Decrease in insulating subcutaneous tissues
   • Decrease in circulating thyroxine
   • Slowed thermogenesis

Neonates

1. The neonate is vulnerable to heat loss because of:
   • Large body surface area relative to body mass
   • Increased basal metabolism rate

- Less adipose tissue for insulation
- Environmental conditions (delivery room, nursery)

2. The neonate with hypoxia or under the influence of drugs (*e.g.*, given to the mother during labor) will have difficulty increasing heat production (Ouimette).
3. The neonate has limited ability to adapt to environmental temperature changes because of:
   - Limited ability to produce heat (brown fat synthesis)
   - Limited shivering ability
4. The newborn loses heat through (Neeson):
   - Evaporation (loss of heat when water on skin changes to vapor)
   - Convection (loss of heat when cool air flows over skin)
   - Conduction (transfer of heat when skin surface is in direct contact with a cool surface)
   - Radiation (transfer of heat from infant to cooler surfaces without direct contact)
5. Nonshivering thermogenesis is a heat-production mechanism located in brown fat (highly vascular adipose tissue), which is found only in infants. When skin temperature begins to drop, thermal receptors transmit impulses to the central nervous system (Neeson). The following sequence illustrates this mechanism:

   Central nervous system → Stimulates sympathetic nervous system → Release of norepinephrine from adrenal gland and at nerve endings in brown fat → Heat production
6. Calorie requirements are high for newborns (approximately 117 calories per kilogram of body weight per day).
7. An increased metabolic rate for heat production results in increased demands for oxygen and glucose. With prolonged cold stress or in compromised neonates, acidosis can result (Klaus).
8. Premature or low-birth-weight infants are more susceptible to heat loss because of the reduced metabolic reserves available (*e.g.*, glycogen).
9. Cooling reduces the amount of glucose as well as oxygenation and circulation, which inhibits the production of surfactant.
10. The newborn can also experience overheating from excessive clothing in hot weather. The full-term infant can sweat in response to overheating, but the premature infant cannot.

Ineffective Thermoregulation
Related to Newborn Transition to Extrauterine Environment

Assessment

Objective

Episodes of Temperature >37° C., or
Episodes of Temperature <36.4° C.

Outcome Criteria

The infant will
- Have a temperature between 36.4° and 37° C.

The parent will
- Explain techniques to avoid heat loss at home

Interventions

A. Assess for contributing factors

Environmental sources of heat loss
Lack of knowledge (caregivers, parents)

B. Reduce or eliminate the sources of heat loss

1. Evaporation
   - In the delivery room, quickly dry skin and hair with a heated towel and place infant in a heated environment.
   - When bathing, provide a warm environment.
   - Wash and dry baby in sections to reduce evaporation.
   - Limit time in contact with wet diapers or blankets.
2. Convection
   - Reduce drafts in delivery room.
   - Avoid drafts on infant (air conditioning, fans, windows, open portholes on Isolette).
3. Conduction
   - Warm all articles for care (stethoscopes, scales, hands of caregivers, clothes, bed linens, cribs).
   - Place infant very close to mother to conserve heat (and foster bonding).
4. Radiation
   - Place infant next to mother in the delivery room.
   - Reduce objects in the room that absorb heat (metal).
   - Place crib or Isolette as far away from walls (outside) or windows as possible.

C. Monitor temperature of newborn (Waechter)

1. Assess axillary temperature initially q ½ hour until stable, then q 4–8 hr.
2. If temperature <36.3° C:
   - Wrap infant in two blankets.
   - Put stockinette cap on.
   - Assess for environmental sources of heat loss.
   - If hypothermia persists over one hour, notify physician.
   - Assess for complications of cold stress: hypoxia, respiratory acidosis, hypoglycemia, fluid and electrolyte imbalances, weight loss.
3. If temperature is >37° C:
   - Loosen blanket.
   - Remove cap, if on.
   - Assess environment for thermal gain.
   - If hyperthermia persists over one hour, notify physician.
4. Assess for signs and symptoms of sepsis every shift:
   - Respiratory function (rate, rhythm, pattern)

- Skin (tone, color, perfusion)
- Poor feeding
- Irritability
- Signs of localized infections (skin, umbilicus, circumcision, eyes, birth lacerations)

D. Initiate health teaching

- Teach caregiver why infant is vulnerable to temperature fluctuations (cold and heat).
- Explain sources of environmental heat loss (see section B).
- Demonstrate how to conserve heat during bathing.
- Instruct that it is not necessary to routinely check temperature at home.
- Teach to check temperature if infant is hot, sick, or irritable as follows:
    Shake down the thermometer
    Place under axilla
    Hold in place for 3 minutes
    Read at eye level
    Report temperature >37.5°C to health care professional

References/Bibliography

Fanaroff A, Martin R (eds): Behrman's Neonatal–Perinatal Medicine. St Louis, CV Mosby, 1983

Klaus M, Fananroff A, Martin R (eds): Care of the High-Risk Neonate. Philadelphia, WB Saunders, 1979

Neeson J, May K: Comprehensive Maternity Nursing, pp 993–995. Philadelphia, JB Lippincott, 1986

Ouimette J: Perinatal Nursing. Boston, Jones and Bartlett, 1985

Ruchala P: The effects of wearing headcoverings on axillary temperature of infants. MCN 10(4):240, 1985

Waechter E, Phillips J, Holaday B: Nursing Care of Children. Philadelphia, JB Lippincott, 1985

Ziegel E, Cranley M: Obstetric Nursing. New York, Macmillan, 1984

Bowel Elimination, Altered*

Constipation

Related to **Painful Defecation**

Colonic Constipation

Related to **Change in Life-Style**
Related to **Immobility**

Perceived Constipation

Related to **(Specify)**

* This diagnostic category is not currently on the NANDA list but has been included for clarity and usefulness.

Diarrhea

Related to **Untoward Side Effects**

Bowel Incontinence

Author's Note: *Altered Bowel Elimination* represents a broad category that is probably too broad for clinical use. It is recommended that more specific categories be used when possible. The three diagnostic categories relating to constipation represent one general constipation category and two specific types. The treatment of colonic constipation differs from the treatment of perceived constipation.

Bowel Elimination, Altered

Definition

Altered bowel elimination: The state in which an individual experiences or is at high risk of experiencing bowel dysfunction resulting in diarrhea or constipation.

Defining Characteristics

Major (must be present)

Reports or demonstrates one or more of the following:
Hard, formed stool
Painful defecation
Habitual use of laxatives/enemas
Bowel movements less than three times a week
Loose liquid stools
Increased frequency (more than three times a day)

Minor (may be present)

Painful defecation
Abdominal discomfort
Rectal fullness
Headache
Anorexia
Urgency
Abdominal cramping
Increased or decreased bowel sounds

Etiological, Contributing, Risk Factors

See Etiological, Contributing, Risk Factors under *Constipation* and *Diarrhea*

Constipation

Related to **Painful Defecation**

Definition

Constipation: The state in which an individual experiences or is at high risk of experiencing stasis of the large intestine resulting in infrequent elimination or hard, dry feces.

Defining Characteristics

Major (must be present)
Hard, formed stool and/or
Defecation occurs less than three times a week

Minor (may be present)
Decreased bowel sounds
Reported feeling of rectal fullness
Reported feeling of pressure in rectum
Straining and pain on defecation
Palpable impaction

Etiological, Contributing, Risk Factors

Pathophysiological
Malnutrition
Sensory/motor disorders
    Spinal cord lesions   Cerebrovascular accident (stroke)
    Spinal cord injury   Neurological diseases
Metabolic and endocrine disorders
    Anorexia nervosa   Hypothyroidism
    Obesity   Hyperparathyroidism
Affective disorders
Pain (upon defecation)
    Hemorrhoids   Back injury
Decreased peristalsis related to hypoxia (cardiac, pulmonary)
Cancer

Treatment-Related
Drug side-effects
    Antacids   Calcium
    Iron   Anticholinergics
    Barium   Anesthetics
    Aluminum   Narcotics (codeine, morphine)
    Aspirin   Diuretics
    Phenothiazines   Anti-Parkinsonian Agents

Surgery
Habitual laxative use

Situational (personal, environmental)

Immobility
Pregnancy
Stress
Lack of exercise
Irregular evacuation patterns
Cultural/health beliefs

Lack of privacy
Inadequate diet (Lack of roughage
thiamine)
Dehydration
Fear of rectal or cardiac pain
Faulty appraisal/dementia

Maturational

Infant: Formula
Child: Toilet training (reluctance to interrupt play)
Elderly: Decreased motility of GI tract

Focus Assessment Criteria

Subjective Data

1. Elimination pattern
   Usual pattern
   Present pattern

   Laxative use (type? how often?)
   Enema use (type? how often?)
2. History of symptoms
   Onset
   Duration
   Location
   Description

   Frequency
   Precipitated by what?
   Relieved by what?
   Aggravated by what?
3. Associated symptoms/complaints of
   Headache
   Weakness
   Lethargy
   Anorexia

   Thirst
   Pain
   Cramping
   Weight loss/gain
4. Life-style
   Activity level
   Occupation
   Exercise (what? how often?)

   Nutrition
      24-hour recall of foods and
         liquids taken
   Usual 24-hour intake
      Carbohydrates
      Fat
      Protein
      Roughage
      Liquids
5. Current drug therapy
   Antibiotics
   Iron
   Steroids

   Antacids
   CNS depressants
6. Medical-surgical history
   Present conditions
   Past conditions

   Surgical history (colostomy?
      ileostomy?)

Objective Data
1. Stool

Color

Brown
Yellow
Yellow-green
Green
Black
Tan (clay-colored)
Red

Odor

Normal
Foul

Consistency

Soft, formed
Soft, bulky
Small, dry
Pasty
Diarrheal
Hard

Size/shape

Narrow
Large caliber
Small caliber
Round

Components

Blood
Mucus
Pus
Parasites
Undigested food

2. Nutrition

Food intake

Type
Amounts

Fluid intake

Type
Amounts

3. GI motility (auscultation, light palpation)

Bowel sounds

High-pitched, gurgling (5 per min)
High-pitched frequent, loud, pushing

Weak and infrequent
Absent

Abdominal distention

None
Slight

Moderate
Severe

Flatulence

None
Occasionally

Frequent

4. Perianal area/rectal exam

Hemorrhoids
Fissures

Irritation
Impaction
Presence/absence of stool in rectum

Principles and Rationale for Nursing Care

General
1. Bowel patterns may be culturally and/or familially determined.
2. Circadian rhythms may be utilized to assist defecation at a regular time.
3. Activity influences bowel elimination by improving muscle tone and stimulating appetite and peristalsis.

4. Factors that influence the characteristics of stool:

Color	Diet	Drugs	Disease
Yellow-yellow green	Breast milk	Antibiotics Senna	Severe diarrhea
Green	Green vegetables	Mercurous chloride Indomethacin Calomel Dithiazanine	Severe diarrhea
Black-dark brown	Cherries	Iron Charcoal Bismuth	Upper GI bleeding Anticoagulants Steroids and salicylates
Pale–whitish	Milk Meat	Antacids	
Clay-colored	Fat		Common bile duct blockage
Red	Beets	Brom sulphalein Tetracyclines (syrup) Phenolphthalein Pyridium	

5. The odor of the stool varies with the pH and the amount of bacterial fermentation.
6. The normalcy of one's bowel patterns is determined by the individual.
7. Psychological discomfort and inadequate coping can produce elimination alterations.

Physiology

1. Intestinal elimination is controlled by neural innervation from the spinal cord and by the stimulation of neural centers in the lower intestinal wall by fecal contents.
2. Bowel evacuation can be delayed by voluntarily inhibiting the urge to defecate.
3. The gastrocolic reflex and duodenocolic reflex stimulate mass peristalsis two or three times a day, most often following meals.
4. Voluntary contraction of the muscles of the abdominal wall aid in the expulsion of feces.

Nutrition

1. Sufficient fluid intake, at least two liters daily, is necessary to maintain bowel patterns and promote proper stool consistency.
2. A well-balanced diet high in fiber content stimulates peristalsis. Foods high in fiber should be avoided during episodes of diarrhea. These include:
    Whole grains and nuts (bran, shredded wheat, brown rice, whole wheat bread)
    Raw and coarse vegetables (broccoli, cauliflower, cucumbers, lettuce, cabbage, turnips, Brussels sprouts)
    Fresh fruits, with skins
3. Bulk and consistency of stool are influenced by dietary and fluid patterns. High vegetable diet produces soft, bulky stools. High meat diet produces small, dry, hard stools.
4. Diets high in unrefined fibrous food produce large soft stools that decrease the colon's susceptibility to disease.
5. Diets low in fiber and high in concentrated refined foods produce small hard stools that increase the colon's susceptibility to disease.
6. Fiber that is not digested absorbs water which adds bulk and softness to the stool, speeds up the passage through the intestines and slows down the rapid transit. (Schuster)
7. Fiber without adequate fluid can aggravate, not facilitate, bowel function.

Laxative Abuse

1. Chronic laxative abuse is one of the major causes of constipation in the elderly. (Schuster)
2. Laxatives and enemas are not components of a bowel management program, but are for emergency use only. (Ellickson)
3. Lactose intolerance can cause gas formation and bloating. These responses may be confused with constipation with a subsequent response of laxative use.

Constipation
Related to Painful Defecation

Assessment

Subjective Data

The person reports:
Pain on defecation
Rectal itching
Straining at stool

Objective Data

Hard consistency of stool
Hemorrhoids
Impaction palpated on rectal exam
Irritated or excoriated perianal area

Outcome Criteria

The person will
- Relate less pain on defecation
- Describe causative factors when known
- Describe rationale and procedure for treatments

Interventions

A. Assess causative factors

Fecal impaction/constipation
Hemorrhoids
Anal fissures
Pregnancy
Surgery that reduces ability to
  bear down

Pilonidal cyst
Anorectal abscess
Lower intestinal obstruction
Enlargement of prostate gland

B. Reduce rectal pain, if possible, by instructing person in corrective measures
- Increase fluid intake
- Increase dietary intake of high-fiber foods
- Increase daily exercise
- Gently apply a lubricant to anus to reduce pain on defecation
- Apply cool compresses to area to reduce itching
- Take sitz bath or soak in tub or warm water (43°–46° C) for 15-minute intervals if soothing
- Take stool softeners or mineral oil as an adjunct to other approaches
- Consult with physician regarding use of local anesthetics and antiseptic agents

C. Protect the surrounding skin from breakdown
- Evaluate the surrounding skin area
- Cleanse properly with nonirritating agent (*e.g.*, use gentle motion; use soft tissues following defecation)
- Suggest a sitz bath following defecation
- Gently apply protective emollient or lubricant

D. Initiate health teaching if indicated
- Teach the methods to prevent rectal pressure that contributes to hemorrhoids
- Avoid prolonged sitting (*e.g.*, stand up every 1 hr for 5–10 min to relieve pressure)
- Avoid straining at defecation
- Soften stools (*e.g.*, low roughage diet, high fluid intake) (see Principles and Rationale for Nursing Care)

Colonic Constipation

Related to **Change in Life-style**

Related to **Immobility**

Definition
Colonic constipation: The state in which an individual experiences or is at risk of experiencing a delay in passage of food residue resulting in dry, hard stool

Defining Characteristics*

Major (80%–100%)
  Decreased frequency
  Hard, dry stool

* Adapted from McLane AM, McShane RE: Empirical validation of defining characteristics of constipation: A study of bowel elimination practices of healthy adults. In Hurley ME (ed): Classification of Nursing Diagnoses: Proceedings of the Sixth Conference, pp 448–455. St. Louis, CV Mosby, 1986

Straining at stool
Painful defecation
Abdominal distention

Minor (50%–79%)

Rectal pressure
Headache, appetite impairment
Abdominal pain

Etiological, Contributing, Risk Factors

Pathophysiological

Malnutrition
Sensory/motor disorders
   Spinal cord lesions
   Spinal cord injury

Cerebrovascular accident (CVA, stroke)
Neurological diseases

Metabolic and endocrine disorders
   Anorexia nervosa
   Obesity

Hypothyroidism
Hyperparathyroidism

Affective disorder
Decreased peristalsis related to hypoxia (cardiac, pulmonary)
Cancer

Treatment-Related

Drug side-effects
   Antacids
   Iron
   Barium
   Aluminum
   Calcium
   Anticholinergics
   Anesthetics
   Narcotics (codeine, morphine)
   Aspirin
   Phenothiazines
   Diuretics
   Anti-Parkinsonian Agents
Surgery
Habitual laxative use

Situational (personal, environmental)

Immobility
Pregnancy
Stress
Lack of exercise
Irregular evacuation patterns

Lack of privacy
Inadequate diet (lack of roughage/thiamine)
Dehydration
Fear of rectal or cardiac pain

Maturational

Infant
   Formula

Child
    Toilet training (reluctance to interrupt play)
Elderly
    Decreased motility of gastrointestinal tract

Colonic Constipation
Related to Change in Life-style

Assessment

Subjective Data

The person reports:
    Hard dry stools less than three times a week
    A change in living patterns (*e.g.*)

Altered daily routine	Inadequate fluid intake
Decreased activity	Recent illness or hospitalization
Lack of privacy	Change in regular schedule of
Diet reported lacking in sufficient	elimination
roughage	

Objective Data

Hard formed stools
Palpable impaction

Outcome Criteria

The person will
  • Describe contributing factors when known
  • Describe methods to prevent constipation

Interventions

A. Assess for causative factors
   Stress
       Occupation
       Family responsibilities
       Financial considerations
   Sedentary life-style
   Hospitalization
   Drug side-effect
   Debilitation
   Lack of privacy (at work or at school)

Recent or frequent travel
Lack of time

B. Promote corrective measures

1. Regular time for elimination
   - Identify normal defecation pattern prior to constipation
   - Review daily routine
   - Advise that time for defecation be included as part of daily routine
   - Discuss suitable time (based on responsibilities, availability of facilities, etc.)
   - Provide stimulus to defecation (*e.g.,* coffee, prune juice)
   - Advise that an attempt to defecate should be made about an hour or so following meal and that it may be necessary to remain in bathroom a suitable length of time
   - Utilize bathroom instead of bedpan if possible
   - Offer bedpan or bedside commode if unable to use bathroom
   - Assist into position on bedpan or commode
   - Provide for privacy (close door, draw curtains around bed, play television or radio to mask sounds, have room deodorizer available)
   - Provide for comfort (reading material as diversion) and safety (call bell available)
   - Allow suitable position (sitting if not contraindicated)
2. Adequate exercise
   - Review current exercise pattern
   - Provide for moderate physical exercise on a frequent basis (if not contraindicated)
   - Provide frequent ambulation of hospitalized patient when tolerable
   - Perform range of motion exercises for person who is bedridden
   - Teach exercises for increased abdominal muscle tone (unless contraindicated)
     a. Contract abdominal muscles several times frequently throughout day
     b. Do sit-ups keeping heels on floor with knees slightly flexed
     c. While supine, raise lower limbs, keeping knees straight

C. Eliminate or reduce contributing factors

1. Untoward side-effects of current medical regimen
   - Administer mild laxative following oral administration of barium sulfate*
   - Assess elimination status while on antacid therapy (may be necessary to alternate magnesium-type antacid with other types)*
   - Encourage increased intake of high-roughage foods and increased fluid intake as adjunct to iron therapy (*e.g.,* fresh fruits and vegetables with skins; bran, nuts, and seeds; whole wheat bread)
   - Encourage early ambulation, with assistance if necessary, to counter effects of anesthetic agents
   - Assess elimination status while receiving certain narcotic analgesics (morphine, codeine) and alert physician if experiencing difficulty with defecation
2. Laxative abuse
   - See *Perceived Constipation*
3. Stress
   - See Appendix X for relaxation techniques for stress reduction
4. Inadequate dietary and fluid intake: see *Altered Nutrition: Less Than Body Requirements*

---

* May require a physician's order.

D. Conduct health teaching as indicated
- Explain to person and family the relationship of life-style changes to constipation
- Explain interventions that relieve symptoms
- Explain techniques to reduce the effects of stress and immobility

Colonic Constipation
Related to Immobility

Assessment

Subjective Data

The person reports:
    Hard stools less than three times a week
    Inability or difficulty moving bowels

Objective Data

Immobility (*e.g.,* casts, traction, paralysis)
Altered state of consciousness
Altered body position (*e.g.,* legs elevated)

Multiple support equipment (*e.g.,* catheters, IV, arterial lines, respirator)
Body restraints
Forced bedrest

Outcome Criteria

The person will
- Describe therapeutic bowel regimen
- Relate or demonstrate improved bowel elimination
- Explain rationale for interventions

Interventions

A. Assess causative factors of immobility

Musculoskeletal (*e.g.,* fractures, sprain, contractures, hip replacement)
Reliance on life-support systems
Chronic or acute illness
Trauma (*e.g.,* burns, head injury)
Physical handicap
Inappropriate coping mechanisms
Bedrest
Psychosomatic illness
Degenerative joint changes (arthritis)
Surgery

B. Promote corrective measures
  1. Balanced diet
    • Review list of foods high in bulk
        Fresh fruits with skins
        Bran
        Nuts and seeds
        Whole grain breads and cereals
        Cooked fruits and vegetables
        Fruit juices
    • Discuss dietary preferences
    • Take into account any food intolerances or allergies
    • Include approximately 800 g of fruits and vegetables (about four pieces of fresh fruit and large salad) for normal daily bowel movement
    • Suggest use of bran in moderation at first (may irritate GI tract, produce flatulence, cause diarrhea or blockage)
    • Gradually increase amount of bran as tolerated (may add to cereals, baked goods, etc.). Explain the need for fluid intake with bran
    • Consider financial limitations (encourage the use of fruits and vegetables in season)
  2. Adequate fluid intake
    • Encourage intake of at least 2 liters—8 to 10 glasses—unless contraindicated
    • Discuss fluid preferences
    • Set up regular schedule for fluid intake
    • Recommend a glass of hot water to be taken one-half hour before breakfast that may act as stimulus to bowel evacuation
  3. Regular time for elimination
    • Identify normal defecation pattern prior to constipation
    • Review daily routine
    • Include time for defecation as part of regular routine
    • Discuss suitable time (based on responsibilities, availability of facilities, etc.)
    • Provide stimulus to defecation (*e.g.*, coffee, prune juice)
    • Suggest that person attempt defecation about an hour or so following meal and remain in bathroom suitable length of time
    • Utilize bathroom instead of bedpan if possible
    • Offer bedpan or bedside commode if unable to use bathroom
    • Assist into position on bedpan or commode
    • Provide for privacy (close door, draw curtains around bed, play television or radio to mask sounds, make room deodorizer available)
    • Provide for comfort (reading material as diversion) and safety (call bell available)
  4. Optimal position
    • Assist patient to normal semi-squatting position to allow optimum usage of abdominal muscles and effect of force of gravity
    • Assist onto bedpan if necessary and elevate head of bed to high Fowler's position or elevation permitted
    • Use fracture bedpan for comfort if preferred
    • Stress the avoidance of straining
    • Encourage exhaling during straining
    • Place call bell within easy reach
    • Maintain safety (siderails)
    • Provide privacy
    • Chart results (color, consistency, amount)

C. Eliminate or reduce contributing factors

1. Fecal impaction
   - If fecal impaction is suspected, perform digital examination of rectum: Have client assume position lying on left side. Don glove, lubricate forefinger, and insert; attempt to break up any hardened fecal mass and remove pieces
   - If impaction is out of reach of gloved finger:
     a. Administer oil retention enema to aid in removal of mass*
     b. Instruct person to retain enema at least 60 minutes or possibly overnight
     c. Follow with cleansing enema* (both enemas may need to be repeated; may need to follow with repeated attempt to break up mass digitally)
   - Make client comfortable and allow to rest
   - Client may require temporary use of stool softener or mild cathartic*
   - Maintain accurate bowel elimination record

2. Severe constipation
   - First day, insert glycerin suppository and have client attempt bowel movement through intermittent straining efforts
   - If ineffective, on second day, insert glycerin suppository and follow same routine
   - If no results, on third day, request prescription for Dulcolax suppository, which if not effective should be followed by enema*
   - To aid in stimulation of reflex, suppository may be followed in 20 to 30 minutes by digital stimulation of anal sphincter
   - Return to first-day routine and follow until pattern is established (may be every 2 to 3 days)

D. Conduct health teaching as indicated

   - Explain to person and significant others the interventions required to prevent vs. treat constipation (*e.g.*, diet, exercise)
   - Refer to Principles and Rationale for Nursing Care for specifics

Perceived Constipation

Related to **(Specify)**

Definition

Perceived constipation: The state in which an individual self-prescribes the daily use of laxatives, enemas, and/or suppositories to ensure a daily bowel movement

---

* May require a physician's order.

Defining Characteristics*

Major (80%–100%)

Expectation of a daily bowel movement with the resulting overuse of laxatives, enemas and suppositories

Expected passage of stool at same time every day

Etiological, Contributing, Risk Factors

Pathophysiological

Altered affect caused by change in:
  Body chemistry
  Tumor
Obsessive-compulsive disorders
Central nervous system deterioration

Situational (personal, environmental)

Cultural/familial health beliefs
Faulty appraisal

Focus Assessment Criteria

See *Altered Elimination*

Principles and Rationale for Nursing Care

See *Altered Elimination*

Perceived Constipation
Related to (Specify)

Assessment

See Defining Characteristics

Outcome Criteria

The person will
  • Verbalize acceptance with BM q 2–3 days
  • Not use laxatives regularly
  • Relate the causes of constipation
  • Describe the hazards of laxative use
  • Relate an intent to increase fiber, fluid, and exercise in daily life as instructed

---

* McLane AM, McShane RE: Empirical validation of defining characteristics of constipation: A study of bowel elimination practices of healthy adults. In Hurley ME (ed): Classification of Nursing Diagnoses: Proceedings of the North American Nursing Diagnosis Association Sixth Conference, pp 448–455. St. Louis, CV Mosby, 1986

Interventions

A. Assess causative or contributing factors
- Painful defecation (see *Constipation* related to *Painful Defecation*
- Inadequate diet, fluids and/or exercise
- Cultural/familial belief
- Faulty appraisal

B. Explain that BM are needed every 2 to 3 days, not daily
- Be sensitive to his beliefs
- Be patient

C. Explain the hazards of regular laxative use
- Provide only temporary relief
- Promote constipation by interfering with peristalsis
- In emergencies use rectal suppository instead of oral laxative

D. Plan Corrective Measures
1. Balanced diet
   - Review list of foods high in bulk
     Fresh fruits with skins
     Bran
     Nuts and seeds
     Whole grain breads and cereals
     Cooked fruits and vegetables
   - Discuss dietary preferences
   - Take into account any food intolerances or allergies
   - Include approximately 800 g of fruits and vegetables (about four pieces of fresh fruit and large salad) for normal daily bowel movement
   - Suggest use of bran in moderation at first (may irritate GI tract, produce flatulence, cause diarrhea or blockage)
   - Gradually increase amount of bran as tolerated (may add to cereals, baked goods, etc.). Explain the need for fluid intake with bran
   - Suggest a commercial fiber product if fiber is inadequate in diet
2. Adequate fluid intake
   - Encourage intake of at least 6 to 10 glasses (unless contraindicated)
   - Discuss fluid preferences
   - Set up regular schedule for fluid intake, increase in hot weather
   - Recommend a glass of hot water to be taken one-half hour before breakfast that may act as stimulus to bowel evacuation
3. Regular time for elimination
   - Include time for defecation as part of regular routine (*e.g.*, 15 min after eating breakfast)
   - Discuss suitable time (based on responsibilities, availability of facilities, etc.)
   - Provide stimulus to defecation (*e.g.*, warm drink, prunes)
   - Teach not to ignore the urge to defecate
   - Provide for privacy (close door, draw curtains around bed, play television or radio to mask sounds, make room deodorizer available)
   - Provide for comfort (reading material as diversion) and safety (call bell available)

4. Optimal position
   - Assist patient to normal semi-squatting position to allow optimum usage of abdominal muscles and effect of force of gravity
   - Assist onto bedpan if necessary and elevate head of bed to high Fowler's position or elevation permitted
   - Use fracture bedpan for comfort if preferred
   - Stress the avoidance of straining
   - Encourage exhaling during straining
   - Place call bell within easy reach
   - Maintain safety (siderails)
   - Provide privacy
   - Chart results (color, consistency, amount)
5. Regular exercise
   - Teach the rationale for increasing activity
   - Suggest walking (refer to *Health Maintenance)*
   - If walking is prohibited
     > Teach to lie in bed or sit on chair and bend one knee at a time to chest (10–20 times) each knee three to four times/day
     > Teach to sit in chair or lie in bed and turn torso from side to side (20–30 times) six to ten times/day

---

Diarrhea

Related to **Untoward Side-effects**

Definition
Diarrhea: The state in which the individual experiences or is at risk of experiencing frequent passage of liquid stool or unformed stool.

Defining Characteristics

Major (must be present)
Loose, liquid stools and/or
Increased frequency (more than three times a day)

Minor (may be present)
Urgency
Cramping/abdominal pain
Increased frequency of bowel sounds
Increase in fluidity or volume of stools

Etiological, Contributing, Risk Factors

Pathophysiological

Nutritional disorders and malabsorptive syndromes

Kwashiorkor
Gastritis
Peptic ulcer
Diverticulitis
Ulcerative colitis

Crohn's disease
Lactose intolerance
Spastic colon
Celiac disease (sprue)
Irritable bowel

Metabolic and endocrine disorders

Diabetes mellitus
Addison's disease

Thyrotoxicosis

Dumping syndrome

Infectious process

Trichinosis
Dysentery
Cholera
Malaria

Shigellosis
Typhoid fever
Infectious hepatitis

Cancer
Uremia
Tuberculosis
Arsenic poisoning
Fecal impaction

Treatment-related

Surgical intervention of the bowel

Loss of bowel

Ileal bypass

Drug side-effects

Thyroid agents
Antacids
Laxatives

Stool softeners
Antibiotics
Chemotherapy

Tube feedings

Situational (personal, environmental)

Stress or anxiety
Irritating foods (fruits, bran cereals)
Travel
Change in bacteria in water
Bacteria, virus, parasite to which no immunity is present
Hot weather
Increased caffeine consumption

Maturational

Allergies
Infant: Breast-fed babies
Elderly: Decreased sphincter reflexes

Focus Assessment Criteria

Refer to criteria for *Potential Altered Bowel Elimination: Constipation*

Principles and Rationale for Nursing Care

1. Rapid transit of feces through the large intestine results in less water absorption and an unformed, liquid stool.
2. Dehydration and electrolyte imbalance occur if diarrhea continues.
3. Malabsorption results in an increase in the bulk of the colon and stimulates intestinal motility.
4. Diarrheal stool can cause excoriation of the anal area because it is usually acidic and contains digestive enzymes.
5. Hyperperistalsis is the motor response to intestinal irritants.
6. High-solute tube feedings may cause diarrhea if not followed by sufficient amounts of water.
7. Diarrhea may be related to an inflammatory process in which the intestinal mucosal wall becomes irritated, resulting in increased moisture content in the fecal masses.
8. Refer to Principles and Rationale for Nursing Care for *Constipation*.

Diarrhea
Related to Untoward Side-effects

Assessment

Subjective Data

The person reports:

Loose stools more than three times daily

Pain

Cramps

Weakness

Objective Data

Observable signs of dehydration

Increased bowel sounds

Liquid stools

Frequent stools (more than three times daily)

Outcome Criteria

The person will
- Describe contributing factors when known
- Explain rationale for interventions
- Report less diarrhea

Interventions

A. Assess causative contributing factors

Tube feedings

Dietary indiscretions/contaminated foods

Food allergies

Foreign travel

B. Eliminate or reduce contributing factors

1. Administration of tube feeding
   - Control infusion rate (depending on delivery set)
   - Administer smaller, more frequent feedings*
   - Change to continuous-drip tube feedings*
   - Administer more slowly if signs of GI intolerance occur
   - Control temperature
   - If refrigerated, warm in hot water to room temperature
   - Dilute strength of feeding temporarily*
   - Follow standard procedure for administration of tube feeding
   - Follow tube feeding with specified amount of water to assure hydration
   - Be careful of contamination/spoilage (unused but opened formula should not be used after 24 hr; keep unused portion refrigerated)
2. Contaminated foods (possible sources)
   - Raw seafood
   - Shellfish
   - Excess milk consumption
   - Raw milk
   - Restaurants
   - Improperly cooked/stored food

C. Reduce diarrhea

a. For adults
   - Discontinue solids
   - Ingest clear liquids (fruit juices, Gatorade, broth)
   - Avoid milk products, fat, whole grain, fresh fruits and vegetables
   - Gradually add semi-solids and solids (crackers, yogurt, rice, bananas, apple-sauce)
b. For breast-fed infants
   - Discontinue solids
   - Offer clear liquid supplements
   - Continue breast-feeding
c. For formula-fed infant or milk-fed child
   - Discontinue formula, milk products, and solid foods
   - Offer small amounts of clear fluids (sweetened diluted tea, diluted cola, ginger ale, sugar water, diluted Jell-O water) 15 ml to 30 ml each one half to 1 hour for first 8 hours
   - Increase amount to 60 ml to 90 ml every 1 to 2 hours if number of stools has lessened
   - Add plain solids (Jell-O, bananas, rice, cereal, crackers) after 24 hours, if improved
   - Gradually return to regular diet (except milk products) after 36 to 48 hours; after 3 to 5 days gradually add milk products (half-strength skim to skim milk to half-strength whole milk to whole milk)
   - Gradually introduce formula (half-strength formula to full-strength formula)

---

* May require a physician's order.

D. Replace fluids and electrolytes
- Increase oral intake to maintain a normal urine specific gravity
- Encourage liquids (water, apple juice, flat ginger ale)
- Children may need administration of commercially prepared solution (*e.g.,* Pedialyte)*
- Encourage fluids high in potassium and sodium (orange and grapefruit juices, bouillon)
- Caution against use of very hot or cold liquids
- See *Fluid Volume Deficit* for additional interventions

E. Conduct health teaching as indicated
1. Explain to client and significant others the interventions required to prevent future episodes
2. Explain the effects of diarrhea on hydration
3. Teach precautions to take when traveling to foreign lands (Maresca)
    a. Avoid foods served cold, salads, milk, fresh cheese, cold cuts and salsa
    b. Drink carbonated or bottled beverages, avoid ice
    c. peel fresh fruits and vegetables
4. Consult with primary health care provider for prophylactic use of bismuth subsalicylate (Pepto-Bismol) 30–60 ml qid during travel and two days after return; or antimicrobials, for treatment of traveler's diarrhea.
5. Explain how to prevent transmission of infection
    - hand washing
    - proper storage, cooking and handling of food
    - if sexually transmitted (fecal-oral contamination) explain methods to prevent

Bowel Incontinence

Definition
Bowel incontinence: A state in which an individual experiences a change in normal bowel habits characterized by involuntary passage of stool.

> **Author's Note:** This diagnostic category represents a situation in which nurses have multiple responsibilities. Individuals experiencing *Bowel Incontinence* have various responses that disrupt functioning such as:
> *Fear* related to embarrassment of lack of control of bowels
> *Potential Impaired Skin Integrity* related to irritative nature of feces on skin
> For some spinal-cord injured persons, *Bowel Incontinence* related to lack of voluntary control over rectal sphincter would be descriptive.

* May require a physician's order.

Defining Characteristics

Major (must be present)

Involuntary passage of stool

Etiological, Contributing, Risk Factors

Pathophysiological

Loss of sphincter control
Progressive dementia
Progressive neuromuscular disorder (*e.g.* multiple sclerosis)
Inflammatory bowel disease

Situational

Depression
Cognitive Impairment
Surgery
   Coloncolostomy

References/Bibliography

Aman RA: Treating the patient, not the constipation. Am J Nurs 80:1634–1635, 1980

Brill EL, Kilts DF: Foundations for Nursing, pp 535–562. Appleton-Century-Crofts, New York, 1980

Burkitt DP, Meisner P: How to manage constipation with high fiber diet. Geriatrics 34(2):33–40, 1979

Chow M et al: Handbook of Pediatric Primary Care, pp 632–638. New York, John Wiley & Sons, 1979

Ellickson E: Bowel management plan for the homebound elderly. Gerontol Nurs 14(1):16–19, 1988

Hickey J: The Clinical Practice of Neurological and Neurosurgical Nursing, pp 221–222, 279–280. Philadelphia, JB Lippincott, 1981

John RL: Giardiasis and amebiasis. RN 44(4):52–57, 1981

Krause MV, Mahan LK: Food, Nutrition, and Diet Therapy, pp 485–496. Philadelphia, WB Saunders, 1979

Maresca T: Assessment and management of acute diarrheal illness in adults. Nurse Pract 11(11):15–16, 1986

McShane R, McLane A: Constipation: impact of etiological factors. J Gerontol Nurs 14(4):31–34, 1988

Resnick B: Constipation: common but preventable. Geriatr Nurs 6(4):213–215, 1985

Rodman MJ: Diarrhea: Think twice before giving meds. RN 43(10):73–84, 1980

Rodman MJ, Smith DW: Pharmacology and Drug Therapy in Nursing, pp 928–935. JB Lippincott, Philadelphia, 1979

Schuster, MM: Fiber deficiency in gastrointestinal disease. in Texter EC (ed): The Aging Gut, pp 133–137. New York, Masson Publishing, 1983

Shelter MG: Stool specimens: Key to detecting intestinal invaders. RN 43(10):50–53, 1980

Sorensen K, Luckmann J: Basic Nursing, pp 693–721. Philadelphia, WB Saunders, 1979

Watson J: Medical–Surgical Nursing and Related Physiology, pp 538–544. Philadelphia, WB Saunders, 1979

Wolff L, Weitzel M, Furst E: Fundamentals of Nursing, pp 479–494. Philadelphia, JB Lippincott, 1979

Wright B, Staats D: The geriatric implications of fecal impaction. Nurse Pract, 11:53–66, 1986

Ineffective Breast-Feeding

Related to **(Specify)**

Definition

Ineffective breast-feeding: The state in which a mother, infant of child experiences dissatisfaction or difficulty with the breast-feeding process.

Defining Characteristics

Major (must be present)

Unsatisfactory breast-feeding process

Minor (may be present)

Actual or perceived inadequate milk supply
Infant inability to attach on to maternal breast correctly
No observable signs of oxytocin release
Observable signs of inadequate infant intake
Nonsustained suckling at the breast
Insufficient emptying of each breast per feeding
Persistence of sore nipples beyond the first week of breast-feeding
Insufficient opportunity for suckling at the breast
Infant exhibiting fussiness and crying within the first hour after breast-feeding; unresponsive to other comfort measures
Infant arching and crying at the breast resisting latching on

Etiological, Contributing, Risk Factors

Pathophysiological

Breast anomaly
Infant anomaly/poor sucking reflex
    cleft lip/palate
Prematurity
Previous breast surgery

Situational

Maternal fatigue
Maternal anxiety
Maternal ambivalence
Inadequate nutrition intake
Inadequate fluid intake
History of unsuccessful breast-feeding
Nonsupportive partner/family
Lack of knowledge

Interruption in breast-feeding
   Ill mother
   Ill infant

Focus Assessment Criteria

Subjective Data

1. History of breast-feeding (self, sibling, friend)
2. Supportive persons (partner, friend, sibling, parent)
3. Source of information on breast-feeding
4. Daily intake:
   Calories
   Calcium
   Vitamin supplement
   Basic food groups
   Fluids

Objective Data

Breast condition (soft, firm, engorgement)
   Engorgement
   Soft
Nipples
   Cracks
   Inverted
   Sore

Principles and Rationale for Nursing Care

1. Lactation is the result of a complex process of interacting factors of the health and nutrition status of the mother, the health status of the infant and breast tissue development under the influence of estrogen and progesterone (Panwar)
2. Milk production and the letdown reflex is controlled by pituitary hormones, prolactin, and oxytocin and is stimulated by infant sucking and maternal emotions (Panwar)
3. The nutritional and fluid requirements for a lactating mother are outlined in Table II-3
4. Many medications are excreted in breast milk. Some are harmful to the infant. Advise the mother to consult with a health care professional (nurse, physician, pharmacist) prior to taking a medication (prescribed or over the counter)

Table II-3.   **Nutritional and Fluid Requirements for Lactating Women***

Calorie	500 extra	(2500–3000/day)
Protein	20 g	(4 servings)
Calcium	1200 mg	(5 servings)
Grains		(at least 4 servings)
Vegetables		(at least 5 servings)
rich in Vitamin c		(at least 2 servings)
green		(at least 1 serving)
Fluids		(2–3 qt)
dairy		(at least 1 qt or equivalent in cheese and yogurt)

*See *Altered Nutrition*, Principles and Rationale, for serving equivalents

5. The advantages of breast-feeding are:
   To Infant
       easier to digest
       reduces allergies
       provides antibodies and macrophages for early immunization
       fewer gastrointestinal infections
   To Mother
       hastens uterine involution
       reduces risks for breast cancer
       allows more time to rest during feedings
       less preparation, less cost
       faster bonding
6. The disadvantages of breast-feeding are:
       Someone cannot substitute
       Time-consuming
       Environmental pollutants in breast milk (PCBs, etc.)

Ineffective Breast-Feeding:
Related to (Specify)

Assessment
See Defining Characteristics

Outcome Criteria

The mother will
- Make an informed decision related to method of feeding infant (breast or bottle)
- Identify activities that deter or promote successful breast-feeding

Interventions

A. Assess causative or contributing factors
    Lack of knowledge
    Lack of role model
    Lack of physician's support
    Discomfort
        Leaking
        Engorgement
        Loss of control of bodily fluid
        Nipple soreness
    Partner's influence
    Patient's mother's attitudes and misconceptions

Social pressure against nursing
Change in body image
Change in sexuality
Feelings of being tied down
Presence of stress
Lack of conviction regarding decision to nurse
Sleepy, unresponsive infant
Fatigue

B. Promote open dialogue

1. Assess knowledge:
     Has woman taken a class in breast-feeding?
     Has she read anything on the subject?
     Does she have friends who are nursing their babies?
     Did her mother nurse?
2. Explain myths and misconceptions
     Ask her to list difficulties she is anticipating
     Common myths:
     My breasts are too small
     My breasts are too large
     My mother couldn't nurse
     How do I know my milk is good?
     How do I know the baby is getting enough?
     The baby will know that I'm nervous
     I have to go back to work, so what's the point of nursing for a short time?
     I'll never have any freedom
     Nursing will cause my breasts to sag
     My nipples are inverted, so I can't nurse
     My husband wouldn't like my breasts any more
     I'll have to stay fat if I nurse
     I can't nurse if I have a C-section
3. Build on mother's knowledge
     Clarify misconceptions
     Explain process of nursing
     Offer literature
     Discuss advantages and disadvantages
     Bring nursing mothers together to talk about nursing and their concerns
4. Support her decision to breast-feed or bottle-feed

C. Assist mother during first feedings

1. Promote relaxation
     Position comfortably
     Use pillows for positioning (especially cesarean-section mothers)
     Use relaxation breathing techniques
     If mother ever feels tense, a glass of wine or beer in moderation may help to relax
2. Demonstrate different positions
     Sitting
     Lying
     Football hold: instruct to place supporting hand on baby's bottom and turn his
         body toward mother's (this promotes security in infant)
3. Demonstrate and explain rooting reflex and show how it can be used to help infant
   latch on

Show mother how to grasp breast with fingers under breast and thumbs on top; this way she can point nipple directly at baby's mouth (avoid scissor hold because it constricts milk flow)

Make sure baby grasps a good portion of areola and not just the nipple

4. Advise mother to increase feeding times gradually, to start at 10 minutes per side and build up over next 3 to 5 days
5. Instruct mother to offer both breasts at each feeding, alternating the beginning side each time
6. Demonstrate:

How to use a finger to keep breast tissue from obstructing infant's nose

Use of finger in infant's mouth to break seal before removing from breast

Ways to awaken baby (may be necessary before offering the second breast)

7. Inform mother that burping may not be necessary with breast-fed babies, but if baby grunts and seems full between breasts she should attempt to burp baby, then continue feeding

D. Provide follow-up support during hospital stay

Develop care plan so that other health team members are aware of any problems or needs

Allow for flexibility of feeding schedule

Promote rooming in

Allow for privacy during feedings

Be available for questions

Be positive even if experience is difficult

E. Assist mother with specific nursing problems (may need assistance of lactation consultant)

1. Engorgement

Wear well-fitting support brassiere day and night; apply warm compresses for 15 to 20 minutes before nursing

2. Sore nipple

Decrease nursing time to 5 to 10 minutes per side. Start baby on nontender side first. Allow for more frequent, short feedings. Suggest alternate positions to rotate infant's grasps. Allow breasts to dry after each feeding

Keep nursing pads dry

Use breast cream only after breasts are dry

Use breast shield as last measure and remove after milk has let down

3. Difficulty with baby grasping nipple

Cup breast with fingers underneath

Position baby for mother's and infant's comfort (turn baby's abdomen toward mother's body)

Stroke infant's cheek for rooting reflex

Hand-express some milk into infant's mouth

Roll nipples to bring them out before feeding

Use nipple shield to help pull out inverted nipples only if above does not work. Remove shield after letdown occurs

Assess infant's suck—may need assistance in development of suck. Use lactation consultant if indicated

4. Separation (following C-section for stressed infant, premature infants, jaundiced infants)

Encourage visits and bonding as much as possible

Provide comfortable, private location for nursing during visit

Provide supportive atmosphere (freedom to ask questions, etc.)
Provide breast pump or make patient aware of availability
Rental of electric pump
Battery-operated pump
Cylinder-type hand pump (do not use bicycle horn pump)
Provide instruction in use of pump and assist mother to integrate breast-feeding into life-style

F. Explore feelings regarding changes in body

1. Encourage verbal expression of feelings
   a. Many women dislike leaking and lack of control. Explain that this is temporary. Demonstrate use of nursing pad.
   b. Changes breasts from "sexual objects" to implements of nutrition. This can affect sexual relationship. Husband gets milk if he sucks on nipples. Milk is released with orgasm. Infant suckling is "sensual" feeling—this causes guilt or confusion in woman. Encourage discussion with other mothers. Include partner in at least one discussion to assess his feelings and how they most affect the nursing experience.
   c. Self-consciousness during feedings. Explore woman's feelings about nursing.
      Where?
      Around whom?
      What is husband's reaction to when and where she nurses?
      Demonstrate use of shawl for modesty, allowing women to nurse in public.

G. Assist the family with

1. Sibling reaction
   Explore feelings and anticipation of problems. Older child may be jealous of contact with baby. Mother can use this time to read to older child. Older child may want to nurse.
   Allow him to try—usually does not like it.
   Stress older child's attributes—freedom, movement, and choices.
2. Fatigue and stress
   Explore situation
   Encourage mother to make herself and infant a priority
   Encourage to limit visits from relatives for first 4 weeks
   Needs support and assistance during first 4 weeks
   Encourage support person to help as much as possible
   Explain to mother not to try to be "superwoman"
3. Feelings of being enslaved
   Allow to express feelings
   Seek assistance
   Pump milk to allow others to feed baby
   Husband can change baby and bring to bed to nurse
   Remember that time between feedings will get longer (every 2 hr for 4 wk; then, every 3–4 hr by 3 mo)

H. Initiate referrals as indicated

1. Lactation consultant if indicated
   a. Lack of confidence
   b. Problems with infant suck and latch-on
   c. Can make follow-up home visits

2. Refer to La Leche League
3. Refer to childbirth educator and childbirth class members
4. Refer to other breast-feeding mothers

References/Bibliography

Cahill M: Breast-Feeding and Working? Booklet No. 58, Franklin Park, IL, La Leche League, 1976
La Leche League International: The Womanly Art of Breast-feeding. Franklin Park, IL, Interstate Printers Publishers, 1978
Lawrence R: Breastfeeding: A Guide for the Health Professional, St. Louis, CV Mosby, 1980
Panwar S: The postpartum period. In Buckley K, Kulb N (eds): Handbook of Maternal-Newborn Nursing, pp 458–459. New York, John Wiley and Sons, 1983
Riordan J: Practical Guide to Breastfeeding. St. Louis, CV Mosby, 1983

Decreased Cardiac Output

Definition

Decreased Cardiac Output: A state in which the individual experiences a reduction in the amount of blood pumped by the heart, resulting in compromised cardiac function.

Defining Characteristics

Low blood pressure	Dysrhythmia
Rapid pulse	Oliguria
Restlessness	Fatigability
Cyanosis	Vertigo
Dyspnea	Edema (peripheral, sacral)
Angina	

Author's Note: This diagnostic category represents a situation in which nurses have multiple responsibilities, too. Individuals experiencing decreased cardiac output may present various responses that disrupt functioning, such as

Activity intolerance
Sleep-rest dysrhythm
Anxiety/fear

or may be at risk for developing physiological complications such as

Dysrhythmias
Cardiogenic shock
Congestive heart failure

This author recommends that the nurse not use *Decreased Cardiac Output* but instead select another diagnostic category that better describes the situation.* It is also recommended that the physiological complications that nurses monitor for and collaborate with medicine for treatment for an individual with decreased cardiac output be labeled as collaborative problems,† as in

Potential complication: Dysrhythmias
Cardiogenic shock
Hypoxia

Not using *Decreased Cardiac Output* allows the nurse to more specifically describe the situations that nurses treat, either as nursing diagnoses or co-treat as collaborative problems.

* Refer to *Activity Intolerance related to insufficient oxygenation* secondary to decreased cardiac output.
† Refer to Chapter 2 for a discussion of collaborative problems.

Comfort, Altered:

Pain

Acute Pain*

Related to **(Specify)**
In Children Related to **(Specify)**

Chronic Pain

Related to **(Specify)**

* This diagnostic category is not currently on the NANDA list but has been included for clarity or usefulness.

Pruritus*

Related to **(Specify)**

Nausea/Vomiting*

Related to **(Specify)**

Author's Note: This diagnostic category can represent a variety of uncomfortable sensations such as pruritus, immobility, NPO status. When an individual experiences nausea and vomiting, the nurse should assess if *Altered Comfort* is the appropriate category or *Potential Altered Comfort* is the appropriate category or *Potential Altered Nutrition*. Short-lived episodes of nausea and/or vomiting (*e.g.*, postoperatively) can be best described with *Altered Comfort* related to nausea/vomiting secondary to effects of anesthesia, analgesics. When the nausea/vomiting is at risk to compromise nutritional intake—*Potential Altered Nutrition:* Less than Body Requirements related to nausea and vomiting secondary to (specify).

* This diagnostic category is not currently on the NANDA list but has been included for clarity or usefulness.

Comfort, Altered:

Definition

Altered comfort: The state in which an individual experiences an uncomfortable sensation in response to a noxious stimulus.

Defining Characteristics

Major (must be present)

The person reports or demonstrates a discomfort

Minor (may be present)

Autonomic response in acute pain
    Blood pressure increased
    Pulse increased
    Respirations increased
    Diaphoresis
    Dilated pupils
Guarded position
Facial mask of pain
Crying, moaning
Abdominal heaviness
Cutaneous irritation

Etiological, Contributing, Risk Factors

Any factor can contribute to altered comfort. The most common are listed below.

Pathophysiological

Musculoskeletal disorders
    Fractures   Arthritis
    Contractures   Spinal cord disorders
    Spasms
Visceral disorders
    Cardiac   Intestinal
    Renal   Pulmonary
    Hepatic
Cancer
Vascular disorders
    Vasospasm   Phlebitis
    Occlusion   Vasodilation (headache)
Inflammation
    Nerve   Joint
    Tendon   Muscle
    Bursa
Contagious diseases (rubella, chicken pox)

Treatment-related

Trauma (surgery, accidents)
Diagnostic tests
    Venipuncture   Biopsy
    Invasive scanning (*e.g.*, IVP)
Medications

Situational (personal, environmental)

    Immobility/improper positioning   Pregnancy (prenatal, intrapartum,
    Overactivity   postpartum)
    Pressure points (tight cast, Ace band-   Allergic response
      ages)   Chemical irritants
                                    Stress

Focus Assessment Criteria

Author's Note: This nursing assessment of pain is designed to acquire data in order to assess the individual adaptation to pain, not to determine the cause of pain or whether it exists.

Subjective Data

1. "Where is your discomfort located; does it radiate?" (Ask child to point to place)
2. "When did it begin?"
3. "Can you relate the cause of this discomfort?" or "What do you think is the cause of your discomfort?"
4. Ask person to describe the discomfort and its pattern
   Time of day
   Duration
   Frequency (constant, intermittent, transient)
   Quality/intensity
5. Ask person to rate his pain using a scale of 0–10 (0 = absence of pain; 10 = worst pain ever experienced)
   Rate at its best
   Rate after pain relief measures
   Rate at its worst
   For children, select a scale appropriate for age
   - Use pictures of faces (Oucher Scale) ranging from smiling to frown to crying with a numerical scale (Beyer)
   - Use four white chips and ask child to indicate how many pieces of hurt he is feeling. (Hester)
6. "How do you usually react to pain (crying, anger, silence)?"
7. "Are there any other symptoms associated with your discomfort (nausea, vomiting, numbness)?"
8. "What helps you when you have discomfort (medications [what, dosage, how often], heat, cold, activity, rest)?"
9. "Do you talk to others about your discomfort (spouse, friends, doctor, nurse)?"
10. Have person indicate the effect of each of the following factors on his discomfort by noting if there is an increase, a decrease, or no effect*

* Adapted from the McGill Pain Questionnaire.

Liquor
Stimulants (*e.g.*, caffeine)
Eating
Heat
Cold
Damp
Weather changes
Massage

Vibration
Pressure
No movement
Movement/activity
Sleep, rest
Lying down
Distraction (*e.g.*, TV)
Urination

Defecation
Tension
Bright lights
Loud noises
Going to work
Intercourse
Mild exercise
Fatigue

11. Ask person what effect pain has had on the following areas or what effect is anticipated
    Work/activity pattern (work/home activities, leisure/play)
    Sleep pattern (difficulty falling asleep/staying asleep)
    Eating pattern (appetite, weight gain/loss)
    Elimination patterns (bowel, constipation/diarrhea, bladder)
    Menses
    Sexual pattern (libido, function)
12. History of pruritus
    Onset
    Precipitated by what
    Site(s)
    Relieved by what
13. History of allergy (individual, family)
14. History of nausea/vomiting
    Onset, duration
    Frequency
    Vomitus (amount, appearance)
    Associated with?
        Medications
        Meals (specific foods)
        Position
    Relief measures?

Activity
Time of day
Pain

Objective Data (acute/chronic pain)

1. Behavioral manifestations

    Mood

    Calmness
    Moaning
    Crying
    Grimacing
    Pacing
    Restlessness
    Withdrawn

    Eye Movements

    Fixed
    Searching
    Open
    Closed
    Perception
    Oriented to time and place

2. Musculoskeletal manifestations

    Mobility of Painful Part

    Full
    Limited/guarded
    No movement

    Muscle Tone

    Spasm
    Tenderness
    Tremors (in effort to hide pain)

3. Dermatologic manifestations
    Color (redness)
    Temperature

    Moisture/diaphoresis
    Edema

4. Cardiorespiratory manifestations

Cardiac	*Respiratory*
Rate	Rate
Blood pressure	Rhythm
Palpations present	Depth

5. Neurologic manifestations
   Sensory alterations
     Paresthesia
     Dysesthesias
6. Cognitive manifestations
   Thought processes

Appropriate	Combative
Inappropriate	Confused
Cooperative	

Principles and Rationale for Nursing Care

Pain

1. Each individual experiences and expresses pain in his own manner, utilizing various sociocultural adaptation techniques.
2. All pain is real, regardless of its causes. Pure psychogenic pain is probably rare, as is pure organic pain. Most bodily pain is a combination of mental events (psychogenic) and physical stimuli (organic).
3. Pain has two components—a sensory component, which is neurophysiological, and a perceptual or experiential dimension with cognitive and emotional origins. The interaction of these two components determines the amount of suffering. (Schechter)
4. Pain tolerance is the duration and intensity of pain that an individual is willing to endure. Pain tolerance differs in individuals and may vary in one individual in different situations.
5. Personal factors that influence pain tolerance are:
     Knowledge of pain and its cause
     Meaning of pain
     Ability to control pain
     Energy level (fatigue)
     Stress level
6. Social and environmental factors that influence pain are:
     Interactions with others
     Response of others (family, friends)
     Secondary gains
     Sensory overload or deprivation
     Stressors
7. If a person must try to convince health care providers that he has pain, he will experience increased anxiety that increases the pain. Both of these are energy depleting.
8. Persons who are prepared for painful procedures by explanations of the actual sensations that will be felt experience less stress than individuals who receive vague explanations of the procedure.
9. Drug tolerance is a physiological phenomenon in which, after repeated doses, the prescribed dose begins to lose its effectiveness.
10. Drug dependence is a physiological state that results from repeated administration of a drug. Withdrawal is experienced if the drug is abruptly discontinued. Tapering down the drug dosage will manage the withdrawal symptoms.

11. Addiction is a behavioral pattern of drug use characterized by overwhelming involve-ment with the use of the drug, the securing of its supply, and the high tendency to relapse after withdrawal. (Jaffe)

12. Studies have shown that the human brain secretes endorphins, which have opiatelike properties that relieve pain. The release of endorphins may be responsible for the positive effects of placebos and noninvasive pain relief measures.

13. Studies have shown that diagnosed physiological pain does respond to placebos, so a positive response to placebos cannot be used to diagnose pain as psychogenic.

14. The use of noninvasive pain relief measures (*e.g.*, relaxation, massage, distraction) can enhance the therapeutic effects of pain-relief medications.

15. Adults and children who are experiencing pain feel their bodies and their lives are out of control. Attempts must be made to provide some choice or control during their day. (Schechter)

16. Inadequate sleep decreases one's ability to tolerate pain and depletes the energy needed to participate in social activities (distraction). (Eland)

17. Nurses' fear of precipitating respiratory depression often makes them reluctant to use intravenous medications. Yet a study reported that only three of 3,263 patients developed respiratory depression from narcotics during an acute hospitalization. (Miller)

18. Nurses' fear of precipitating addiction often makes them reluctant to administer narcotics. Porter and Jack identified that four addicts out of 11,000 reported they received Demerol in the hospital.

Medications

1. The preventive approach to pain is to establish a regular schedule for medication administration to treat the pain before it becomes severe rather than follow the PRN approach.

2. The preventive approach may reduce the total 24-hour dose as compared to PRN approach; it provides a constant blood level of the drug, it reduces craving for the drug, and it reduces the anxiety of having to ask and wait for PRN relief.

3. The oral route of administration is preferred when possible. Liquid medications can be given to individuals who have difficulty swallowing.

4. If frequent injections are necessary, the IV route is preferred because it is not painful and absorption is guaranteed, but the side-effects ($\downarrow$ respirations, $\downarrow$ B.P.) may be more profound.

Acute Pain Compared with Chronic Pain

1. Pain can be classified as acute or chronic pain, according to cause and duration, not intensity.

2. Acute pain is an episode of pain that has a duration of one second to less than six months. The cause is usually organic disease or injury. With healing, the pain subsides and eventually disappears.

3. Chronic pain is a pain experience that lasts for six months or longer. Chronic pain can be described as limited, intermittent, or persistent. *Limited pain* is pain caused by known physical pathology, and an end of the pain will come (*e.g.*, burns). *Intermittent pain* is pain that provides the person with pain-free periods. The cause may or may not be known (*e.g.*, headaches). *Persistent pain* is pain that usually occurs daily. The cause may or may not be known and is usually not a threat to life (*e.g.*, low back pain).

4. The visible signs of pain (physical and behavioral) are determined by the individual's pain tolerance and the duration of the pain, not the pain intensity.

5. The person may respond to acute pain physiologically and behaviorally: physi-

ologically by diaphoresis, an increased heart rate, an increased respiratory rate, and increased blood pressure; behaviorally by crying, moaning, or showing anger.
6. The person with chronic pain usually has adapted to pain, both physiologically and behaviorally, so that visible signs of pain may not be present.
7. The inability to manage pain produces feelings of frustration and inadequacy in the health care providers.
8. The person with chronic pain may respond with withdrawal, depression, anger, frustration, and dependency, all of which can affect the family in the same way.

Pain in Children

1. Several studies reported that when adults and children undergo the same surgery, the children are undermedicated. (Eland, Beyer) In one study, 52% of the children received no analgesic postoperatively, while the remaining 48% received aspirin or acetaminophen predominantly.
2. The response to pain in children is influenced by maturational age, cultural-ethnic background, previous experience with pain, and response from others to the pain.
3. The child's maturational and chronological age will influence this response to pain.
   A child less than 3 years old responds with tense body posture, irritability, rolling of the head, rubbing or pulling the affected body part, and physical resistance to painful procedure.
   A preschool child responds in the same way as a younger child and may verbalize about location of pain.
   A school-age child is influenced by cultural and parental influences. He can control the pain response, can clearly describe the pain, and may conceal or exaggerate pain for personal gain.
4. Verbal communication is usually not sufficient or reliable for explaining pain or painful procedures to children under seven. The nurse can explain by demonstrating with pictures or dolls. The more senses that are stimulated in the explanations to children, the greater the communication.
5. Even though children usually respond more openly to pain when their parents are present, the parents should be encouraged to be present in order to promote trust.
6. The weight of the child, not the age, should be considered when calculating analgesic relief.
7. Children will often deny pain to avoid injections (Eland). O'Brien and Knosler found that 40% of medication for postoperative pain were administered intramuscularly.

Pruritus

1. Pruritus [itching] is the most common skin alteration. It can be a response of the skin to an allergen or it can be a sign or symptom of a systemic disease such as cancer, liver or renal dysfunction, or diabetes mellitus.
2. Pruritus is aggravated by excessive warmth, excessive dryness, rough fabrics, fatigue or stress, and monotony (lack of distractions).
3. Pruritus arises as a result of subepidermal nerve stimulation by proteolytic enzymes. These enzymes are released from the epidermis as a result of either primary irritation or secondary allergic responses.
4. The same unmyelinated nerves that act for burning pain also serve for pruritus.
5. Clinically, burning and pain are allied sensations. As a pruritic sensation increases in intensity, the sensation may become burning.
6. Methods that interrupt pain also will interrupt pruritus. Local anesthetics, cold, or peripheral nerve resection eliminate both pain and pruritus.
7. Damage to the subepidermal network abolishes itch selectively because deep receptors do not exist for itch as they do for pain. If dermatitic skin is severely damaged, there may be damage to the itch receptor. As the skin heals, pruritis may return.

High-risk Elderly

1. Pain is omnipresent in the elderly and may be accepted by elders and professionals as a normal and unavoidable accompaniment to aging. Unfortunately, many chronic diseases that are common in the elderly, such as osteoarthritis and rheumatoid arthritis, may not be adequately managed regarding pain.
2. Elderly persons may not demonstrate objective signs and symptoms of pain because of years of adaptation and increased pain tolerance. The individual may eventually accept the pain, thereby lowering expectations for comfort and mobility. Pain coping mechanisms cultivated throughout life are important to identify and reinforce in pain management. Effective pain management can greatly improve the overall physical functioning and emotional well-being of the individual.
3. The effects of narcotic analgesics are prolonged in the elderly, because of decreased metabolism and clearance of the drug. Also, side effects seem to be more frequent and pronounced in the elderly, especially anticholinergic effects, extrapyramidal effects, and sedation. It is advised that drugs be started at a lower dosage, and because elderly persons often take multiple drugs, drug interactions should be monitored.

Nausea/Vomiting

1. Nausea and vomiting, when determined to have emotional origins, may be the result of developmental adjustment and adaption. A child learns that vomiting is unacceptable and thus learns to control vomiting. The child receives approval for not vomiting. Should childhood situations or conflicts resurface, the adult may experience nausea and vomiting. This adult may use nausea and vomiting to control or get attention. (Norris)
2. Vomiting serves as a first line defense against injurious agents ingested. Nausea may precede vomiting. (Norris)
3. Nausea and vomiting may be a signal of disease, injury, or the normal physiological adjustment to pregnancy.
4. Fifty to eighty percent of all pregnant women experience "morning sickness." (Fairweather)
5. Fatigue has been reported to precipitate nausea/vomiting in pregnant women. (Voda)
6. Voda reported that eating a high-protein snack before going to bed at night decreases morning nausea in some pregnant women.
7. Cotanch and Strum reported that progressive muscle relaxation was most effective in decreasing vomiting in individuals receiving chemotherapy.

Pain

Definition

Pain: The state in which an individual experiences and reports the presence of severe discomfort or an uncomfortable sensation.

Author's Note: This diagnostic category represents an individual who is experiencing pain. Clinically, it is more useful to differentiate acute pain from chronic pain in order to prescribe nursing interventions. Refer to *Acute Pain or Chronic Pain* for specific nursing interventions.

Defining Characteristics

Subjective
Communication (verbal or coded) of pain descriptors

Objective
   Guarding behavior, protective
   Self-focusing
   Narrowed focus (altered time perception, withdrawal from social contact, impaired
      thought processes)
   Distraction behavior (moaning, crying, pacing, seeking out other people and/or
      activities, restlessness)
   Facial mask of pain (eyes lackluster, "beaten look," fixed or scattered movement,
      grimace)
   Alteration in muscle tone (may span from listless to rigid)
   Autonomic responses not seen in chronic stable pain (diaphoresis blood pressure and
      pulse change, pupillary dilation, increased or decreased respiratory rate)

Acute Pain

Related to **(Specify)**

Definition
Acute pain: The state in which an individual experiences pain that can last from one
second to as long as six months. It subsides with healing or when the stimulus is
removed.

Defining Characteristics

Major (must be present)
The person reports or exhibits pain (may be the only assessment data present)

Minor (may be present)
   Fear of pain
   Inability to concentrate
   Guarded positioning
   Muscle spasm
   Increase in pulse, blood pressure, and respiration
   Evidence of inflammation (redness, heat, swelling)
   Rubbing or pulling of body part
   Tense body posture

Acute Pain
Related to (Specify)

Assessment

Subjective Data
The person reports:
    Pain (may be the only sign of pain)
    Fear of pain
    Inability to concentrate

Objective Data
    Guarded positioning
    Muscle spasm
    Increase in pulse, blood pressure, and respiration
    Evidence of inflammation (redness, heat, swelling)
    Rubbing or pulling of body part
    Tense body posture

Outcome Criteria

The person will
- Convey that others validate that the pain exists
- Relate relief after a satisfactory relief measure as evidenced by (specify)

Interventions

A. Assess for factors that decrease pain tolerance
    Disbelief on the part of others
    Lack of knowledge
    Fear (*e.g.*, of addiction or loss of control)
    Fatigue
    Monotony

B. Reduce or eliminate factors that increase the pain experience
 1. Disbelief on the part of others
    a. Relate to the individual your acceptance of his response to pain
      - Acknowledge the presence of his pain
      - Listen attentively to him concerning his pain
      - Convey to him that you are assessing his pain because you want to better understand it (not determine if it is really present)
    b. Assess the family for the presence of misconceptions about pain or its treatment
      - Explain the concept of pain as an individual experience
      - Discuss the reasons why an individual may experience increased or decreased pain (*e.g.*, fatigue [increased] or presence of distractions [decreased])

- Encourage family members to share their concerns privately (*e.g.*, fear that the person will use his pain for secondary gains if they give him too much attention)
- Assess whether the family doubts the pain and discuss the effects of this on the person's pain and on the relationship
- Encourage the family to give attention also when pain is not exhibited

2. Lack of knowledge
   - Explain causes of the pain to the person, if known
   - Relate how long the pain will last, if known
   - Explain diagnostic tests and procedures in detail by relating the discomforts and sensations that will be felt and approximate the length of time involved (*e.g.*, "During the intravenous pyelogram you might feel a momentary hot flash through your entire body")
   - Allow person to see and handle equipment if possible

3. Fear
   a. Provide accurate information to reduce fear of addiction
      - Explore with him the reasons for the fear
      - Explain the difference between drug tolerance and drug addiction (refer to Principles and Rationale for Nursing Care)
   b. Assist in reducing fear of losing control
      - Provide him with privacy for his pain experience
      - Attempt to limit the number of health care providers who provide care to him
      - Allow him to share how intense his pain is and express to him how well he tolerated the pain
   c. Provide information to reduce fear that the medication will gradually lose its effectiveness
      - Discuss drug tolerance with him
      - Discuss the interventions for drug tolerance with the physician (*e.g.*, changing the medication, increasing the dose, decreasing the interval)
      - Discuss the effect of relaxation techniques on medication effects

4. Fatigue
   - Determine the cause of fatigue (sedatives, analgesics, sleep deprivation)
   - Explain that pain contributes to stress, which increases fatigue
   - Assess the person's present sleep pattern and the influence of his pain on his sleep
   - Provide him with opportunities to rest during the day and with periods of uninterrupted sleep at night (must rest when pain is ↓)
   - Consult with physician for an increased dose of pain medication at bedtime
   - Refer to *Sleep Pattern Disturbance* for specific interventions to enhance sleep

5. Monotony
   a. Discuss with the person and family the therapeutic uses of distraction, along with other methods of pain relief
   b. Emphasize that the degree an individual can be distracted from his pain is not at all related to the existence of or the intensity of the pain
   c. Explain that distraction usually increases pain tolerance and decreases pain intensity, but after the distraction ceases the individual may experience increased awareness of pain and fatigue
   d. Vary the environment if possible. If on bed rest:
      - Encourage personnel to wear seasonal pins and bright-colored apparel
      - Encourage family to decorate room with flowers, plants, pictures
      - Provide the person with music
      - Consult with recreational therapist for an appropriate task

   e. If at home:
- Encourage individual to plan an activity for each day, preferably outside the home
- Discuss the possibility of learning a new skill (*e.g.*, a craft, a musical instrument)

   f. Teach a method of distraction during an acute pain (*e.g.*, painful procedure) that is not a burden (*e.g.*, count items in a picture, count anything in the room, such as patterns on wallpaper or count silently to self); breathe rhythmically; listen to music and increase the volume as the pain increases

C. Collaborate with the individual to determine what methods could be utilized to reduce the intensity of his pain

   a. Consider the following prior to selecting a specific pain relief method:
- The individual's willingness to participate (motivation), ability to participate (dexterity, sensory loss), preference, support of significant others for method, contraindications (allergy, health problem)
- The method's cost, complexity, precautions, and convenience

   b. Explain the various noninvasive pain relief methods to the individual and his family and why they are effective (see Appendix VI)

D. Collaborate with the individual to initiate the appropriate noninvasive pain relief measures (refer to Appendix VI for specific instructions on each method)

1. Relaxation
- Instruct on techniques to reduce skeletal muscle tension, which will reduce the intensity of the pain
- Utilize pillows and blankets to support the painful part to reduce the amount of muscle tension
- Promote relaxation with a back rub, massage, or warm bath (*e.g.*, for a person with a fractured limb, rub the opposite limb over the fractured site)
- Teach a specific relaxation strategy (*e.g.*, slow, rhythmic breathing or deep breath—clench fists—yawn)
- Enlist the aid of the family as coaches

2. Cutaneous stimulation
- Discuss with the person the various methods of skin stimulation and their effects on pain (see Appendix VI)
- Discuss the use of heat applications*: their therapeutic effects and when indicated
- Discuss each of the following methods and the precautions
     Hot water bottle
     Electric heating pad
     Warm tub
     Moist heat pack
     Hot summer sun
     Thin plastic wrap over painful area to retain body heat (*e.g.*, knee, elbow)
- Discuss the use of cold applications*: their therapeutic effects and when indicated
- Discuss each of the following methods and the precautions of each
     Cold towels (wrung out)
     Cold-water immersion for small body parts

* May require a physician's order.

Ice bag
Cold gel pack
Ice massage
- Explain the therapeutic uses of menthol preparations and massage/back rub

E. Provide the person with optimal pain relief with prescribed analgesics

- Determine preferred route of administration: po, IM, IV, rectal (refer to Principles and Rationale for Nursing Care)
- Assess vital signs, especially respiratory rate, prior to administering medication
- Consult with pharmacist for possible adverse interactions with other medications (*e.g.*, muscle relaxants, tranquilizers)
- Use a preventive approach
    a. Medicate prior to an activity (*e.g.*, ambulation) to increase participation, but evaluate the hazard of sedation
    b. Instruct the person to request PRN pain medication before the pain is severe
    c. Collaborate with physician to order meds on a 24-hour basis rather than PRN (refer to Principles and Rationale for Nursing Care for information on the preventive approach)

F. Assess the response to the pain-relief medication

- After administering a pain-relief medication, return in one-half hour to assess effectiveness
- Ask person to rate the severity of his pain, prior to the medication, and the amount of relief received
- Ask him to indicate when the pain began to increase
- Consult with physician if a dosage or interval change is needed; the dose may be increased by 50% until effective (Twycross)

G. Reduce or eliminate common side-effects of narcotics

1. Sedation
    - Assess if the cause is the narcotic, fatigue, sleep deprivation, or other drugs (sedatives, antiemetics)
    - Inform person that drowsiness usually occurs the first 2 to 3 days and then subsides
    - If drowsiness is excessive, consult with physician to try a slight dose reduction
2. Constipation
    - Explain the effect of narcotics on peristalsis
    - Consult with physician on the use of a stool softener with long-term drug use
    - Refer to *Constipation* for additional interventions
3. Nausea and vomiting (See also *Nausea/Vomiting.*)
    - Instruct person that nausea will usually subside after a few doses
    - Refrain from withholding narcotic doses because of nausea; rather, secure an order for an antiemetic
    - Instruct individual to take deep breaths and to voluntarily swallow to decrease vomiting reflex
    - If nausea persists, consult with physician for the appropriate antiemetic or for a change of narcotic that produces less nausea (*e.g.*, morphine)
4. Dry mouth
    - Explain that narcotics decrease saliva production

- Instruct person to rinse mouth often, suck on sugarless sour candies, eat pineapple chunks or watermelon, if permissible, and drink liquids often
- Explain the necessity of good oral hygiene and dental care

H. Assist the family to respond positively to the individual's pain experience

- Assess the family's knowledge of and response to the pain experience
- Give accurate information to correct family misconceptions (*e.g.*, addiction, doubts about pain)
- Provide individuals with opportunities to discuss their fears, anger, and frustrations in private; acknowledge the difficulty of the situation
- Incorporate family members in the pain relief modality if possible (*e.g.*, stroking, massage)
- Praise their participation and their concern

I. Assist the person with the aftermath of pain

- Inform him when the cause of the pain has been removed or decreased (*e.g.*, spinal tap)
- Encourage him to discuss his pain experience
- Praise him for his endurance and convey to him that he handled his pain well, regardless of how he behaved
- Allow person to keep souvenir of his pain, if desired (*e.g.*, gallstones), or a record of repeated procedures (*e.g.*, venipunctures)

J. Initiate health teaching as indicated

- Discuss with the person and the family noninvasive pain relief measures (relaxation, distraction, massage)
- Teach the techniques of choice to the person and his family
- Explain the expected course of the pain (resolution) if known (*e.g.*, fractured arm, surgical incision)

Acute Pain (in Children)
Related to (Specify)

Assessment

Subjective Data

Whimpering	Reduced appetite (poor feeder)
Crying	Does not want to be left alone
Moaning	Inability to be comforted

Objective Data

Tense body posture	Rubbing or pulling body part
Irritability	Refusal to move body part
Restlessness	Strained facial expression

Outcome Criteria

The child will, according to age and ability
- Identify the source of his pain
- Identify activities that increase and decrease pain
- Describe comfort from others during the pain experience

Interventions

A. Assess for pain experience

1. Assess the child's pain experience
   - Determine the child's concept of the cause of pain, if feasible
   - Ask child to point to the area that hurts
   - Determine the intensity of the pain at its worst and best
   - For children under four to five use Oucher Scale of five faces from very happy (1) to crying (5)
   - For children over four, ask child to rate his pain using a scale of 0–5 (0 = no pain and 5 = worst pain)
       "What number is your pain when it hurts the least?"
       "What time of day (morning, afternoon, evening)?"
   - Use the same scale each time for consistency; indicate on care plan which scale to use
   - Ask the child what makes the pain better and what makes it worse
   - Assess if fear or loneliness are contributing to pain
2. Assess the child and his family for the presence of misconceptions about pain or its treatment
   - Explain the pain source to the child using verbal and sensory (visual, tactile) explanations (*e.g.*, allow child to handle equipment or perform treatment on doll) (refer to Appendix IX for specific techniques of play therapy)
   - Explicitly explain and reinforce to the child that he is not being punished
   - Explain to the parents the necessity of good explanations to promote trust
   - Explain to the parents that the child may cry more openly when they are present but that their presence is important for promoting trust

B. Promote security with honest explanations and opportunities for choice

1. Promote open, honest communications
   - Tell the truth; explain
       How much it will hurt
       How long it will last
       What will help the pain
   - Do not threaten (*e.g., do not* tell the child, "If you don't hold still you won't go home")

- Explain to the child that the procedure is necessary so he can get better and it is important to hold still so it can be done quickly
- Discuss with the parents the importance of truth-telling; instruct parents to
    Tell child when they are leaving and when they will return
    Relate to the child that they cannot take away his pain but that they will be with him (except in circumstances when parents are not permitted to remain)
- Allow the parents opportunities to share their feelings about witnessing their child's pain and their helplessness

2. Prepare the child for a painful procedure
    - Discuss the procedure with the parents; determine what they have told the child
    - Explain the procedure in words suited to the child's age and developmental level (See *Altered Growth and Development* for age-related needs)
        Allow a two-year-old to watch you taking out sutures from a doll or stuffed animal
        Permit the child to hold instruments
    - Relate the discomforts that will be felt (*e.g.*, what the child will feel, taste, see or smell)
        "You will get an injection that will hurt for a little while and then it will stop"
        Be sure to explain when an injection will cause two discomforts: the prick of the needle and the absorption of the drug
    - Encourage the child to ask questions before and during the procedure; ask the child to share with you what he thinks is going to happen and why
    - Share with the child (who is old enough—over $3^{1}/_{2}$) that
        You expect that he will hold still and that it will please you if he can
        It is all right to cry or squeeze your hand if it hurts
    - Arrange to have parents present for procedures (especially for children 18 months to 5 years)

3. Reduce the pain during treatments when possible
    a. If restraints must be utilized, have sufficient personnel available in order not to delay the procedure
    b. When administering injections
        - Expect the child (over $2^{1}/_{2}$ or 3) to hold still
        - Have the child participate by holding the Band-Aid for you
        - Tell the child how pleased you are that he helped
        - Pull the skin surface as taut as possible (for IM)
        - Comfort the child after the procedure
        - Tell child step-by-step what is going to happen right before it is done
    c. Explain to the child that he can be distracted from the procedure if he wants (the use of distraction without the child's knowledge of the impending discomfort is not advocated because the child will learn to mistrust)
        - Tell a story with a puppet
        - Ask the child to name or count objects in a picture
        - Ask the child to look at the picture and to locate certain objects ("Where is the dog?")
        - Ask child to tell you about his pet
        - Ask child to count your blinks
    d. Avoid rectal temperatures in preschoolers; if possible, use electronic oral probes
    e. Provide the child with privacy during the painful procedure; utilize a treatment room rather than the child's bed

- The child's bed should be a "safe" place
- No procedures should be done in the playroom or schoolroom

4. Provide the child optimal pain relief with prescribed analgesics
   - Medicate child prior to painful procedure or activity (*e.g.*, ambulation)
   - Consult with physician for a change of the IM route to the IV route.
   - Assess for visual signs of pain, since child may not request pain medication because of fear of needle

5. Reduce or eliminate the common side-effects of narcotics
   a. Sedation
      - Assess if the cause is the narcotic, fatigue, sleep deprivation, or other drugs (sedatives, antiemetics)
      - If drowsiness is excessive, consult with physician to try a slight dose reduction
   b. Constipation
      - Explain to older children why pain medications cause constipation
      - Increase roughage in diet (*e.g.*, ask child what fruits he likes; sprinkle 1 teaspoon of bran on cereal)
      - Encourage child to drink eight to ten (8 oz) glasses of liquids each day
      - Teach child how to do abdominal isometric exercises if activity is restricted (*e.g.*, "Pull in your tummy; now relax your tummy; do this ten times each hour during the day")
      - Instruct child to keep a record of his exercises (*e.g.*, make a chart with a star sticker placed on it whenever the exercises are done)
      - Refer to *Constipation* for additional interventions
   c. Dry mouth
      - Explain to older children that narcotics decrease saliva production
      - Instruct to rinse mouth often, suck on sugarless sour candies, eat pineapple chunks and watermelon, drink liquids often
      - Explain the necessity of brushing his teeth after every meal

6. Assist the child with the aftermath of pain
   - Tell the child when the painful procedure is over
   - Pick up the small child to indicate it is over
   - Encourage the child to discuss his pain experience (draw or act out with dolls)
   - Encourage the child to perform the painful procedure using the same equipment on a doll under supervision (See Appendix IX for specific interventions)
   - Praise the child for his endurance and convey to him that he handled the pain well regardless of how he behaved (unless he was violent to others)
   - Give the child a souvenir of his pain (Band-Aid, badge for bravery)
   - Teach the child to keep a record of painful experiences and to place a star next to those he held still for (*e.g.*, gold stars on a paper for each injection or venipuncture)

7. Collaborate with child to initiate appropriate noninvasive pain relief modalities
   - Encourage mobility as much as indicated, especially when pain is at its lowest level
   - Discuss with child and parents activities that are liked and incorporate them in daily schedule (*e.g.*, clay modeling, painting)
   - Discuss with the child (over 7) that the pain can be less if the child thinks about something else and demonstrate the effects
      a. Ask child to count to 100 (or count your eye blinks)
      b. As child is counting, apply gentle pressure to Achilles tendon (pinch back of heel)
      c. Gradually increase the pressure

    d. Ask child to stop counting but keep pressure on heel

    e. Ask child if he can feel the discomfort in his heel now and if he felt it when he was counting

- Refer to guidelines for noninvasive pain relief measures (Appendix VI)

8. Assist the family to respond optimally to the child's pain experience

- Assess the family's knowledge of and response to the pain experience (*e.g.,* does the parent support the child who has pain?)
- Assure the parents that they can touch or hold their child, if feasible (*e.g.,* demonstrate that touching is possible even in the presence of tubes and equipment)
- Give accurate information to correct misconceptions (*e.g.,* the necessity of the treatment even though it causes pain)
- Provide parents with opportunities to discuss their fears, anger, frustrations in private
- Acknowledge the difficulty of the situation
- Incorporate the parents in the pain relief modality if possible (*e.g.,* stroking, massage, distraction)
- Praise their participation and their concern

C. Initiate health teaching and referrals if indicated

- Provide child and family with ongoing explanations
- Utilize the care plan to promote continuity of care for hospitalized child
- Refer parents to pertinent literature for themselves and children (See Bibliography)

Chronic Pain

Related to **(Specify)**

Definition

Chronic pain: The state in which an individual experiences pain that is persistent or intermittent and lasts for more than six months.

Defining Characteristics

Major (must be present)

The person reports that pain has existed for more than six months (may be the only assessment data present)

Minor (may be present)

    Discomfort

    Anger, frustration, depression because of situation

    Facial mask of pain

Anorexia, weight loss
Insomnia
Guarded movement
Muscle spasms
Redness, swelling, heat
Color changes in affected area
Reflex abnormalities

Chronic Pain
Related to (Specify)

Assessment

Subjective Data
The person reports that the following signs have existed for more than six months
Pain (may be the only assessment data present)
Discomfort
Anger, frustration, depression about situation

Objective Data
Facial mask of pain
Anorexia, weight loss
Insomnia
Guarded movement
Muscle spasms
Redness, swelling, heat
Color changes in affected area
Reflex abnormalities

Outcome Criteria

The person will
- Relate that others validate that the pain exists
- Practice selected noninvasive pain relief measures to manage his pain
- Relate improvement of pain and an increase in daily activities as evident by (specify)

Interventions

A. Assess the person's pain experience; determine the intensity of the pain at its worst and best

- Ask person to rate his pain using a scale of 0–10 (0 = absence of pain; 10 = worst pain) or a 0–5 scale

Rate it at its best
Rate it after a pain-relief measure
Rate it at its worst
- Collaborate with the individual to determine what methods could be utilized to reduce the intensity

B. Assess for factors which decrease pain tolerance

Disbelief on the part of others
Fear
Fatigue
Monotony

C. Reduce or eliminate factors that increase the pain experience

1. Disbelief of others
   a. Relate to the individual your acceptance of his response to pain
      - Acknowledge the presence of his pain
      - Listen attentively to him concerning his pain
      - Convey to him that you are assessing his pain because you want to better understand it, not determine if it is really present
   b. Assess the family for the presence of misconceptions about pain or its treatment
      - Explain the concept of pain as an individual experience
      - Discuss the reason why an individual may experience increased or decreased pain (*e.g.*, fatigue [increased] or presence of distractions [decreased])
      - Encourage family to share these concerns privately (*e.g.*, fear that the person will use his pain for secondary gains if they give him too much attention)
      - Assess if the family doubts the pain
      - Discuss the effects of this on the person's pain and on the relationship
      - Encourage family to give him attention also when he does not exhibit the pain
2. Provide person with accurate information to reduce his fears
   a. Fear of addiction
      - Explore with him the reasons for the fear
      - Explain the difference between drug tolerance and drug addiction
   b. Fear of losing control
      - Provide privacy for his pain experience
      - Attempt to limit the number of health care providers who provide care to him
   c. Fear that the medication will gradually lose its effectiveness
      - Discuss drug tolerance with him
      - Explain the use of combining noninvasive pain relief measures with medications
   d. Fear of family that the person will use his pain for secondary gains
      - Encourage family to share these concerns privately
      - If the family doubts the pain, discuss the effects of this on the person's pain experience and on their relationship
      - Encourage family to give him attention also when he does not exhibit pain
3. Fatigue
   - Determine the cause of fatigue (sedatives, analgesics, sleep deprivation)
   - Explain that pain contributes to stress, which increases fatigue
   - Assess the person's present sleep pattern and the influence of pain on his sleep
   - Provide opportunities to rest during the day and periods of uninterrupted sleep at night
   - Refer to *Sleep Pattern Disturbance* for specific interventions to enhance sleep

4. Monotony
   a. Discuss with the person and family the therapeutic uses of distraction, along with other methods of pain relief
   b. Emphasize that the degree to which an individual can be distracted from his pain is not at all related to the existence of or the intensity of the pain
   c. Explain that distraction usually increases pain tolerance and decreases pain intensity, but after the distraction ceases the individual may experience increased awareness of pain and fatigue
   d. Vary the environment if possible. If on bed rest:
      • Encourage personnel to wear seasonal pins and bright-colored apparel
      • Encourage family to decorate the room with flowers, plants, pictures
      • Provide the person with music
      • Consult with recreational therapist for an appropriate task
   e. If at home:
      • Encourage individual to plan an activity for each day, preferably outside the home
      • Discuss the possibility of learning a new skill (*e.g.*, a craft, a musical instrument)

D. Assess the effects of chronic pain on the individual's life, utilizing the person and his family

Performance (job, role responsibilities)
Social interactions
Finances
Activities of daily living (sleep, eating, mobility, sexuality)
Cognition/mood (concentration, depression)
Family unit (response of members)

E. Assist the person and his family to reduce the effects of depression on lifestyle
   • Encourage verbalization of individual and family concerning difficult situations
   • Listen carefully
   • Explain the relationship between chronic pain and depression
   • See *Ineffective Individual Coping* for additional interventions

F. Consult with the individual to determine what methods could be utilized to reduce the intensity of his pain
   • Before selecting a specific noninvasive pain relief method, consider the person's
      Willingness to participate (motivation)
      Ability to participate (dexterity, sensory loss)
      Preference
      Support of significant others for method
      Contraindications (allergy, health problem)
   • Consider the method's cost, complexity, precautions, and convenience
   • Explain the various noninvasive pain relief methods to the individual and his family and why they are effective (Appendix VI)

G. Collaborate with the individual to initiate the appropriate noninvasive pain relief measures (refer to Appendix VI for specific instructions on each method)

1. Relaxation techniques to reduce skeletal muscle tension that will reduce the intensity of the pain

- Utilize pillows and blankets to support the painful part to reduce the amount of muscle tension
- Promote relaxation with a back rub, massage, or a warm bath* (*e.g.*, for a person with a fractured limb, rub the opposite limb over the fractured site)
- Teach a specific relaxation strategy (*e.g.*, slow, rhythmic breathing or deep breath—clench fists—yawn)
- Enlist the aid of the family as coaches
- Discuss other techniques that can be learned (meditation, yoga, biofeedback, guided imagery)

2. Cutaneous stimulation
   - Discuss with the person the various methods of skin stimulation and their effects on pain (Appendix VI)
   - Discuss the use of heat applications,* their therapeutic effects and when indicated
   - Discuss each of the following methods and their precautions
         Hot water bottle
         Electric heating pad
         Electric light bulb
         Warm tub
         Moist heat pack
         Hot summer sun
         Thin plastic wrap over painful area to retain body heat (*e.g.*, knee, elbow)
   - Discuss the use of cold applications,* their therapeutic effects and when indicated
   - Discuss each of the following methods and their precautions
         Cold towels (wrung out)
         Cold-water immersion for small body parts
         Ice bag
         Cold gel pack
         Ice massage
   - Explain the therapeutic uses of
         Menthol preparations
         Massage/back rub
         Pressure
         Vibration
         Transcutaneous electric nerve stimulation (TENS)

3. Discuss with the person and the family the therapeutic uses of distraction along with other methods of pain relief
   - Emphasize that the degree to which an individual can be distracted from his pain is not at all related to the existence or intensity of the pain
   - Explain that distraction usually increases pain tolerance and decreases pain intensity, but after the distraction ceases the individual may experience increased awareness of pain and fatigue
   - If possible, use modalities that stimulate one or more of the major senses in a rhythmic manner
     a. Hearing: music, counting silently to self, being read to
     b. Vision: television, counting items in a picture or patterns on wallboard, reading (or telling) a story
     c. Touch and movement: massage, rocking, rhythmic breathing, stroking
   - Encourage the person to participate in activities that are pleasurable and time-consuming (*e.g.*, arts and crafts)

* May require a physician's order.

H. Provide the individual pain relief with prescribed analgesics*

1. Determine preferred route of administration: po, IM, IV, rectal (refer to Principles and Rationale for Nursing Care)
2. Assess the response to the medication
   a. For admitted persons
      - After administering a pain relief medication, return in one-half hour to assess effectiveness
      - Ask him to rate the severity of his pain prior to the medication and the amount of relief received
      - Ask him to indicate when the pain began to increase
      - Consult with the physician if a dosage or interval change is needed
   b. For outpatients
      - Ask him to keep a record of when he takes his medication and what kind of relief was received
      - Instruct him to consult his physician with questions concerning medication dosage
3. Encourage the use of po medications as soon as possible
   - Consult with physician for a schedule to change from IM to po
   - Explain to individual and family that oral medications can be as effective as IM
   - Explain how the transition will occur:
      a. Begin po medication at a larger dose than necessary (loading dose)
      b. Continue PRN IM medication
      c. Gradually reduce po medication dose
      d. Use the person's account of pain to regulate doses
   - Consult with physician for the possibility of adding aspirin or acetaminophen to the medication regime

I. Reduce or eliminate common side-effects of narcotics

1. Sedation
   - Assess if the cause is the narcotic, fatigue, sleep deprivation, or other drugs (sedatives, antiemetic)
   - Inform individual that drowsiness usually occurs the first 2 to 3 days then subsides
   - If drowsiness is excessive, consult with physician to try a slight dose reduction
2. Constipation
   - Explain the effect of narcotics on peristalsis
   - Consult with physician for the use of a stool softener with long-term drug use
   - Instruct person to always use the toilet or commode to have a bowel movement, in order to assume the correct position for defecation
   - Teach to increase roughage in diet (e.g., add 1 to 2 teaspoons of bran to food and increase fruit, whole grain breads, and cereal in diet)
   - Encourage to drink 8 to 10 glasses (8 oz) of liquids each day
   - Encourage daily exercises (e.g., walking, teach isometric exercises to individuals in bed)
   - Refer to Constipation for additional interventions
3. Nausea and Vomiting
   - Consult with physician for the appropriate antiemetic or for a change of narcotic that produces less nausea (e.g., morphine)
   - Instruct person that nausea will usually subside after a few doses

---

* May require a physician's order.

- Refrain from withholding narcotic dose because of nausea; rather, secure an order for an antiemetic.
- Encourage small, frequent amounts of ice chips or cool, clear liquids (dilute tea, Jell-O water, flat ginger ale, or Coke) unless vomiting continues (*e.g.*, adults 30–60 cc q ½–1 hr; children, 15–30 cc q ½–1 hr).
- Consider giving medications by suppository rather than by mouth
- Decrease the stimulation of the vomiting center by reducing unpleasant sights and odors and providing good mouth care after vomiting
- Instruct person to
  Practice deep breathing and voluntary swallowing to suppress the vomiting reflex
  Sit down after eating but not lie down
  Eat smaller meals; eat slowly
  Restrict liquids with meals to avoid overdistending the stomach; avoid drinking fluids 1 hour before and after meals
  If possible, avoid the smell of food preparation
  Try eating cold foods because they have less odor
  Avoid sweets and fried or fatty foods
  Eat salty foods if not contraindicated
  Loosen clothing
  Sit in fresh air
4. Dry mouth
   - Explain that narcotics decrease saliva production
   - Instruct to rinse mouth often, suck on sugarless sour candies, eat pineapple chunks or watermelon, and drink liquids often
   - Explain the necessity of good oral hygiene and dental care

J. Assist the family to respond optimally to the individual's pain experience
- Assess the family's knowledge of pain and of responses to the pain experience
- Give accurate information to correct family misconceptions (*e.g.*, addiction, doubt about pain)
- Provide individuals with opportunities to discuss their fears, anger, frustrations in private; acknowledge the difficulty of the situation
- Incorporate the family in the pain relief method if possible (*e.g.*, coaching relaxation, massaging)
- Encourage family to seek assistance if needed for specific problems, such as coping with chronic pain: family counselor; financial and service agencies (*e.g.*, American Cancer Society)

K. Promote optimal mobility
- Discuss the value of exercise to strengthen and stretch muscles, decrease stress, and promote sleep
- Assist individual to plan daily activities when pain is at its lowest level

L. Initiate health teaching and referrals as indicated; discuss with the individual and family the various treatment modalities available
  Family therapy
  Group therapy
  Behavior modification
  Biofeedback
  Hypnosis
  Acupuncture
  Exercise program

Pruritus

Related to **(Specify)**

Definition
Pruritus: The state in which an individual experiences an unpleasant, irritating cutaneous sensation of itching/burning that causes a desire to scratch.

Defining Characteristics
See *Altered Comfort*

Pruritus
Related to (Specify)

Assessment

Subjective Data

>The person reports itching/burning sensations and an urge to claw, scratch, or dig at body parts.
>
>The person reports fatigue.

Objective Data

>Scratch marks/redness (erythema)
>Dermographic streaks
>Restlessness, irritability
>Rubbing or scratching of body parts
>Rash or lesions/thickened skin

Outcome Criteria

The person will
- Verbalize decreased pruritus
- Describe causative factors when known
- Describe rationale and procedure for treatment

Interventions

A. Assess causative and contributing factors
- Skin care habits (home remedies)
- Exposure to a contagious disease (rubella, fungus)
- Exposure to chemical irritant (paints, oils, cleaning agents, cosmetics)
- Systemic disease (liver disease, diabetes, thyroid dysfunction, collagen disease, renal disease, leukemia, Hodgkin's disease)
- Parasites (pinworms, chiggers, ringworm)
- Hypersensitivity to drug, food, insect bite
- Psychogenic stress (acute or chronic)

B. Reduce or eliminate causative and contributing factors if possible
1. Maintain hygiene without producing dry skin
   - Baths should be given frequently
   - Use cool water when acceptable
   - Use mild soap (castile, lanolin) or a soap substitute
   - Blot skin dry; do not rub
   - Apply cornstarch lightly to skin folds by first sprinkling on hand (to avoid caking of powder); in bacterial or fungal conditions, use antifungal or antiyeast powder preparations
2. Prevent excessive dryness
   - Lubricate skin with Alpha Keri lotion unless contraindicated; pat on by hand or with gauze
   - Apply lubrication after bath to help moisture retention
   - Apply wet dressings continuously or intermittently to relieve itching and remove crusts and exudate
   - Provide 20- to 30-minute tub soaks with temperature of 32° to 38° C; water can contain oatmeal powder, Aveeno, cornstarch, or baking soda
3. Promote comfort and prevent further injury
   - Advise against scratching; explain the scratch-itch-scratch cycle
   - Secure order for topical corticosteroid cream for local inflamed pruritic areas; occlude area with plastic wrap at night to increase effectiveness of cream and prevent further scratching
   - Secure an antihistamine order if itching is unrelieved
   - Utilize mitts (or cotton socks) if necessary on children and confused adults
   - Maintained trimmed nails to prevent injury; file after trimming
   - Remove particles from bed (food crumbs, caked power)
   - Use old, soft sheets and avoid wrinkles in bed; if bed protector pads are used, place draw sheet over them to eliminate direct contact with skin
   - Avoid using perfumes and scented lotions
   - Avoid contact with chemical irritants/solutions
   - Wash clothes in a mild detergent and put through a second rinse cycle to reduce residue, avoid use of fabric softeners
   - Prevent excessive warmth by use of cool room temperatures and low humidity, light covers with bed cradle; avoid overdressing
   - Apply ointments with gloved or bare hand, depending on type, to lightly cover skin; rub creams into skin
   - Utilize frequent, thin applications of ointment rather than one thick application
4. In children
   - Explain to child why he shouldn't scratch

- Dress child in long sleeves, long pants, or a one-piece outfit to prevent scratching
- Avoid overdressing child, which will increase warmth
- Give child a tepid bath, before bedtime, add two cupsful of cornstarch to bath water
- Apply caladryl lotion to weeping pruritic lesions
- Use cotton blankets or sheets next to skin
- Remove furry toys that may increase lint and pruritus
- Teach child to press area that itches but not to scratch, or to put cool cloth on the area if permitted

C. Proceed with health teaching when indicated

- Explain causes of pruritus and possible methods to avoid causative factors
- Explain interventions that relieve symptoms
- Explain factors that increase symptoms
- Teach person to avoid fabrics that irritate skin (wool, coarse textures)
- Teach person to wear protective clothing (rubber gloves, apron) when using chemical irritants
- Refer for allergy-testing if indicated
- Provide opportunity to discuss frustrations
- For further interventions, refer to *Ineffective Individual Coping* if pruritus is stress-related.

Nausea/Vomiting

Related to **(Specify)**

Definition

Nausea: The state in which an individual experiences a sensation of abdominal heaviness, uneasiness with an inclination to vomit.

Author's Note: Acute nausea/vomiting is always a state of discomfort but not always a nutritional problem. When nausea/vomiting is persistent, the diagnostic category of *Altered Nutrition:* Less than body requirement related to nausea/vomiting would be indicated.

Defining Characteristics

Major (must be present)

Complains of "sickness of the stomach" or queasiness and an inclination to vomit

Minor (may be present)

Anorexia
Flushed or chills

Diaphoresis
Pallor
Increased salivation

Etiological, Contributing, Risk Factors

Pathophysiological
Fever
Infections (viral, bacterial, parasitic)
   GI
   Renal
   Infuenza
CNS disorders
   Meniere's Syndrome
   Labyrinthitis
Increased intracranial pressure
Cardiac disorders
   Acute myocardial infarction
Gastrointestinal/hepatic disorders
   Hiatal hernia
   Cholelithiasis
   Gastritis
   Pancreatitis
   Hepatitis
Endocrine disorders
   Diabetic acidosis
   Adrenal insufficiency
Anorexia nervosa, bulimarexia
Electrolyte imbalance
Cancer (biliary, hepatic, pancreatic)

Treatment-related
Side-effects of medications
   e.g.,
      Corticosteroids
      Cardiac glycosides
      Opitates
      Narcotics
      Chemotherapy
Radiation
Alcohol
Anesthesia

Situational (personal, environmental)
Pain
Noxious stimuli
   Odors
   Sights
Motion (car, airplane, boat)
Contaminated foods

Sounds
Tastes

Maturational
>   Children—fever, childhood diseases, *e.g.*, measles
>   Adolescents/adults—pregnancy

Focus Assessment Criteria

See *Altered Comfort*

Nausea/Vomiting
Related to (Specify)

Assessment

See Defining Characteristics

Assessment

Subjective Data

Person complains of feeling nauseated ("sick to my stomach"), vomiting

Objective Data

Vomiting

> **Outcome Criteria**
>
> The individual will
> • report decreased symptoms
> • describe relief measures during episodes

Interventions

A. Assess nausea and vomiting episodes
   • Duration
   • Frequency
   • Vomitus (amount/appearance)
   • Associated with
        Medications
        Meals
        Position
        Activity
        Time of day
        Pain (headache, earache, constipation)
        Specific foods
   • Relief measures (medications, food)

B. Institute measures to protect and comfort individual

1. Protect persons at risk for aspiration (immobile, children)
2. Address the cleanliness of the person and environment
3. Provide opportunity for oral care after each episode
4. Apply cool damp cloth to person's forehead, neck and wrists

C. Reduce or eliminate noxious stimuli

Pain
   • Plan care so that unpleasant or painful procedures do not take place before meals
   • Medicate individual for pain one-half hour before meals according to physician's orders
   • Provide pleasant, relaxed atmosphere for eating (no bedpans in sight; don't rush); try a "surprise" (*e.g.*, flowers with meal)
   • Arrange plan of care to decrease or eliminate nauseating odors or procedures near mealtimes

Fatigue
   • Teach or assist individual to rest before meals
   • Teach individual to spend minimal energy in food preparation (cook large quantities and freeze several meals at a time; request assistance from others)

Odor of food
   • Teach him to avoid cooking odors—frying foods, brewing coffee—if possible (take a walk; select foods that can be eaten cold)
   • Suggest using foods that require little cooking during periods of nausea

D. Decrease the stimulation of the vomiting center

• Reduce unpleasant sights and odors
• Provide good mouth care after vomiting
• Teach person to practice deep breathing and voluntary swallowing to suppress the vomiting reflex
• Instruct him to sit down after eating but not to lie down
• Encourage him to eat smaller meals and eat slowly
• Restrict liquids with meals to avoid overdistending the stomach; also avoid fluids 1 hour before and after meals
• If possible, avoid the smell of food preparation
• Try eating cold foods, which have less odor
• Loosen clothing
• Sit in fresh air
• Avoid lying down flat for at least two hours after eating (an individual who must rest should sit or recline so head is at least 4 in higher than feet)

E. Promote foods that stimulate eating and increase protein consumption

1. During acute episodes:
      Encourage frequent small amounts of ice chips or cool clear liquids (dilute tea, Jell-O water, flat ginger ale or cola) unless vomiting continues (adults 30–60 cc q ½–1 hr; children 15–30 cc q ½–1 hr)
      Consider giving medications by suppository rather than by mouth
2. Maintain good oral hygiene (brush teeth, rinse mouth) before and after ingestion of food
3. Offer frequent small feedings (six per day plus snacks) to reduce the feeling of a distended stomach
4. Allow individual to choose food items as close to actual eating time as possible

5. Arrange to have highest protein/calorie nutrients served at the time individual feels most like eating (*e.g.*, if chemotherapy is in early morning, serve in late afternoon)
6. Encourage significant others to bring in favorite home foods
7. Instruct person to
   - Eat dry foods (toast, crackers) upon arising
   - Eat salty foods if permissible
   - Avoid overly sweet, rich, greasy, or fried foods
   - Try clear, cool beverages
   - Sip slowly through straw (*e.g.*, soda water)
   - Take whatever he feels he can tolerate
   - Eat small portions, low in fat, and eat more frequently
   - Drink peppermint, spearmint, or raspberry tea
   - Eat yogurt or milk at night or before arising

F. Initiate health teaching and referrals as indicated

1. Teach techniques to individual and family for home food preparation to increase nutritional intake
   - Add powdered milk or egg to milkshakes, gravies, sauces, puddings, cereals, meatballs, or milk to increase protein-calorie content
   - Add blenderized or baby foods to meat juices or soups
   - Use fortified milk (*e.g.*, 1 c instant nonfat milk to 1 qt fresh milk)
   - Use milk or half and half instead of water when making soups and sauces; soy formulas can also be used
   - Add cheese or diced meat whenever able
   - Add cream cheese or peanut butter to toast, crackers, celery sticks
   - Add extra butter or margarine to soups, sauces, vegetables
   - Spread toast while hot
   - Use mayonnaise (100 cal/T) instead of salad dressing
   - Add sour cream or yogurt to vegetables or as dip
   - Use whipped cream (60 cal/T)
   - Add raisins, dates, nuts, and brown sugar to hot or cold cereals
   - Have extra food (snacks) easily available
   - Try commercial supplements available in many forms (liquid, powder, pudding); keep switching brands until some are found that are acceptable to individual in taste and consistency
2. Teach individuals experiencing chemotherapy to practice progressive relaxation twice a day and when receiving therapy. (Cotanch)
3. Teach that a variety of interventions have been reported to be helpful to control nausea when pregnant
   - Avoidance of fatigue
   - High-protein meals and snack before retiring
   - Carbohydrates (crackers) on arising
   - Carbonated beverages, coke syrup, orange juice, ginger ale and herbal teas
   - Lying down to relieve symptoms
4. Instruct the pregnant woman to try one food- or beverage-type relief measure at a time (*e.g.*, high-protein meals/bedtime snack); if nausea is not relieved, try another measure

References/Bibliography

Anderson J: Nursing management of the cancer patient in pain: A review of the literature. Cancer Nursing 5:33–41, 1982

Barber J: Hypnosis as a psychological technique in the management of cancer pain. Cancer Nursing 1:361–363, 1978

Beyerman K: Flawed perceptions about pain. Am J Nurs 82:302–304, 1982

Bray CA: Postoperative pain: Altering the patient's experience through education. AORN J 43(3):672, 674–5, 1986

Copley IJ: No matter what you call it, it's still pain to the patient. RN 41(2):64, 1978

Copp L: Pain coping model and typology. Image: J Nurs Schol 17(3)69–71, 1985

Davis AJ: Brompton's cocktail: Making good-byes possible. Am J Nurs 78:610–612, 1978

Dernham P: Phantom limb Pain, Geriat Nurs 7(1):34–37, 1986

Eland J: Pain management and comfort. J Gerontol Nurs 14(4):10–15, 1988

Evans M, Hansen B: Administering injections to different-age children. Matern Child Nurs J 6:194–199, 1981

Fagerbaugh S, Strauss A: How to manage your patient's pain . . . and how not to. Nursing 10(6):44–47, 1980

Foley K: The treatment of cancer pain. N Engl J Med 313(2):84–95, 1985

Hansen B, Evans M: Preparing a child for procedures. Matern Child Nurs J 6:392–397, 1981

Jacox AK (ed): Pain: A Source Book for Nurses and Other Professionals. Boston, Little, Brown & Co, 1977

Jacox AK: Assessing pain. Am J Nurs 79:895–900, 1979

Johnson JA, Repp EC: Nonpharmacologic pain management in arthritis. Nurs Clin North Am 19(4):583–591, 1984

Klisch ML: The Simonton method of visualization. Cancer Nurs 3:295–300, 1980

Krieger D: Therapeutic touch: The imprimatur of nursing. Am J Nurs 75:784–787, 1975

Kwentus J, Harkins S, Lignon N, Silverman J: Current concepts of geriatric pain and its treatment. Geriatrics 40(4):48–57, 1985

Lasagna L: The influences of age on analgesic pain relief. JAMA 218:1831–1833, 1971

Leuner H: Guided affective imagery. Am J Psychother 23:4–22, 1969

Lipman AJ: Drug therapy in cancer pain. Cancer Nurs 10:26–31, 1980

McCafferty M: Understanding your patient's pain. Nurs 10(4):26–31, 1980

McCafferty M: Nursing Management of the Patient with Pain, 2nd ed. Philadelphia, JB Lippincott, 1980

McGuire DB: Assessment of pain in cancer inpatients using the McGill Pain Questionnaire, Oncol Nurs Forum 11(6):32–7, Nov–Dec 1984

McGuire DB: Selecting an instrument to measure cancer related pain. Oncol Nurs Forum 11(6):85–87, 1984

Miller RR, Jick H: Clinical effects of meperidine in hospitalized medical patients. J Clin Pharmacol 18(4):180–189, 1978

Moseley JR: Alterations in comfort related to terminal illness. Nurs Clin North Am 20(2):427–438, 1985

Perry S, Heidrich G: Placebos. Am J Nurs 81:721–725, 1981

Porter J, Jick H: Addiction rate in patients treated with narcotics. N Engl J Med 302:123, 1980

Saunders C: Care of the dying: Control of pain in terminal cancer. Nurs Times 72:1133–1135, 1976

Silman J, Diblasi M, Washburn CJ: The management of pain. Am J Nurs 79:74–78, 1979

Storlie F: Pointers for assessing pain. Nursing 8(3):37–39, 1978

Wilson R, Elmassian B: Endorphins. Am J Nurs 81:722–725, 1981

Pruritus

Bruno P: Skin problems. In Carnevali D, Patrick M (eds): Nursing Management for the Elderly, pp 457–478. Philadelphia, JB Lippincott, 1979

Bulechek G, McCloskey J: Nursing Interventions: Treatments for Nursing Diagnoses. Philadelphia, WB Saunders, 1985

Callen JP, Starviski MA, Voorhees JJ: Cutaneous manifestations of systemic illness. In Manual of Dermatology, pp 129–161. Chicago, Year Book Medical Publishers, 1980

Jacobs M, Geels W: Signs and Symptoms in Nursing: Interpretation and Management. Philadelphia, JB Lippincott, 1985

Lever WF, Schaumburg-Lever G: Histopathology of the Skin. Philadelphia, JB Lippincott, 1983

Lisanti P: Altered integumentary functioning. In Mahoney EA, Flynn JP (eds): Handbook of Medical–Surgical Nursing, pp 203–209. New York, John Wiley and Sons, 1983

Pillsbury DM: A Manual of Dermatology. Philadelphia, WB Saunders, 1971

Sauer G: Manual of Skin Diseases, 4th ed. Philadelphia, JB Lippincott, 1980

Sutton RL, Waisman M: The Practitioners' Dermatology. Tampa, FL, Medical Books, 1975

Tucker S, Key M: Occupational skin disease. In Rom WM (ed): Environmental and Occupational Medicine, pp 301–311. Boston, Little, Brown & Co, 1983

Twycross RG, Lack SA: Symptom Control in Far Advanced Cancer: Pain Relief. Baltimore, Urban and Schwarzenberg, 1983

Nausea/Vomiting

Cotanch P, Strum S: Progressive muscle relaxation as antiemetic therapy for cancer patients. Oncol Nurs 14(1):33–37, 1987

Iorio C: The management of nausea and vomiting in pregnancy. Nurse Pract 13(5):23–28, 1988

Voda A, Randall M: Nausea and vomiting of pregnancy. In Norris C (ed): Concept Clarification in Nursing, Maryland, Aspen System, 1982

Children

Beyer JE, et aI: Patterns of postoperative analgesic use with adults and children following cardiac surgery. Pain 17(9):71–81, 1983

Ellis J: Using pain scales to prevent undermedication. Matern Child Nurs J 13(3):180–182, 1988

Eland JM, Anderson J: The experience of pain in children. In Jacox AK (ed): Pain; A Sourcebook for Nurses and Other Health Professionals, pp 453–473. Boston, Little, Brown & Co, 1977

O'Brien S, Konsler G: alleviating children's postoperative pain. Matern Child Nurs 13(3):183–186, 1988

Schechter N: Pain; Acknowledging it, assessing it, treating it. Contemp Pediatrics 4(7):16–46,1987

Communication, Impaired*

Related to **Hearing Loss**
Related to **Aphasia**
Related to **Foreign Language Barrier**

Communication, Impaired Verbal

Related to **Impaired Ability to Articulate Words**

> **Author's Note:** This diagnostic category represents communication problems that involve both sending and receiving messages (talking and listening).

Communication, Impaired*

Related to **Hearing Loss**
Related to **Aphasia**
Related to **Foreign Language Barrier**

Definition

Impaired communication: The state in which the individual experiences, or could experience, a decreased ability to send or receive messages (*i.e.,* he has difficulty exchanging thoughts, ideas, or desires).

* This diagnostic category is not currently on the NANDA list but has been included for clarity or usefulness.

Defining Characteristics

Major (must be present)
Inappropriate or absent speech or response

Minor (may be present)
>   Stuttering
>   Slurring
>   Problem in finding the correct word when speaking
>   Weak or absent voice
>   Decreased auditory comprehension
>   Deafness or inattention to noises or voices
>   Confusion
>   Inability to speak dominant language

Etiological, Contributing, Risk Factors

Pathophysiological
>   Cerebral impairment
>>   Expressive or receptive aphasia
>>   Cerebrovascular accident
>>   Brain damage (*e.g.*, birth/head trauma)
>>   CNS depression/increased intracranial pressure
>>   Tumor (of the head, neck, or spinal cord)
>>   Mental disabilities
>>   Chronic hypoxia/decreased cerebral blood flow
>   Neurologic impairment
>>   Quadriplegia
>>   Nervous system diseases (*e.g.*, myasthenia gravis, multiple sclerosis)
>>   Vocal cord paralysis
>>   Auditory nerve damage
>   Respiratory impairment (*e.g.*, shortness of breath)
>   Auditory impairment (decreased hearing)
>   Laryngeal edema/infection
>   Oral deformities
>>   Cleft lip or palate
>>   Malocclusion or fractured jaw
>>   Missing teeth

Treatment-related
>   Surgery
>>   Endotracheal intubation
>>   Tracheostomy/tracheotomy/laryngectomy
>>   Surgery of the head, face, neck, or mouth
>>   Pain (especially of the mouth or throat)
>>   Drugs (*e.g.*, CNS depressants, anesthesia)

Situational (personal, environmental)
>   Fatigue (affecting ability to listen)
>   No access to hearing aid/malfunction of hearing aid

Speech pathology
Stuttering
Lisping
Ankyloglossia ("tongue-tie")
Voice problems
Language barrier (unfamiliar language or dialect)
Psychological barrier (*e.g.*, fear, shyness)
Lack of privacy
Lack of support system
Loss of recent memory recall

Maturational

Elderly (auditory losses)
Infants
Children

Focus Assessment Criteria

Subjective Data

1. Note the usual pattern of communication as described by the person or his family

Very verbal	Speaks only when spoken to
Sometimes verbal	Does not speak/respond
Sign language	Responds inappropriately
Writes only	Gestures only

- Does the person feel he has difficulty hearing or has he ever worn a hearing aid?
- Does the person feel he is communicating normally today?
- If not, what does he feel may help him to communicate better?
- Is there a specific person he would like to talk with or have present to help him express ideas?

2. Does the person feel he can usually express himself well?
3. Does the person feel there are barriers hindering his ability to communicate?
   Lack of privacy
   Fear of uncertain origin
   Fear of being inappropriate or "stupid"
   Not enough time to gather his thoughts and ask questions
   Need for presence of significant other or familiar face
   Language, dialect, or cultural barrier (specify)
   Lack of knowledge of subject being discussed
   Pain, stress, or fatigue

Objective Data

1. Describe the person's ability to form words

Good	Weak (whisper)
Slurred	Absent
Lisping	Language barrier
Stuttering	Difficulty breathing and talking
Slow	

2. Describe the person's ability to comprehend
   Understands simple commands or ideas
   Able to follow complex instructions or ideas

Sometimes able to follow instructions or ideas
Not able to follow simple instructions or ideas
Understands only if hearing aid is working
Understands only if he can see your mouth (lip-reads)
3. What is the person's developmental age?

Infant	Child	Adult
Toddler	Adolescent	Aged

4. Describe the person's ability to make sentences

Good	Unclear ideas	Can make short,
Slow	Nonsensical or	simple sentences
Weak	confused	Language barrier

5. How does the person's affect or manner appear to you?

Nervous	Fearful	Pained
Anxious	Withdrawn	Uncomfortable
Attentive	Flat	Comfortable

6. Does the person maintain eye contact?

Good	Occasional	None

7. Are there contributing factors that may inhibit the person's ability to communicate?
Alterations in thought processes (*e.g.*, memory deficit, psychosis)
Pain, stress, or fatigue
Oral, facial, or neck deformity (or surgery)
Breathing impairment
Auditory impairment
Visual impairment
CNS depression
Vocal cord paralysis
Muscle paralysis
Expressive aphasia
Receptive aphasia

Principles and Rationale for Nursing Care

General

1. Speech is man's fundamental way of expressing needs, desires, and feelings. Poor communication can cause feelings of frustration, anger, hostility, depression, fear, confusion, and isolation.
2. Communication is affected by eye contact, loudness and intonation of voice, facial expression, and proximity of the communicators.
3. Communication may be hampered by lack of privacy.
4. Good communicators are also good listeners, who listen for both facts and feelings.
5. Silence may signify either acceptance, defiance, a delay in wishing to comment, or a needed break to gather thoughts. Allowing silence may enhance communication.
6. To be sure a message is understood, one should have the receiver repeat what has been said. A reply of "Yes" or "I understand" may not be enough.
7. People should overcome the human tendency to shout or "talk down" to a person who is verbally handicapped. Impaired verbal speech does not necessarily signify impairment of intelligence or of the ability to hear and understand.
8. Dysarthria is a disturbance in the voluntary muscular control of speech caused by conditions such as Parkinson's disease, multiple sclerosis, myasthenia gravis, cere-

bral palsy and CNS damage. The same muscles are used in eating and swallowing. Persons with dysarthria usually do not have problems with comprehension.

Hearing Loss

1. Lip-reading takes a great deal of skill and concentration. Pain, stress, or fatigue may impair the individual's ability to read lips.
2. People who suffer from deafness are prone to social isolation because of their difficulty in communicating with people who can hear normally.
3. Many people over 65 suffer from some sort of hearing loss.
4. Using written communication frequently offers a good alternative method of communicating for the person who is hard of hearing.
5. Hearing aids magnify *all* sounds. Therefore extraneous sounds (*e.g.,* rustling of papers, minor squeaks, etc.) can inhibit understanding of voiced messages.

Aphasia

1. Aphasia is an altered ability to communicate because of cerebral damage. The alterations can be verbal, gestural, visual, or graphic.
2. Expressive aphasia is a disturbance in the ability to speak, write, or gesture understandably.
3. Receptive aphasia is a disturbance in the ability to comprehend written and spoken language.
4. The person with receptive aphasia may have intact hearing but cannot process or is unaware of his own sounds.
5. People with head trauma or aphasia may have difficulty with retention and memory recall. Old memories may return first, with memory recall of recent events returning last.
6. Emotional lability (swings between crying and laughing) is common to persons with aphasia. This behavior is not intentional and declines with recovery.

Cultural or Foreign Language Barriers

1. Knowledge of a foreign language depends upon four elements: The knowledge of how to speak the language in conversation, the ability to understand the language in conversation, the ability to read the language, and the ability to write the language.
2. An answer of "yes" from a foreigner may be an effort to please rather than a sign of understanding what has been said.
3. Even though the nurse cannot speak another's language, she can convey a climate of acceptance by talking in a pleasant tone of voice and using actions to demonstrate meaning (*e.g.,* smiling and motioning to sit down, while saying, "Sit down, please.")
4. An attempt on the nurse's part to communicate over a language barrier encourages a foreign individual to do the same.
5. People should overcome the human tendency either to ignore or shout at people who do not speak the dominant language.
6. Appropriate distance between communicators varies from culture to culture. Some may normally stand face to face, while others must stand several feet apart to be comfortable.
7. Communicating through the use of touch or holding varies from culture to culture. For example, some cultures view touching as an extremely familiar gesture, some cultures shy away from touching a given part of the body (a pat on the head may be offensive), and some cultures consider it appropriate for men to kiss each other and for women to hold hands.

Impaired Communication
Related to Hearing Loss

Assessment

Subjective Data

> The person reports that he has difficulty hearing.
> The person reports that he should be wearing a hearing aid.
> The person uses sign language/gestures only.

Objective Data

> The person wears a hearing aid.
> The person does not respond to sound/voices.
> The person responds inappropriately to spoken words.
> The person is inattentive much of the time.
> The person shouts much of the time.

Outcome Criteria

The person will
- Wear a hearing aid (if appropriate)
- Receive messages through alternative methods (*e.g.*, written communication, sign language, speaking distinctly into "good" ear)
- Relate/demonstrate an improved ability to communicate

Interventions

A. Assess the person's ability to receive verbal messages

1. If he can hear with a hearing aid, make sure that it is on and functioning.
   - Check batteries by turning volume all the way up until it whistles. (If it does not whistle, new batteries should be inserted.)
   - Make sure volume is at a level that enhances hearing. (Many people with hearing aids turn the volume down from time to time for peace and quiet.)
   - Make a special effort to have the patient wear his hearing aid on off-the-unit visits. (For example, the hearing aid should be on when the patient goes for special studies, or to the operating room, and the chart should be flagged so that everyone is aware of this.)
2. If he can hear with only one ear, speak slowly and *clearly* directly into the good ear. (It is more important to speak *distinctly* than to speak loudly.)
   - If the person is admitted to the hospital, place him so that his good ear faces the door.
   - Approach the person from the side on which he hears best (*i.e.*, if he hears better with his left ear, approach him from the left).
3. If the person can lip-read:
   - Look directly at the person and talk slowly and clearly.

- Avoid standing in front of light—have the light on your face so that the person can see your lips.
- Minimize distractions that may inhibit the person's concentration.
  - Minimize conversations if the person is fatigued, or use written communication.
  - Reinforce important communications by writing them down.
4. If he can read and write, provide pad and pencil at all times (even when he goes to the radiology department, etc.)
5. If he can understand only sign language, have an interpreter with him as much as possible.
6. If the person is in a group (*e.g.*, diabetes class), place him in the front of the room near the teacher.

B. Utilize factors that promote hearing and understanding

1. Talk distinctly and clearly, facing the person.
2. Minimize unnecessary sounds in the room:
   - Have only one person talk.
   - Be aware of background noises (*e.g.*, close the door, turn off the television or radio).
3. Repeat, then rephrase a thought, if the person does not seem to understand the whole meaning.
4. Use touch and gestures to enhance communication.
5. Encourage the person to maintain contact with other deaf people to minimize feelings of social isolation.

Impaired Communication
Related to Aphasia

Aphasia is a communication impairment—a difficulty in expressing, a difficulty in understanding, or a combination of both—resulting from cerebral impairments.

Outcome Criteria

The person will
- Demonstrate increased ability to understand
- Demonstrate improved ability to express himself
- Relate decreased frustration with communication

Assessment

Subjective Data
The person reports:
   An inability to express self

A difficulty in responding verbally
History of
 Cerebrovascular accident
 Tumor
 Cerebral trauma/increased intracranial pressure

Objective Data
Slurred speech
Unintelligible speech
Inappropriate responses to questions

Interventions

A. Identify a method the person can use to communicate basic needs
1. Assess ability to comprehend, speak, read, and write
2. Provide alternative methods of communication
   - Use pad and pencil, alphabet letters, hand signals, eye blinks, head nods, bell signals
   - Make flash cards with pictures or words depicting frequently used phrases (*e.g.*, "Wet my lips," "Move my foot," glass of water, bedpan)
   - Encourage person to point, use gestures, and pantomime
   - Consult with speech pathologist for assistance in acquiring flash cards

B. Identify factors that promote communication
1. Create atmosphere of acceptance and privacy
2. Provide a non-rushed environment
   - Use normal loudness level and speak unhurriedly, in short phrases
   - Encourage the person to take his time talking and to enunciate words carefully with good lip movements
   - Decrease external distractions
   - Delay conversation when the person is tired
3. Assess the individual's frustration level and do not push beyond it
   - Estimate 30 seconds of passed time before providing the individual with the word he may be trying to find (except when the person is frustrated or needs the request immediately, *e.g.*, bedpan)
   - Provide cues through pictures or gestures
4. Utilize techniques to increase understanding
   - Face the individual and establish eye contact if possible
   - Use uncomplicated one-step commands and directives
   - Have only one person talk (it's more difficult to follow a multisided conversation)
   - Encourage the use of gestures and pantomime
   - Match words with actions; use pictures
   - Terminate conversation on a note of success (*e.g.*, move back to an easier item)

C. Utilize techniques that enhance verbal expression
1. Make a concerted effort to understand when the person is speaking
   - Allow enough time to listen if the person speaks slowly
   - Rephrase his message aloud to him in order to validate it
   - Respond to all attempts at speech even if they are unintelligible (*e.g.*, "I do not know what you are saying. Can you try to say it again?")

- Acknowledge when you understand, and do not be concerned with imperfect pronunciation at first
- Ignore mistakes and profanity
- Don't pretend you understand if you don't
- Observe the person's nonverbal cues for validation (*e.g.*, he answers yes and shakes his head no)
- Allow the person time to respond; do not interrupt; supply words only occasionally

2. Teach techniques to improve speech
   - Ask the person to slow speech down, and say each word clearly, while providing the example
   - Encourage the person to speak in short phrases
   - Explain to the person that his words are not clearly understood (*e.g.*, "I can't understand what you are saying")
   - Suggest a slower rate of talking, or taking a breath prior to speech
   - Encourage the person to take his time and concentrate on forming his words
   - Ask the person to write down his message, or to draw a picture, if verbal communication is difficult
   - Encourage the person to speak in short phrases
   - Ask questions that can be answered with a yes or no
   - Focus on the present; avoid topics that are controversial, emotional, abstract, or lengthy

D. Acknowledge the individual's frustration

1. Verbally address the problem of frustration over inability to communicate, and explain that patience is needed for both the nurse and the person who is trying to talk
2. Maintain a calm, positive attitude (*e.g.*, "I can understand you if we work at it")
3. Use reassurance (*e.g.*, "I know it's hard, but you'll get it"); use touch if acceptable
4. Maintain a sense of humor
5. Allow tears (*e.g.*, "It's OK. I know it's frustrating. Crying can let it all out")
6. For the person who has a limited ability to talk (*i.e.*, can make simple requests, but not lengthy statements), encourage writing letters or keeping a diary to ventilate feelings and share concerns
7. Give the person opportunities to make decisions about his care (*e.g.*, "Do you want a drink? Would you rather have orange juice or prune juice?")
8. Provide alternative methods of self-expression
   - Humming/singing
   - Dancing/exercising/walking
   - Writing/drawing/painting/coloring
   - Helping (tasks such as opening mail, choosing meals)

E. Identify factors that promote comprehension

1. Assess hearing ability and use of functioning hearing aids
2. Assess ability to see, and encourage the person to wear his glasses
   - Explain to the person that seeing better will increase understanding of what is happening around him
   - Even if the person is blind, look at him when talking to "throw" voice in his direction
3. Provide sufficient light and remove distractions (see *Sensory-Perceptual Alterations*)
4. Speak when the person is ready to listen

- Achieve eye contact, if possible
- Gain the person's attention by a gentle touch on the arm and a verbal message of "Listen to me" or "I want to talk to you"
5. Modify your speech
   - Speak slowly, enunciate distinctly
   - Use common adult words
   - Do not change subjects or ask multiple questions in succession
   - Repeat or rephrase requests
   - Do not increase volume of voice unless person has hearing deficit
   - Match your nonverbal behavior with your verbal actions—to avoid misinterpretation (*e.g.*, do not laugh with a coworker while performing a task)
   - Try to use the same words with the same task (*e.g.*, bathroom vs. toilet, pill vs. medication)
   - Keep a record at bedside of the words to maintain continuity
   - As the person improves, allow him to complete your sentences (*e.g.*, "This is a ... [pill]")
6. Utilize other methods of communication besides verbal
   - Use pantomime
   - Point
   - Use flash cards
   - Show him what you mean (*e.g.*, pick up a glass)
   - Write key words on a card, so he can practice them while you show the object (*e.g.*, paper, toilet)

F. Show respect when providing care

1. Avoid discussing the person's condition in his presence; assume he can understand despite his deficits
2. Monitor other health care providers
3. Talk to the person whenever you are with him

G. Initiate health teaching and referrals if indicated

1. Teach techniques to significant others and repetitive approaches to improve communications
2. Encourage the family to share feelings concerning communication problems
   - Explain the reasons for labile emotions and profanity
   - Explain the need to include the person in family decision-making
3. Seek consultation with a speech pathologist early in treatment regime

---

Impaired Communication
Related to Foreign Language Barriers

Assessment

Subjective Data
The person states
    "I don't understand ... [name of language]"
    "I don't speak ... [name of language]"

Objective Data

Foreign accent
Absence of speech
Body language only means of communication (person only nods or gestures)

Outcome Criteria

The person will
- Be able to communicate basic needs
- Relate feelings of acceptance, reduced frustration and isolation

---

Interventions

A. Assess the individual's ability to communicate in English*

1. Assess what language the person speaks best
2. Assess the person's ability read, write, speak, and comprehend English

B. Identify factors that promote communication through a language barrier when a translator is not present

1. Face the person and give a pleasant greeting, in a normal tone of voice
2. Talk clearly and somewhat slower than normal (do not overdo it)
3. If the person does not understand or speak (respond), use alternative method of communication
   - Try writing down message
   - Use gestures or actions
   - Use pictures or drawings
   - Make flash cards that translate words or phrases
4. Encourage the person to also use the aforementioned methods of communication (try to overcome shyness)
5. Encourage the person to teach others some of the words or greetings of his own language (this helps to promote a feeling of acceptance and a willingness to learn)

C. Be cognizant of possible cultural barriers

1. Be careful when touching the person, for it may not be appropriate in some cultures
2. Be aware of the different ways that men and women are expected to be treated (cultural differences may influence whether a man speaks to a woman about certain matters, or vice versa)
3. Make a conscious effort to be nonjudgmental about another's cultural differences
4. Make note of what seems to be a comfortable distance from which to speak

D. Initiate referrals when needed

1. Use a *fluent* translator when discussing matters of importance (such as taking a health history or signing an operation permit)
2. If possible, allow the translator to spend as much time as the person wishes (be flexible with visitor's rules and regulations)
3. If a translator is not available, try to plan a daily visit from someone who has some

---

* English will be used as an example of the dominant language.

knowledge of the person's language (many hospitals and social welfare offices keep a "language" bank with names and phone numbers of people who are willing to translate)

Communication, Impaired Verbal

Related to **Impaired Ability to Articulate Words**

Definition

Impaired verbal communication: The state in which the individual experiences, or could experience, a decreased ability to speak but can understand others.

Defining Characteristics

Major (one must be present)
 Inability to speak words but can understand others
 Articulation or motor planning deficits

Minor (may be present)
 Shortness of breath

Etiological, Contributing, Risk Factors

See *Impaired Communication*

Focus Assessment Criteria

See *Impaired Communication*

Principles and Rationale for Nursing Care

See *Impaired Communication*

Impaired Verbal Communication
Related to Impaired Ability to Articulate Words

Assessment

Subjective Data

The person reports inability or difficulty in pronouncing words

Objective Data

Difficulty in pronouncing words
Inability to use voice
    Post-laryngectomy   Tracheostomy
    Intubation   Decreased ventilatory capacity

Outcome Criteria

The person will
- Demonstrate improved ability to express self
- Relate decreased frustration with communication

Interventions

A. Identify a method by which person can communicate his basic needs

1. Assess ability to comprehend, speak, read, and write
2. Provide alternative methods of communication
   - Use pad and pencil, alphabet letters, hand signals, eye blinks, head nods, bell signals
   - Make flash cards with pictures or words depicting frequently used phrases (*e.g.,* "Wet my lips," "Move my foot," glass of water, bedpan)
   - Encourage the person to point, use gestures, and pantomime
   - Consult with speech pathologist for assistance in acquiring flash cards

B. Identify factors that promote communication

1. For individuals with dysarthria
   - Reduce environmental noise to increase the caregiver's ability to listen to words (*e.g.,* radio, TV)
   - Do not alter your speech or messages, since his comprehension is not affected; speak on an adult level
   - Encourage the person to make a conscious effort to slow down his speech and to speak louder (*e.g.,* "Take a deep breath between sentences")
   - Ask him to repeat words that are unclear; observe for nonverbal cues to help understanding
   - If he is tired, ask questions that require only short answers
   - If speech is unintelligible, teach the person to use gestures, written messages, and communication cards
2. For individuals who cannot speak (*e.g.,* endotracheal intubation, tracheostomy)
   - Reassure that his speech will return, if it will
   - If not, explain what alternatives are available (*e.g.,* esophageal speech, sign language)
   - Do not alter your speech, tone, or type of message, since the person's ability to understand is not affected; speak on an adult level
   - Read lips for cues

C. Promote continuity of care to reduce frustration

1. Observe for signs of frustration or withdrawal
   - Verbally address the problem of frustration over inability to communicate, and

explain that patience is needed for both the nurse and the person who is trying to talk

- Maintain a calm, positive attitude (*e.g.,* "I can understand you if we work at it")
- Use reassurance (*e.g.,* "I know it's hard, but you'll get it")
- Maintain a sense of humor
- Allow tears (*e.g.,* "It's OK. I know it's frustrating. Crying can let it all out")
- For the person who has a limited ability to talk (*e.g.,* can make simple requests, but not lengthy statements), encourage writing letters or keeping a diary to ventilate feelings and share concerns
- Anticipate needs and ask questions that need a simple yes or no answer

2. Maintain a specific care plan
   - Write the method of communication that is used (*e.g.,* "Uses word cards," "Points to night stand for bedpan")
   - Record directions for specific measures to reduce communication problems (*e.g.,* allow him to keep urinal in bed)

D. Initiate health teaching and referrals as indicated

- Teach significant others techniques and repetitive approaches to improve communications
- Encourage the family to share feelings concerning communication problems
- Seek consultation with a speech pathologist early in treatment regime

References/Bibliography

Communication, Impaired

Auvil C: Reflections: The sound of silence. Am J Nurs (84)8:1072, 1984
Bushweller E: Bridging the communication gap. Nursing (14)9:112, 1984
Campbell S: Some sound advice for managing a hearing impaired patient. Nursing (14)12:46, 1984
Conture E: Stuttering. Englewood Cliffs, NJ, Prentice-Hall, 1982
DeVilleous L: What to do when you just can't communicate. Nurs Life 2(2):34–32, 1982
Dreher B: Overcoming speech and language disorders. Geriatr Nurs 2:345–349, 1981
Freemaond C, Hefferin C: Are you out of touch with your patients? RN (47)4:51–53, 1984
Forbes B: Let your actions do the talking. Nursing (14)3:112, 1984
Giarratona C: Reach out and touch Henry. Nursing (14) 12:47–49, 1984
Hanawalt A, Troutman K: If your patient has a hearing aid. Am J Nurs (84)7:900–901, 1984
Jungman L: When your feelings get in the way. Am J Nurs 79:1074–1075, 1979
Kyes J: Pseudocommunication is the nurse–patient game. Nursing Life: 2(1)50–54, 1982
Leonard R: Speak for yourself. Nursing 15(11):30–31, 1985
Patry-Lahey R: Helping a laryngectomy patient go home. Nursing 15(3):63–64, 1985
Ragnakers MJ: Communications blocks revisited. Am J Nurs 79:1079–1081, 1979
Santopietro M: How to get through to a refugee patient. Nursing 11(1):43–48, 1981
Steffe D: More than a touch: Communicating with a blind and deaf patient. Nursing 15(8):36–39, 1985
Van Riper C: Speech Correction 6 E. Englewood Cliffs, NJ, Prentice-Hall, 1982
Watkins S et al: Clearing impacted ears. Am J Nurs 84(9):1107, 1984
Weinhouse I: Speaking to the needs of your aphasic patient. Nursing 11(3):34–36, 1981

Resources for the Consumer

Organizations

Agency for Hearing Loss:
Write: Alexander Graham Bell Association
3417 Volta Place N.W.
Washington D.C. 20007

Coping, Ineffective Individual

Related to **Depression in Response to Identifiable Stressors**

Defensive Coping

Related to **(Specify)**

Ineffective Denial

Related to **(Specify)**

Author's Note: This diagnostic category can be used to describe a variety of situations in which an individual does not adapt effectively to stressors. Examples can be isolating behaviors, aggression, destructive behavior, etc. If the response is inappropriate use of the defense mechanism, denial or defensiveness, the diagnosis *Ineffective Denial* or *Defensive Coping* can be used instead of *Ineffective Individual Coping*.

Coping, Ineffective Individual

Definition

Ineffective individual coping: A state in which the individual experiences or is at risk of experiencing an inability to manage internal or environmental stressors adequately due to inadequate resources (physical, psychological, behavioral and/or cognitive).

Defining Characteristics*

Major (one must be present)

Change in usual communication patterns (if acute)
Verbalization of inability to cope
Inappropriate use of defense mechanisms
Inability to meet role expectations

Minor (may be present)

Anxiety
Reported life stress
Inability to problem-solve
Alteration in social participation
Destructive behavior towards self or others
High incidence of accidents
Frequent illnesses
Verbalization of inability to ask for help
Verbal manipulation
Inability to meet basic needs

Etiological and Contributing Factors

Pathophysiological

Changes in body integrity
   Loss of body part
   Disfigurement secondary to trauma
Altered affect caused by changes in body chemistry
   Tumor (brain)
   Injection of mood-altering substance
Physiological manifestations of persistent stress

Situational (personal, environmental)

Changes in physical environment
   War
   Natural disaster
   Relocation
   Seasonal work (migrant worker)
   Poverty

* Adapted from Vincent (see Bibliography)

Disruption of emotional bonds due to
- Death
- Separation or divorce
- Desertion

- Relocation
- Incarceration

Unsatisfactory support system

Institutionalization
- Jail
- Foster home
- Orphanage

- Educational institution
- Maintenance institution for disabled

Sensory overload
- Factory environment

- Urbanization: crowding, noise pollution, excessive activity

Inadequate psychological resources
- Poor self-esteem
- Excessive negative beliefs about self

- Helplessness
- Lack of motivation to respond

Culturally related conflicts with life experiences
- Premarital sex
- Abortion

Treatment-related

Separation from family and home (*e.g.*, hospitalization, nursing home)
Conflict between need for medical treatment and culture
Disfigurement due to surgery
Altered in appearance due to drugs, radiation, or other treatment
Altered affect due to hormonal therapy
Sensory overload due to medical technology (*e.g.*, critical care units)

Maturational

Child
- Developmental tasks (independence vs. dependence)
- Entry into school

- Competition among peers
- Peer relationships

Adolescent
- Physical and emotional changes
- Independence from family
- Heterosexual relationships

- Sexual awareness
- Educational demands
- Career choices

Young adult
- Career choices
- Educational demands
- Leaving home

- Marriage
- Parenthood

Middle adult
- Physical signs of aging
- Career pressures
- Child-rearing problems

- Problems with relatives
- Social status needs
- Aging parents

Elderly
- Physical changes
- Changes in financial status
- Change in residence

- Retirement
- Response of others to older people

Focus Assessment Criteria

Ineffective coping can be manifested in a variety of ways. A person or family may respond with an alteration in another life process (*e.g.,* spiritual distress, altered parenting, potential for violence). The nurse should be aware of this and use assessment data to ascertain the dimensions affected.

Subjective Data

Self-concept
>   "How would you describe yourself?"
>   "What do you like (dislike) about yourself?"

Support system
>   "To whom do you turn or usually go for help when you have a problem?" (See *Altered Family Processes* for additional data)

Emotional status
>   "How would you describe your usual emotional state?"
>   "What can cause a change in your usual state of mind?"
>   "How would you describe your current life situation?"

Problem-solving abilities
>   "When you have a problem, how do you usually deal with it?"

Presence of stress-related symptoms:
>   Cardiovascular
>> Headache

Fainting (blackouts, spells)

>   Gastrointestinal
>> Nausea
>> Vomiting
>> Abdominal pain
>>   (cramps, stomach ache)

Change in appetite
Change in stool

>   Respiratory
>> Shortness of breath

Chest discomfort
  (pain, tightness, ache)

>   Musculoskeletal
>> Pain
>> Weakness

Fatigue

>   Genitourinary
>> Menstrual changes
>> Urinary discomforts (pain,
>>   burning, urgency, hesitancy)

Sexual difficulty (pain,
  impotence, altered libido,
  anorgasmia)

>   Dermatological
>> Itching
>> Rash

"Sweats"

>   Psychiatric
>> Anxiety
>> Panic

"The blues"
"Bad nerves"

Objective Data

>   Appearance
>> Altered affect ("Poker" face)
>> Appropriate

Poor grooming
Inappropriate dress

>   Behavior
>> Calm

Tearful

Hostile	Sudden mood swings
Withdrawn	

Cognitive function
  Altered orientation to time, place, person
  Impaired concentration
  Altered ability to problem-solve
Presence of stress-related disorders (common examples):
  Cardiovascular—migraine headache
  Gastrointestinal—irritable bowel syndrome, obesity
  Respiratory—COPD associated with tobacco use, asthma
  Musculoskeletal—chronic low back pain syndrome, muscle tension headache
  Genitourinary—psychogenic impotence in males
  Dermatological—idiopathic urticaria (hives), eczema
  Psychiatric—chronic depression, anxiety disorder, panic attack disorder
Abusive behaviors
  To self
    Excessive smoking
    Excessive alcohol intake
    Excessive food intake
    Drug abuse
    Reckless driving
  To others
    Doesn't care
    Neglects needs of dependent family members
    Is unwilling to listen
    Doesn't communicate
    Imposes physical harm on family member (bruises, burns, broken bones)

Principles and Rationale for Nursing Care

Concepts Related to the Nature of Coping

1. Coping refers to psychological and behavioral activities made to master, tolerate, or minimize external or internal demands and conflicts (Lazarus).
2. Coping effectively requires successful management of many tasks: maintenance of self-concept, maintenance of satisfying relationships with others, maintenance of emotional balance, and management of stress.
3. There is no one way to cope with all situations.
4. There are two basic types of coping behavior (Lazarus): problem-focused—manipulation of the persons and environmental factors inducing stress—and emotion-focused—the management of stress-related emotions. Examples follow:

Problem-focused	*Emotion-focused*
1. Make appointment with the boss to discuss pay raise	1. Play basketball three times per week
2. Write out time schedule for homework and adhere to it	2. Allow myself to cry when I get home
	3. Practice yoga daily

5. Appraisal is the thought process that evaluates the situation. Constructive realistic appraisal strategies can be facilitated with the following questions: What is at stake? What are the choices? Where is there help?

Stress

1. Stress may be defined as the nonspecific response of the body to any demand (Selye).
2. Stress has physiological manifestations. (See "stress-related symptoms" and "stress-related disorders" under Focus Assessment Criteria.)

Depression

1. Reactive depression occurs as a response to a situational stressor.
2. Endogenous depression, possibly somatic in origin, is a maladaptive response to often unidentifiable causes.

Reactive vs. Endogenous Depression

Element	Reactive Depression	Endogenous Depression
Precipitating event	Identifiable	Unclear
Family history	Unrelated	Familial tendency
Symptoms	Related to grief and anxiety; worse at night	Seemingly unrelated to events; worse in morning
Activity	Diminished motor and cognitive behavior	Agitated, restless
Emotion	Client feels sad	Alternates between sadness and manic gaiety
Cognitive abilities	May be slightly diminished	Retarded psychomotor performance
Orientation	Oriented and responsive to environment	May not be oriented or responsive
Treatment	Responds well to counseling and environmental change	Requires somatic treatment

Ineffective Individual Coping
Related to Depression in Response to Identifiable Stressors

Assessment

Subjective Data

The personal verbalizes feelings of
  Failure ("I should have . . .)
  Sadness, blues
  Loneliness
  Worry, fear
The person describes symptoms of
  Fatigue
  Constipation or diarrhea
  Insomnia or excessive sleep

Vague confusion
Helplessness ("I can't . . . ")
Hopelessness, apathy
Preoccupation with self

General pain
Stiffness
Menstrual changes

Anorexia
Headache
Dry mouth

Dizziness, numbness
Frequent crying episodes (or
    desire to cry)

Objective Data

Physical symptoms
    Rashes
    Tachycardia
Emotional symptoms
    Distressed, tearful, sad
Altered cognitive ability
    Inability to concentrate
    Poor memory
Physical appearance
    Poor personal hygiene
    Lack of grooming

Lusterless eyes
Weight changes

Altered affect

Difficulty with problem-solving
Inability to make decisions

Poor nutrition

Outcome Criteria

The person will
- Verbalize feelings related to his emotional state
- Identify his coping patterns and the consequences of the behavior that results
- Identify personal strengths and accept support through the nursing relationship
- Make decisions and follow through with appropriate actions to change provocative situations in personal environment

---

Interventions

A. Assess causative and contributing factors

- Negative self-concept
- Moral or ethical conflict (see *Spiritual Distress*)
- Disapproval by others
- Inadequate problem-solving
- Loss-related grief (see *Grieving*)
- Sudden change in life pattern
- Recent change in health status of self or significant other
- Inadequate support system

B. Assess individual's present coping status

1. Determine onset of feelings and symptoms and their correlation with events and life changes
2. Assess ability to relate facts
3. Listen carefully as client speaks, to collect facts and observe facial expressions, gestures, eye contact, body positioning, tone and intensity of voice
4. Determine risk of client's inflicting self-harm and intervene appropriately
   a. Assess for signs of potential suicide
      - History of previous attempts or threats (overt and covert)

- Changes in personality, behavior, sexual life, appetite, sleep habits
- Preparations for death (putting things in order, making a will, giving away personal possessions, acquiring a weapon)
- A sudden elevation in mood

b. Demonstrate to client that you believe him and desire to help
  - Avoid challenging him, minimizing his feelings, arguing, or trying to reason with him
  - Listen attentively and stay close until the danger has passed or help is secured

c. Offer support as client talks
  - Reassure him that the feelings he has must be difficult
  - When client is pessimistic, attempt to provide a more hopeful, realistic perspective

d. See *Potential for Self-harm* for additional information on suicide prevention

C. Teach constructive problem-solving techniques

1. Assist the person to problem-solve in a constructive manner
   - What is the problem?
   - Who or what is responsible for the problem?
   - What are his options? (Make a list)
   - What are the advantages and disadvantages of each option?
2. Discuss possible alternatives, (*i.e.*, talk over the problem with those involved, try to change the situation, or do nothing and accept the consequences)
3. Assist the individual to identify problems that he cannot control directly and help him to practice stress-reducing activities for control (*e.g.*, exercise program, yoga); see Appendix VII for problem-solving techniques
4. Instruct client in relaxation techniques; emphasize the importance of setting 15 to 20 minutes aside each day to practice relaxation. Write down the following guidelines (see Appendix X for additional relaxation techniques)
   - Find a comfortable position in chair or on floor
   - Close eyes
   - Keep noise to a minimum (only very soft music if desired)
   - Concentrate on breathing slowly and deeply
   - Feel the heaviness of all extremities
   - If muscles are tense, tighten, then relax, each one from toes to scalp

D. Assist client to develop appropriate strategies based upon his personal strengths and previous experiences

1. Have client describe previous encounters with conflict and how he managed to resolve them
2. Encourage client to evaluate own behavior
   - "Did that work for you?"
   - "How did it help?"
   - "What did you learn from that experience?"
3. Be supportive of functional coping behaviors
   - "Your way of handling this situation two years ago worked well for you then, can you do it now?"
   - Give options; however, the decision-making must be left to the client
4. Mobilize the client into a gradual increase in activity
   - Identify activities that were previously gratifying but have been neglected: personal grooming or dress habits, shopping, hobbies, athletic endeavors, arts and crafts

- Encourage client to include these activities in daily routine for a set time span ("I will play the piano for 30 minutes every afternoon")
- Stress importance of activity in helping one recover from depression; state that depression is immobilizing and that client must make a conscious effort to fight it in order to recover
5. Find outlets that foster feelings of personal achievement and self-esteem
   - Make time for relaxing activities (*e.g.*, dancing, exercising, sewing, woodworking)
   - Find a helper to take over responsibilities from time to time (get a babysitter)
   - Learn to compartmentalize (don't carry problems around with you all the time; enjoy free time)
   - Take longer vacations (not just a few days here and there)
   - Provide opportunities to learn and use stress management techniques (*e.g.*, jogging, yoga; see also Appendix X)
6. Correct lack of support systems
   - Establish a network of people who understand your situation
   - Decide who is best able to act as a support system (don't expect empathy from people who themselves are overwhelmed with their own problems)
   - Make time to share personal feelings and concern with coworkers (encourage ventilation; frequently people who share the same circumstances are helpful to one another)
   - Maintain a sense of humor
   - Allow tears

E. Initiate health teaching and referrals as indicated

- For depression-related problems beyond the scope of nurse generalists, refer to appropriate professional (marriage counselor, psychiatric nurse therapists, psychologist, psychiatrist)

Defensive Coping

Related to **(Specify)**

Definition

Defensive coping: The state in which an individual repeatedly projects falsely positive self-evaluation as a defense against underlying perceived threats to positive self-regard.

Defining Characteristics*

Major (80%–100%)

Denial of obvious problems/weaknesses
Projection of blame/responsibility

* Source: Norris J, Kunes-Connell M: Self-esteem disturbance: A clinical validation study. In McLane A (ed): Classification of Nursing Diagnoses: Proceedings of the Seventh Conference, St. Louis, CV Mosby, 1987

Rationalizes failures
Hypersensitive to slight criticism
Grandiosity

Minor (50%–79%)

Superior attitude toward others
Difficulty in establishing/maintaining relationships
Hostile laughter or ridicule of others
Difficulty in testing perceptions against reality
Lack of follow through or participation in treatment or therapy

Etiological, Contributing, Risk Factors

See *Chronic Low Self-esteem*

Focus Assessment Criteria

See *Ineffective Individual Coping*

Principles and Rationale for Nursing Care

See *Ineffective Individual Coping*

Defensive Coping
Related to (Specify)

Assessment

See Defining Characteristics

Outcome Criteria

The person will:
- Verbalize a realistic perception of self with strengths and limitations
- Identify consequences of his behavior

Interventions

A. Provide opportunities to channel emotional and physical energy
- Provide paper and pen for writing thoughts and feelings
- Encourage noncompetitive activities, avoid activities that require concentration and attention to rules
- Use brief, one-to-one interactions during time when person is easily distracted; increase time as attention span increases

B. Decrease environmental stimuli
- Be aware of how person is responding to stimuli (*e.g.*, increase in loudness, activity, irritability)

- Decrease noise, visitors and other persons in environment
- Avoid group activities when individual is easily distractible

C. Assist in appropriate expression of thoughts and feelings

- Clarify what is being said (*e.g.*, "Who are 'they'?")
- Validate your interpretation ("Is this what you mean?")
- Refocus conversation so that only one topic at a time is discussed
- Let the person know when you are unable to follow the flow of conversation

D. Assist person to realistically evaluate his behavior

- Direct conversation from a delusional orientation to a reality-based one
- Tactfully express doubt about reality distortions
- Have person examine the consequences of his grandiose/ambitious acts

E. Provide positive socialization experiences

See *Altered Thought Processes* related to *Inability to Evaluate Reality* for interventions

F. Be aware of your own reactions

- Don't take verbal abuse personally; respond in a matter-of-fact attitude
- Talk over with team members to prevent manipulation
- Be consistent in your approach
- Define acceptable behavior
- Enforce established limits

G. Maintain physical safety and health

- Ensure adequate rest periods
- Ensure adequate elimination pattern
- Provide high-calory, high-protein foods
- Monitor for weight loss
- Use foods and liquids that are easily digested
- Observe for signs and symptoms of infections or illness
- Assist with grooming

H. Initiate health teaching

1. Teach
    - The importance of taking medication even when the patient feels good
    - Medication side-effects, toxic effects and associated care such as routine blood levels
2. Explain that feelings of grandiosity may lead to overspending and personal risks
3. Describe clues that will indicate the need for professional help (*e.g.*, promiscuity, alcohol/drug overuse, insomnia, euphoria, overspending)

Ineffective Denial

Related to **Acknowledgement of Substance Abuse/Dependency**

Definition

Ineffective denial: The state in which an individual minimizes or disavows symptoms or a situation to the detriment of his health.

Author's Note: This type of denial differs from the denial in response to a loss. The denial in response to an illness or loss is necessary to maintain psychological equilibrium and is beneficial. Ineffective denial is not beneficial when the individual will not participate in regimens to improve health or the situation (*e.g.*, denial of substance abuse). If the cause of the ineffective denial is not known, *Ineffective Denial related to unknown etiology* can be utilized; for example, *Ineffective Denial related to unknown etiology* as manifested by repetitive refusal to admit barbiturate use is a problem.

Defining Characteristics*

Major (80%–100%)

Delays seeking or refuses health care attention to the detriment of health
Does not perceive personal relevance of symptoms or danger

Minor (50%–79%)

Uses home remedies (self-treatment) to relieve symptoms
Does not admit fear of death or invalidism
Minimizes symptoms
Displaces source of symptoms to other areas of the body
Unable to admit impact of disease on life pattern
Makes dismissive gestures or comments when speaking of distressing events
Displaces fear of impact of the condition
Displays inappropriate affect

Etiological, Contributing, Risk Factors

Pathophysiological
Any chronic and/or terminal illness

Treatment-related
Prolonged treatment with no positive results

* Source: Norris J, Kunes-Connell M: Self-esteem disturbance: A clinical validation study. In McLane A (ed): Classification of Nursing Diagnoses: Proceedings of the Seventh Conference, St. Louis, CV Mosby, 1987

Situational/Psychological

Loss of job
Loss of spouse/significant other
Financial crisis
Feelings of negative self-concept, inadequacy, guilt, loneliness, despair, sense of failure
Feelings of increased anxiety/stress need to escape personal problems, anger and frustration
Feelings of omnipotence
Culturally permissive attitudes toward alcohol/drug use
Religious sanctions

Maturational

Adolescence: peer pressure
Adulthood: job stress, expectation of alcohol/drug use, losses (job, spouse, children)
Elderly: losses (spouse, function, financial), retirement

Biological/Genetic

Family history of alcoholism

Focus Assessment Criteria

See *Ineffective Individual Coping*

Principles and Rationale for Nursing Care

See *Ineffective Individual Coping*

Ineffective Denial
Related to Acknowledgement of Substance Abuse/Dependency

Assessment

Subjective Data

The person will:
Deny that alcohol/drug use is problematic
Justify his use of alcohol/drugs
Blame others for his use of alcohol/drugs
Verbalize need of daily use
Report unsuccessful attempts to reduce or stop use
Express grandiosity, inflated self-esteem
Express suspiciousness
Report need for increased amount to achieve same effect (tolerance)

Objective Data

The person will demonstrate interference in:
  Occupational functioning
    Absenteeism
    Daytime fatigue
    Failed assignments
    Loss of job
  Social Functioning
    Arguments with mate/friends
    Violence while intoxicated
    Traffic accidents
    Legal difficulties
    Boisterousness/talkativeness
    Impulsiveness
    Poor judgement
    Apathy
  Physiological Functioning
    Alcohol Abuse
      Blackout
      Memory impairment
      Decreased sensation in lower extremities
      Malnutrition
      Impatience
      Unsteady gait
      Liver damage
      Gout symptoms
      Gastritis/gastric ulcers
      Pancreatitis
      Cardiomyopathy
      Withdrawal symptoms (*e.g.*, tremors, nausea, vomiting, increased blood pressure, pulse, sleep disturbances, disorientation, hallucinations, agitation, seizures)
    Opiate Abuse
      Drowsiness
      Slurred speech
      Pupillary constriction
      Impaired memory
      Slowed motor movements
      Malnutrition
      Infections (*e.g.*, pneumonia, TB, skin abscesses)
      Liver disease
      Low testosterone levels
      Gastric ulcers
      Respiratory depression
      Constipation
      Tetanus
      Decreased response to pain
      Withdrawal symptoms (*e.g.*, tearing, runny nose, dilated pupils, mild hypertension, tachycardia, nausea, vomiting, restlessness, joint pain)
    Amphetamine and Cocaine abuse
      Increased alertness

    Decreased appetite
    Increased heart rate
    Dilated pupils
    Chills
    Nausea and vomiting
    Hepatitis
    Tetanus
    Infections and abscesses associated with self-injections
    CVA
    Hallucinations
    Cardiac arrhythmias
    Seizures
    Respiratory depression
Hallucinogen Abuse
    Increased heart rate
    Sweating
    Palpitations
    Blurred vision
    Tremors
    Incoordination
    Hallucinations
    Flashbacks
Cannabis Abuse
    Increased heart rate
    Conjunctival infection
    Increased appetite
    Bronchitis
    Sinusitis
    Possible impaired sperm production and chromosomal damage
Barbiturates/Sedative/Hypnotics Abuse
    Drowsiness
    Impaired memory
    Cellulitis
    Hepatitis
    Endocarditis
    Pneumonia
    Respiratory depression
    Signs of intoxication and withdrawal similar to alcohol abuse

---

Outcome Criteria

The person will:
- Admit to an alcohol/drug abuse problem
- Explain the psychological and physiological effects of alcohol and/or drug use
- Abstain from alcohol/drug use
- State recognitions of the need for continued treatment
- Express a sense of hope
- Use alternative coping mechanisms to cope with stress

Interventions

A. Assist to improve self-esteem
- Be nonjudgmental
- Assist person in gaining an intellectual understanding that this is an illness not a moral problem
- Provide opportunities to perform successfully; gradually increase responsibility
- Provide educational information about progressive nature of substance abuse and its effects on the body and interpersonal relationships
- Refer to *Self-esteem Disturbance* for further interventions

B. Instill a sense of hope
- Maintain a positive attitude
- Communicate the expectation that person can overcome problems
- Set realistic, short-term goals
- Facilitate interactions with persons who have recovered or are recovering
- Refer to *Hopelessness* for further interventions

C. Assist in identifying and altering patterns of substance abuse
- Identify situations when the user is expected to use alcohol/drugs (*e.g.*, at home with TV, after work with friends)
- Encourage avoidance of situations when alcohol/drugs are being used
- Assist person in replacing drinking/smoking buddies with nonusers (AA/NA are helpful alternatives here. Each AA/NA group is unique; encourage person to find a group he is comfortable with.)
- Assist in organizing and adhering to a daily routine
- Have person chart their alcohol/drug use (amount, time, situation); useful with early-stage substance abusers who are resistant to treatment (Metzger)

D. Assist in meeting physiological and safety needs
1. Observe for signs of withdrawal
2. Provide supportive care through the detoxification period
3. Prevent access to abused substances. Monitor visitors and belongings
4. Assess for presence of medical consequences of alcohol/drug use
   - Prostatitis
   - Fetal alcohol syndrome (mental retardation, malformations, hyperactivity, growth deficiency, cardiac problems)
   - WBC, RBC, platelet deficiencies
   - Bleeding tendencies (decreased Vitamin K production)
   - Peripheral neuropathy, myopathy
   - Hypertension
   - Cardiac tissue damage, cardiomyopathy
   - Gastritis, pancreatitis
   - Hepatitis (alcoholic) cirrhosis
   - Vitamin metabolism defects
   - Esophageal varices, hemorrhoids, ascites
5. Assess potential for violence, refer to *Potential for Violence* for further interventions
6. Assess for suicide potential, refer to *Potential for Self-harm* for further interventions
7. Teach side effects and appropriate interventions associated with medications (*e.g.*, Antabuse [disulfiram], methadone, antianxiety drugs [Librium]

E. Assist person to identify effects of substance abuse on his life and significant others

- In early stages of abstinence, blaming alcohol for problems may be helpful: avoids guilt and blame (Metzger, 1988)
- As abstinence becomes more secure, assist person to take responsibility for own choices
- Discuss reasons for drug/alcohol use
- Explore problems that have resulted from substance abuse (marriage, relationships, work)
- Assess motivation to stop abuse (*e.g.*, What areas of life are important enough to change for—job, family, health? From his point of view, what does he gain/lose? How does he see life in a few years? Will substance abuse interfere?)

F. Discuss alternative coping strategies

1. Teach relaxation techniques and meditation. Encourage use when he recognizes anxiety. Refer to Appendix X for stress management techniques.
2. Teach thought-stopping techniques to use when thoughts about drinking/ substance use occur. Instruct him to say vocally or subvocally "STOP, STOP" and to replace that thought with a positive one. The technique must be practiced and the individual may need assistance in identifying replacement thoughts.
3. Assist in anticipating stressful events (*e.g.*, job, family, social situations) where alcohol/drug use is expected; role-play alternative strategies.
   - Teach assertiveness skills

G. Assist person to achieve abstinence

- Set goals that are short term (*e.g.*, stopping one day at a time versus insisting never to drink/use again).
- Be direct in questioning about alcohol/drug use (*e.g.*, Have you used alcohol/ drugs since . . . ? Where? When? In what situation?).
- Assist in recognizing stressors that lead to substance abuse.
- Assist person in evaluating the negative consequences of the behavior. Visualization may be helpful.
- When person denies alcohol/drug use, look for nonverbal clues to substantiate facts (*e.g.*, is there congruence verbal and nonverbal, deteriorating appearance, job performance or social skills?).
- When on firm ground and a trusting relationship has been established, confront his denial.
- Discourage person from attempting to correct other problems such as obesity and smoking during this time.
- Don't attempt to probe past history in early abstinence.

H. Assist in resocialization

- Involve in groups and in establishing an alcohol/drug-free network
- Establish a trusting relationship
- Involve the family in the treatment process

I. Initiate referral as indicated

- Alcoholics Anonymous
- AlAnon
- Treatment facility

References/Bibliography

General

Bennett A: Recognizing the potential suicide. Geriatrics 22(3):175–181, 1967

Carlson C, Blackburn B: Behavioral Concepts and Nursing Interventions. Philadelphia, JB Lippincott, 1978

Donnelly G: Can self-hypnosis conquer stress? RN 68(1):63–64, 1981

Dorin A: Adolescent sexuality, adolescent depression. Pediatric Nursing 3(4):49–50, 1978

Faulk L, Bellack J: Intrapersonal and interpersonal assessment. In Bellack J (ed): Nursing Assessment, pp 142–170. Bradford, PA, Wadsworth Health Sciences, 1984

Fontana AF, Dowds BN, Marcus JL et al: Coping with interpersonal conflict through life events and hospitalization. Nerv Ment Dis 162:88–98, 1976

Halton C: Suicide: Assessment and Intervention. New York, Appleton-Century-Crofts, 1977

Hymovich DP: Development of the Chronicity Impact and Coping Instrument: Parent Questionnaire (C1C1: PQ). Nurs Res 33(4):218–222, 1984

Jalowiec A, Murphy E, Marjorie J: Powers Psychometric Assessment of the Jalowiec Coping Scale. Nurs Res 33(3):157–161, 1984

Lazarus R, Folkman S: An analysis of coping in a middle-aged community sample. J Health Soc Behav 21:219–239, 1980

Martin RA, Poland EY: Learning to Change: A Self-Management Approach to Adjustment. New York, McGraw-Hill, 1980

Maxwell M: Cancer and suicide. Cancer Nurs 3(2):33–38, 1980

Metzger L: From Denial to Recovery. San Francisco, Jossey-Bass, 1988

Pender N: Health Promotion in Nursing Practice, Part 3. New York, Appleton-Century-Crofts, 1982

Rosenbaum M: Depression: What to do, what to say. Nursing 10(8):64–66, 1980

Selye H: Stress Without Distress. Philadelphia, JB Lippincott, 1974

Tobachnick N, Farberow N: The assessment of self-destructive potentiality. In Farberow NL, Shneidman ES (eds): The Cry for Help, pp 61–77. New York, McGraw-Hill, 1961

Vincent KG: The validation of a nursing diagnosis. Nurs Clin North Am 20(4):631–639, 1985

Substance Abuse

Finley B: Counseling the alcoholic client. J Psychiatr Nurs 19(6):32–34, 1981

Kurose K, Anderson T, Bull W et al: A standard care plan for alcoholism. Am J Nurs 81:1001–1006, 1981

Lecues J, Dana R, Blenius G: Substance Abuse Counseling: An Individualized Approach. Pacific Grove, CA, Brooks/Cole Publishing, 1988

Leporatic N, Chychula L: How you can really help the drug-abusing patient. Nursing 12(6):46–49, 1982

Marks VL: Health teaching for recovering alcoholic patients. Am J Nurs 80:2058–2061, 1980; 81:755–757, 1981

Richard E, Shephard AC: Giving up smoking: A lesson in loss theory. Am J Nurs 81:755–757, 1981

Waititz J: Adult Children of Alcoholics. Pompano Beach, FL, Health Communications, 1983

Wieczorek R, Natapoff J: Alcoholism-drug abuse. In A Conceptual Approach to the Nursing of Children, pp 1239–1251. Philadelphia, JB Lippincott, 1981

Wilson J: The plight of the elderly alcoholic. Geriatrics 2(2):114–118, 1981

Resources for the Consumer

Literature

Girdano D, Everly G: Controlling Stress and Tension. Englewood Cliffs, NJ, Prentice Hall, 1979

Selye H: Stress Without Distress. Philadelphia, JB Lippincott, 1974

Newman M, Berkowitz B: How to Be Your Own Best Friend. Ballantine Books, New York, 1971

Mace D, Mace V: How to Have a Happy Marriage. Nashville, Festival Books, 1977

Simonton OC, Simonton S, Creighton J: Getting Well Again. New York, St. Martin's Press, 1978

Woititz J: Adult Children of Alcoholics. Pompano Beach, FL, Health Communications, 1983

Organizations

Drug and Alcohol Nursing Association, Inc., Box 371, College Park, MD 20740

Alcohol, Drug Abuse and Mental Health Administration, Office of Communications and Public Affairs, 5600 Fishers Lane, Room 6C-15, Rockville, MD 20857

National Clearinghouse for Mental Health Information, Public Inquiries Section, 5600 Fishers Lane, Room 11A-21, Rockville, MD 20857

American Cancer Society, 777 3rd Avenue, New York, NY 10017

American Heart Association, 7320 Greenville Avenue, Dallas, TX 75231

American Lung Association, 1740 Broadway, New York, NY 10019

National Interagency Council on Smoking and Health, 291 Broadway, Room 1005, New York, NY, 10007

Coping, Ineffective Family: Disabling

Related to **(Specify)** as manifested by **Domestic Abuse (Adults)**
Related to **(Specify)** as manifested by **Child Abuse**

Definition

Ineffective family coping, disabling: The state in which a family demonstrates destructive behavior in response to an inability to manage internal or external stressors due to inadequate resources (physical, psychological, cognitive, and/or behavioral).

> **Author's Note:** The diagnostic category *Ineffective Family Coping: Disabling* describes a family that has a history of demonstrating destructive overt or covert behavior or has adapted detrimentally to a stressor. This category differs from *Altered Family Processes,* which describes a family that usually functions constructively but is challenged by a stressor that has altered or may alter its functioning. *Sustained Altered Family Processes* may progress to *Ineffective Family Coping.*

Defining Characteristics

Major (one must be present)

Neglectful care of the client
Decisions/actions which are detrimental to economic and/or social well-being
Neglectful relationships with other family members

Minor (may be present)

Distortion of reality regarding the client's health problem
Intolerance
Rejection
Abandonment
Desertion
Psychosomaticism
Taking on illness signs of client
Agitation
Depression
Aggression
Hostility
Impaired restructuring of a meaningful life for self
Prolonged over-concerns for client
Client's development of helpless inactive dependence

Etiological, Contributing, Risk Factors

The following describes those individuals or families who are at high risk for contributing to a family's destructive coping behavior.

Parent(s)	*Child*
Single	Of unwanted pregnancy
Adolescent	Of undesired gender or of forced intercourse
Abusive	With undesired characteristics
Emotionally disturbed	Physically handicapped
Alcoholic	Mentally handicapped
Drug addict	Hyperactive
Terminally ill	Terminally ill
Acute disability/accident	Adolescent rebellion
Elderly dependent	

Pathophysiological

Any condition that challenges one's ability for self care, for fulfilling role responsibilities, and finances can contribute to *Ineffective Family Coping*. See *Altered Family Processes* for specific situations.

Other

History of ineffective relationship with own parents
History of abusive relationships with parents
Unrealistic expectations of child by parent
Unrealistic expectations of self by parent
Unrealistic expectations of parent by child
Unmet psychosocial needs of child by parent
Unmet psychosocial needs of parent by child

Focus Assessment Criteria

Owing to the complexity and variability of this diagnostic category, the nurse must determine the type and extent of the assessment needed with each family.

1. Individual coping patterns of adult members: refer to assessment criteria for *Ineffective Individual Coping*
2. Family coping patterns: refer to assessment criteria for *Altered Family Processes*
3. Parenting patterns: refer to assessment criteria for *Altered Parenting*
4. Violence potential: refer to assessment criteria for *Potential for Violence*
5. Potential Stressors
   - Employment status
     Unemployed
     Job satisfaction
   - Housing
     Physical space: adequate, crowded   Privacy
     Cleanliness
   - Transportation
     Car   Shared
     Bus
     Dependency on other
     Proximity to work/school/shopping
   - Financial
     Resources   Medical expenses
     Additional expenses
   - Child/elder care provisions
     Who shares burden
   - Change in job/school status

• Legal history
History of criminal/delinquent
Offenses

Principles and Rationale for Nursing Care

General

Refer to *Altered Family Processes* for principles of the family.

1. Domestic violence/abuse is one expression of a dysfunctional family system. There are numerous other ways dysfunction can be expressed, and this will need to be assessed by nurse.
2. Abuse can take several forms: physical assault may or may not result in injury; verbal attacks; isolation; theft of money or property; violation of rights including eviction from own home; forced sexual activity; social and emotional neglect.
3. A dysfunctional system is one in which there is interference with mutual need attainment.
4. Abusive families are characterized by:
   • Poor differentiation of individuals within the family
   • Lack of autonomy
   • Family is insulated from the influence of others; socially isolate
   • Desperate competition for affection and nurturance among members
   • Feelings of helplessness and hopelessness
   • Abuse/violence learned as a way to reduce tension
   • Low frustration tolerance; poor impulse control
   • Closeness and caring confused with abuse/violence
   • Communication patterns are characterized by mixed and double messages
   • High level of conflict surrounding family tasks
   • Parental coalition is nonexistent
5. Impulse control can be diminished by neurological impairment or alcohol/drug abuse.
6. The role of the victim is a critical factor in the occurrence of child and spouse abuse. The role is socially learned and characterized by helplessness. This occurs when victims learn over time that they cannot control their lives (Shapiro).
7. The process of generational inversion creates problems in that some parents have difficulty accepting that their children are adults.
8. Elderly are increasingly vulnerable to abuse as they become economically, physically, socially, and emotionally more dependent and resources of the caretakers are limited.
9. The intensity of the reaction to an abusive experience indicates the degree of critical life issues and may be compounded by previous unresolved conflicts.
10. Guilt reactions are common among victims. They frequently feel responsible for the incident. This helps to protect them against feelings of powerlessness.
11. Elderly individuals are reluctant to report abuse for fear of retaliation, exposure of their child to legal/community censure, and fear of removal from the home.

Spouse Abuse

1. Spouse abuse in the form of beatings occur in 1% of all families. Fifty percent of American families are disrupted by some form of violence. Fifteen percent of all homicides are spouse killings; 50% of the victims are women. Women usually kill their husbands with guns and knives, while husbands usually beat wives to death.
2. The battered wife syndrome has three major concepts—the cycle of violence (Figure II–1), learned helplessness and anticipatory fear. (Blair)

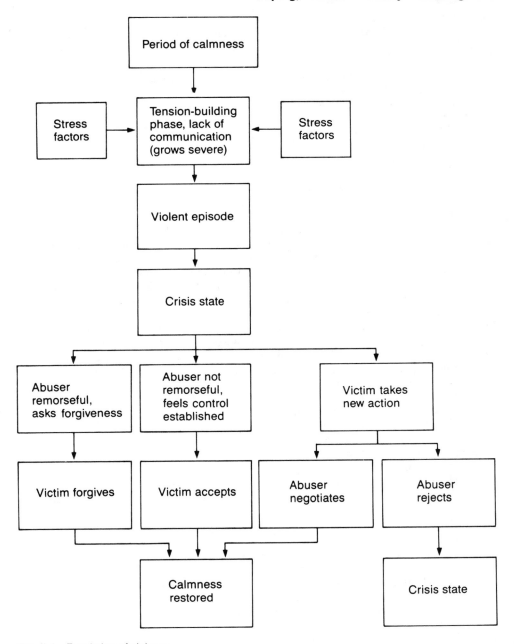

Fig. II-1   Escalation of violence.

3. Learned helplessness can be the result of childhood experiences, witnessing or receiving abuse or the outcome of the battering relationship. (Blair)
4. Victims of abuse are "brainwashed by terror." The victim of abuse uses denial and rationalization when she remains in the battering relationship. (Blair)

5. Battered women rarely report the incident to the health care provider, but instead seek assistance with psychosomatic conditions (chest pain, choking sensations, abdominal pain, fatigue, GI disorders and pelvic pain) or with injuries with inappropriate explanations for them. (Greany)
6. The victims seldom report abuse because of: (Blair)
   - Feelings of guilt and shame
   - Fear of social stigmatization
   - Fear of the abuser
   - View of violence as normal
   - Lack of alternative resources
7. Violent episodes
   Escalate in frequency and severity over time
   Require less and less provocation to trigger them
   Include verbal as well as physical abuse
   Are made more brutal by alcohol use
8. Battering has a distinct cycle, as indicated in Figure II–1.
9. Women who attempt to defend themselves during the tension-building phase often are successful in preventing the beating, while women who attempt to defend themselves during the assaultive phase often sustain a more brutal beating.
10. The abuser's ability to control his spouse directly increases his feelings of autonomy and esteem. Therefore, the fear of loss (and control) of his spouse directly influences his feelings about himself.
11. Battered women who did not witness abuse as children usually remain in the marriage twice as long as women who witnessed abuse as children.
12. Factors contributing to a battered woman's remaining in the marriage are
    Belief that children need a two-parent family
    Lack of financial support
    Lack of a place to go
    Belief that the abuse will stop
    Fear for her life or her children's lives
    Fear of unknown future
13. Personal characteristics of the abuser
    No dominant ethnic or socioeconomic characteristics
    History of abuse from caregivers or witnessed abuse as a child
    Blames outside factors for everything that goes wrong; blames wife for causing him to get angry
    Denies the violence or minimizes its severity
    Impulsive
    Excessively dependent on and jealous of spouse (spouse is usually the only significant relationship he has)
    Fears losing her, which can contribute to suicide, homicide, depression, or anger
    When not hitting, is often a good, loving husband
14. Personal characteristics of the battered woman
    Low self-esteem
    Easily upset
    Belief that she has incited her husband to beat her and is to blame
    Raised in families that restricted emotional expression (*e.g.*, anger, hugging)
    Subscribes to the feminine sex-role stereotype
    Frequently marries to escape restrictive, confining family
    Becomes extremely resourceful and self-sufficient in order to survive

Usually was not abused as a child and did not witness abuse

Views herself as a victim with no option but to appease her spouse

15. The likelihood of a woman seeking and utilizing assistance for abuse is increased if (Sammons)

She has been in the relationship less than 5 years

She is employed

She has friends or relatives who live nearby (within a few miles)

She discussed the abuse with others

The abuse is frequent (daily, weekly), severe (required medical treatment/hospitalization), or increasing in frequency

Child Abuse and Neglect

1. Approximately 1 million cases of suspected abuse and neglect were reported in 1978. Of these cases, 38% were substantiated. (AHA) The estimated number of cases of actual abuse and neglect was 2–4 million.
2. The discrepancy between the reported cases of child abuse and the estimated number is related to the failure of professionals to report suspected cases, the misdiagnosis of inflicted injuries as accidental, and the lack of listing of child abuse in the International Classification of Disease.
3. The nurse should consult the legislation mandating the reporting of child abuse for the specifics of legal definition, penalties for failure to report, reporting procedure, and legal immunity for reporting.
4. The nurse may come in contact with an abused child in an emergency room, school, or physician's office or in her personal life.
5. The identification of child abuse is dependent on the nurse's recognizing the physical signs, specific parent behavior, specific child behavior, inconsistencies in the history of the injury, and contributing factors (familial, environmental).
6. In order to minimize misdiagnosing child abuse, Wong suggests that health care professionals:
   • Be aware that false allegations of abuse are common
   • Child abuse may be mistaken for diseases as hemophilia, erythema multiforme or accidental injuries as car seat burns.
   • Child abuse may be used as a charge in custody battles.
   • Anatomically correct dolls and drawings are tools to help confirm, but they are not confirmation in themselves.
   • Parents or accused persons may not have been given adequate opportunity to present their account of the incident.
7. The first priority of care for the abused child is preventing further injury.
8. Reporting child abuse is a means of getting help to the child and the family. The purpose of protective services is to preserve the family. Only after all other possibilities have failed is the child removed from the home. All states have laws regarding child abuse; everyone who comes in contact with children in their normal working day has a legal responsibility to report suspected child abuse.
9. Child abuse is a symptom of a family in crisis or a family dysfunction. The crisis can be illness, financial difficulties, or any recent change in the family unit (new members, loss of a member, relocation).
10. Separation of the infant from its parents, as in the case of prematurity, can reduce the attachment and nurturing behaviors of the mother toward her child. A disproportionate number of abused children were premature or ill at birth.
11. Children are usually abused by someone they know: a parent, a babysitter, a relative,

or a friend of the family. It must be remembered that the majority of people who abuse a child are well-intentioned adults who know the child and care about its welfare. Their intent was to punish or teach the child a lesson. The abusing parent usually feels extremely guilty and is often relieved when help is offered. The child also may feel guilt, sensing that he is "bad" and therefore required the discipline.

12. Factors that contribute to child abuse are:
   - Lack of or unavailability of the extended family
   - Economic conditions (inflation, unemployment)
   - Lack of role model as a child
   - High-risk children (unwanted, of undesired sex or appearance, physically or mentally handicapped, hyperactive, or terminally ill)
   - High-risk parents (single, adolescent, emotionally disturbed, alcoholic, drug addicted, or physically ill)

13. Characteristic personal patterns of abusers are:
   - No dominant ethnic or socioeconomic characteristics
   - History of abuse by their parents and lack of warmth and affection from them
   - Social isolation (few friends or outlets for tensions)
   - Marked lack of self-esteem, with low tolerance for criticism
   - Emotional immaturity and dependency
   - Distrust of others
   - Inability to admit the need for help
   - High expectations for/of child (perceiving child as a source of emotional gratification)
   - Desire for the child to give them pleasure

14. The nonabusing parent, who is usually passive and compliant in the abuse, must be included in the treatment plan.

Ineffective Family Coping: Disabled
Related to (Specify) as manifested by Domestic Abuse

Domestic abuse is defined as any action that is intended to harm another person (physical, emotional, financial, social, sexual).

Assessment

Subjective Data

The person relates
   Punishments that inflict physical, emotional, financial, social, or sexual harm
   Statements indirectly suggesting abuse
      "I need help"
      "I can't go home"
      "I need a friend"
   A family history of violence/abuse
      Verbal assaults/threats
      Reports of neglect—elderly without adequate physical care, grooming, nutrition

Social isolation
History of forced sexual activity
Failure to receive medical care—eyeglasses, medications

Objective Data
Bruises or welts
 On face, buttocks, thighs, or upper body
 May appear patterned (by rope, belt, or palm)
 May be different colors from different episodes
 Incompatible with normal injuries
Burns
 From cigarettes (on palms, soles, hands, back, or buttocks)
 Oval-shaped (from immersion in scalding liquids)
 From rope (around neck or extremity)
Fractures or dislocations
Lacerations and abrasions
Miscellaneous injuries
 Nausea and abdominal swelling (from being punched in abdomen)
 Bald patches (from having hair pulled)
 Poisoning
 Gunshot wound
 Malnutrition
 Poor hygiene

Outcome Criteria

The person will
- Discuss the physical assaults
- Identify factors that contribute to violence
- Seek assistance for abusive behavior
- Relate community resources available when help is desired

Interventions
The interventions needed to address the complexity and the magnitude of the problems inherent in domestic violence are usually out of the scope of a nurse generalist. The interventions provided here are to assist the nurse who has a short-term interaction with the individual.

A. Assess for the presence of factors that inhibit victims from seeking aid
1. Personal beliefs
 Fear for safety of self or children
 Fear of embarrassment
 Low self-esteem
 Guilt (punishment justified)
 Myths ("It is normal;" "It will stop")
2. Lack of knowledge of
 The severity of the problem

Community resources
Legal rights
3. Lack of financial independence
4. Lack of support system

B. Reduce or eliminate factors if possible

1. Personal beliefs
   - Provide an opportunity to validate abuse and talk about feelings; (if the acutely injured person is accompanied by spouse/caregiver, who is persistent about staying, make an attempt to see the person alone *e.g.*, tell her you need a urine specimen and accompany her to the bathroom).
   - Be direct and nonjudgmental (Blair)
        How do you handle stress?
        How does your partner or caregiver handle stress?
        How do you and your partner argue?
        Are you afraid of him?
        Have you ever been hit, pushed, or injured by your partner?
   - Provide options but allow them to make a decision at their own pace
   - Encourage a realistic appraisal of the situation; dispel guilt and myths
        Violence is not normal for most families
        Violence may stop but it usually becomes increasingly worse
        The victim is not responsible for the violence
2. Lack of knowledge
   - Provide a list of community agencies available to victim and abuser (emergency and long-term)
        Hotlines
        Legal services
        Shelters
        Counseling agencies
   - Discuss the availability of the social service department for assistance
   - Consult with the legal resources in the community and familiarize the victim with the state laws regarding:
        Eviction of abuser
        Counseling
        Temporary support
        Protection orders
        Criminal law
        Types of police interventions
3. Lack of financial independence
   - Refer to social service (agency or community)
4. Lack of support system
   - Assess the availability and quality of the support system (relatives, neighbors)
   - Discuss the importance of regular social contacts to provide opportunities to share and to prevent isolation
   - Assist in arranging respite care and other home health services (hot meals, patient aides) for the elderly.

C. Document findings and dialogue for possible future court use (Blair)

   - Occurrence, frequency
   - Type of injury

- Record suspicious injuries where "the pattern of injuries is inconsistent with the history"

D. Initiate health teaching and referrals if indicated

1. Teach the community about the problem of spouse/elder abuse
   Parent–school organizations
   Women's clubs
   Programs for schoolchildren
2. Instruct caregivers in how to properly manage an elderly client at home, transferring to chair, modified appliances, how to maintain orientation.
3. Refer for financial assistance and transportation arrangements
4. Refer for assertiveness training (see Appendix X).
5. Inform family of senior citizen centers or daycare programs.
6. Refer the abuser to the appropriate community service (only refer men who have asked for assistance or admitted their abuse, for revealing the wife's confidential disclosure may trigger more abuse)
7. To secure additional information, contact:
   National Clearinghouse on Domestic Violence
   P.O. Box 2309
   Rockville, MD 20852

Ineffective Family Coping: Disabled
Related to (Specify) as manifested by Child Abuse/Neglect

Child abuse is an action or inaction that brings injury to a child, including physical and psychological injury, neglect, and sexual abuse.

Assessment

Subjective Data (Kempe, Heifer)

The parent or caretaker
 Cannot explain the source of injury
 Gives an explanation that is in conflict with the developmental ability of the child (*e.g.,* six-month-old spilled pot on stove)
 Gives an explanation that is inconsistent with injury (*e.g.,* concussion and broken leg from falling out of bed)
 Has delayed seeking medical attention
 Describes frequent injuries and accidents
 Blames someone else for causing the injury
 Verbalizes family discord, feelings of inadequacy; says that the child is different in some way or that his anger cannot be controlled
The child
 Reports an incident of abuse
 Tells a story that conflicts with the caretaker's story

Objective Data

The parent or caretaker
    Does not comfort the child
    Is detached
    Is out of control or highly controlled
The child
    Has a developmental lag
    Appears poorly cared for
    Is fearful of adults
    Seeks to comfort the parent
    Remains stoic during painful procedures
    Has a lack of social initiative

Findings and reports

Of abuse
    Multiple injuries in various stages of healing
    Injury to genital area
    Gonorrhea
    Marks on skin from straps, buckles, rope, cigarette burns
    Subdural hematoma
    Bruising around the eye
    Contusions
    Ruptured abdominal organs
    Early pregnancy (underage 12–14)
Of neglect
    Malnourished
    Unbathed
    Inadequately dressed for weather
    Frequently left unsupervised

Outcome Criteria

The child will
  • Seek comfort from the nurse
  • Be free from injury or neglect
The parent will
  • Seek assistance for his abusive behavior
  • Demonstrate nurturing behavior toward the child

Interventions

A. Identify families at risk for child abuse
  • Refer to Principles and Rationale for Nursing Care

B. Intervene prior to abuse with families at risk
  • Establish a relationship with parents that encourages them to share difficulties ("Being a parent is sure hard [frustrating] work, isn't it?")
  • Provide parents with access to information about parenting and child development (see *Altered Growth and Development*)

- Provide anticipatory guidance relative to growth and development (*e.g.*, the need to cry in early months; toilet training)
- Stress the importance of support systems (*e.g.*, encourage parents to exchange experiences with other parents)
- Encourage parents to allow time for their own needs (*e.g.*, attend an exercise class three times a week)
- Discuss with parents how they respond to parental frustrations (share feelings with other parents?) and instruct them not to discipline children when very angry
- Explore other methods of discipline aside from physical punishment
- Refer parents to exert help
- Inform parents of community services (telephone hotlines, clergy)

C. Identify suspected cases of child abuse

1. Assess for and evaluate
   a. Evidence of maltreatment (refer to Assessment data)
   b. History of incident or injury
      Conflicting stories
      Story improbable for age of child
      Story not consistent with injury
   c. Parental behaviors
      Care sought for a minor complaint (*e.g.*, cold) when other injuries are seen
      Exaggerated or absent emotional response to the injury
      Unavailable for questioning
      Fails to show empathy for child
      Angry or critical of child for being injured
      Demands to take child home if pressured for answers
   d. Child behaviors
      Does not expect to be comforted
      Adjusts inappropriately to hospitalization
      Defends parents
      Blames self for inciting parents to rage

D. Report suspected cases of child abuse

1. Know your state's child abuse laws and procedures for reporting child abuse (*e.g.*, Bureau of Child Welfare, Department of Social Services, Child Protective Services)
2. Maintain an objective record
   Description of injuries
   Conversations with parents and child in quotes
   Description of behaviors, not interpretation (*e.g.*, avoid "angry father;" instead, "Father screamed at child, 'If you weren't so bad this wouldn't have happened'")
   Description of parent–child interactions (*e.g.*, shies away from mother's touch)
   Nutritional status
   Growth and development compared to age-related norms

E. Promote a therapeutic environment during hospitalization for child and parent

1. Provide the child with acceptance and affection
   - Show child attention without reinforcing inappropriate behavior
   - Use play therapy to allow child self-expression
   - Provide child with consistent caregivers and reasonable limits on behavior; avoid pity
   - Avoid asking too many questions and criticizing parent's actions

- Ensure that play and educational needs are met
- Explain in detail all routines and procedures

2. Assist child with grieving if foster home placement is necessary
   - Acknowledge that child will not want to leave parents despite how severe the abuse was
   - Allow opportunities for child to ventilate feelings
   - Explain the reasons for not allowing child to return home; dispel belief that this is a punishment
   - Encourage foster parents to visit child in hospital

3. Provide interventions that promote parent's self-esteem and sense of trust
   - Tell them it was good that they brought the child to the hospital
   - Welcome parents to the unit and orient them to activities
   - Promote their confidence by presenting a warm, helpful attitude and acknowledging any competent parenting activities
   - Provide opportunities for parents to participate in their child's care (*e.g.,* feeding, bathing)

F. Initiate health teaching and referrals as indicated

1. Provide anticipatory guidance for families at risk
   - Assist individuals to recognize stress and to practice techniques to manage stress; See Appendix X (*e.g.,* planning for time alone away from child)
   - Discuss the need for realistic expectations of the child's capabilities
   - Teach child development and constructive methods for handling developmental problems (enuresis, toilet training, temper tantrums); refer to literature in Bibliography
   - Discuss methods of discipline other than physical (*e.g.,* deprive the child of his favorite pastime: "May not ride your bike for a whole day;" "May not play your stereo")
   - Emphasize rewarding positive behavior

2. Refer abusive parents to community agencies and professionals for counseling

3. Disseminate information to the community about the problem of child abuse (*e.g.,* parent–school organizations, radio, television, newspaper)
   - Discuss with parents and parents-to-be the problems of parenting
   - Teach those who are at risk of being future abusers
   - Discuss constructive stress management
   - Teach the signs and symptoms of abuse and the method for reporting
   - Focus on abuse as a problem that results from child-rearing difficulties, not parental deficiencies
   - Relay your understanding of stresses but do not condone abuse
   - Focus on the parent's needs; avoid an authoritative approach
   - Take opportunities to demonstrate constructive methods for working with children (give the child choices; listen carefully to the child)

4. Consider developing parenting classes for parents (preventive, corrective) to increase their skills as nurturers and teachers. Weekly topic examples:
   What is parenting?
   Child development and play
   Discipline and toiling training
   Play and nutrition
   Safety and health
   Discipline and common problems
   Parental needs
   Expectations versus realities (Soditus, Mock)

Compromised Family Coping

Definition

Compromised family coping: That state in which a usually supportive primary person (family member or close friend) is providing insufficient, ineffective, or compromised support, comfort, assistance, or encouragement which may be needed by the client to manage or master adaptive tasks related to his or her health challenge.

> **Author's Note:** This diagnostic category describes situations that are similar to the diagnostic categories *Impaired Adjustment* and *Altered Family Processes*. Until clinical research differentiates this category from the aforementioned categories use *Impaired Adjustment* and/or *Altered Family Processes*.

Defining Characteristics

Subjective

Client expresses or confirms a concern or complaint about significant other's response to his or her health problem

Significant person describes preoccupation with personal reactions (*e.g.*, fear, anticipatory grief, guilt, anxiety) to client's illness, disability, or to other situational or developmental crises

Significant person describes or confirms an inadequate understanding or knowledge base, which interferes with effective assistive or supportive behaviors

Objective

Significant person attempts assistive or supportive behaviors with less than satisfactory results

Significant person withdraws or enters into limited or temporary personal communication with the client at time of need

Significant person displays protective behavior disproportionate (too little or too much) to the client's abilities or need for autonomy

Etiological, Contributing, Risk Factors

See *Altered Family Processes*

Coping, Family: Potential for Growth

Definition

Family coping, potential for growth: Effective managing of adaptive tasks by family member involved with the client's health challenge, who now is exhibiting desire and readiness for enhanced health and growth in regard to self and in relation to the client.

Author's Note: This diagnostic category describes components that are found in *Altered Family Processes* and *Health-Seeking Behaviors*. Until clinical research differentiates the category from the aforementioned category, use *Altered Family Processes* or *Health-Seeking Behaviors* depending on the data presented.

Defining Characteristics

Family member attempting to describe growth impact of crisis on his or her own values, priorities, goals or relationships

Family member moving in direction of health-promoting and enriching life-style which supports and monitors maturational processes, audits and negotiates treatment programs, and generally chooses experiences which optimize wellness

Individual expressing interest in making contact on a one-to-one basis or on a mutual-aid group basis with another person who has experienced a similar situation

Etiological, Contributing, Risk Factors

See *Health-Seeking Behaviors* and *Altered Family Processes*

References/Bibliography

Allen J, Allen B: Violence in the family, Family and Community Health 4(2):19–33, 1981

Blair K: The battered woman: Is she a silent partner? Nurse Pract 11(6):38, 1986

Harris C: Women and violence. In Fogel C, Woods N (eds): Health Care of Women: A Nursing Perspective, pp 139–145. St. Louis, CV Mosby, 1981

Fleming J: Stopping Wife Abuse. Garden City, NY, Doubleday and Co. 1979

Friedman MM: Family Nursing: Theory and Assessment. New York, Appleton-Century-Crofts, 1981

Greany G: Is she a battered woman? A guide for emergency response. Am J Nurs 84(5):725–727, 1984

Greenland C: Violence and the family. Can J Public Health 7(1): 19–24, 1980

Hymovich D, Barnard M (ed): Family Health Care, 2 Vols. New York, McGraw-Hill, 1979

Lieberknecht K: Helping the battered wife. Am J Nurs 78:654–656, 1978

Martin D: Battered Wives. San Francisco, Glide Publications, 1976

Melichar M: Using crisis theory to help parents cope with a child's temper tantrums. Matern Child Nurs J 5(3): 181–185, 1980

Mercer RT: Teenage motherhood: The first year. J Obstet Gynecol Nurs 9(1):16–29, 1980

Moore ML: Newborn, Family and Nurse. Philadelphia, WB Saunders, 1981

Nelms B: What is a normal adolescent? Matern Child Nurs J 6(6):402–406, 1981

Petrillo M, Sagay S: Emotional Care of the Hospitalized Child. Philadelphia, JB Lippincott, 1980

Roy M (ed): Battered Women: A Psychosociological Study of Domestic Violence. New York, Van Nostrand Reinhold, 1977

Sammons L: Battered and pregnant. Matern Child Nurs J 6:246–250, 1981

Star B: Battered Women. In McNall LK (ed): Contemporary Obstetric and Gynecologic Nursing, pp 121–135. St. Louis, CV Mosby, 1980

Steinmet S: Violence between family members. Marriage Family Review 1:1–16, 1978

Shapiro R: Therapy with violent families. In Saunders S, Anderson A, Hart C et al (eds): Violent Individuals and Families: A Handbook for Practitioners, Springfield, IL, CC Thomas, 1984

Steinmetz S: Family violence toward elders. In Saunders S, Anderson A, Hart C et al (eds): Violent Individuals and Families: A Handbook for Practitioners. Springfield IL, CC Thomas, 1984

Stranik MK, Hogberg, BL: Transition into parenthood. Am J Nurs 79:90–93, 1979

Stuart G, Sundeen S: Principles and Practice of Psychiatric Nursing. St Louis, CV Mosby, 1983

Waley L, Wong D: Nursing Care of Infants and Children. St. Louis CV Mosby, 1963

Walker L: The Battered Woman. New York, Harper & Row, 1979

Woolery L, Barkley N: Enhancing couple relationship during prenatal and postnatal classes. Matern Child Nurs J 6(3):184–188, 1981

Abuse

Anderson CL: Assessing parenting potential for child abuse risk. Pediatr Nurs 13(5):323–327, 1987

American Humane Association (AHA): Highlights of Official Child Neglect and Abuse Reporting 1985. AHA, Denver, CO, 1987

Elvik SL: From disclosure to court: The facets of sexual abuse. J Pediatr Health Care 1(6):136–140, 1987

Elvik SL, Berkowitz C, Greenberg C: Child sexual abuse: The role of the nurse practitioner. Nurse Pract 11(1):15, 1986

Helfer RE, Kempe CH: Helping the Battered Child and His Family. Philadelphia, JB Lippincott, 1972

Hurwitz A, Castells S: Misdiagnosed child abuse and metabolic diseases. Pediatr Nurs 13:33–36, 1987

Mulvihill D: Between parent and child. The Canadian Nurse 83(2):12–15, 1987

Olson RJ: Index of suspicion: Screening for child abusers. Am J Nurs 76:108–110, 1976

Soditus C, Mock D: Interrupting the cycle of child abuse. Matern Child Nurs J 13(3): 196–98, 1988

Symposium on child abuse and neglect. Nurs Clin North Am 16(2), 1981

Tagg PI: Nursing interventions for the abused child and his family. Pediatr Nurs 2(5):36–39, 1976

Wegmann M, Lancaster J: Child neglect and abuse. Family and Community Health 11(2):11–17, 1981

Wong D: False allegations of child abuse: The other side of tragedy. Pediatr Nurs 13(5):329–333, 1987

Bonding

Dean P, Morgan P, Towle JM et al: Making baby's acquaintance a unique attachment. Strategy 7(1):37–41, 1982

Jenkins R, Westhus NK: The nurse role in parent-infant bonding: Overview, assessment, intervention. J Obstet Gynecol Nurs 10(2):114–118, 1981

Josten L: Prenatal assessment guide for illuminating possible problems with parenting. Matern Child Nurs J 6(2):113–117, 1981

Klaus MH, Kennell JH: Maternal/Infant Bonding. St. Louis, CV Mosby, 1976

Mercer R: Nursing Care for Parents at Risk. Thorofare, NJ, Charles B Slack, 1977

Resources for the Consumer

Literature

Child Care Manual.
ROCOM Press, P.O. Box 1577, Newark, NJ 07101

Christophersen ER: Little People: Guidelines for Common Sense Childrearing. Lawrence, KS, H & H Enterprises, 1977

Forward S: Men Who Hate Women and the Women Who Love Them. New York, Bantam Books, 1986

Salk L, Kramer R: How to Raise a Human Being. New York, Warner Books, 1973
Your Child From 1 to 6. U.S. Department of Health, Education, and Welfare, Children's Bureau, Publication No. 30, Washington, D.C. 20014.

Organizations
Parents Without Partners, 7910 Woodmount Avenue, #1000 Washington, D.C. 20014; also local chapters
LaLeche League International, 9616 Minneapolis Avenue, Franklin Park, IL 60131; also local chapters
Parent Effectiveness Training, 531 Stevens Avenue, Solana Beach, CA 92075

Local Counseling Services
Catholic Charities, Jewish Family Services, Christian Family Services, community agencies, and mental health centers

Decisional Conflict

Definition

Decisional conflict: The state in which an individual/group experiences uncertainty about a course of action when the choice involves risk, loss, or challenge.

Defining Characteristics*

Major (80%–100%)

Verbalized uncertainty about choices
Verbalization of undesired consequences of alternative actions being considered
Vacillation between alternative choices
Delayed decision-making

Minor (50%–79%)

Verbalized feeling of distress while attempting a decision
Self-focusing
Physical signs of distress or tension (increased heart rate, increased muscle tension, restlessness, etc.) whenever the decision comes within focus of attention
Questioning personal values and beliefs while attempting to make a decision

Etiological, Contributing, Risk Factors

Many situations can contribute to decisional conflict, particularly those that involve complex medical interventions of great risk. Any decisional situation can precipitate conflict for an individual, thus the examples listed below are not exhaustive, but reflective of situations that may be problematic and possess factors that increase the difficulty.

Treatment-related

Surgery
    Tumor removal
    Cataract
    Laminectomy
    Orchiectomy
    Cosmetic
    Joint replacement
    Hysterectomy
    Transplant
Diagnostics
    Amniocentesis
    Ultrasound
    X-rays
Chemotherapy

* Hiltunen E: Diagnostic content validity of the nursing diagnosis: decisional conflict. Unpublished raw data, 1987

Radiation
Dialysis
Mechanical ventilation
Enteral feedings
Intravenous hydration

Situational

Personal
   Marriage
   Separation
   Divorce
   Parenthood
   Birth control
   Artificial insemination
   Adoption
   Foster home placement
   Institutionalization (child, parent)
   Breast vs. bottle feeding
   Abortion
   Sterilization
   Nursing home placement
Work/task
   Career change
   Relocation
   Business investments
   Professional ethics
Lack of relevant information
Confusing information
Disagreement within support systems
Inexperience with decision-making
Unclear personal values/beliefs
Conflict with personal values/beliefs
Resignation
Family history of poor prognosis
Hospital environment—loss of control
Ethical dilemmas—quality of life
                    cessation of life-support systems
                    do not resuscitate

Maturational

Adolescent
   Peer pressure
   Sexual activity
   Alcohol/drug use
   Illegal/dangerous situations
   Use of birth control
   Whether to continue a relationship
   College
   Career choice
Adult
   Career change

        Marriage
        Parenthood
    Older adult
        Retirement
        Nursing home placement

Focus Assessment
Decisional conflict is a subjective state that the nurse must validate with the individual. The nurse will assess each individual to determine the person's level of decision-making within the present conflict situation. Some of the same cues may be seen in persons with diagnoses of *Powerlessness, Spiritual Distress* and *Hopelessness.*

Subjective Data
1. Decision-making patterns
    "Tell me about the decision you need to make."
    "How would you describe your usual method of making decisions?"
    "In the past, how did you arrive at decisions that had a positive outcome?"
    "What decisions have you made that you felt confident about?"
    "When you make a decision, do you do it alone or do you like to involve other people? If so, whom do you consult for advice?"
    Person may say:
    "I simply cannot decide."
    "What should I do?"
    "What would you do if you were me?"
    "Why don't you just tell me what I should do?"
2. Perception of the conflict
    "How does it make you feel when you think about the decision you have to make?"
    "Why is this a stressful decision for you?"
    "What things make you uncomfortable about deciding?"
    "Has there been a change in your sleep patterns, appetite, activity level?"
    Person may state:
    "The risk is too great for me to decide."
    "This whole situation makes me very anxious."
    "I can't believe I got myself into this predicament."
    "I feel so uptight every time I think about the decision I have to make."
    "I feel like I have no control over the decision that needs to be made."

Objective Data
1. Body language
    Posture (relaxed, rigid)
    Facial expression (calm, annoyed, tense)
    Hands (relaxed, rigid, wringing)
    Eye contact (appropriate, darting)
2. Motor activity
    Within normal limits
    Immobile
    Increased
    Pacing
    Agitation
3. Affect
    Within normal limits

Labile
Controlled
Flat
Inappropriate

Principles and Rationale for Nursing Care

General

1. Making decisions is a way of life.
2. An antecedent condition of decision-making is a problem. Problems exist when there is a discrepancy between what is and what could or should be.
3. Making a decision is a systematic process—a means, rather than an end. Decision-making is a sequential process where each step builds on the previous one.
4. Optimal decision making is more likely to occur when done in a systematic manner, but it does not necessarily have to be a rigid, step-by-step process.
5. People are not usually taught a systematic method for making a decision, so frequently they rely on past experiences and intuition.
6. There are essentially three decision-making models in health care.
   A. Paternalism
      • Health-care providers make all of the decisions concerning patient care.
      • Locus of control is external to the client and significant others.
      • Client's values and life-style are not taken into consideration.
   B. Consumerism
      • Health-care providers put aside their own values and only provide the client and significant others with the information they request.
      • The locus of control is internal for the client and significant others.
      • Health-care providers do nothing to influence the decision made—abandonment.
   C. Humanism/Advocacy
      • This is a collaborative process where everyone's values (client, significant others, health-care providers) are taken into consideration.
      • The locus of control is shared and all participants have an equal role in decision-making.
      • This generates a mutual respect for individual dignity and worth.
      • Information and support are provided so that the client can make his own decision.
7. The most important right that a person possesses is the right of self-determination, the right to make the ultimate decision concerning what will or will not be done to his body (Marsh).
8. Choice is facilitated when an individual is free to make it.
9. Values provide one foundation for decision-making. Experience is a major source for value development. Values involve choice.
10. In a crisis situation, decisions are influenced more by values than consideration of possible outcomes.
11. Health-care providers' own values will shape their interaction with families facing ethical decisions.
12. Value conflicts often lead to confusion, indecision, and inconsistency.
13. Decision-making is more complicated for a person when his goals conflict with those of his significant others.
14. People may decide contradictory to their values if the need to please others is greater than the need to please themselves.

15. The decision-making process is complicated when there is a need for a rapid decision. When there is less time, there is less ability to make a good decision.
16. Mastering content for effective decision-making requires time. Time allows a person to choose the option that provides the most benefit with the least amount of risk.
17. Difficult decisions create stress and conflict. Conflict occurs when values and actions are not in congruence.
18. Conflict can create fears and anxieties that negatively impact the ability to make an effective decision.
19. Decisional conflict occurs when there are simultaneous opposing tendencies within an individual to accept or reject a course of action (Janis).
20. Decisional conflict becomes more intense when it involves a threat to status and self-esteem.
21. Decisional conflict is greater when none of the alternatives are good.
22. External resources become very important for the person in decisional conflict that has a low level of confidence in his ability to make a beneficial decision.

End-of-Life Decisions

1. Intense stress is experienced when families and health-care providers are faced with decisions regarding either the initiation or discontinuation of life-support systems. (Johnson)
2. When there is no indication of the person's wishes or choices for his/her end of life or the family disagrees, the stress increases. (Johnson)
3. Individuals and families should be encouraged to provide directions (documented) that can be used to guide future clinical decisions if they are incompetent or unable to make them. (Johnson)
4. Johnson and Justin reported the following in a sample of 400 persons who had no current life-threatening disease:
   - 43% had discussed their feelings regarding end-of-life decisions with others
   - 95% did not desire to be kept alive if they would be mentally incompetent
   - 93% always wanted to be told the truth about their condition

---

Outcome Criteria

The individual/group will
- Relate the advantages and disadvantages of choices
- Share their fears and concerns regarding choices and responses of others
- Make an informed choice

Interventions

A. Assess causative/contributing factors

Lack of experience with or ineffective decision-making
Value conflict
Fear of outcome/response of others
Insufficient/inconsistent information
Controversy with support system
Unsatisfactory health-care environment

B. Reduce or eliminate causative or contributing factors

Internal

1. Lack of experience with or ineffective decision-making
   a. Review past decisions made by the person and what steps were taken to help him decide. Focus on major life events and what the final outcome was. Capitalize on past decisions that have served the person well.
   b. Facilitate a logical decision-making process.
      - Assist the person in recognizing what the problem is and clearly identify the decision that needs to be made.
      - Have him make a list of all the possible alternatives or options.
      - Help identify the probable outcomes of the various alternatives.
      - Aid in evaluating the alternatives based on actual or potential threats to beliefs/values.
      - Encourage the person to make a decision.
   c. Assess the person's usual locus of control (see *Powerlessness,* page 591) and support his decision-making patterns.
   d. Encourage the person's significant others to be involved in the entire decision making process.
   e. Suggest that the person utilize his significant others as a sounding board when considering the decision alternatives.
   f. Respect the person as a competent decision maker—treat his decisions and desires with respect.
   g. Be available to review the decision that needs to be made and the various alternatives.
   h. Teach and assist with patient relaxation techniques (see Appendix X) when the decision causes anxiety and stress.
   i. Facilitate refocusing on the decision that needs to be made when the person experiences fragmented thinking during periods of high anxiety.
   j. Encourage the person to take time in deciding.
   k. With adolescents, focus on the present—what will happen versus what will not. Help identify the important things in their life as they do not have extensive past experiences upon which to base decisions.
2. Value Conflict (also refer to *Spiritual Distress,* page 710)
   a. Explore the whys of how the person is feeling.
   b. Assist the individual in exploring personal values and relationships that may have an impact on the decision.
   c. Explore obtaining a referral with the person's spiritual leader.
   d. Utilize values clarification techniques to assist the person in reviewing the parts of his life that reflect what he believes in.
      - Have the person identify his most prized and cherished activities in his life.
      - Ask reflective statements that lead to further clarification.
      - Review past decisions where the person has needed to make public affirmation of opinions and beliefs.
      - Evaluate stands the person has taken on controversial subjects. Does he view them in black and white terms, or various shades of gray?
      - Identify values the person is proud of. Have him rank them in order of importance.
   e. Encourage the person to base decision upon his most important values.
   f. Support individual making informed decision—even if decision conflicts with own values
      - Consult own spiritual leader

- Change patient assignments so person can be cared for by nurse with compatible beliefs
- Arrange for discussions among health care team to share feelings

3. Fear of outcome/response of others (also refer to *Fear,* page 324)
- Provide clarification regarding potential outcomes and correct misconceptions.
- Explore with the person what the risks of not deciding would be.
- Encourage expression of feelings.
- Promote self-worth.
- Encourage the person to face what he fears.
- Encourage the person to share what he fears with significant others.
- Actively reassure the person that the decision is his to make and that he has the right to do so.
- Assist the person in recognizing that it is his life; if he feels comfortable with the decision, others will respect his conviction.
- Reassure the person that individuality is acceptable.

External

4. Insufficient or inconsistent information
- Provide information in a comprehensive and sensitive manner.
- Correct misinformation.
- Give concise information that covers the major points when the decision must be made quickly.
- Inform the person of his right to know.
- Enable the person to determine the amount of information that he desires to obtain.
- Encourage verbalization to determine the person's perception of choices.
- Assure that the person clearly understands what is involved concerning the decision and the various alternatives—informed choice.
- Encourage the person to seek second professional opinions regarding health.
- Collaborate with other health-care members/significant others to determine appropriate timing for truthfulness.

5. Controversy with support system
- Assure the person that he does not have to give in to pressure from others, be it family, friends or health professionals.
- Do not allow others to undermine the person's confidence in making the decision for himself.
- Identify leaders within the support system and provide information.

6. Unsatisfactory healthcare environment
- Establish a trusting and meaningful relationship that promotes mutual understanding and caring.
- Provide a quiet environment for thought; reduce sensory stimulation.
- Allow uninterrupted periods with significant others.
- Promote accepting, nonjudgmental attitudes.
- Reduce the number of small decisions that the person needs to make to facilitate focusing on the decision in conflict.
- Avoid using paternalistic/maternalistic attitudes and actions. Foster acceptance of responsibility for the person's own decisions.

C. Initiate health teaching and referrals when indicated.

1. Explore with individual and family if they have discussed and recorded their end-of-life decisions.
2. Describe the possible future dilemmas when these discussions are avoided.

3. Instruct the individual and family members to provide directives in the following areas:

> Person to contact in emergency
> Person individual most trusts with personal decisions
> Decision to be kept alive if individual will be mentally incompetent
> Preference to die at home, hospital, no preference
> Desire to sign a living will
> Decision on organ donation
> Funeral arrangements, burial, cremation
> Circumstances when information should be withheld from individual

4. Document these decisions and make two copies (retain one and give one to the person who is designated to be the decision-maker in an emergency).
5. Discuss the purpose of a living will. Provide information when requested. To obtain a copy of your state's living will, write to the Society for the Right to Die, 250 West 57th Street, New York, NY 10107.

References/Bibliography

Aberman S, Kirchhoff K: Infant-feeding practices: mothers' decision making. J Obstet Gynecol Neonatal Nurs 14(5): 394–397, 1985

Bailey JT, Hendricks DE: Decisions made easy. Nurs Life 7(4): 18–19, 1987

Bedell SE: "Do you want to be resuscitated?" Hosp Pract 21(3):6–9, 1986

Bille DA: Locus of decision making in patient and family education: Its effect on promoting wellness. Nurs Adm Quarterly 2(3): 62–65, 1987

Bulechek G, McCloskey J: Nursing Interventions: Treatments for Nursing Diagnosis. Philadelphia, WB Saunders, 1985

Coletta SS: Values Clarification in Nursing: Why? Am J Nurs 78(12): 2057–2063, 1978

Gadow S: Advocacy: An ethical model for assisting patients with treatment decisions. In Wong CB, Swazey JP (ed): Dilemmas of Dying: Policies and Procedures for Decisions Not to Treat. Boston, GK Hall Medical Publishers, 1981

Janis IL, Mann L: Decision Making: A Psychological Analysis of Conflict, Choice and Commitment. New York, The Free Press, 1977

Johnson RA, Justin R: Documenting patients' end of life decisions. Nurse Pract 13(6):41, 1988

Kohnke MF: The nurse as advocate. Am J Nurs 80(11): 2038–2040, 1980

Lancaster W, Lancaster J: Rational decision making: managing uncertainty. J Nurs Adm 12(2):23–28, 1982

Mapanga M: Deciding factors. Nurs Mirror 161(12): 31–32, 1985

Marsh FL: Refusal of treatment. Clin Geriatr Med 2(3): 511–520, 1986

Minogue JP, Reedy NJ: Companioning parents in perinatal decision making. J Perinat Neonatal Nurs 1(3): 25–35, 1988

Nugent PS: Management and Modes of Thought. J Nurs Adm 12(2):19–25, 1982

Schoene-Seifert B, Childress JF: How much should the cancer patient know and decide?. CA-A Cancer Journal for Clinicians 36(2):85–94, 1986

Simon SB, Howe LW, Kirschenbaum H: Values Clarification: A Handbook of Practical Strategies for Teachers and Students. New York, Hart Publishing Company, 1978

Tauer KM: Promoting effective decision making in sexually active adolescents. Nurs Clin North Am 18(2): 275–292, 1983

Valanis BG, Rumpler CH: Helping women to choose breast cancer treatment alternatives. Cancer Nurs 8(3): 167–175, 1985

Resources for the Consumer

Literature

Life Support: Families Speak About Hospitals, Hospice and Home Care for the Fatally Ill, The Institute for Consumer Policy Research, 256 Washington St., Mt. Vernon, NY 10553

Morra M, Potts E: Choices: Realistic Alternatives in Cancer Treatment, New York, Avon, 1987
Scully T, Scully C: Playing God, New York, Simon and Schuster, 1987
Thinking of Having Surgery, Department of Health and Human Services, Washington, D.C., 20201
    800-638-6833 (Free)
Questions and Answers on Organ Transplantation, Health Resources and Services Administration,
    5600 Fishers Lane, Room 17-60, Rockville, MD 20857 (Free)

Organizations

Cancer Information Services 1-800-4Cancer

Society For Right to Die
250 West 57th St.
New York, NY 10107
Information on living will

National Genetics Foundation Inc.
555 West 57th St.
New York, NY10019

Friends and Relatives of Institutionalized Aged, Inc.
440 East 26th St.
New York, NY 10010
212-481-4422

National Information Center for Handicapped Children and Youth
P.O. Box 1492
Washington, DC 20013
703-522-3332

Potential for Disuse Syndrome

Definition

Potential for disuse syndrome: The state in which an individual is at risk for deterioration of body systems as the result of prescribed or unavoidable musculoskeletal inactivity.

Author's Note: This diagnostic category can be used to describe an individual who is at high risk for the adverse effects of immobility. It is no longer necessary to use separate categories as *Potential Altered Respiratory Function* or *Potential Impaired Skin Integrity,* for they are incorporated into this syndrome category. However, if an individual who is immobile manifests the signs or symptoms of impaired skin integrity or another diagnosis, the specific diagnosis should be used. The nurse should continue to use *Potential for Disuse Syndrome* so that deterioration of the other body systems does not occur.

Defining Characteristics

Presence of risk factors (see Etiological, Contributing, Risk Factors)

Etiological, Contributing, Risk Factors

Pathophysiological

Decreased sensorium
Unconscious
Neuromuscular impairment
    Multiple sclerosis   Muscular dystrophy
    Parkinsonism   Partial/total paralysis
    Guillain–Barré Syndrome   Spinal cord injury
Musculoskeletal
    Fractures
    Rheumatic diseases
End-stage disease
    AIDS   Cardiac
    Renal   Cancer
Psychiatric/mental health disorders
    Major depression   Severe phobias
    Catatonic state

Treatment-related

Surgery (amputation, skeletal)
Traction/casts/splints
Prescribed immobility
Mechanical ventilation
Invasive vascular lines

Situational
   Depression
   Fatigue
   Debilitated state
   Pain

Maturational
   Newborn/infant/child/adolescent
      Down syndrome
      Legg–Calve–Perthes disease
      Osteogenesis imperfecta
      Cerebral palsy
      Spina bifida
      Risser–Turnbuckle jacket
      Juvenile arthritis
      Autism
      Mental/physical disability
   Elderly
      Decreased motor agility
      Muscle weakness
      Presenile dementia

Focus Assessment Criteria

Subjective Data
   1. History of systemic disorders
      Neurologic
         CVA, head trauma, increased intracranial pressure
         Multiple sclerosis, polio, Guillain–Barré, myasthenia gravis
         Spinal cord injury, tumor, birth defect
      Cardiovascular
         Myocardial infarction
         Congential heart anomaly
         Congestive heart failure
      Musculoskeletal
         Osteoporosis
         Fractures
         Arthritis
      Respiratory
         Chronic obstructive pulmonary disease (COPD)
         Orthapnea
         Pneumonia
         Dyspnea on exertion
      Debilitating diseases
         Cancer
         Endocrine disease
         Renal disease
   2. History of symptoms (complaints of)
      Pain
      Muscle weakness
      Fatigue

3. History of recent trauma or surgery
Fractures
Head injury
Abdominal surgery or injury

Objective Data

1. Dominant hand
   Right   Left   Ambidextrous
2. Motor function

Right arm	Strong	Weak	Absent	Spastic
Left arm	Strong	Weak	Absent	Spastic
Right leg	Strong	Weak	Absent	Spastic
Left leg	Strong	Weak	Absent	Spastic

3. Mobility

Ability to turn self	Yes	No	Assistance needed (specify)
Ability to sit	Yes	No	Assistance needed (specify)
Ability to stand	Yes	No	Assistance needed (specify)
Ability to transfer	Yes	No	Assistance needed (specify)
Ability to ambu-late	Yes	No	Assistance needed (specify)

   Weight-bearing (assess both right and left sides)
   　　Full   As tolerated
   　　Partial   Non-weight bearing
   Gait
   　　Stable   Unstable
   Assistive devices
   　　Crutches   Walker   Prosthesis
   　　Cane   Wheelchair   Other
   　　Braces
   Restrictive devices
   　　Cast or splint   Ventilator   IV
   　　Traction   Drain   Monitor
   　　Braces   Foley   Dialysis
   Range of motion (shoulders, elbows, arms, hips, legs)
   　　Full   Limited (specify)   None
4. Motivation (as perceived by nurse and/or reported by person)
   　　Excellent   Satisfactory   Poor

Principles and Rationale for Nursing Care

General

1. "Immobility is inconsistent with human life." Mobility provides one control over one's environment; without mobility, one is at the mercy of one's environment. (Christian)
2. Activity, mobility and flexibility are integral to one's life-style. Immobility has a serious impact on one's self-concept and life-style. (Christian)
3. Society values youthfulness, energy, and productivity. Immobility is contradictory to these values.

4. Immobility restricts the person's ability to seek out sensory stimulation. In contrast, immobile persons may be unable to remove themselves from an environment that is too stressful or noisy. (Christian)
5. Musculoskeletal inactivity or immobility has adverse effects on all the body systems. Table II–4 outlines the effects of immobility on body systems.
6. A muscle loses about 3% of its original strength each day it is immobilized. (Millen)
7. Prolonged immobility has adverse effects on psychological health, learning, socialization, and ability to cope. Table II–5 illustrates these effects.
8. The more portions of the body immobilized and the longer the immobilization, the greater the adverse effects.
9. Joints without range of motion will develop contractures in 3–7 days because flexor muscles are stronger then extensor muscles.
10. Increased serum calcium resulting from bone destruction caused by lack of motion and weight-bearing increases the coagulability of the blood. This, in addition to circulatory stasis, makes the person vulnerable to thrombosis formation.
11. The peristaltic contractions of the ureters are insufficient when in a reclining position, thus there is stasis of urine in the kidney pelvis.

Table II-4. **Adverse Effects of Immobility on Body Systems**

System	Effect
Cardiac	Decrease in myocardial performance Decreased heart rate and stroke volume Decreased oxygen uptake
Circulatory	Venous Thrombosis Dependent edema Reduced venous return Increased intravascular pressure
Respiratory	Stasis of secretions Impaired cilia Drying of sections of mucous membranes Slower, more shallow respirations
Musculoskeletal	Muscle atrophy Shortening of muscle fiber (contracture) Decreased strength/tone Osteoporosis Joint degeneration Fibrosis of callogen fibers (joints)
Metabolic	Nitrogen excretion Hypercalcemia Anorexia Decreased metabolic rate Obesity Elevated creatine levels
Gastrointestinal	Constipation
Genitourinary	Urinary stasis Urinary calculi Urinary retention
Integumentary	Decreased capillary flow Tissue acidosis to necrosis
Neurosensory	Reduced innervation of nerves damaged by pressure or compromised blood supply

Table II-5.   **Psychosocial Effects of Immobility
(Zubek and McNeil, Hammer and Kenan)**

	Effect
Psychological	Increased tension Negative change in self-concept Fear, anger
Learning	Decreased motivation Decreased ability to retain, transfer learning Decreased attention span
Socialization	Change in roles Social isolation
Growth and Development	Dependency

12. Compression of nerves by casts, restraints, or improper positions can result in ischemia and nerve degeneration. Compression of the personal nerve results in footdrop; compression of the radial nerve results in wrist drop.

Children/adolescents

1. Mobility is integral in achieving developmental tasks. Refer to Table II–8: Age-related Developmental Tasks in the diagnostic category *Altered Growth and Development*. Examine how restricted movement can thwart achievement of developmental tasks.
2. Physical activity serves as a vehicle for communication and expression for children. Children respond to anxiety with increased activity. (Waley p 1530)
3. Adolescent developmental requirements include
     Acquisition of an appropriate body image
     Forming a sense of identity (*e.g.*, sexual)
     Establishing peer relationships
     Redefining roles
     Engaging in physical activity (Erikson)
4. Adolescents require mobility to manage stress effectively and to reduce tension (Christian)
5. Immobilization has a negative impact on the adolescent's ability to interact with peers and to participate in peer-related activities.
6. Sibinaga and Freedman reported that children who are restrained (casts, splints, straps) during their first 3 years of life have more difficulty with language than other children who are not restricted.
7. Children react to immobility with anger, aggressive behavior, or passivity.
8. Hypercalcemia can occur within 10 days in completely immobilized children. (Waley p 1529)
9. Immobilization causes isolation from peers, disruption of one's sense of time and space and changes in one's perception of the future. (Smith)
10. Children substitute the following for their inability to move: (Kalafatich)
     • Focusing on their past abilities
     • Watching the activity of others
     • Increased speech
     • Increased fantasy
     • Moving a limb that is not affected or rhythmic rocking

Outcome Criteria

The person will demonstrate continued
- Intact skin/tissue integrity
- Maximum pulmonary function
- Maximum peripheral blood flow
- Full range of motion
- Bowel, bladder, and renal functioning
- Use of social contacts and activities when possible

The person will
- Explain rationale for treatments
- Make decisions regarding care when possible
- Share feelings regarding immobile state

Interventions

A. Identify causative and contributing factors

- Pain; refer also to *Altered Comfort*
- Fatigue; refer also to *Fatigue*
- Decreased motivation; refer also to *Impaired Adjustment*
- Depression; refer also to *Ineffective Individual Coping*

B. Promote optimal respiratory function

- Vary the position of the bed, thus gradually changing the horizontal and vertical position of the thorax, unless contraindicated
- Assist to reposition, turning frequently from side to side (hourly if possible)
- Encourage deep breathing and controlled coughing exercises five times every hour
- Teach individual to use blow bottle or incentive spirometer every hour when awake (with severe neuromuscular impairment, the person may have to be awakened during the night as well)
- For child, use colored water in blow bottle; have him blow up balloons, blow soap bubbles, blow cotton balls with straw
- Auscultate lung fields every 8 hours; increase frequency if altered breath sounds are present
- Encourage small frequent feedings to prevent abdominal distention

C. Maintain usual pattern of bowel elimination. Refer to Constipation related to immobility for specific interventions

D. Prevent pressure ulcers

1. Utilize repositioning schedule that relieves vulnerable area most often (*e.g.,* if vulnerable area is the back, turning schedule would be left side to back, back to right side, right side to left side, and left side to back); post "turn clock" at bedside
2. Turn person or instruct him to turn or shift weight every 30 minutes to 2 hours, depending on other causative factors present and the ability of the skin to recover from pressure

3. Frequency of turning schedule should be increased if any reddened areas that appear do not disappear within 1 hour after turning
4. Position person in normal or neutral position with body weight evenly distributed
5. Keep bed as flat as possible to reduce shearing forces; limit Fowler's position to only 30 minutes at a time
6. Use foam blocks or pillows to provide a bridging effect to support the body above and below the high-risk or ulcerated area so that affected area does not touch bed surface; do not use foam donuts or inflatable rings, since this will increase the area of pressure
7. Alternate or reduce the pressure on the skin surface with:
   Foam mattresses
   Air mattresses
   Air-fluidized beds
   Vascular boots to suspend heels
8. Utilize enough personnel to lift person up in bed or chair rather than pull or slide skin surfaces; use Heelbo protectors to reduce friction on elbows and heels
9. To reduce shearing forces, support feet with footboard to prevent sliding
10. Promote optimum circulation when person is sitting
    • Limit sitting time for person at high risk for ulcer development
    • Instruct person to lift self using chair arms every 10 minutes if possible or assist person in rising up off the chair every 10 to 20 minutes, depending on risk factors present
11. Inspect areas at risk of developing ulcers with each position change
    Ears
    Occiput
    Heels
    Sacrum
    Scrotum
    Elbows
    Trochanter
    Ischia
    Scapula
12. Observe for erythema and blanching and palpate for warmth and tissue sponginess with each position change
13. Massage vulnerable areas with each position change
14. Refer to *Impaired Skin Integrity* for additional interventions

E. Promote factors that improve venous blood flow

Elevate extremity above the level of the heart (may be contraindicated if severe cardiac or respiratory disease is present)

Avoid standing or sitting with legs dependent for long periods of time

Consider the use of Ace bandages or below-knee elastic stocking to prevent venous stasis

Reduce or remove external venous compression which impedes venous flow
   Avoid pillows behind the knees, or get bed that is elevated at the knees
   Avoid leg crossing
   Change positions, move extremities, or wiggle fingers and toes every hour
   Avoid garters and tight elastic stockings above the knees

Measure baseline circumference of calves and thighs daily if individual is at risk for deep venous thrombosis, or if it is suspected

F. Maintain limb mobility and prevent contractures
  1. Increase limb mobility
     • Perform range-of-motion exercises (frequency to be determined by condition of the individual)
     • Support extremity with pillows to prevent or reduce swelling
     • Encourage the person to perform exercise regimens for specific joints as prescribed by physician or physical therapist
  2. Position the person in alignment to prevent complications
     • Avoid pillows under knee; support calf instead
     • Point toes and knees toward ceiling when the client is in a supine position
     • Use footboard to prevent foot drop
     • Avoid prolonged periods of hip flexion (*i.e.,* sitting position)
     • To position hips, place rolled towel lateral to hip to prevent external rotation
     • Arms abducted from the body with pillows
     • Elbows in slight flexion
     • Wrist in a neutral position, with fingers slightly flexed, and thumb abducted and slightly flexed
     • Position of shoulder joints changed during the day (*e.g.,* abduction, adduction, range of circular motion)

G. Prevent urinary stasis and calculi formation
  • Provide a daily intake of fluid of 2000 ml or greater a day (unless contraindicated) refer to *Fluid Volume Deficit* for specific interventions
  • Main urine *p*H below 6.0 (acidic) to reduce the formation of calcium calculi with acid ash foods (cereals, meats, poultry, fish, cranberry juice, apple juice)
  • Teach to avoid foods high in calcium and oxalate (*) as:
      milk, milk products, cheese
      bran cereals
      *spinach, cranberries, plums, raspberries, gooseberries
      sardines, shrimp, oysters
      legumes, whole-grain rice
      *chocolate
      asparagus, rhubarb, kale, Swiss chard, turnip greens, mustard greens, broccoli, beet greens
      peanut butter, ripe olives

H. Reduce and monitor bone demineralization
  1. Monitor for hypercalcemia
     • serum levels
     • nausea/vomiting, polydipsia, polyuria, lethargy
  2. Provide weight-bearing when possible
     • tilt-table
  3. Maintain vigorous hydration
     • adult 2000 ml/day
     • adolescents 3000–4000 ml/day

I. Promote sharing and a sense of well-being
  1. Encourage to share feelings and fears regarding restricted movement
  2. Utilize play therapy (Appendix IX) to encouarge child to share feelings (*e.g.,* put cast on doll)

3. Encourage to wear own clothes rather than pajamas
   - encourage the wearing of unique adornments as an expression of individuality (*e.g.,* baseball caps, colorful socks)

J. Reduce the monotony of immobility

1. Vary daily routine when possible (*e.g.,* give bath in the afternoon, so that the person can watch a special show or talk with a visitor who drops in to see him)
2. Include the individual in planning schedule for daily routine
   - Allow the person to make as many decisions as possible
   - Make daily routine as normal as possible (*e.g.,* have the person wear street clothes during the day if feasible)
3. Plan time for visitors
   - Encourage person to make a schedule for visitors so everyone does not come at once or at an inconvenient time
   - Spend quality time with the person (*i.e.,* not time that is task-oriented; rather, sit down and talk)
4. Be creative; vary the physical environment and daily routine when possible
   - Update bulletin boards, change the pictures on the walls, move the furniture within the room
   - Maintain a pleasant, cheerful environment (*i.e.,* plenty of light, flowers, conversation pieces)
   - Place the person near a window if possible
   - Provide reading material, radio, television, "books on tape" (if person is visually impaired)
   - Plan an activity daily to give person something to look forward to; always keep your promises
   - Discourage the use of television as the primary source of recreation unless it is highly desired
   - Consider using a volunteer to spend time reading to the person or helping with an activity
   - Encourage suggestions and new ideas (*e.g.,* "Can you think of things you might like to do?")
5. Plan appropriate activities for children
   - Provide an environment with accessible playthings that suit the child's developmental age and see that they are well within reach
   - Encourage family to bring in child's favorite playthings, including items from nature that will keep the real world alive (*e.g.,* goldfish, leaves in fall)

K. Provide opportunities for individual to control decisions

- Allow person to manipulate surroundings, such as deciding what is to be kept where (shoes under bed, picture on window)
- Keep needed items within reach (call bell, urinal, tissues)
- Discuss daily plan of activities and allow person to make as many decisions as possible about it
- Increase decision-making opportunities as person progresses
- Respect and follow individual's decision if you have given him options
- Record person's specific choices on care plan to ensure that others on staff acknowledge preferences ("Dislikes orange juice," "Takes shower," "Plan dressing change at 7:30 prior to shower")
- Keep promises
- Provide opportunity for person and family to express feelings

- Provide opportunities for person and family to participate in care
- Plan a care conference to allow staff to discuss methods of individualizing care; encourage each nurse to share at least one action that she discovered a particular individual liked
- Shift emphasis from what one cannot do to what one can do
- Set goals that are short-term, behavioral, practical, and realistic

References/Bibliography

Baird S: Development of a nursing assessment tool to diagnose altered body image in immobilized patients. Orthop Nurs 4(3):47–54, 1985

Bohachick PA: Pulmonary embolism in neurological and neurosurgical patients. J Neurosci Nurs 19(4): 191–197, 1987

Brower P, Hicks D: Maintaining muscle function in patients on bed rest. Am J Nurs 72(7): 1250–1253, 1972

Carnevali D, Brueckner S: Immobilization—reassessment of a concept. Am J Nurs 70(7): 1502–1507, 1970

Christian BJ: Immobilization: Psychosocial Aspects. In Norris C (ed): Concept Clarification in Nursing. Rockville, MD, Aspen Publications, 1982

Downs F: Bedrest and sensory disturbances. Am J Nurs 74(3): 434–438, 1974

Drayton-Hargrove S, Reddy MA: Rehabilitation and long-term management of the spinal cord injured adult. Nurs Clin North Amer 21(4): 599–610, 1986

Erikson E: Identity and the life cycle: Selected papers, Psychol Issues 1(6):118–146, 1959

Hammer R, Kenan E: The psychological aspects of immobilization. In Steinberg FU (ed): The Immobilized Patient: Functional Pathology and Management. New York, Plenum, 1980

Houk NG: The disabled adolescent: Promoting a positive self-concept by achievement of developmental tasks. In Chinn PL, Leonard KB (eds): Current Practice in Pediatric Nursing, St. Louis, CV Mosby, 1980

Kalafatich A: Immobilization in adolescents. In Norris C (ed): Concept Clarification in Nursing, Rockville, MD, Aspen Publications, 1982

Kelly M: Exercises for bedfast patients. Am J Nurs 66(10): 2209–2213, 1986

Lentz: Selected aspects of deconditioning secondary to immobilization. Nurs Clin North Amer 16(4): 729–737, 1981

Maklebust J: Pressure Ulcers: Etiology and Prevention. In Mondoux L (ed): Pressure Ulcers. Philadelphia, WB Saunders, 1987

Ng L, McCormick K: Position changes and their physical consequences. ANS 4(4): 13–25, 1982

Olson E et al: The hazards of immobility. Am J Nurs 67: 780–797, 1967

O'Neil R: Problems associated with disuse syndromes—including the integument. In Beland IL, Passos JY (eds): Clinical Nursing, 4th ed, pp1107–1123. New York, Macmillan, 1981

Schaupner C: Impaired mobility. In Jacobs M, Geels W (eds): Signs and Symptoms in Nursing. Philadelphia, JB Lippincott, 1985

Smith KV, Henry JP: Cybernetic foundations for rehabilitation. Am J Phys Med 46(2):379–467, 1967

Tyler M: The respiratory effects of body positioning and immobilization. Respir Care 29: 472–481, 1984

Zubek JP, McNeil M: Perceptual deprivation phenomena: Role of the recumbent position. J Abnorm Psychol 72:147, 1967

Diversional Activity Deficit

Related to **Monotony of Confinement**

Related to **Post-Retirement Inactivity (Change in Life-Style)**

Definition

Diversional activity deficit: The state in which the individual or group experiences or is at risk of experiencing decreased stimulation from or interest in leisure activities.

Defining Characteristics

Major (must be present)

Observed and/or statements of boredom/depression due to inactivity

Minor (may be present)

Constant expression of unpleasant thoughts or feelings
Yawning or inattentiveness
Flat facial expression
Body language (shifting of body away from speaker)
Restlessness/fidgeting
Immobile (on bedrest or confined)
Weight loss or gain
Hostility

Etiological, Contributing, Risk Factors

Pathophysiological

Communicable disease
Pain

Treatment-related

Long or frequent treatments

Situational (Personal, environmental)

No peers or friends
Monotonous environment
Long-term hospitalization or confinement
Lack of motivation
Loss of ability to perform usual or favorite activities
Excessively long hours of stressful work
No time for leisure activities
Career changes (*e.g.,* teacher to housewife, retirement)
Children leaving home ("empty nest")
Immobility
Decreased sensory perception (*e.g.,* blindness, hearing loss)

Maturational
    Infants/children (lack of appropriate toys/peers)
    Elderly (sensory/motor deficits)

Focus Assessment Criteria

Subjective Data

Perception of person's current activity level
    Too busy (not enough time for relaxing activities)
    Busy but able to find time to do relaxing activities
    Bored, trapped, wishes there was more recreational activity
Past activity patterns (type, frequency)
    Work
    Leisure
Activities the person desires
        Availability   Assistance needed
        Feasibility   Support system

Objective Data

Developmental age
Motivation
        Interested   Withdrawn
        Disinterested   Hostile
Presence of barriers to recreational activities
    Physical
        Immobility   Pain
        Altered level of consciousness   Sensory deficits (visual, auditory)
        Fatigue   Equipment (traction, IVs)
        Altered hand mobility
    Psychological/cognitive
        Lack of motivation   Depression
        Lack of knowledge   Embarrassment
    Socioeconomic
        Lack of available support system   Financial limitations
        Previous patterns of inactivity   Transportation difficulties

Principles and Rationale for Nursing Care

1. All humans need stimulation. In the adult, lack of stimulation results in boredom and depression. In the infant or child it causes "failure to thrive" and may stunt growth severely.
2. Boredom paralyzes an individual's productivity and causes a feeling of stagnation. It is often a major contributing factor to substance abuse (overeating, drug abuse, alcoholism, and smoking).
3. The bored person has introspective feelings of being oppressed and trapped, which give rise to conscious or unconscious anger or hostility.
4. Being aware that one is bored allows one to redirect activities to increase stimulation.
5. Nurses who understand the concept of boredom and are aware of their own patterns of reacting to and dealing with boredom are better able to deal with boredom in others.

6. Taking responsibility for doing something about a boring situation is a positive means of dispelling boredom.
7. Children in a strange environment need permission to be themselves and to play.
8. Immobilized children especially need play activity to make them feel less victimized.

Diversional Activity Deficit
Related to Monotony of Confinement

Assessment

Subjective Data

The person states
  "I'm bored; there's nothing to do"
  "I feel trapped"
  "I can't do anything"
  "I'm tired of being here"
  "I have no friends or family"
  "I have no one to play with"
  "I feel restless"

Objective Data

  Inability to move
  Confinement to room or building
  Limited or no support system
  Flat affect or facial expression
  Lethargy or sleepiness
  Restlessness/fidgeting
  Hostility/anger

Outcome Criteria

The person will
  • Relate feelings of boredom and discuss methods of finding diversional activities
  • Related methods of coping with feelings of anger or depression caused by boredom
  • Engage in a diversional activity

Interventions

A. Assess causative factors

  Monotony
  Inability to make decisions concerning his own plan of care (see *Powerlessness*)

Diminished socialization (see *Social Isolation*)
Lack of motivation/depression

B. Reduce or eliminate causative factors

1. Monotony
   a. Vary daily routine when possible (*e.g.*, give bath in the afternoon, so that the person can watch a special show or talk with a visitor who drops in to see him)
   b. Include the individual in planning schedule for daily routine
      - Allow the person to make as many decisions as possible
      - Make daily routine as normal as possible (*e.g.*, have the person wear street clothes during the day if feasible)
   c. Plan time for visitors
      - Encourage person to make a schedule for visitors so everyone does not come at once or at an inconvenient time
      - Spend quality time with the person (*i.e.*, not time that is task oriented; rather, sit down and talk)
   d. Be creative, vary the physical environment and daily routine when possible
      - Update bulletin boards, change the pictures on the walls, move the furniture within the room
      - Maintain a pleasant, cheerful environment (*i.e.*, plenty of light, flowers, conversation pieces)
      - Place the person near a window if possible
      - Provide reading material, radio, television "books on tape" (if person is visually impaired)
      - Plan an activity daily to give person something to look forward to and always keep your promises
      - Discourage the use of television as the primary source of recreation unless it is highly desired
      - Consider using a volunteer to spend time reading to the person or helping with an activity
      - Encourage suggestions and new ideas (*e.g.*, "Can you think of things you might like to do?")
2. Lack of motivation
   a. Stimulate motivation by showing interest and encouraging sharing of feelings and experiences
      - Discuss the person's likes and dislikes
      - Encourage sharing of feelings of present and past experiences
      - Spend time with the person purposefully talking about other topics (*e.g.*, "I just got back from the shore. Have you ever gone there?")
   b. Help the person to work through feelings of anger and grief
      - Allow him to ventilate
      - Take the time to be a good listener
      - See *Anxiety* for additional interventions
   c. Plan appropriate activities for children
      - Provide an environment with accessible playthings that suit the child's developmental age and see that they are well within reach
      - Keep toys in all waiting areas
      - Encourage family to bring in child's favorite playthings, including items from nature that will help to keep the real world alive (*e.g.*, goldfish, leaves in fall)

Diversional Activity Deficit
Related to Post-Retirement Inactivity (Change in Life-Style)

Assessment

Subjective Data

The person reports
    "There's nothing to do"
    "I'm too old"
    "I feel useless"
    "No one needs me anymore"
Recent retirement
Empty nest (children gone from home)
Career terminated
Loss of significant others

Objective Data
    Flat affect
    Lethargy
    Anger

Outcome Criteria

The person will
- Relate feelings of improved self-esteem and productivity
- Relate available community services and agencies that can be used for hobbies or recreational activities
- Use his strengths to contribute to himself and others
- Redirect energy toward interests that are personally fulfilling and provide diversional activity

---

Interventions

A. Assess causative factors

    Lack of significant others (loneliness, "empty nest")
    Loss of independence (*e.g.,* inability to drive, climb stairs)
    Fear of being unwanted or not needed
    Retirement
    Career termination or changes

B. Identify factors that promote activity and socialization

  1. Encourage socialization with peers and all age groups (frequently the very young and the very old mutually benefit from interaction with each other)

2. Acquire assistance to increase the person's ability to travel
   - Arrange transportation to activities if necessary
   - Acquire aids for safety (*e.g.,* wheelchair for going to shopping center, a walker for ambulating in hallways)
3. Increase the person's feelings of productivity and self-worth
   - Encourage person to use his strengths to help others and himself (*e.g.,* give him tasks to perform in a general project)
   - Acknowledge efforts made by the person (*e.g.,* "You look nice tonight" or "Thank you for helping Mr. Jones with his dinner")
   - Encourage open communication; value the person's opinion ("Mr. Jones, what do you think about _____?")
   - Encourage the person to challenge himself with learning a new skill or pursuing a new interest
   - Refer to *Social Isolation* for additional interventions

C. Initiate referrals if indicated

1. Suggest joining AARP (American Association of Retired Persons)
2. Write the local Health and Welfare Council
3. Provide a list of associations with senior citizen activities
   YMCA
   Churches
   Golden Age Club
   Encore Club
   MORA (Men of Retirement Age)
   Gray Panthers
   Sixty Plus Club
   XYZ Group (Extra Years of Zest)
   Young at Heart Club
   SOS (Senior Outreach Services)
   Leisure Hour Group

References/Bibliography

Books

Bulechek G, McCloskey J: Nursing Interventions. Philadelphia, WB Saunders, 1985
Burnside I: Psychosocial Nursing Care of the Aged. New York, McGraw-Hill, 1973
Carlson C: Behavioral Concepts in Nursing. Philadelphia, JB Lippincott, 1979
Carnevali D, Patrick M: Nursing Management of the Elderly. Philadelphia, JB Lippincott, 1986
Carpenito L: Handbook of Nursing Diagnosis. Philadelphia, JB Lippincott, 1985
Jacobs M, Geels W: Signs and Symptoms in Nursing. Philadelphia, JB Lippincott, 1985
Travelbee M: Interpersonal Aspects of Nursing. Philadelphia, FA Davis, 1971
Weiner M: Working with the Aged. Englewood Cliffs, NJ, Prentice-Hall, 1978

Articles

Ames B: Art and the dying patient. Am J Nurs 80:1094–1096, 1980
Billings C: Emotional first aid. Am J Nurs 80:2005–2009, 1980
Brooten D: Career guide: To change what needs changing . . . doesn't take Wonder Woman. Nursing 11(3):81–83, 1981
Clark C: Burnout: Assessment and intervention. J Nurs Adm 10(9):39–43, 1980
Kauffman M: Sharing the patient experience. Am J Nurs 78:860–862, 1978

Koch K: Teaching poetry writing to the old and the ill. Milbank Memorial Fund Quarterly/Health and Society 56(1):113–125, 1978

Kovesces J: Burnout doesn't have to happen. Nursing 10(10):105–110, 1980

Lore A: Supporting the hospitalized elderly person. Am J Nurs 79:496–499, 1979

Martin D: Enjoyable activity for everyone. Geriatric Nursing 2:210–213, 1981

McGoran S: On developing empathy: Teaching students self-awareness. Am J Nurs 78:859–860, 1978

Piche J: Tell a story. Am J Nurs 78:1189–1193, 1978

Resources for the Consumer

Literature

American Association of Retired Persons, 1909 K Street NW, Washington, DC

Dysreflexia

Related to **(Specify): Potential**

Definition

Dysreflexia: The state in which an individual with a spinal cord injury at T7 or above experiences a potential life-threatening uninhibited sympathetic response of the nervous system to a noxious stimulus.

> **Author's Note:** This represents a situation that the nurse and/or client can prevent or treat. If the nurse's initial treatment does not abate the symptoms, medical treatment is imperative. Thus, Potential Dysreflexia may better describe a clinical situation than does Dysreflexia.

Defining Characteristics

Major (must be present)

Individual with spinal cord injury (T7 or above) with:
- Paroxysmal hypertension (sudden periodic elevated blood pressure where systolic pressure is over 140 mmHg and diastolic is above 90 mmHg)
- Bradycardia or tachycardia (pulse rate of less than 60 or over 100 beats per minute)
- Diaphoresis (above the injury)
- Red splotches on skin (above the injury)
- Pallor (below the injury)
- Headache (a diffuse pain in different portions of the head and not confined to any nerve distribution area)

Minor (may be present)

- Chilling
- Conjunctival congestion
- Horner's Syndrome (contraction of the pupil, partial ptosis of the eyelid, enophtalmos and sometimes loss of sweating over the affected side of the face
- Paresthesia
- Pilomotor reflex
- Blurred vision
- Chest pain
- Metallic taste in mouth
- Nasal congestion

Etiological, Contributing, Risk Factors

Pathophysiological

Visceral stretching and irritation
- Bowel
    - Constipation
    - Fecal impaction

Bladder
  Distended bladder
  Urinary calculi

Infection

Stimulation of skin (abdominal, thigh)
Acute abdominal conditions
Spastic sphincter

Treatment-related

Removal of fecal impaction
Clogged or nonpatent catheter
Surgical incision

Situational

Lack of knowledge

Focus Assessment Criteria

Subjective Data

1. History of dysreflexia
   a. Triggered by:
            Bladder distention
            Bowel distention
            Tactile stimulation
            Skin lesion
            Sexual activity
            Menstruation
   b. Initial symptoms
            Headache
            Sweating, where?
            Chills
            Metallic taste in mouth
            Nasal congestion
            Blurred vision
            Numbness
            Other _____
   c. Medications used? What?
2. Bladder program (type, problems)
3. Bowel program (type, problems)
4. Knowledge of dysreflexia
   • Cause
   • Self-treatment
   • Medical treatment
   • Prevention

Principles and Rationale for Nursing Care

1. The autonomic nervous system, sympathetic and parasympathetic, is located in the cerebrum, hypothalamus, medulla, brain stem, and spinal cord. With spinal cord injury, the cord activity below the injury is deprived of the controlling effects from the higher centers, which results in poorly controlled responses. (Hickey)

2. When sensory receptors are stimulated below a spinal lesion, sympathetic discharge, medicated by the spinothalamic tract and posterior columns, results. This reflex stimulation of the sympathetic nervous system causes spasms of the pelvic viscera and the arterioles. These spasms cause vasoconstriction below the level of the injury. Baroreceptors in the aortic arch and carotid sinus respond to the hypertensive state with superficial vasodilatation, flushing, diaphoresis, and piloerection (gooseflesh) above the level of the spinal lesion. Vagal stimulation slows the heart rate, but because the cord is severed, vagal impulses to dilate vessels are prohibited. (Hickey)
3. Intravenous pharmocologic intervention may be warranted if the noxious stimuli cannot be removed and/or the hypertension is not reduced. Some medications are: diazoxide (Hyperstat), hydralazine (Apresoline), sodium nitroprusside (Nipride), and ganglionic blocking agents such as phenoxybenzamine (Dibenzyline) and guanethidine sulfate (Ismelin).
4. Failure to reverse dysreflexia can result in status epilepticus, stroke, and death.

Potential Dysreflexia
Related to (Specify)

Assessment

See Defining Characteristics

Outcome Criteria

The individual/family will
- State factors that cause dysreflexia
- Describe the treatment for dysreflexia
- Relate when emergency treatment is indicated

Interventions

A. Assess for the presence of causative or contributing factors.

See Etiological, Contributing, Risk Factors

B. If signs of dysreflexia occur, *raise the head of the bed* and remove the noxious stimuli

1. Bladder distention
   a. Check for distended bladder
   b. If catheterized
      - check catheter for kinks or compression
      - irrigate with only 30 ml of saline very slowly
      - replace catheter if it will not drain
   c. If not catheterized, insert catheter using Nupercaine ointment and remove 500 ml, then clamp for 15 minutes; repeat cycle until bladder is drained.

2. Fecal impaction
   - First apply dibucaine hydrochloride ointment (Nupercaine) to the anus and into the rectum for 1 inch (2.54 cm)
   - Gently check rectum with a well-lubricated glove
   - Insert rectal suppository or gently remove impaction
3. Skin irritation
   - Spray skin lesion that is triggering dysreflexia with a topical anesthetic agent

C. Continue to monitor blood pressure every 3–5 minutes

D. Immediately consult physician for pharmacological treatment if symptoms or noxious stimuli are not eliminated

E. Initiate health teaching and referrals as indicated

1. Teach signs and symptoms and treatment of dysreflexia to person and family.
2. Teach when immediate medical intervention is warranted.
3. Explain what situations can trigger dysreflexia (menstrual cycle, sexual activity, bladder or bowel routines)
4. Teach to watch for early signs and to intervene immediately.
5. Teach to observe for early signs of bladder infections and skin lesions (pressure ulcers, ingrown toenails).
6. Advise consultation with physician for long-term pharmocologic management if individual is very vulnerable.

References/Bibliography

Guttman L, Whitteridge D: Effects of bladder retention on autonomic mechanisms after spinal cord injuries. Brain, 70(4): 361–404, 1947

Head H, Riddoch G: The autonomic bladder, excessive sweating and some other reflex conditions in gross injuries of the spinal cord. Brain 40: 188–263, 1917

Hickey J: Neurological and Neurosurgical Nursing, 2nd ed, pp 411–412, Philadelphia, JB Lippincott, 1986

Kewalramani LS: Autonomic dysreflexia in traumatic myelopathy. Am J Phys Med 59 (1):1–19, 1980

Kurnick NB: Autonomic hyperreflexia and its control in patients with spinal cord lesions. Ann Intern Med 44: 678–686, 1956

Lindan R et al: Incidence and clinical features of autonomic dysreflexia in patients with spinal cord injury. Paraplegia 18: 285–292, 1980

Mathias C J et al: Plasma catecholamines during paroxysmal neurogenic hypertension in quadriplegic man. Circ Res 39 (2): 204–208, 1976

Naftchi N E et al: Hypertensive crisis in quadriplegic patients Circulation 57 (2): 336–341, 1978

Niederpruem M S: Autonomic dysreflexia. Rehabil Nurs 9: 29–31, 1984

Family Processes, Altered

Related to **an Ill Family Member**

Definition

Altered family processes: The state in which a normally supportive family experiences a stressor that challenges its previously effective functioning ability.

> **Author's Note:** The nursing diagnosis *Altered Family Processes* describes a family that usually functions optimally but is challenged by a stressor that has altered or may alter the family's function. This diagnosis differs from *Ineffective Family*, which describes a family that has a pattern of destructive behavioral responses. Unsuccessful resolution of a problem can change *Altered Family Processes* to *Coping: Disabled.*

Defining Characteristics

Family system cannot or does not:

Major (must be present)

Adapt constructively to crisis
Communicate openly and effectively between family members

Minor (may be present)

Meet physical needs of all its members
Meet emotional needs of all its members
Meet spiritual needs of all its members
Express or accept a wide range of feelings
Seek or accept help appropriately

Etiological, Contributing, Risk Factors

Any factor can contribute to altered family processes. Some common factors are listed below.

Pathophysiological

Illness of family member
    Discomforts related to the   Change in the family member's
      illness's symptoms   ability to function
Trauma
    Surgery   Loss of body part or function

Treatment-related

Disruption of family routines due to time-consuming treatments (*e.g.,* home dialysis)
Physical changes due to treatments of ill family member
Emotional changes in all family members due to treatments of ill family member
Financial burden of treatments for ill family member
Hospitalization of ill family member

Situational (personal, environmental)
  Loss of family member
    Death
    Going away to school
    Separation
    Divorce
      Incarceration
      Desertion
      Hospitalization
  Gain of new family member
    Birth
    Adoption
      Marriage
      Elderly relative
  Poverty
  Disaster
  Relocation
  Economic crisis
    Unemployment
      Financial loss
  Change in family roles
    Working mother
      Retirement
  Birth of child with defect
  Conflict
    Goal conflicts
    Moral conflict with reality
      Cultural conflict with reality
      Personality conflict in family
  Breach of trust between members
    Dishonesty
      Adultery
  History of psychiatric illness in family
  Social deviance by family member (including crime)

Focus Assessment Criteria
1. Character of family
     Age and sex of members
     Ethnic background
     Religious background
       What is the religious affiliation?
       Does the family participate in religious activity?
       How often?
2. Health status
     What is the current health status of each member?
     Are children within the appropriate range for growth and development?
     What is the health history of each family member?
       Illness
       Surgery
         Accidents
         Allergies
     What preventive measures are practiced?
       Immunizations
       Health Exams
         Dental
         General
           Eye
           Gynecological
       Health practices
         Family planning
         Regular exercise (2–3 times
           a week for 30 minutes)
         Weight control
         Abstention from smoking
           Abstention from or moderate use
             of alcohol
           Daily dental care
           Self-breast exam (for women)
           Testes exam (for men)

Constructive responses
    Relies on each other   Seeks knowledge and resources
    Shares feelings, thoughts   Utilizes support systems
    Appraises problem accurately
Destructive responses
    Denial   Abandonment
    Exploitation of members   Authoritarianism
      (threats, violence, neglect,
      scapegoating)
Do any adults have a history of ineffective coping patterns (depression, violence, substance abuse)?
What are the strengths of the family?
What are the limitations of the family?

Principles and Rationale for Nursing Care

The Nature of the Human Family
1. Each family has a personality to which each member contributes.
2. The family unit may be viewed as a system with
    Interdependency between members
    Interactional patterns that provide structure and support for members
    Boundaries between the family and the environment and between members with varying degrees of permeability
3. Families change with time. They must accomplish specific tasks that originate from the needs of their members. Table II-6 illustrates the tasks of the family.
4. Each family responds to life challenges in ways that reflect experiences in the past and goals for the future.
5. Within a family, members interact in a variety of roles, which result from individual and group needs: parent, spouse, child, sibling, friend, teacher, and so on. Illness of a family member may cause great changes, putting the family at high risk for maladaptation (Fife).
6. Communication patterns of the family determine the quality of the family life.
7. Each family member influences the family unit. Thus, the health of an individual will influence the health of the family.

Crisis and Family Coping
1. Stress is defined as the body's response to any demand made on it. Stress has the potential for becoming a crisis when the person or family cannot cope constructively.
2. A crisis is an event that occurs when the person's usual problem-solving methods are inadequate to resolve the situation.
3. The family in response to crisis will do one of the following: return to pre-crisis functioning, develop a more optimal level of functioning (higher level), or develop a destructive form of functioning (lower level).
4. The goal of crisis management is to assist the family to return to its pre-crisis functioning. If the pre-crisis functioning was destructive (*e.g.,* alcoholism), the goal would be to develop a more optimal level of functioning. (See Appendix VII for guidelines for crisis management.)
5. Common sources of family stress are (Minuchin)
    External sources of stress that one member is experiencing (*e.g.,* job- or school-related)

Table II-6.   **Stage-Critical Family Developmental Tasks Through the Family Life Cycle**

Stage of the Family Life Cycle	Positions in the Family	Stage-critical Family Developmental Tasks
1. Married couple	Wife Husband	Establishing a mutually satisfying marriage Adjusting to pregnancy and the promise of parenthood Fitting into the kin network
2. Childbearing	Wife-mother Husband-father Infant daughter or son or both	Having, adjusting to, and encouraging the development of infants Establishing a satisfying home for both parents and infant(s)
3. Preschool-age	Wife-mother Husband-father Daughter-sister Son-brother	Adapting to the critical needs and interests of preschool children in stimulating growth-promoting ways Coping with energy depletion and lack of privacy as parents
4. School-age	Wife-mother Husband-father Daughter-sister Son-brother	Fitting into the community of school-age families in constructive ways Encouraging children's educational achievement
5. Teenage	Wife-mother Husband-father Daughter-sister Son-brother	Balancing freedom with responsibility as teenagers mature and emancipate themselves Establishing postparental interests and careers as growing parents
6. Launching center	Wife-mother-grandmother Husband-father-grandfather Daughter-sister-aunt Son-brother-uncle	Releasing young adults into work, military service, college, marriage, etc., with appropriate rituals and assistance Maintaining a supportive home base
7. Middle-aged parents	Wife-mother-grandmother Husband-father-grandfather	Rebuilding the marriage relationship Maintaining kin ties with older and younger generations
8. Aging family members	Widow/widower Wife-mother-grandmother Husband-father-grandfather	Coping with bereavement and living alone Closing the family home or adapting it to aging Adjusting to retirement

(Duvall EM: Marriage and Family Development, 5th ed. Philadelphia, JB Lippincott, 1977; reproduced with permission)

External sources of stress that influence the family unit (*e.g.,* finances, relocation)

Developmental stressors (*e.g.,* child-bearing, new baby, child-rearing, adolescence, new member or members—arrival of older grandparent, marriage of
single parents—or loss of spouse)

Situational stressors (*e.g.,* illness, hospitalization, separation)

6. Constructive or functional coping mechanisms of families faced with a stress crisis
are (Friedman)

Greater reliance on each other

Maintenance of a sense of humor

Increased sharing of feeling and thoughts

Promotion of each member's individuality

Accurate appraisal of the meaning of the problem

Search for knowledge and resources about the problem

Utilization of support systems

7. Destructive or dysfunctional coping mechanisms of families faced with a stress or
crisis are (Friedman)

Denial of the problem

Exploitation of one or more of the family members (threats, violence, neglect,
scapegoating)

Separation (hospitalization, institutionalization, divorce, abandonment)

• Authoritarianism (no negotiation)

• Preoccupation of family or members (who lack affection) to appear close

8. Parenthood is a crisis. Some common problems are

Increase in mate arguments

Fatigue resulting from schedule

Disrupted social life

Diminished sexual life

Multiple losses—actual or perceived (*e.g.,* independence, career, beauty, attention)

9. Characteristics of families prone to crisis include

Apathy (resigned to state in life)

Poor self-concept

Low income

Inability to manage money

Unrealistic preferences (materialistic)

Lack of skills and education

Unstable work history

Frequent relocations

History of repeated inadequate problem-solving

Lack of adequate role models

Lack of participation in religious or community activities

Environmental isolation (no telephone, inadequate public transportation)

Illness in the Family

1. Successful coping with illness requires the family to complete the following tasks:
acknowledge the problem and seek help, accept the problem and its implications,
and adjust as the member begins reconstruction.

2. The family acknowledges the problem by identifying the symptoms as serious
enough to warrant investigation, and gaining knowledge of accessible resources.

3. There exists a time lag between identification of symptoms and help-seeking behavior, which may vary between families, depending upon previous experience with the health care system, cultural interpretations of health and illness, and financial concerns.
4. The family must face the diagnosis and its implications. This task is multidimensional, including

Experiencing the initial shock
Engaging in open communication between members
Minimizing anxiety and its disabling consequences
Preventing prolonged despair, guilt, blame, hostility
Accepting a valid diagnosis

5. The family must adjust, as the member begins to recover, by

Adapting to new ways of living and making appropriate changes as recovery ensues
Fostering independence of recovering member
Accepting residual disability and making any necessary accommodations
Recognizing depression and anxiety in family member during change from "sick role" to "well role"

6. The family must return to normalcy by returning to previous activities as much as possible and incorporating the recovered member back into the flow of family activities and responsibilities.

Alterations in Family Processes
Related to an Ill Family Member*

Assessment

Subjective Data

Family members verbalize fear, anxiety, and anger
Family members engage in destructive bickering
Individual family members make direct or subtle appeal for help, such as
"I can't cry but feel like I need to" (asking for permission to cry)
"I don't want her to know how worried I am" (asking for help with communication)
"I haven't eaten anything since this morning" (asking permission to leave the bedside of ill family member)
"I don't know where I went wrong" (requesting reassurance that illness is not his fault)
Family members are unable to make a decision together
One or more family members refuse to assist with ill member's care

Objective Data

Absence of family interaction (both verbally and nonverbally)

* This specific diagnosis applies to most illnesses. For families experiencing a terminal illness, see *Grieving Related to Anticipated Loss* for specific interventions

Tendency of family members to interfere with necessary nursing and medical interventions

Sudden outburst of emotions without apparent cause and/or emotional liability of family members

---

Outcome Criteria

The person (family members) will
- Frequently verbalize feelings to professional nurse and each other
- Participate in care of ill family member
- Facilitate return of ill family member from sick role to well role
- Maintain functional system of mutual support for each member
- Seek appropriate external resources when needed

Interventions

A. Assess causative and contributing factors

1. Illness-related factors
    Sudden, unexpected nature of illness
    Burdensome problems of a chronic nature
    Potentially disabling nature of illness
    Symptoms creating disfiguring change in physical appearance
    Social stigma associated with illness
    Financial burden
2. Factors related to behavior of ill family member
    Refuses to cooperate with necessary interventions
    Engages in socially deviant behavior associated with illness: suicide attempts, violence, substance abuse
    Isolates self from family
    Acts out or is verbally abusive to health professionals and family members
3. Factors related to the family as a whole
    Presence of unresolved guilt, blame, hostility, jealousy
    Inability to problem-solve adequately
    Ineffective patterns of communication among members
    Changes in roled expectations and resulting tension
4. Factors related to illness in family
    Absence of caring
    Lack of family members available for support
5. Factors related to health care environment
    Intervening professionals lack expertise in crisis intervention, counseling, or basic communication skills
    Not enough health professionals can spend time with the family
    Lack of continuity of care
    Lack of physical facilities in institution to ensure privacy or individualized care
6. Factors related to the community
    Lack of support from spiritual resources (philosophical and/or religious)
    Lack of relevant health education resources
    Lack of supportive friends

Lack of adequate community health care resources (*e.g.,* long-term follow-up care, hospice, respite agency)

B. Acknowledge your feelings about the family and their situation
- Attempt to resolve these feelings
    Pity
    Identifying with own family
    Blaming ill person and/or family for circumstances
    Judgmental attitude toward family
    Practicing punishing behavior (*e.g.,* ignoring people involved)
- Gain experience in crisis intervention and communication skills
- Approach the family with warmth, respect, and support
- Avoid vague and confusing advice and clichés such as "Take it easy, everything will be OK"
- Reflect family emotions to confirm these feelings ("This is very painful for you"; "You are very frightened")
- Keep family members abreast of changes in ill member's condition when appropriate

C. Create a private and supportive hospital environment for family
- Keep client's door closed if possible
- Provide family members with a meeting place alternative to client's room
- Make sure family members are oriented to visiting hours, bathrooms, vending machines, cafeteria, etc.
- If possible, provide pillows/blankets for family members spending the night

D. Facilitate family strengths
- Acknowledge these strengths to family when appropriate
    "I can tell you are a very close family"
    "You know just how to get your mother to eat"
    "Your brother means a great deal to you"
- Involve family members in care of ill member when possible (feeding, bathing, dressing, ambulating)
- Involve family members in patient care conferences when appropriate
- Encourage family to acquire substitutes to care for the ill person, to provide the family with time away
- Promote self-esteem of individual family members ("Your daughter may respond to your drawings if we place them in her crib") (see *Self-Concept Disturbance . . .*)

E. Intervene when family weaknesses dominate
- Facilitate communication
- Encourage verbalization of guilt, anger, blame, and hostility and subsequent recognition of own feelings in family members
- Enlist help of other professionals when problems extend beyond realm of nursing (*e.g.,* social worker, clinical psychologist, nurse therapist, clinical specialist, psychiatrist, child care specialist)

F. Facilitate understanding, in other family members, of how ill member feels
- Discuss stresses of hospitalization
- Describe implications of "sick role" and how it will return to "well role"
- Aid family members to change their expectations of the ill member in a realistic manner

G. Assist family with appraisal of the situation

- What is at stake? Encourage family to have a realistic perspective by providing accurate information and answers to questions
- What are the choices? Assist family to reorganize roles at home and set priorities to maintain family integrity and reduce stress
- Where is there help? Direct family to community agencies, home health care organizations, and sources of financial assistance as needed (see *Impaired Home Maintenance Management* for additional interventions)

H. Provide the family with anticipatory guidance as illness continues

- Inform parents of the effects of prolonged hospitalization on children (appropriate to developmental age)
- Prepare family members for signs of depression, anxiety, and dependency, which are a natural part of the illness experience
- If the ill family member is an elderly parent undergoing surgery, inform the children that the patient may be confused or disoriented for a limited period of time following surgery

I. Initiate health teaching and referrals as necessary

- Include family members in group education sessions
- Refer families to lay support and self-help groups
  - Al-Anon
  - Syn-Anon
  - Alcoholics Anonymous
  - Sharing and Caring (American Hospital Association)
  - Ostomy Association
  - Reach for Recovery
  - Lupus Foundation of America
  - Arthritis Foundation
  - National Multiple Sclerosis Society
  - American Cancer Society
  - American Heart Association
  - American Diabetes Association
  - American Lung Association
- Facilitate family involvement with social supports
  - Assist family members to identify reliable friends (clergy, significant others, etc.) and encourage seeking help when appropriate

References/Bibliography

Burr B, Good BJ, Good MD: The impact of illness on the family. In Taylor RB (ed): Family Medicine: Principles and Practice, pp 221–232. New York, Springer-Verlag, 1978

Christensen KE: Family epidemiology: An approach to assessment and intervention. In Hymovich DP, Barnard MV (eds): Family Health Care, 2nd ed, vol 1, pp 17–30. New York, McGraw-Hill, 1979

Duvall EM: Marriage and Family Development, 5th ed. Philadelphia, JB Lippincott, 1977

Fife BL: A model for predicting the adaptation of families to medical crisis: An analysis of role integration. Image: The Journal of Nursing Scholarship 18(4):108–112, 1985

Friedman M: Family Nursing: Theory and Assessment. New York, Appleton-Century-Crofts, 1981

Geary MC: Supporting family coping. Supervisor Nurse 10(3):57–59, 1979

Giacquinta B: Helping families face the crisis of cancer. Am J Nurs 77:1585–1588, 1977

Hymovich DP, Barnard MV (eds): Family Health Care, 2nd ed. New York, McGraw-Hill, 1979

Johnson SH: High-Risk Parenting. Philadelphia, JB Lippincott, 1979

McCubbin, M: Nursing Assessment of Parental Coping with Cystic Fibrosis. Western J Nurs Res 6(4):407–418, 1984

Miller S, Winstead-Fry P: Family Systems Theory in Nursing Practice. Norwalk, CT, Reston Publishing, 1982

Minuchin A: Families and Family Therapy. Cambridge, MA, Harvard University Press, 1974

Fatigue

Related to **(Specify)**

Definition

Fatigue: The self-recognized state in which an individual experiences an overwhelming sustained sense of exhaustion and decreased capacity for physical and mental work that is not relieved by rest.

> **Author's Note:** Fatigue is different from tiredness. Tiredness is a transient, temporary state (Rhoten) caused by lack of sleep, improper nutrition, sedentary life-style, or a temporary increase in work or social responsibilities. Fatigue is a pervasive, subjective, drained feeling that cannot be eliminated, but the individual can be assisted to adapt to fatigue. Activity intolerance is different from fatigue in that the person with activity intolerance will be assisted in increasing endurance to progress and will increase his or her activity. The person with chronic fatigue will not return to his or her previous level of functioning.

Defining Characteristics*

Major (80%–100%)

Verbalization of an unremitting and overwhelming lack of energy
Inability to maintain usual routines

Minor (50%–79%)

Perceived need for additional energy to accomplish routine tasks
Increase in physical complaints
Emotionally labile or irritable
Impaired ability to concentrate
Decreased performance
Lethargic or listless
Distinterest in surroundings/introspection
Decreased libido
Accident prone

Etiological, Contributing, Risk Factors

Many factors can cause fatigue. Some common factors are:

Pathophysiological

Acute infections
    Mononucleosis
    Hepatitis
    Viral
Fever

* Voith AM, Frank AM, Pigg JS: Validations of fatigue as a nursing diagnosis. In Classification of Nursing Diagnoses: Proceedings of the Seventh National Conference, p 280. St. Louis, CV Mosby, 1987

Chronic infection
  Hepatitis
  Endocarditis
Impaired oxygen transport system
  Congestive heart failure
  Chronic obstructive lung disease
  Anemia
  Peripheral vascular disease
Endocrine/metabolic disorders
  Diabetes mellitus
  Hypothyroidism
  Pituitary disorders
  Addison's disease
Chronic diseases
  Renal failure
  Cirrhosis
Neuromuscular disorders
  Parkinson's disease
  Arthritis
  Myasthenia gravis
  Multiple sclerosis
Obesity
Electrolyte imbalances
Cancer
Nutritional disorders
Gait disorders
Acquired immunodeficiency syndrome (AIDS)

Treatment-related

Chemotherapy
Radiation therapy
Antidepressants
Drug withdrawal

Situational

Depression
Extreme stress
Crisis (personal, developmental, career, family, financial)
Sensory overload (noise, illumination, etc.)
Extreme temperatures
Prolonged excessive role demands

Maturational

Adult
  Pregnancy (first trimester)
  Caregiver (ill child, aging parent)

Focus Assessment Criteria

Subjective Data

1. History of fatigue
    Onset?

Precipitated by what?
Pattern:
    morning, evening, transient, unfading
Relieved by rest?
2. Associated signs and symptoms

Fever	Dyspnea
Weight loss	Sleep disorders
Sleep-seeking behavior	Decreased motivation
Irritability	

3. Medical history (recent illnesses, chronic disease)
4. Medications
5. Effects of fatigue on:

Concentration	Family
Finances	Marriage
Occupation	Recreation
Role responsibilities	

Objective Data

Proceed with physical assessment based on the subjective data collected, *e.g.,* general appearance, speech affect, vital signs, range of motion, etc.

Principles and Rationale for Nursing Care

General

1. Fatigue can be a simple or complex problem. It is a subjective experience with physiological, situational, and psychological components.
2. Normal fatigue is an expected response to physical exertion, change in daily activities, additional stress, or inadequate sleep. (Kellum)
3. Fatigue can be (Morris)
   - Psychologically caused with resulting psychological and physiological manifestations
   - Physiologically caused with resulting psychological and physiological manifestations
   - A warning sign of a health disorder
   - Relieved by prescribed rest (physical and psychological)
4. American society values energy and productivity. Those without energy are viewed as sluggish or lazy. Energy and vitality are valued positively, while fatigue and tiredness are viewed negatively (Rhoten)
5. Fatigue can result from pathophysiology such as:
   Decreased cardiac output
   Prolonged circulatory time
   Accumulation of metabolic wastes
   Decreased oxygen transport
6. Fatigue can be manifested in areas of cortical inhibition such as: (Rhoten)
   Decreased attention
   Slowed and impaired perception
   Impaired thinking
   Decreased motivation
   Decreased performance in physical and mental activities
   Loss of fine coordination
   Poor judgment
   Indifference to one's surroundings

7. Rest is not defined as lying in bed. Rest is described as a person in an environment where one can relax, mentally and physically. The person replenishes his or her energy supply during this period. (Morris)
8. Depression slows one's thought processes and produces a decrease in physical activities. Work output decreases, and endurance is reduced. The effort to continue activity produces fatigue.
9. Anxiety can interfere with one's thought processes, increase movements, and disturb gastrointestinal function, thus causing fatigue.
10. Hargreaves described a high incidence of "fatigue syndrome" in young married women in moving to a new town. Factors that contributed to the fatigue were increased physical work, changes in support systems, and other stresses in relocation.
11. Reciprocity or returning support to one's support system is vital for balanced and healthy relationships (Tilden). Individuals who are fatigued have difficulty with reciprocity.

Cancer and Fatigue

1. Prolonged stress may be the main cause of chronic fatigue in persons with cancer. (Aistars)
2. The stressors (pathophysiological, situational, treatment-related) contributing to fatigue in cancer clients are illustrated in Table II-7

Fatigue

Related to **(Specify)**

Assessment

See Defining Characteristics

Outcome Criteria

The person will:
- Discuss the causes of fatigue
- Share feelings regarding the effects of fatigue on his/her life
- Establish priorities for daily and weekly activities
- Participate in activities that stimulate and balance physical, cognitive, affective, and social domains

---

Interventions

The nursing interventions for this diagnostic category are interventions for individuals with fatigue with etiologies that cannot be eliminated. The focus of nursing care is to assist the individual and family to adapt to the fatigue state.

A. Assess causative or contributing factors

1. Lack of sleep, refer to *Sleep Pattern Disturbance*
2. Poor nutrition, refer to *Altered Nutrition*
3. Sedentary life-style, refer to *Health-Seeking Behaviors*
4. Inadequate stress management, refer to *Health-Seeking Behaviors*
5. Physiological impairment

Table II-7.   **Fatigue-Contributing Factors in Cancer Clients**

Pathophysiological (Aistars)
Hypermetabolic state associated with active tumor growth
Competition between the body and the tumor for nutrients
Chronic pain
Organ dysfunction (*e.g.,* hepatic, respiratory, gastrointestinal)

Treatment-related (Aistars)
Accumulation of toxic waste products secondary to radiation, chemotherapy
Inadequate nutritional intake secondary to nausea, vomiting
Anemia
Analgesics, antiemetics
Diagnostic tests
Surgery

Situational (personal, environmental)
Uncertainty about future
Fear of death, disfigurement
Social isolation
Losses (role responsibilities, occupational, body parts, function, appearance, economic)
Separation for treatments

6. Treatment (chemotherapy, radiation, medications)
7. Chronic excessive role or social demands

B. Explain the causes of his/her fatigue (see Principles for explanations)

C. Allow expression of feelings regarding the effects of fatigue on his/her life
  • Identify those activities that are difficult
  • Interfere with role responsibilities
  • Frustrations
  • Refer to *Impaired Adjustment* if individual expresses nonacceptance of limitations

D. Assist the individual to identify strengths, abilities, interests (refer to *Hopelessness* for specific interventions)

E. Assist individual to identify energy patterns and the need to schedule activities
  1. Instruct individual to record fatigue levels q1 hour during a 24-hour period (select a usual day) (Aistars)
    • Ask to rate his fatigue 0–10 using the Rhoten fatigue scale (0 = not tired, peppy; 10 = total exhaustion) (Rhoten)
    • Record the activities at the time of each rating
  2. Analyze together the 24-hour fatigue levels
    • Times of peak energy
    • Times of exhaustion
    • Activities associated with increasing fatigue

F. Assist individual to identify what tasks can be delegated
  • Explore what activities are viewed as important for the individual to maintain self-esteem
  • Attempt to divide the vital activities or tasks into components; delegate parts of the task but retain certain components, *e.g.*:

> meal preparation
>> shopping
>> storing
>> preparing food for cooking
>> cooking
>> serving
>> cleaning up

- Plan the important tasks during periods of high energy, *e.g.,* prepare all the day's meals in the morning

G. Explain the purpose of pacing and prioritization (Brunner)
- Assist individual to identify priorities and to eliminate nonessential activities
- Plan each day to avoid energy- and time-consuming nonessential decision-making
- Organize work with work items within easy reach
- Distribute difficult tasks throughout the week
- Rest before difficult tasks and stop before fatigue ensues

H. Teach energy conservation techniques
1. Modify the environment
   - Replace steps with ramps
   - Install grab rails
   - Elevate chairs 3–4 inches
   - Organize kitchen or work areas
   - Reduce trips up and down stairs, *e.g.,* put a commode on first floor
2. Plan small frequent meals to decrease energy required for digestion
3. Use taxi instead of driving self
4. Delegate housework, *e.g.,* employ a high school student for a few hours after school

I. Explain the effects of conflict and stress on energy levels
- Refer to *Ineffective Individual Coping* for problem-solving strategies

J. Explain the psychological and physiological benefits of exercise and discuss what is realistic
- Refer to *Health-Seeking Behaviors* for specific information

K. Provide significant others opportunities to discuss their feelings in private regarding:
- Changes in the person with fatigue
- Their care-taking responsibilities
- Financial issues
- Changes in life-style, role responsibilities, relationships
- Refer to *Impaired Home Maintenance Management* for additional strategies for caregivers

L. Initiate health teaching and referrals as indicated
- Counseling
- Community services (Meals-On-Wheels, housekeeper)
- Financial assistance

References/Bibliography

Aistars J: Fatigue in the cancer patient: A conceptual approach to a clinical problem. Oncol Nurs Forum 14 (6d): 25–30, 1987

American Psychiatric Association Diagnostic and Statistical Manual of Mental Disorders, Washington, DC, APA, 1980

Brunner L, Suddarth D: Textbook of Medical Surgical Nursing, 6th Ed, p 214. Philadelphia, JB Lippincott, 1988

Freal JE, Kraft GH, Coryell JK: Principles of prioritizing symptomatic fatigue in multiple sclerosis. Arch Phys Med Rehabil March 1963, pp 135–137

Hargreaves M: The fatigue syndrome. Practitioner 218:841–843, 1977

Kellum MD: Fatigue. In Jacobs MM, Geels W (eds): Signs and Symptoms in Nursing. Philadelphia, JB Lippincott, 1985

Miller JF: Energy deficits in the chronically ill: The patient with arthritis. In Coping with Chronic Illness: Overcoming Powerlessness, p 203. Philadelphia, FA Davis,

Monroe LF: Psychological and physiological differences between good and poor sleepers. J Abnorm Psychol 72(3):255–264

Morris M: Tiredness and fatigue. In Norris C (ed): Concept Clarification in Nursing, pp 263–275. Rockville, MD, Aspen Systems Corp, 1982

Potempa K, Lopez M, Reid C, Lawson L: Chronic fatigue. Image, 18(4): 165–169, 1986

Rhoten D: Fatigue and the postsurgical patient. In Norris C (ed): Concept Clarification in Nursing. Rockville, MD, Aspen Systems Corp, 1982

Riddle PK: Chronic fatigue and women: A description and suggested treatment. Women Health, 7(1): 37–47, 1982

Tilden VP, Weinert C: Social support and the chronically ill individual. Nurs Clin North Am 22(3): 613–620, 1987

Fear

Related to **(Specify)**

Definition

Fear: A state in which an individual or group experiences a feeling of physiological or emotional disruption related to an identifiable source that is perceived as dangerous.

> **Author's Note:** Fear differs from anxiety in that the person can identify the threat, while in anxiety the threat cannot be accurately identified. Although it is possible for fear to be present without anxiety, clinically, fear and anxiety usually coexist.

Defining Characteristics

Major (must be present)

Feeling of dread, fright, apprehension and/or
Behaviors of
 Avoidance
 Narrowing of focus on danger
 Deficits in attention, performance, and control

Minor (may be present)

Verbal reports of panic, obsessions
Behavioral acts of
 Aggression   Dysfunctional immobility
 Escape   Compulsive mannerisms
 Hypervigilance   Increased questioning/verbalization
Visceral-somatic activity

Musculoskeletal	*Genitourinary*
Muscle tightness	Urinary frequency
Fatigue	

Cardiovascular	*Skin*
Palpitations	Flush/Pallor
Rapid pulse	Sweating
Increased blood pressure	Paraesthesia

Respiratory	*CNS/perceptual*
Shortness of breath	Syncope
Increased rate	Insomnia
	Lack of concentration
	Irritability
	Absentmindness
	Nightmares
	Pupil dilation

Gastrointestinal

Anorexia
Nausea/vomiting
Diarrhea

Etiological, Contributing, Risk Factors

Fear can occur as a response to a variety of health problems, situations, or conflicts. Some common sources are indicated below.

Pathophysiological

Loss of body part
Loss of body function
Disabling illness

Long-term disability
Terminal disease

Treatment-related

Hospitalization
Surgery and its outcome
Anesthesia
Invasive procedures
Radiation

Situational (personal, environmental)

Influences of others
Pain
New environment
New people

Lack of knowledge
Change or loss of significant other
Divorce
Success
Failure

Maturational

Children: age-related fears (dark, strangers), influence of others
Adolescent: school adjustments, social and intellectual competitiveness, independence, authorities
Adult: marriage, pregnancy, parenthood
Elderly: retirement, relinquishing roles, functional losses

Focus Assessment (Subjective/Objective)

1. Onset
    Have the person tell you his "story" about his fearfulness
2. Manner of communication
    Verbal reports of distress?
    Fear-related behavioral acts?
    Visceral or somatic activity?
3. Thought process and content
    How does person organize his thoughts?
    Are thoughts clear, coherent, logical, confused, or forgetful?
    Can he concentrate, or is he preoccupied?
    Do misperceptions interfere with reality testing?
4. Control behaviors
    Does fear interfere with life-style?
    Can the person use several control behaviors or only one persistent behavior?
    What understanding does the person have about his fear?

Do coping mechanisms help solve problems (functional) or do they contribute to further problems (maladaptation)?
5. Emotional state

Is emotional feeling tone appropriate or inappropriate to the situation?

Do facial expressions, voice tone, and body posture correspond to the intensity of the person's verbal expression of fear?
6. Perception and judgment

Is fear still present after stressor is eliminated?

Do only major events lead to fearfulness, or do minor events trigger fears?

Can the person comprehend the present and focus on his actions, or is he overwhelmed by future anticipations?

Is the fear a response to a present stimulus, or is it distorted by influences in the past?
7. Relatedness to others

Does the person's intensity of fear cause movement away from others?

What or who are his support systems?

Can he accept support from the nurse or others?
8. Children

Is the child's fear normal and expected for his age group?

What actions of the parents contribute to the fear?

What actions of the parents reduce the fear?
9. Assess for the presence of visceral-somatic activity

Musculoskeletal	*Genitourinary*
Muscle tightness Fatigue	Urinary frequency
Cardiovascular	*Skin*
Palpitations Rapid pulse Increased blood pressure	Flush/Pallor Sweating Paresthesia
Respiratory	*CNS/perceptual*
Shortness of breath Increased rate	Syncope Insomnia Lack of concentration Irritability Absentmindness Nightmares
Gastrointestinal	*Visual*
Anorexia Nausea/vomiting Diarrhea	Pupil dilation

Principles and Rationale for Nursing Care

General

1. Psychological defense mechanisms are distinctly individual and can be adaptive or maladaptive.
2. Fear differs from anxiety in that fear is the feeling aroused when there is an accurate perception of an external threat; anxiety is a feeling aroused when the perception is of an imagined danger in response to internal beliefs.

3. Both fear and anxiety lead to disequilibrium.
4. Activity uses energy and dissipates the physical reaction to fear.
5. Anger may be an adaptive response to certain fears.
6. Safety feelings increase when a person identifies with another person who has successfully dealt with a similar fearful situation.
7. A sense of adequacy in confronting danger reduces fear. Fear disguises itself. The expressed fear may be a substitute for other fears that are not socially acceptable. Awareness of factors that cause intensification of fears enhances controls and prevents heightened feelings. Fear is reduced when the safe reality of a situation is confronted.
8. Fear can become anxiety (*e.g.,* fear becomes internalized and serves to disorganize instead of becoming adaptive).
9. Chronic physical reactions to stressors lead to susceptibility and chronic disease.
10. Physiological responses are manifested throughout the body primarily from the hypothalamus's stimulation of the autonomic and endocrine systems.
11. Individuals interpret the degree of danger from a threatening stimulus. The physiological and psychological systems react with equal intensity to the perceived threat ($\uparrow$ BP, $\uparrow$ heart rate, $\uparrow$ respiratory rate).
12. Fear is adaptive and is a healthy response to danger.

Children
1. A child learns fear from unpleasant direct experiences with people and things or from adults or other children who communicate their fears to him.
2. Adults increase fears in children when they utilize fear to encourage obedience (*e.g.,* "If you don't wear your boots you'll get sick and have to get a needle at the hospital"; "If you are bad, that policeman will get you and put you in jail")
3. Preschool children (2 to 5 years) with their egocentric thinking and their limited ability for conceptual thinking experience distress when they witness another person hurting. For example, a 3-year-old child who witnesses another child receive an injection may cry as violently as the child who actually received the injection.
4. Fears throughout childhood follow a developmental sequence.
5. Fear behaviors are *consistent* and *immediate* upon exposure or mention of a specific stressor; if the response is erratic, the diagnosis might more accurately be anxiety.

Birth–2 Years
Fears evolve from physical stimuli, *e.g.*
    Loud noises (thunder)
    Strange people
    Strange places
    Sudden movements
    Flashes of light

2–5 Years
Fears evolve from real and imagined situations, *e.g.*
    Injury or mutilation
    Ghosts, devils, monsters
    Dark
    Bathtub and toilet drains
    Being alone
    Dreams
    Robbers

6 Years
Fears are numerous, *e.g.*
    Loud noises
    Ghosts, devils, monsters
    Large animals
    Imagined unseen persons (outside window, under bed)
    Fire, thunder, lightning, water
    Being lost
    Being hurt
    Something will happen to parents

7 Years
Fears are still numerous, *e.g.*
    Dark, cellar, attic
    Burglars
    Imagined unseen persons (outside window, under bed)
    Failure (with friends; in school, sports)
    Not being liked
    Various subjects presented by radio or on television

8–9 Years
Fears and worries are fewer, *e.g.*
    Things that cannot be explained or proved nonexistent (death, pain)
    Poor achievement (grades, being late)

10 Years
Fears are many but child worries less, *e.g.*
    Animals (snakes, wild animals)
    High places
    Fires, ghosts
    Dark, blood
    Poor achievement (grades, sports)

11 Years
This is the most worried and fearful stage, *e.g.*
    Strong fear of being alone
    Worry about school, money, parents' welfare, illness
    Rejection by opposite sex
    Strange animals
    Pain, disease, and loss of mother (by girls)

12 Years
This is a less fearful time, *e.g.*
    The dark
    Noises at night
    Intruders

Fear
Related to (Specify)

Assessment
See Defining Characteristics

Outcome Criteria

The adult will
- Relate increase in psychological and physiological comfort
- Differentiate real from imagined situations
- Describe effective and ineffective coping patterns
- Identify his own coping responses

The child will
- Discuss his fears
- Relate an increase in psychological comfort

Interventions
The nursing interventions for the diagnosis *Fear* represent interventions for any individual with fear regardless of the etiological or contributing factors.

A. Assess possible contributing factors
1. Perception of threatening stimulus (realistic)
   Unfamiliar environment (new home, admission, new people)
   Intrusion on personal space
   Life-style change (promotion, marriage, retirement)
   Biological change (dysfunction, rejection)
   Self-esteem threat (abandonment, rejection)
2. Distorted perceptions of dangerous stimulus
3. Age-related fears

B. Reduce or eliminate contributing factors
1. Unfamiliar environment
   - Orient to environment using simple explanations
   - Speak slowly and calmly
   - Avoid surprises and painful stimulus
   - Use soft lights and music
   - Remove threatening stimulus
   - Plan one-day-at-a-time familiar routine
   - Encourage gradual mastery of a situation
   - Provide transitional object with symbolic safeness (security blanket, religious medals)
2. Intrusion on personal space
   - Allow personal space
   - Move person away from stimulus
   - Remain with him until fear subsides (listen, use silence)

- Later, establish frequent and consistent contacts; utilize family members and significant others to stay with him
- Use touch as tolerated (sometimes holding person firmly will help him maintain control)

3. Threat to self-esteem
   - Support preferred coping style when adaptive mechanisms are used (some prefer details; others, general explanations)
   - Initially, decrease the person's number of choices
   - Use simple direct statements (avoid detail)
   - Give direct suggestion to manage everyday events
   - Encourage expression of feelings (helplessness, anger)
   - Give feedback about his expressed feelings (support realistic assessments)
   - Refocus interaction on areas of capability rather than dysfunction
   - Encourage normal coping mechanisms
   - Encourage sharing common problems with others
   - Give feedback of effect his behavior has on others
   - Encourage him to face the fear

4. Distorted perceptions
   - Encourage responses that reflect reality
   - Ask straightforward questions ("Do you feel pain?" "Does my asking you about your feelings make you uncomfortable?")
   - Provide information to reduce distortions ("No, I will not harm you" "That was only a shadow and not the bogey man")
   - Encourage specifics and discourage generalizations; have him give details, not vague general assumptions ("Who are you referring to when you say 'they' are trying to kill you?")
   - Explore superficial interactions
     a. Examine the person's reason for avoiding feelings
     b. Allow him to know that it is OK to feel
     c. Share your reaction to the event ("I can see why you're upset; if that happened to me I would have felt like screaming")
   - Provide an emotionally nonthreathening atmosphere
     a. Provide situations that are predictable
     b. Allow for consistency in personnel to enhance comfort and familiarity
     c. Announce changes in the environment

5. Age-related fears (Refer to Principles and Rationale for Nursing Care)
   - Provide child with opportunities to express his fears and to learn healthy outlets for anger or sadness, *e.g.*, play therapy (see Appendix IX for Guidelines for Play Therapy)
   - Acknowledge illness, death, pain as real and refrain from protecting children from the reality of its existence; encourage open, honest sharing
   - Accept the child's fear and provide him with an explanation, if possible, or some form of control; share with child that these fears are okay
     a. Fear of imaginary animals, intruders ("I don't see a lion in your room, but I will leave the light on for you, and if you need me again, please call")
     b. Fear of parent being late (establish a contingency plan, *e.g.*, "If you come home from school and Mommy is not here, go to Mrs. S. next door")
     c. Fear of vanishing down a toilet or bathtub drain
        Wait until child is out of tub before releasing drain
        Wait until child is off the toilet before flushing
        Leave toys in bathtub and demonstrate how they do not go down the drain

    d. Fear of dogs, cats

        Allow child to watch a child and a dog playing from a distance

        Do not force child to touch the animal

    e. Fear of death

        See Principles and Rationale for Nursing Care for *Grieving*

    f. Fear of pain

        See *Acute Pain in Children*

- Discuss with parents the normalcy of fears in children; explain the necessity of acceptance and the negative outcomes of punishment or of forcing the child to overcome the fear
- Provide child with opportunity to observe other children cope successfully with feared object

C. Initiate health teaching and referrals as indicated

1. When intensity of feelings has decreased, bring behavioral cues into the person's awareness
   - Teach signs that indicate increased fear ("Your face flushes and you clench your fists when we discuss your discharge")
   - Indicate adaptiveness of behavior
2. Explain how expressed fear of one thing may be hidden fear of something else
3. Teach how to problem-solve

   What is the problem?

   Who or what is responsible for the problem?

   What are the options?

   What are advantages and disadvantages of each option?
4. Teach ways for enhancing control
   - Include the person in the treatment process ("Please raise your hand if the procedure causes pain")
   - Share test results when appropriate
     a. Inform ahead of time about tests (time interval depends on ability to cope)
     b. Identify activities that rechannel emotional energy to diffuse intensity
     c. Use nightlight or flashlight to diffuse fear (child with fear of dark can be given a flashlight to use ad lib)
     d. Before tests or surgery, prepare patient as to what to expect, especially sensations, and define this role and how to participate in the role (*e.g.,* breathing exercises postoperatively may take mind off of fears and dissipate physical reaction)
5. Recommend or instruct concerning methods that increase comfort or relaxation (see Appendix X for Guidelines)

   Progressive relaxation technique

   Reading, music, breathing exercises

   Desensitization, self-coaching

   Thought stopping, guided fantasy

   Yoga, hypnosis, assertiveness training
6. Participate in community functions to teach parents age-related fears and constructive interventions, *e.g.,* parent–school organizations, newsletters, civic groups

References/Bibliography

Bowlby J: Children, mourning and its implications for psychiatry. Am J Psychiatry 118:481–498, 1961

Burke S: A developmental perspective on the nursing diagnosis of fear and anxiety. Nursing Papers 13(4):20, 59–64, 1981

McFarland G, Wasli E: Nursing Diagnosis and Process in Psychiatric Mental Health Nursing. Philadelphia, JB Lippincott, 1986

Petrillo M, Sanger S: The Emotional Care of the Hospitalized Child. Philadelphia, JB Lippincott, 1980

Ross D: Thought-stopping: A coping strategy for impending feared events. Issues Comprehen Pediatr Nurs 7:83–89, 1984

Sadler A: Assertiveness training. In Bulechek G, McCloskey J (eds): Nursing Interventions: Treatements for Nursing Diagnoses, pp 234–235. Philadelphia, WB Saunders, 1985

Scandrett S, Uecker S: Relaxation training. In Bulechek G, McCloskey J (eds): Nursing Interventions: Treatments for Nursing Diagnoses, pp 22–48. Philadelphia, WB Saunders, 1985

Yanni M: Perceptions of parents' behavior and children's general fearfulness. Nurs Res 31(2):79–82, 1982

Yocum C: The differentiation of fear and anxiety. In Kim M, McFarland G, McLane A (eds): Classification of Nursing Diagnoses: Proceeding of Fifth National Conference. St. Louis, CV Mosby, 1984

Wass H, Cason L: Fears and anxieties about death. Issues Compreh Nurs 8(1/6):25–45, 1985

Whaley L, Wong D: Nursing Care of Infants and Children, pp 429–777, 952–955. St. Louis, CV Mosby, 1979

Wieczorek R, Natapoff J: A Conceptual Approach to Nursing of Children: Health Care From Birth Through Adolescence. Philadelphia, JB Lippincott, 1981

Fluid Volume Deficit

Related to **Decreased Oral Intake**

Related to **Abnormal Fluid Loss**

Definition

Fluid volume deficit: The state in which an individual who is not NPO experiences or is at risk of experiencing vascular, interstitial, or intracellular dehydration.

> **Author's Note:** This diagnostic category represents situations in which nursing can prescribe definitive treatment to prevent fluid depletion or to reduce or eliminate contributing factors such as insufficient oral intake. Situations that represent hypovolemia caused by hemorrhage or NPO states should be considered collaborative problems, not nursing diagnoses. Nursing monitors to detect for these situations and collaborates with medicine for treatment. These situations can be labeled *Potential Complication: Hemorrhage* or *Potential Complication: Hypovolemia.*

Defining Characteristics

Major (must be present)

Output greater than intake
Dry skin/mucous membranes

Minor (may be present)

Increased serum sodium
Increased pulse rate (from baseline)
Decreased urine output or excessive urine output
Concentrated urine or urinary frequency
Decreased fluid intake
Decreased skin turgor
Thirst/nausea/anorexia

Etiological, Contributing, Risk Factors

Pathophysiological

Excessive urinary output
    Uncontrolled diabetes
    Diabetes insipidus (inappropriate antidiuretic hormone)
Burns (post-acute)
Fever or increased metabolic rate
Infection
Abnormal drainage
    Wound
    Excessive menses
    Other
Peritonitis
Diarrhea

Situational (personal, environmental)

    Vomiting/Nausea

    Decreased motivation to drink liquids

        Depression

        Fatigue

    Dietary problems

        Fad diets/fasting

        Anorexia

        High solute tube feedings

    Difficulty swallowing or feeding self

        Oral pain

        Fatigue

    Climate exposure

        Extreme heat/sun

        Excessive dryness

    Hyperpnea

    Extreme exercise effort/diaphoresis

    Excessive use of

        Laxatives or enemas

        Diuretics or alcohol

Maturational

    Infant/child: Decreased fluid reserve, decreased ability to concentrate urine

    Elderly: Decreased fluid reserve, decreased sensation of thirst

Focus Assessment Criteria

Subjective Data

    1. History of symptoms

        The person complains of

Nausea/vomiting/anorexia	Thirst
Weight loss	Polyuria/dysuria
Diarrhea/loose stool	Fever/diaphoresis

    2. History of contributing and causative factors

        Diabetes mellitus (diagnosed, family history)/diabetes insipidus

        Cardiac disease

        Renal disease

        Blood loss

        Gastrointestinal disorders or surgery

        Alcohol use

        Medications

Laxatives/enemas	Side-effects that are GI irritants
Diuretics	(antibiotics)

        Allergies (food, milk)

        Extreme heat/humidity

        Extreme exercise effort accompanied by sweating

        Depression

        Pain

    3. Current drug therapy

Type, dosage	Frequency (last dose taken when?)

Objective Data

1. Assess for presence of contributing factors
    Abnormal or excessive fluid loss
        Liquid stools
        Vomiting or gastric suction
        Diuresis or polyuria
        Diaphoresis
    Decreased fluid intake related to
        Fatigue
        Decreased level of con-
            sciousness

    Abnormal or excessive drainage
        (*e.g.,* fistulas, drains)
    Loss of skin surfaces (*e.g.,* burns)
    Fever

    Depression/disorientation
    Nausea or anorexia
    Physical limitations (*e.g.,* unable
        to hold glass)

2. Assess for signs of dehydration
    Skin
        Mucosa (lips, gums) (dry)
        Tongue (furrowed/dry)
        Turgor (decreased)
        Color (pale or flushed)
        Moisture (dry or diaphoretic)
        Fontanelles of infants (depressed)
        Eyeballs (sunken)
    Urine output
        Amount (varied; very large or minimal amount)
        Color (amber; very dark or very light)
        Specific gravity (increased or decreased)
        Intake vs. output (less intake than output)
    Weight (loss/gain)
    Neck veins (collapsed when lying flat)
3. Diagnostic studies
    Hemoglobin/hematocrit
    Electrolytes
    Blood urea nitrogen (BUN)
    Urinalysis
    Creatinine

Principles and Rationale for Nursing Care

General

1. Fluid intake is primarily regulated by the sensation of thirst. Fluid output is primarily regulated by the kidneys' ability to concentrate urine.
2. The average daily fluid loss for the normal individual is urine, 1500 ml; stool, 200 ml; and perspiration/respiration ("insensible water loss"), 1000–1300 ml.
3. The body gains water in two ways: from food and drink absorbed through the gastrointestinal tract (this is the major source) and from the cellular oxidation of nutrients.
4. Excreted body fluids pull electrolytes with them, resulting in electrolyte loss:
    Urine (K^+ Na^+)
    Gastric juices (K^+, H^+)
    Perspiration (Na^+ Cl^-)
    Stool (K^+)

5. Normal serum electrolytes are

Cations (positive ions)	Sodium (137–148 mEq/liter)
	Potassium (3.5–5 mEq/liter)
	Calcium (8.5–10.5 mg/dl)
	Magnesium (1.5–2.5 mEq/liter)
Anions (negative ions)	Chloride (95–106 mEq/liter)
	Bicarbonate (21–28 mEq/liter)
	Protein (6.0–8.5 gm/dl)
	Organic acids (2.4–4.5 mg/dl)
	Phosphate (2.5–4.8 mg/dl)
	Sulfate (minuscule)

6. A balance of water and sodium is necessary for normal body fluid levels. Water provides 90% to 93% of the volume of body fluids, while sodium provide 90% to 95% of the solute of extracellular fluid.

7. Excessive fluid loss can be expected during

Fever or increased metabolic rate
Extreme exercise or diaphoresis
Climate extremes (heat/dryness)
Excessive vomiting or diarrhea
Burns, tissue insult, fistulas

8. Blood is the cooling fluid of the body. Dehydration (and resulting decrease in blood volume) causes an increased body temperature, pulse, respirations.

9. Water can normally be found in three spaces of the body—within the blood vessels, within the interstitial spaces (extracellular), and within the cell itself (intracellular).

10. Dehydration may occur within the vascular tree, while water within the interstitial spaces may be excessive (edema). Abnormal shifts between body compartments may cause fluid excess or deficit.

11. The specific gravity of the urine reflects the kidney's ability to concentrate urine; the range of urine specific gravity varies with the state of hydration and the solids to be excreted. (Specific gravity is elevated when dehydration is present, signifying concentrated urine.) Values are

Normal: 1.010–1.025
Concentrated: >1.025
Diluted: <1.010

12. Serum electrolytes serve four major functions

Assisting in regulating fluid balance
Assisting in enzyme reactions
Participating in acid-base regulation to maintain normal pH
Playing an essential role in nervous and muscular activity

13. A normal balance of cations (positive ions), anions (negative ions), and buffers is necessary for normal blood pH. (Normal arterial pH is 7.37–7.45.) *A very slight variation in these normals can cause death.*

14. Potassium is the major cation of the intracellular fluid-influencing acid–base balance and cellular hydration. High or low potassium interferes with the conduction of nerve impluses through skeletal, smooth, and cardiac muscle. *This may be manifested by cardiac and muscular irritability or flaccidity, which can cause life-threatening arrhythmias.*

15. Conditions that increase the incidence of hypokalemia (low potassium) are

Diuretic therapy (K^+ loss in urine)
Ascites (K^+ loss to accumulation of fluid in the abdomen)
Poor dietary habits (poor K^+ intake)
Extreme diaphoresis (Na^+ and K^+ loss)

Prolonged diarrhea/malabsorption syndrome (K^+ loss via stool)
Prolonged gastric suction (K^+ loss from gastric contents)
Surgery/tissue trauma (cellular loss of K^+)

16. Persons undergoing lengthy abdominal or chest surgery lose large amounts of fluid through direct evaporation from the open surgical cavity to the air in the operating room. (This additional insensible loss may account for immediate postoperative fluid deficit.)

Fluid Intake

1. The average adult requires 2,000 ml–3,000 ml of fluid intake per day. Under normal conditions, a nonperspiring adult needs 1500 ml of fluids daily. An additional 1000 ml of fluids comes from solid foods and oxidation during metabolism.
2. To correctly assess a person's potential for fluid imbalance, close examination of the previous 24 to 72 hours' intake and output is necessary. (In renal or cardiac disease, it may be necessary to consider intake and output for the previous 5 to 7 days, as well as body weight.)
3. People at high risk for fluid imbalance include
    People on medication for fluid retention, high blood pressure, seizures, or "anxiety" (tranquilizers)
    People who suffer from diabetes, cardiac disease, excessive alcohol intake, malnourishment, obesity, or GI distress
    Adults over 60, and children under 6
    People who are confused, depressed, comatose, or lethargic (no sensation of thirst)
4. In determining the 24-hour intake requirement for an infant or child, both caloric and fluid intake should be measured. The following calculations can be utilized:

Calorie Intake

For a child up to 10 kg of body weight: 100 cal/kg
For a child between 11 kg and 20 kg: 1000 cal plus 50 cal/kg for each kg above 20

Fluid Intake (for maintenance)

Approximately 120 ml per 100 cal of metabolism
Abnormal fluid loss must be replaced in addition to the above.

5. With inadequate caloric intake, metabolism of the body's stores of fat and muscle may provide a significant increase in total body water, resulting in weight gain that may hide malnutrition (*e.g.,* the "bloating" of terminal malnutrition).
6. Adequate protein intake is necessary to maintain normal osmotic pressures. Foods that have a high protein content are meats, fish, fowl, soybeans, eggs, legumes, and cheese.
7. Large amounts of sugar, alcohol, and caffeine act as diuretics that increase urine production and may cause dehydration.
8. People receiving tube feedings are at high risk for dehydration, because the high solute concentration of the tube feeding may cause diarrhea and diuresis. *Tube feedings must be supplemented with specific amounts of water to maintain adequate hydration.*
9. A high intake of sodium causes increased retention of water.
    Foods with high sodium content include salted snacks, bacon, cheddar cheese, pickles, soy sauce, processed luncheon meats, MSG (monosodium glutamate), canned vegetables, catsup, and mustard. Some over-the-counter drugs such as bicarbonate of

soda, antacids, cough suppressants, and many oral hygiene products also have a high sodium content.

Foods with moderate sodium content include eggs, milk, hamburger, canned corn, and canned tomato juice.

Foods with low sodium content include fruits, chicken, liver, fresh vegetables, unsalted bread, and unsalted crackers.

10. Foods with a high potassium content include bananas, dates, raisins, oranges, tomatoes, puffed wheat cereal, potatoes, liver, Pepsi, and Gatorade.

Edema

1. People with cardiac pump failure are at high risk for both vascular and tissue fluid excess (*i.e.,* pulmonary and peripheral edema). Acute pulmonary edema should be considered a medical emergency.
2. The most frequent vascular cause of tissue edema is increased venous pressure, which causes increased capillary blood pressure.
3. Edema inhibits blood flow to the tissue, resulting in poor cellular nutrition and increased susceptibility to injury.
4. Edema is often seen as a result of

   Venous obstruction (pressure point, such as sitting with legs crossed) and resulting venous pooling

   Heart failure (decreased cardiac output) resulting in backup of blood in the heart, lungs, and vessels

   Lymphatic obstruction (*e.g.,* after a lymph node dissection)

   Trauma (tissue injury that releases histamines, causing vasodilation and increased permeability and movement of fluid); examples are burns, sprains, fractures

   Hypoxia of the cell

   Vitamin C deficiency or extreme malnutrition

   Prolonged steroid therapy

High-Risk Elderly

1. Phillips reported a decrease in thirst as one ages.
2. The elderly are more susceptible to fluid loss and dehydration because of:
   - Decreased renal blood flow
   - Decreased glomerular filtration
   - Impaired ability to regulate temperature
   - Decreased ability to concentrate urine
   - Increase in physical disabilities decreases access to fluids
   - Self-limiting of fluids for fear of incontinence
3. Seventy-five percent of the fluid intake in the elderly occurs between 6 AM and 6 PM. (Adams)

Fluid Volume Deficit
Related to Decreased Oral Intake

Assessment

Subjective Data
The person reports
>Nausea and vomiting/anorexia
>Altered ability to drink or swallow (sore throat, dysphagia)
>Upper limb limitations
>Decreased motivation to obtain fluids (weakness, depression, fatigue)

Objective Data
>Decreased urine output
>Increased specific gravity of urine
>Dry skin or dry mucous membranes
>Decreased lacrimal secretions and decreased saliva
>Poor skin turgor
>Furrowed tongue

Outcome Criteria

The person will
- Increase intake of fluids to a minimum of 2,000 ml (unless contraindicated)
- Relate the need for increased fluid intake during stress or heat
- Maintain a urine specific gravity within a normal range
- Demonstrate no signs and symptoms of dehydration

Interventions

A. Assess causative factors
>Inability to feed self
>Dislike of available liquids
>Sore throat
>Extreme fatigue or weakness
>Lack of knowledge (of the need for increased fluid intake)

B. Reduce or eliminate causative factors
1. Inability to feed self
    See *Self-Care Deficit*
2. Dislike of available liquids
    - Assess likes and dislikes; provide favorite fluids within dietary restrictions
    - Plan an intake goal for each shift (*e.g.,* 1000 ml during day; 800 ml during evening; 300 ml at night)

- For children, offer
  a. Appealing forms of fluids (popsicles, frozen juice bars, snow cones, water, milk, Jell-O with vegetable coloring added; let child help make it)
  b. Unusual containers (colorful cups, straws)
  c. A game or activity
- Read a book to child and have him drink a sip when a page is turned, or have a tea party
- Have child take a drink when it is his turn in a game
- Make a set schedule for supplementary liquids to promote the habit of in-between meal fluids (*e.g.,* juice or Kool-Aid at 10 AM and 2 PM each day)

3. Sore throat
- Offer warm or cold fluids; consider frozen ices
- Consider warm saline gargle or anesthetic lozenges before fluids

4. Extreme fatigue or weakness
- Give smaller amounts more frequently
- Provide for periods of rest prior to meals

5. Lack of knowledge
- Assess the person's understanding of the reasons for maintaining adequate hydration, and methods for reaching goal of fluid intake
- Include significant others
- See Principles and Rationale for Nursing Care under *Health-Seeking Behaviors*

C. Have person maintain a written record (log) of fluid intake and urinary output (if necessary)

D. Prevent dehydration in high-risk individuals (see Principles for high-risk persons)

- Monitor intake; assure at least 1500 ml of oral fluids q24 hours.
- Monitor output; assure at least 1000–1500 ml per 24 hours.
- Offer fluids in large glasses, 120 or 240 ml. (Adams)
- Weigh daily in same clothes, at same time. A 2–4% weight loss indicates mild dehydration (Metheny); 5–9% weight loss indicates moderate dehydration.
- Monitor serum electrolytes, blood urea nitrogen, urine and serum, osmolality, creatinine, hematocrit, and hemoglobin.
- For persons scheduled for fasting prior to diagnostic studies, increase their fluid intake eight hours before fasting.
- Review client's medications. Do they contribute to dehydration (*e.g.,* diuretics)? Do they require increased fluid intake (*e.g.,* lithium)?
- Teach that coffee, tea, and grapefruit juice are diuretics and can contribute to fluid loss.
- Consider the additional fluid losses associated with vomiting, diarrhea, fever.

E. Initiate health teaching as indicated

- Give verbal and written directions for desired fluids and amounts
- Include the person/family in keeping a written record of fluid intake
- Provide a list of alternative fluids (*e.g.,* ice cream, pudding)
- Explain the need to increase fluids during exercise, fever, infection, and hot weather
- Teach the person how to observe for dehydration (especially in infants) and to intervene by increasing fluid intake (see Objective and Subjective Data for signs of dehydration)
- Seek medical consultation for continued dehydration

Fluid Volume Deficit
Related to Abnormal Fluid Loss

Abnormal fluid loss describes fluid loss by vomiting, diarrhea, excessive diaphoresis, or drains, not hemorrhage or acute burns.

Assessment

Subjective Data

The person reports
    "I keep going to the bathroom all the time"
    "I have to get up several times a night to urinate"
    "I have loose bowels [diarrhea]"
    "I've been vomiting a lot"
    "I break out in a cold sweat"
    "I'm thirsty all the time"

Objective Data

    Extreme diaphoresis
    Increased body drainage
        Vomitus/nasogastric suction
        Chest tubes/thoracentesis
        Sump drains/paracentesis
        T-tubes
        Liquid or loose stools
        Polyuria
        Wound drainage (pus, serous, etc.)
    Weight loss
    Output exceeds intake

Outcome Criteria

The person will
- Maintain adequate intake of fluid and electrolytes as evidenced by (specify)
- Identify his abnormal fluid loss and relate methods of decreasing this loss if possible
- Maintain a urine specific gravity within normal range

Interventions

A. **Assess causative factors**
    Vomiting
    Fever
    Gastric suction
    Diarrhea/loose stools

B. Remove or reduce causative factors

1. Vomiting
   - Encourage small, frequent amounts of ice chips or clear liquids such as weak tea or flat cola or ginger ale* (adults 30 ml, children 15 ml; see *Altered Nutrition; Less Than Body Requirements*)
2. Fever (see also *Hyperthermia*)
   a. Maintain temperature lower then 101°F (38.4°C) through tepid water sponging and medication (*e.g.,* A.S.A. or acetaminophen)*
      - Eliminate excessive clothing and bed covers
      - Keep the room temperature cool
      - Encourage cool, clear liquids when medication is at peak effectiveness and temperature is lowest
      - Substitute frozen ices or popsicles if necessary (be resourceful)
      - If the temperature is extremely high, >103°F (39.5°C), apply ice packs to pulse points (groin, axilla)*
   b. Specifically for children under 5 with a sudden rise in temperature ("spiking fever"):
      - Work to attain a temperature <101°F (38.4°C) as soon as possible with medication* (A.S.A., acetaminophen) and sponging
      - Use tepid water (85°–90°F/29.4°–37.7°C) for sponging or bathing the child
      - Caution parents not to cover the child with blankets and to be aware of the increased risk of febrile seizures
      - Give the child small amounts of *clear liquids only* (15 ml)
      - Teach the parents how to protect the child, should a seizure occur, and *instruct them to seek immediate medical consultation*
3. Gastric suction (nasogastric or other)
   - Use only normal saline for irrigation of gastric tubes to minimize electrolyte imbalance
   - Do not allow swallowing of water or ice chips; a "few small sips" can readily add up over a period of time
   - For the thirsty individual with gastric suction, *unless contraindicated by surgery or renal failure,* consult with the physician concerning ingestion of measured sips of Gatorade (1 oz/hr)
   - Always subtract all fluid ingested (via either tube or mouth) from any total gastric drainage to attain net drainage
   - Keep a careful, clear record of intake and output: amount, character, color
   - Offer frequent mouth care
4. Diarrhea/loose stools, see *Diarrhea*
5. Wound drainage
   - Keep careful records of the amount and type of drainage
   - Weigh dressings, if necessary, to estimate fluid loss (weigh the wet dressing; weigh a dry dressing of the same type; compare the difference)
   - Weigh the person daily if the drainage is excessive and difficult to measure (*e.g.,* soaked sheets)
   - Replace fluid loss (may be contraindicated in cardiac failure, renal failure, or head trauma)

C. Initiate health teaching as indicated

1. Assess the person's understanding of the type of fluid loss he is experiencing (what

---

* May require a physician's order.

electrolytes are lost) and the fluids that provide replacement (see Principles and Rationale for Nursing Care)
2. Give verbal and written instructions for fluid replacement (*e.g.,* "Drink at least 3 quarts of liquid a day, including 1 quart of Gatorade")
3. Teach the person to
   - Avoid sudden exposure and overexposure to heat/sun/and exercise
   - Gradually increase exposure and activity in hot weather
   - Eat three balanced meals a day
   - Increase fluid intake during hot days
   - Decrease activity during extreme weather

References/Bibliography

See *Fluid Volume Excess*

Fluid Volume Excess

Related to **(Specify)**

Definition

Fluid volume excess: The state in which an individual experiences or is at risk of experiencing intracellular or interstitial fluid overload.

> **Author's Note:** This diagnostic category represents situations in which nursing can prescribe definitive treatment to reduce or eliminate factors that contribute to edema or teach preventive actions. Situations that represent vascular fluid overload should be considered collaborative problems, not nursing diagnoses. They can be labeled *Potential Complication: Congestive Heart Failure or Potential Complication: Hypervolemia*

Defining Characteristics

Major (must be present)
Edema
Taut, shiny skin

Etiological, Contributing, Risk Factors

Pathophysiological
Renal failure, acute or chronic
Decreased cardiac output
    Myocardial infarction
    Congestive heart failure   Valvular disease
    Left ventricular failure   Tachycardia/arrhythmias
Varicosities of the legs
Liver disease
    Cirrhosis   Cancer
    Ascites
Tissue insult
    Injury to the cell wall   Hypoxia of the cell
Inflammatory process
Hormonal disturbances
    Pituitary   Estrogen
    Adrenal

Treatment-related
Steroid therapy

Situational (personal, environmental)
Excessive sodium intake/fluid intake
Low protein intake
    Fad diets   Malnutrition

Dependent venous pooling/venostasis
    Immobility   Standing or sitting for long
                                              periods of time

Venous pressure point
    Tight cast or bandage
Pregnancy
Inadequate lymphatic drainage

Maturational
Elderly (decreased cardiac output)

Focus Assessment Criteria

Subjective Data
1. History of symptoms
    Complaints of
        Shortness of breath   Weakness/fatigue
        Weight gain   Edema
    Onset/duration
    Location
    Description
    Aggravated by?
    Precipitated by?
    Relieved by?
2. History of contributing and causative factors
    Family or personal history of diabetes
    Pregnancy
    Pre-menses
    Cardiac or renal disease
    Liver disease
    Alcoholism
    Hyper- or hypothyroidism
    Hypertension
    Steroid therapy
    Malnutrition
    Excessive salt intake
    Excessive use of tap-water enemas
    Lymphatic obstruction (*e.g.*, post lymph node dissection)
    Excessive parenteral fluid replacement
3. Current drug therapy
    Type, dosage
    Frequency
    Last dose taken when?
4. Dietary intake
    Estimated protein intake (adequate/inadequate)
    Estimated caloric intake (adequate/inadequate/excess)
        Estimated fluid intake (adequate/inadequate/excess)
        Daily alcohol consumption   Type _____ Amount _____

Objective Data
1. Assess vital signs for signs of fluid overload

Pulse (bounding or dysrhythmic)

Respirations

Rate (tachypnea)

Quality (labored or shallow)

Lung sounds (rales or rhonchi)

Blood pressure (elevated)

2. Palpate for edema

Press thumb for at least 5 seconds into the skin and note any remaining indentations

Note degree and location (feet, ankles, legs, arms, sacral, generalized)

3. Assess for weight gain (weigh daily on the same scale, at the same time)

4. Assess for neck vein distention (distended neck veins at 45° elevation of the head may indicate fluid overload or decreased cardiac output)

5. Diagnostic studies

Electrolytes

Hemoglobin and hematocrit

Blood urea nitrogen (BUN)

Creatinine

Urinalysis

Principles and Rationale for Nursing Care

See *Fluid Volume Deficit*

Fluid Volume Excess
Related to (Specify)

Assessment

Subjective Data

The person reports

"I'm not supposed to eat salt"

"I feel bloated (tired, weak)"

Sudden or abnormal weight gain

History of

Fingers, feet, or ankles swelling

"Bad heart"

"Bad kidneys"

Hypertension

Cancer or lymph node dissection

Liver disease or alcoholism

Immobility or neurological deficit (*e.g.*, stroke or spinal cord injury)

Recent trauma or burn

Objective Data

Pedal or sacral puffiness

Puffing of face and extremities

Shiny, taut skin

Pitting edema (skin, when depressed by thumb, remains indented)

Weight gain
Fluid intake greater than fluid output

Outcome Criteria

The person will
- Relate causative factors and methods of preventing edema
- Exhibit decreased peripheral edema

Interventions

A. Identify contributing and causative factors

Improper diet (excessive sodium intake; inadequate protein intake)
Dependent venous pooling/venostasis
Venous pressure point (*e.g.,* tight cast or bandage)
Inadequate lymphatic drainage
Immobility/neurologic deficit
Lack of knowledge of or compliance with medical regimen

B. Reduce or eliminate causative and contributing factors

1. Improper diet
   - Assess dietary intake and habits that may contribute to fluid retention
     a. Be specific; record daily and weekly intake of food and fluids
     b. Assess weekly diet for adequate protein or excessive sodium intake
        Discuss likes and dislikes of foods that provide protein
        Teach to plan weekly menu that provides protein at a price that is affordable
   - Encourage the person to decrease salt intake
     a. Teach the person to
        Read labels for sodium content
        Avoid convenience foods, canned foods, and frozen foods
        Cook without salt and use spices to add flavor (lemon, basil, tarragon, mint)
        Use vinegar in place of salt to flavor soups, stews, etc. (*e.g.,* 2–3 teaspoons of vinegar to 4–6 quarts, according to taste)
     b. Ascertain with physician whether salt substitute may be used (caution individual that he must use exactly the substitute prescribed)
2. Dependent venous pooling
   - Assess for evidence of dependent venous pooling or venostasis
   - Encourage alternating periods of horizontal rest (legs elevated) with vertical activity (standing) (this may be contraindicated in congestive heart failure)
   - Keep edematous extremity elevated above the level of the heart whenever possible (unless contraindicated by heart failure)
     a. Keep edematous arms elevated on two pillows or with IV pole sling
     b. Elevate legs whenever possible, using pillows under legs (avoid pressure points, especially behind knees)
     c. Discourage leg and ankle crossing
   - Reduce constriction of vessels
     a. Assess wearing apparel for proper fit and constrictive areas

    b. Instruct person to avoid panty girdles/garters, knee highs, and leg crossing and to practice keeping legs elevated when possible
- Consider using antiembolism stockings or Ace bandages; measure legs carefully for stockings/support hose*
  - a. Measure from back of heel to back of knee, or top of thigh, depending on desired stocking length
  - b. Measure circumference of calf and thigh
  - c. Consider both measurements in choosing a stocking, matching measurements with size requirement chart that accompanies the stockings
  - d. Apply stockings while lying down (*e.g.*, in the morning before arising)
  - e. Check extremities frequently for adequate circulation and evidence of constrictive areas

3. Venous pressure points
   - Assess for venous pressure points associated with casts, bandages, tight stockings
     - a. Observe circulation at edges of casts, bandages, stockings
     - b. For casts, insert soft material to cushion pressure points at edges
     - c. Check circulation frequently
   - Shift body weight in cast to redistribute weight within the cast (unless contraindicated)
     - a. Encourage person to do this himself every 15 to 30 minutes during waking hours to prevent venostasis
     - b. Encourage wiggling of fingers or toes, and isometric exercise of unaffected muscles within the cast*
     - c. If the person is unable to do this himself, assist him at least hourly to shift body weight
     - d. See *Impaired Physical Mobility*

4. Inadequate lymphatic drainage
   - Keep extremity elevated on pillows
     - a. If edema is marked, the arm should be elevated, *but not in adduction* (this position may constrict the axilla)
     - b. The elbow should be higher than the shoulder
     - c. The hand should be higher than the elbow
   - Take blood pressures in unaffected arm
   - Do not give injections or start intravenous fluids in affected arm
   - Protect the affected arm from injury
     - a. Teach the person to avoid strong detergents, carrying heavy bags, holding a cigarette, injuring cuticles or hangnails, reaching into a hot oven, wearing jewelry or a wristwatch, or using Ace bandages
     - b. Advise the person to apply lanolin or similar cream several times a day to prevent dry, flaky skin
     - c. Encourage the person to wear a "Medic Alert" tag engraved with *Caution: lymphedema arm—no tests—no needle injections*
     - d. Caution the person to see a physician if the arm becomes red, swollen or unusually hard
   - After a mastectomy, encourage range-of-motion exercises and use of affected arm to facilitate development of a collateral lymphatic drainage system (explain to the person that lymphedema is often decreased within a month, but that she

---

* May require a physician's order.

should continue massaging, exercising, and elevating the arm for 3 or 4 months following surgery)
5. Immobility/neurologic deficit
- Plan passive or active range-of-motion exercises for all extremities every 4 hours, including dorsiflexion of the foot to massage veins
- Change the individual's position at least every 2 hours, utilizing the four positions (left side, right side, back, abdomen), if not contraindicated (see *Impaired Skin Integrity*)
- If the person must be maintained in high Fowler's position, assess for edema of the buttocks and sacral area and help the person to shift body weight every 2 hours to prevent pressure on edematous tissue
6. Lack of knowledge
- Assess the person's knowledge of
    Medical diagnosis (*e.g.,* congestive heart failure, renal failure)
    Diet
    Medications (*e.g.,* diuretics, cardiotonics)
    Activity
    Use of Ace bandages, antiembolus stockings

C. Protect edematous skin from injury

- Inspect skin for redness and blanching
- Reduce pressure on skin areas; pad chairs and footstools
- Prevent dry skin
    Use soap sparingly
    Rinse off soap completely
    Use a lotion to moisten skin
- See *Impaired Skin Integrity* for additional information on preventing injury

D. Initiate health teaching and referrals as indicated

- Give clear instructions verbally and in writing for all medications: what, when, how often, why, side-effects; pay special attention to drugs directly influencing fluid balance (*e.g.,* diuretics, steroids)
- Write down instructions for diet, activity, use of Ace bandages, stockings, etc.
- Have the person demonstrate his understanding of the instructions
- Have the person keep a written record of intake/output
- With severe fluctuations in edema, have the person weigh himself every morning and before bedtime daily; instruct the person to keep a written record of weights
- For less severe illness, the person may need to weigh himself daily only and record
- Caution the person to call physician for excessive edema/weight gain (>2 lb/day) or increased shortness of breath at night or on exertion
- Explain that the above may be indicative of early heart problems and may require medication to prevent them from getting worse
- Consider home care or visiting nurses referral to follow at home
- Provide literature concerning low-salt diets; consult with dietitian if necessary

References/Bibliography

Books

Aspinall MJ, Tanner C: Decision Making and the Nursing Process. New York, Appleton-Century-Crofts, 1981

Brunner LS, Suddarth DS: Textbook of Medical-Surgical Nursing, 5th ed. Philadelphia, JB Lippincott, 1984

Bulechek G, McCloskey J: Nursing Interventions. Philadelphia, WB Saunders, 1985

Carnevali D, Patrick M: Nursing Management for the Elderly. Philadelphia, JB Lippincott, 1985

Carpenito L: Handbook of Nursing Diagnosis. Philadelphia, JB Lippincott, 1984

Fischbach F: A Manual of Laboratory Diagnostic Tests for Nurses. Philadelphia, JB Lippincott, 1985

Jacobs M, Geels W: Signs and Symptoms in Nursing. Philadelphia, JB Lippincott, 1985

Kintzel KC: Advanced Concepts in Clinical Nursing, 2nd ed. Philadelphia, JB Lippincott, 1977

Metheny NM, Snively WD Jr: Nurses' Handbook of Fluid Balance, 5th ed. Philadelphia, JB Lippincott, 1987

Patrick M, Woods S et al: Medical Surgical Nursing. Philadelphia, JB Lippincott, 1985

Porth C: Pathophysiology. Philadelphia, JB Lippincott, 1985

Potter P, Perry A: Fundamentals of Nursing. St Louis, CV Mosby, 1985

Articles

Adams F: How much do elders drink? Geriatr Nurs 9(4):218–221, 1988

Beaumont E: Ascites: When the liver can't cope. RN 47:(10):26–30, 1984

Boylan A, Marbach B: Dehydration: Subtle, sinister . . . preventable. RN 42(8):37–41, 1979

Chambers J: Assessing the dialysis patient at home. Am J Nurs 81:750–754, 1981

Chambers J: Common fluid and electrolyte disorders. Nurs Clin North Am 22(4):749–872, 1987

Dale R: Symposium on fluid, electrolyte, and acid-base balance. Nurs Clin North Am 15(3):535–536, 1980

Felver L: Understanding the electrolyte maze. Am J Nurs 80:1591–1599, 1980

Folk-Lighty C: Solving the puzzles of patients' fluid imbalances. Nursing 14(2):34–41, 1984

Guthrie D, Guthrie R: DKA (diabetic ketoacidosis): Breaking the vicious cycle. Nursing 11(6):54–61, 1981

Huber M, Calliiari D: Hereditary angioedema—The swelling disorder. Am J Nurs 85(10):1090–1092, 1985

Lane G: When persistence pays off: Resolving the mystery of unexplained electrolyte imbalance. Nursing 12(1):44–47, 1982

McConnell E: Urinalysis: A common test, but never routine. Nursing 12(2):108–111, 1982

National Academy of Sciences, Food and Nutrition Board: Recommended Dietary Allowances, 9th ed rev. Washington DC, The Academy, 1980

Phillips PA et al: Reduced thirst after water deprivation in healthy elderly men. N Engl J Med 311:753–759, 1984

Quinlan M: Edema: What really causes it and how to control it. RN 47(4):54–57, 1984

Reedy D: How you can prevent dehydration. Geriatr Nurs 9(4):224–226, 1988

Stewarts ML: When the patient has the "other" diabetes. RN 47(5):54–58, 1985

Twombly M: The shift into third space. Nursing 8(1):38–46, 1978

Urrows ST: Physiology of body fluids. Nurs Clin North Am 15:603–615, 1980

Grieving*

Related to **An Actual or Perceived Loss**

Grieving, Anticipatory

Related to **(Specify)**

Grieving, Dysfunctional

Related to **(Specify): Potential**

Definition

Grieving: A state in which an individual or family experiences an actual or a perceived loss (person, object, function, status, relationship), or the state in which an individual or family responds to the realization of a future loss (anticipatory grieving).

Anticipatory grieving: The state in which the individual/ group experiences feelings in response to an expected significant loss.

Dysfunctional grieving: The state in which an individual/group experiences prolonged unresolved grief and engages in detrimental activities.

> **Author's Note:** This diagnostic category represents individuals or groups that have sustained a loss. Because it may be problematic and hazardous to label *Grieving* as either anticipatory or dysfunctional, the *Grieving* category provides a useful alternative to describe individuals experiencing the normal process of grieving.

Defining Characteristics

Major (must be present)

The person

Reports an actual or perceived loss (person, object, function, status, relationship) or Anticipates a loss

* This diagnostic category is not currently on the NANDA list but has been included for clarity or usefulness.

Minor (may be present)

Denial	Worthlessness	Hallucinations
Guilt	Suicidal thoughts	Delusions
Anger	Crying	Phobias
Despair	Sorrow	Anergia

Inability to concentrate

Visual, auditory, and tactile hallucinations about the deceased

Etiological, Contributing, Risk Factors

Many situations can contribute to feelings of loss. Some common situations are:

Pathophysiological

Loss of function (actual or potential) related to a disorder

Neurological	Musculoskeletal	Respiratory
Cardiovascular	Digestive	Renal
Sensory		

Loss of function or body part related to
    Trauma

Treatment-related

Dialysis

Surgery (mastectomy, colostomy, hysterectomy)

Situational (personal, environmental)

Chronic pain

Terminal illness

Death

Changes in life-style

Childbirth	Child leaving home (*e.g.,* college
Marriage	or marriage)
Separation	Loss of career
Divorce	

Type of relationship (with the person who is leaving or is gone)

Multiple losses or crises

Lack of social support system

Maturational

Loss associated with aging

Friends	Function
Occupation	Home

Focus Assessment Criteria

Subjective Data

1. Family

    Previous coping patterns for crisis

    Quality of the relationship of the ill or deceased person to each family member

    Position or role responsibilities of the ill or deceased person

Sociocultural expectations for bereavement
Religious expectations for bereavement
2. Individual family members
    Previous experiences with loss or death (as child, adolescent, or adult)
        Did family talk out their grief?
        Did they practice any particular religious rituals associated with bereavement?
    Present interactions between or among family members
        Adults
        Children
            Maturational level
            Understanding of crisis
            Degree of participation
    Knowledge of expected grief reactions
    Relationship to ill or deceased person
3. Expressions of
    Ambivalence   Anger
    Denial   Depression
    Fear   Guilt
    Concerns
4. Report of
    Gastrointestinal disturbances
        Indigestion   Weight gain or loss
        Nausea or vomiting   Constipation or diarrhea
        Anorexia
    Insomnia
    Preoccupation with sleep
    Fatigue (decreased or increased activity level)
    Inability to carry out self-care, social and work responsibilities

Objective Data

1. Normative
    Shock   Sorrow
    Disbelief, denial   Withdrawal
    Anger   Preoccupation with lost object
    Crying   Hopelessness
2. Pathological pattern (profound; increases in intensity; continuous over 12 months)
    Anger   Denial
    Depression   Regression
    Isolation   Obsession
    Despair   Hallucinations
    Worthlessness   Delusions
    Guilt   Phobias
    Suicidal thoughts
    Stoic

Principles and Rationale for Nursing Care

General

1. American culture is devoted to youth and life. Even though death surrounds each person, it is viewed as pertaining to someone else, not oneself.

2. Loss can be viewed as consisting of four components: dying, death, grief, and mourning.
3. Loss can occur without death; when a person experiences any loss (object, relationship), grief and mourning ensue.
4. Grief is the emotional response to loss; grief work is the adaptive process of mourning. It can be identified as

Emancipation from bondage to the deceased
Readjustment to the environment
Formation of new relationships

5. An individual's grief is affected by many factors, such as personality, previous losses, intimacy of relationship, and personal resources.
6. Staging (of grieving process) can create problems if the nurse applies the stages universally to all persons, disregarding individual differences. Staging also may encourage the nurse to focus on the symptoms as opposed to the strength of the person/family.
7. The following stages (Engle) are specific enough to assist the nurse to intervene and broad enough to prevent labeling.

I. Shock and disbelief
 Initial denial   Decreased activity
 Numbed feelings   Sporadic periods of despair
II. Developing awareness of loss
 Sadness   Guilt
 Anger   Crying
III. Restitution (usually requires at least a year)
 The work of mourning   Preoccupation with thoughts
 Painful void in life   of loss
IV. In the months to follow
 Beginning to put the lost rela-
  tionship in perspective (its
  positive and negative qualities)

---

8. "The notion that grief is a neat, orderly, linear process completed at some arbitrary point in time" has been refuted. (Haylor)
9. Unresolved grief is a pathological response of prolonged denial of the loss or a profound psychotic response. Examples of such responses are

Progressively deeper regression, depression
Progressively deeper isolation
Somatic manifestations (prolonged)
Obsessions, phobias
Delusions, hallucinations
Attempted suicide

10. Factors that contribute to unresolved grief are

Quality of the individual's attachment to the loved object
Presence of ambivalence toward the loved object

Presence of lowered self-esteem
Inability to grieve

11. Grief work cannot begin until the loss is acknowledged. Nurses can encourage this acknowledgment by open honest dialogue and by providing the family with an opportunity to view the dead person.

12. Life review is a process whereby a dying person reminisces about the past, especially unresolved conflicts, in an attempt to resolve them. Life review also provides the person with an opportunity to evaluate his successes and failures.

13. Terminal illness with its concurrent treatments and its progression produces a multitude of losses

Loss of function (all systems)
Loss of financial independence
Change in appearance
Loss of friends
Loss of self-esteem
Loss of self

14. Divorce presents many losses for the partners, children, grandparents, etc. The losses are roles, relationships, homes, possessions, finances, control, routines, and patterns.

Children

1. The child responds to death depending on his developmental age (see table) and the response of significant others.

Developmental Understanding of Death

Age	Degree of Understanding
<3 years	Cannot comprehend death, fears separation
3 to 5	Views illness as a punishment for real or imagined wrongdoing Has little concept of death as final because of immature concept of time May view death as a kind of sleep May feel he caused the event to happen (magical thinking) (*e.g.*, by bad thoughts about person)
6 to 10	Begins to fear death Attempts to put meaning to the event (*e.g.*, devil, ghost, God) Associates death with mutilation and punishment Can feel responsibility for the event
10 to 12	Usually has an adult concept of death (inevitable, irreversible, universal) Attitudes greatly influenced by reactions of parents and others Very interested in postdeath services and rituals
Adoles-cence	Has priorities for group acceptance and independence Illness threatens both sets of priorities

2. Children may learn early that discussions about death are taboo.

3. Children may utilize symbolic or nonverbal language to communicate their awareness of death and dying.

4. Children can be encouraged to communicate symbolically through writing or telling stories or by drawing pictures (see Appendix for play therapy guidelines).

5. Children need to feel the joys and sorrows of life in order to begin to incorporate both in their lives appropriately.

6. Children can feel rejected/unloved if parents or a significant other is unable to offer emotional support/nurturing because of their own grief.

Grieving
Related to an Actual or Perceived Loss

Assessment

Subjective Data

The person expresses

Sadness	Fear	Anergia; anxiety
Depression	Denial	Visual, auditory,
Shock	Guilt	and/or tactile hal-
		lucinations about
		the deceased

Objective Data

Crying
Inability to cry
Withdrawn behavior
Apathetic behavior
Changes in grooming, hygiene, weight or health status

Outcome Criteria

The individual will
- Express his grief
- Describe the meaning of the death or loss to him
- Share his grief with significant others (children, spouses)

Interventions

A. Assess for causative and contributing factors that may delay the grief work

Unavailable or lack of
support system
Denial
Shock
Anger
Depression
Guilt
Fear
Dependency
Multiple losses
Uncertainty of loss
(*e.g.,* MIA, missing children)
Failure to grieve prior losses

Inability to grieve (cultural,
social, age-related)
History of previous emotional
illness
Personality structure
Early object loss
Nature of the relationship with
the lost person or object

B. Reduce or eliminate causative or contributing factors if possible

1. Promote a trust relationship
   - Promote feelings of self-worth through one-on-one and/or group sessions
   - Allow for established time to meet and discuss feelings
   - Communicate clearly, simply, and to the point
   - Assess what the person and the family are learning by the use of feedback
   - Offer support and reassurance
   - Create a therapeutic milieu
   - Establish a safe, secure, and private environment
   - Demonstrate respect for the person's culture, religion, race, and values

2. Support the person and the family's grief reactions
   - Explain grief reactions
     Shock and disbelief
     Developing awareness
     Restitution
   - Describe varied acceptable expressions
     Elated or manic behavior as a defense against depression
     Elation and hyperactivity as a reaction of love and protection from depression
     Various states of depression
     Various somatic manifestations (weight loss or gain, indigestion, dizziness)
   - Assess for past experiences with loss
     Loss of significant other in childhood
     Losses in later life

3. Promote family cohesiveness
   - Support the family at its level of functioning
   - Encourage self-exploration of feelings with family members
   - Explain the need to discuss behaviors that interfere with relationships
   - Recognize and reinforce the strengths of each family member
   - Encourage the family to evaluate their feelings and support one another

4. Promote grief work with each response
   a. Denial
      - Recognize that this is a useful and necessary response
      - Explain the use of denial by one family member to the other members
      - Do not push client to move past denial without emotional readiness
   b. Isolation
      - Convey a feeling of acceptance by allowing grief
      - Create open, honest communications to promote sharing
      - Reinforce the person's self-worth by allowing privacy
      - Encourage client/family to gradually increase social activities (support groups, church groups, etc.)
   c. Depression
      - Reinforce the person's self-esteem
      - Identify the level of depression and develop the approach accordingly
      - Use empathetic sharing; acknowledge grief ("It must be very difficult")
      - Identify any indications of suicidal behavior (frequent statements of intent, revealed plan)
      - See *Potential for Self-harm* for additional information
   d. Anger
      - Understand that this feeling usually replaces denial
      - Explain to family that anger serves to try to control one's environment more closely because of inability to control loss

- Encourage verbalization of the anger
- See *Anxiety* for additional interventions for anger

e. Guilt
  - Acknowledge the person's expressed self-view
  - Encourage client to identify positive contributions/aspects of the relationship
  - Avoid arguing and participating in the person's system of shoulds and should nots
  - Discuss the person's preoccupation with him and attempt to move verbally beyond the present

f. Fear
  - Focus on the present and maintain a safe and secure environment
  - Help the person to explore reasons for a meaning of the behavior
  - Consider alternative ways of expressing his feelings

g. Rejection
  - Reassure the person by explaining what is happening
  - Explain this response to family members

h. Hysteria
  - Reduce environmental stresses (*e.g.,* limit personnel)
  - Provide person with a safe, private area to display grief

5. Promote grief work in children
   - Encourage parents and staff to be truthful and offer explanations that can be understood
   - Encourage parents and/or significant others to nurture children during the grieving process
   - Explore with child his concept of death in the context of his maturational level
     "What does death mean to you?"
     "Have you ever known a person or a pet that died?"
     "What happens when someone dies?"
   - Correct misconceptions about death, illness, and rituals (funerals)
     Person was not bad
     Person is not asleep
     Body does not go to God but soul does
   - Prepare the child for grief responses of others
     Explain that people are sad and cry when someone dies
     Explain the need to cry and how helpful it is
     Discuss with the family the inclusion of the child in postdeath services
   - If the child plans to attend the funeral or visit the funeral home, a thorough explanation of the setting, rituals, and expected behaviors of mourners is necessary before (the family can plan the visit of the child to be short and also before the other mourners arrive)
   - Reduce the fear of separation and feelings of guilt
     Allow child to share fears
     Allow child to remain with significant others while they grieve at home
     Reinforce to child that they are not responsible for the sadness
     Provide child with close contact and holding
     Discuss with the child feelings of sadness/guilt because he/she argued or talked badly about the deceased person once. Stress all friends or relatives argue sometimes
   - Provide accurate explanations for sibling illness or death
     Prepare child if sibling is terminal
     Explain the illness to the child in terms he can understand

Stress that the illness or death did not result from being bad or because the well child wished it

6. Assist parents of a deceased infant (newborn, stillbirth, miscarriage) with grief work (Mina):
   - Provide parents with access to hospital chaplain and/or own religious leader
   - Encourage parents to see and hold their infant to validate the reality of the loss
   - Design a method to communicate to auxiliary departments that the parents are in mourning (*e.g.,* rose sticker on door, chart)
   - Prepare a memory packet (wrapped in clean baby blanket) (photograph [Polaroid], ID bracelet, footprints with birth certificate, lock of hair, crib card, fetal monitor strip, infant's blanket)
   - Encourage parents to take memory packet home. If they prefer not to, keep the packet on file in case parents change their minds later.
   - Encourage parents to share the experience with siblings at home (refer to pertinent literature for consumers)
   - Provide for follow-up support and referral services after discharge (*e.g.,* social service, support group)

7. Identify persons who are at high risk for potential pathological grieving reactions
   Absence of any emotion
   Previous conflict with deceased person
   History of ineffective coping patterns

8. Teach individual/family signs of pathological grieving, especially persons who are at risk
   Prolonged hallucinations
   Continued searching for the deceased (frequent moves/relocations)
   Delusions
   Isolation
   Egocentricity
   Overt hostility (usually toward a family member)

C. Provide health teaching and referrals as indicated

- Teach the person and the family signs of resolution
  Griever no longer lives in the past but is future oriented and establishing new goals
  Griever breaks ties with lost object/person after approximately 6 to 12 months of grieving
  Griever begins to resocialize
- Identify agencies that may be helpful
  Community agencies
  Religious groups

Grieving, Anticipatory

Definition

Anticipatory grieving: The state in which an individual/group experiences feelings in response to an expected significant loss.

Defining Characteristics

Major (must be present)

Expressed distress at potential loss

Minor (may be present)

Denial
Guilt
Anger
Sorrow
Change in eating habits
Change in sleep patterns
Change in social patterns
Change in communication patterns
Decreased libido

Etiological, Contributing, Risk Factors

See *Grieving*

Anticipatory Grieving
Related to (Specify)

Assessment

Subjective Data

The person expresses

Sadness	Fear	Anorexia
Depression	Denial	
Shock	Guilt	
Anger	Anergia	

Objective Data

Crying
Inability to cry
Withdrawn behavior
Apathetic behavior

Outcome Criteria

The person will
- Express his grief
- Participate in decision-making for the future
- Share his concerns with significant others

Interventions

A. Assess for causative and contributing factors of anticipated or potential loss

Terminal illness	Socioeconomic status
Separation, (divorce,	Alteration in body image
hospitalization, marriage,	Alteration in self-esteem
relocation, job)	Aging

B. Assess individual response

Denial	Shock
Rejection	Anger
Bargaining	Depression
Isolation	Guilt
Helplessness	Fear

1. Encourage the person to share concerns
   - Utilize communication techniques of open-ended questions and reflection ("What are your thoughts today?" "Are you sad?")
   - Acknowledge the value of the person and his grief by using touch and by sitting with him and verbalizing your concern ("This must be a very difficult time for you")
   - Recognize that some individuals may choose not to share their concerns, but convey that you are available if they desire to do so later
2. Assist the person and the family to identify strengths
   "What do you do well?"
   "What are you willing to do to improve your life?"
   "Is religion a source of strength for you?"
   "Do you have close friends?"
   "Who do you turn to in times of need?"
   "What does this person do for you?"
3. Promote the integrity of the person and the family by acknowledging strengths
   "Your brother looks forward to your visit"
   "Your family is so concerned for you"
4. Support person and family with grief reactions
   - Prepare person and family for grief reactions
   - Explain grief reactions to person and family
   - Focus on the present life situation until the person or family indicates the desire to discuss future
5. Promote family cohesiveness
   - Identify availability of a support system
     a. Meet consistently with family members
     b. Identify family member roles, strengths, weaknesses

- Assess communication patterns
  a. Listen and clarify the messages being sent
  b. Identify the patterns of communication within the family unit by assessing positive and negative feedback, verbal and nonverbal communications, and body language
- Provide for the concept of hope by
  Supplying accurate information
  Resisting the temptation to give false hope
  Discussing concerns willingly
- Promote group decision-making to enhance group autonomy
  a. Establish consistent times to meet with person and family
  b. Encourage members to talk directly with each other and to listen to each other

6. Promote grief work with each response
  a. Denial
     - Initially support and then strive to increase the development of awareness (when individual indicates readiness for awareness)
  b. Isolation
     - Listen and spend designated time consistently with person and family
     - Offer the person and the family opportunity to explore their emotions
     - Reflect on past losses and acknowledge loss behavior (past and present)
  c. Depression
     - Begin with simple problem solving and move toward acceptance
     - Enhance self-worth through positive reinforcement
     - Identify the level of depression and indications of suicidal behavior or ideas
     - Be consistent and establish times daily to speak with person and family
  d. Anger
     - Allow for crying to release this energy
     - Listen to and communicate concern
     - Encourage concerned support from significant others as well as professional support
  e. Guilt
     - Listen and communicate concern
     - Allow for crying
     - Promote more direct expression of feelings
     - Explore methods to resolve guilt
  f. Fear
     - Help person and family recognize the feeling
     - Explain that this will help cope with life
     - Explore person's and family's attitudes about loss, death, etc.
     - Explore person's and family's methods of coping
  g. Rejection
     - Allow for verbal expression of this feeling state in order to diminish the emotional strain
     - Recognize that expression of anger may create a rejection of self to significant others

7. Provide for expression of grief
  - Encourage emotional expressions of grieving
  - Caution the use of sedatives and tranquilizers, which may prevent and/or delay emotional expressions of loss

- Encourage verbalization of clients and families of all age groups
  a. Support family cohesiveness
  b. Promote and verbalize strengths of the family group
- Encourage person and family to engage in life review
  a. Focus and support the social network relationships
  b. Reevaluate past life experiences and integrate them into a new meaning
  c. Convey empathetic understanding

8. Identify potential pathological grieving reactions

Delusions
Hallucinations
Phobias
Obsessions
Isolations
Conversion hysteria
Agitated depression
Delay in grief work
Suicidal indications

Difficulty crying or controlling crying
Loss of control of environment leading to hopelessness, helplessness
Intense reactions lasting longer than 6 months with few signs of relief
Restrictions of pleasure

9. Refer individual with potential for pathological grieving responses for counseling (psychiatrist, nurse therapist, counselor, psychologist)

C. Provide health teaching and referrals as indicated

- Explain what to expect

Sadness
Feelings of aloneness
Guilt
Emotions will be very labile initially and become more stable as grief work is accomplished

Fear
Rejection
Anger

- Teach person and family signs of resolution
  a. Griever no longer lives in past but is future oriented, establishing new goals
  b. Griever breaks ties with lost object/person after approximately 6 to 12 months of grieving
  c. Griever begins to resocialize
- Teach signs of pathological responses and referrals needed
  a. Defenses used in uncomplicated grief work that become exaggerated or maladaptive responses
  b. Persistent absence of any emotion
  c. Prolonged intense reactions of anxiety, anger, fear, guilt, helplessness
- Identify agencies that may enhance grief work

Self-help groups
Widow-to-widow groups
Parents of deceased children
Single parent groups
Bereavement groups

Grieving, Dysfunctional

Related to **(Specify): Potential**

Definition

Dysfunctional grieving: The state in which an individual or group experiences prolonged unresolved grief and engages in detrimental activities.

> **Author's Note:** How one responds to loss is highly individual. Responses to acute loss should not be labeled *Dysfunctional* regardless of the severity. Dysfunctional grieving is characterized by its sustained or prolonged detrimental response. The validation of dysfunctional grieving cannot occur until several months to a year after the loss. In many clinical settings, the diagnosis of *Potential Dysfunctional Grieving* for individuals at high risk for unsuccessful reintegration after a loss may be more useful.

Defining Characteristics

Major (must be present)

> Unsuccessful adaptation to loss
> Prolonged denial, depression
> Delayed emotional reaction

Minor (may be present)

> Social isolation or withdrawal
> Failure to develop new relationships/interests
> Failure to restructure life after loss

Etiological, Contributing, Risk Factors

See *Grieving*

Potential Dysfunctional Grieving
Related to (Specify)

Assessment

Subjective Data

Reported:

> History of ineffective coping
> Poor or ambivalent feelings toward the lost person/object
> Inadequate support system
> Unexpected death

Multiple losses
Absence of any emotion

Outcome Criteria

The individual/group will
- Share grief with significant others
- Describe feelings expected with loss
- Verbalize an intent to seek professional assistance if there are no signs of resolution

---

Interventions

A. Assess for causative and contributing factors that may contribute to dysfunctional grieving
- Unavailable (or lack of) support system
- Emotionally bland or cheerful and stoic behavior
- History of a difficult relationship with the lost person or object
- Multiple past losses
- Ineffective coping strategies
- Unexpected death

B. Promote a trust relationship
- Promote feelings of self-worth through one-on-one and/or group sessions
- Allow for established time to meet and discuss feelings
- Communicate clearly, simply, and to the point
- Assess what the person and the family are learning by the use of feedback
- Offer support and reassurance
- Create a therapeutic milieu
- Establish a safe, secure, and private environment
- Demonstrate respect for the person's culture, religion, race, and values

C. Support the person and the family's grief reactions
1. Explain grief reactions
     Shock and disbelief
     Developing awareness
     Restitution
2. Describe varied acceptable expressions
     Elated or manic behavior as a defense against depression
     Elation and hyperactivity as a reaction of love and protection from depression
     Various states of depression
     Various somatic manifestations (weight loss or gain, indigestion, dizziness)
3. Assess for past experiences with loss
     Loss of significant other in childhood
     Losses in later life
4. Promote family cohesiveness
   - Support the family at its level of functioning
   - Encourage self-exploration of feelings with family members

- Explain the need to discuss behaviors that interfere with relationships
- Recognize and reinforce the strengths of each family member
- Encourage the family to evaluate their feelings and support one another

D. Promote grief work with each response

1. Denial
   - Recognize that this is a useful and necessary response
   - Explain the use of denial by one family member to the other members
   - Do not push client to move past denial without emotional readiness
2. Isolation
   - Convey a feeling of acceptance by allowing grief
   - Create open, honest communications to promote sharing
   - Reinforce the person's self-worth by allowing privacy
   - Encourage client/family to gradually increase social activities (support groups, church groups, etc.)
3. Depression
   - Reinforce the person's self-esteem
   - Identify the level of depression and develop the approach accordingly
   - Use empathetic sharing; acknowledge grief ("It must be very difficult")
   - Identify any indications of suicidal behavior (frequent statements of intent, revealed plan)
   - See *Potential for Self-harm* for additional information
4. Anger
   - Understand that this feeling usually replaces denial
   - Explain to family that anger serves to try to control one's environment more closely because of inability to control loss
   - Encourage verbalization of the anger
   - See *Anxiety* for additional information for anger
5. Guilt
   - Acknowledge the person's expressed self-view
   - Role play to allow person to "express" to the dead person what he wants to say or how he feels
   - Encourage client to identify positive contributions/aspects of the relationship
   - Avoid arguing and participating in the person's system of shoulds and should nots
   - Discuss the person's preoccupation with him and attempt to move verbally beyond the present
6. Fear
   - Focus on the present and maintain a safe and secure environment
   - Help the person to explore reasons for a meaning of the behavior
   - Consider alternative ways of expressing his feelings
7. Rejection
   - Reassure the person by explaining what is happening
   - Explain this response to family members
8. Hysteria
   - Reduce environmental stresses (*e.g.,* limit personnel)
   - Provide person with a safe, private area to display grief

E. Provide health teaching and referrals as indicated

- Teach the person and the family signs of resolution
  Griever no longer lives in past but is future oriented and establishing new goals

       Griever breaks ties with lost object/person after approximately 6 to 12 months of
          grieving
       Griever begins to resocialize, seeks new relationships, experiences
- Teach individual/family signs of pathological grieving, especially persons who are at
  risk, and to seek professional counseling
      Prolonged depression
      Denial
      Lives in past
      Prolonged hallucinations
      Continued searching for the deceased (frequent moves/relocations)
      Delusions
      Isolation
      Egocentricity
      Over hostility (usually toward a family member)
- Identify agencies that may be helpful
      Community agencies
      Religious groups

References/Bibliography

Books

Backer BA, Hannon N, Russell N: Death and Dying Individuals and Institutions. New York, John
Wiley & Sons, 1982

Battin D, Aakin A, Gerber I et al: Coping and vulnerability among the aged bereaved. In
Schroenber B, Gerber I, Wiener A et al (eds): Bereavement: Its Psychosocial Aspects. New York,
Columbia University Press, 1975

Barton D (ed): Dying and Death: A Clinical Guide for Caregivers. Baltimore, Williams and Wilkins,
1977

Beitler R: 1968. The life review: An interpretation of reminiscence in the aged. In Neugarten BL
(ed): Middle Life and Aging. Chicago, University of Chicago Press, 1968

Caughill R (ed): The Dying Patient: A Supportive Approach. Boston, Little, Brown, 1976

Fulton R (ed): Death and Identity. Bowie, MD, Charles Press, 1976

Hamilton M, Reid H (eds): A Hospice Handbook: A New Way to Care for the Dying. Grand Rapids,
Wm B Eerdmans, 1980

Kastenbaum R: Death, Society, and Human Experience. St. Louis, CV Mosby, 1977

Kastenbaum R: Psychological death. In Pearson L (ed): Death and Dying. Cleveland, Case Western
Reserve University Press, 1969

Kennedy E: Crisis Counseling: The Essential Guide for Nonprofessional Counselors. New York,
Continuum, 1981

Kyes JJ, Hofling CK: Basic Psychiatric Concepts in Nursing, 4th ed. Philadelphia, JB Lippincott,
1980

Kübler-Ross, E: Death: The Final Stage of Growth. Englewood Cliffs, NJ, Prentice-Hall, 1975

Packes C: Bereavement: Studies of Grief in Adult Life. New York, International Universities Press,
1972

Rando TA: Grief, Dying, and Death: Clinical Interventions for Caregivers. Champaign, IL, Research
Press, 1984

Werner-Beland, JA: Grief Responses to Long-Term Illness and Disability. Virginia, Reston Publishing, 1980

Periodicals

Benoliel JQ: Loss and adaptation: Circumstances, contingencies and consequences. Death Studies
9:217–233, 1985

Benoliel JQ: Loss and terminal illness. Nurs Clin North Am 20(2):439–448, 1985

Butler RN: The life review. Psychiatry 26:65–76, 1963

Domming J, Stackman J, O'Neill P et al: Experiences with dying patients. Am J Nurs 73:1058–1064, 1973

Engle G: Grief and grieving. Am J Nurs 64:93–97, 1964

Friedmann-Campbell M, Hart CA: Theoretical strategies and nursing interventions to promote psychosocial adaption to spinal cord injuries and disability. J Neurosurg Nurs 16(6):335–342, 1984

Haylor M: Human response to loss. Nurse Pract 12(5):63, 1987

Hutton L: Annie is alone: The bereaved child. Matern Child Nurs J 6:274–277, 1981

Kowalsky E: Grief, a lost life-style. Am J Nurs 78(3):418–420, 1978

Kowalski K, Osborn MR: Helping mothers of stillborn infants to grieve. Matern Child Nurs J 2:29–32, 1977

Lake C, Marian B et al: The role of a grief support team following stillbirth. Am J Obstet Gynecol 146:877–881, 1983

Mina C: A program for helping grieving parents. Matern Child Nurs J 10:118–121, 1985

Philpot T: St. Joseph's Hospice: Death—a part of life. Nursing Mirror 151(16):20–23, 1980

Oehler J: The frog family books: Color pictures sad or glad. Matern Child Nurs J 6:281, 1981

Radford C: Nursing care to the end. Nursing Mirror 150(2):30–31, 1980

Ross-Alaolmolki K: Supportive care for families of dying children. Nurs Clin North Am 20(2): 457–466, 1985

Schultz CA: The dynamics of grief. J Emerg Nurs 15(5):26–30, 1979

Sheer BL: Help for parents in a difficult job: Broaching the subject of death. Matern Child Nurs J 5:320–324, 1977

Wass H, Corr C (eds): Childhood and death. Issues Compr Pediatr Nurs 8(1–6):1–383

Willans JH: Appetite in the terminally ill patient. Nursing Times 76(10):875–876, 1980

Williams H, Rivara FP, Rothenberg MB: The child is dying: Who helps the family? Matern Child Nurs J 6:261–265, 1981

Wong D: Bereavement: The empty mother syndrome. Matern Child Nurs J 5:384–389, 1980

Wooten B: Death of an infant. Matern Child Nurs J 6:257–260, 1981

Resources for the Consumer

Literature

Newborn Death ($2.35)
Miscarriage ($2.35)
Where's Jess ($3.00)
Centering Corporation
Box 3367
Omaha, NE 68103-0367

Answers to a Child's Questions About Death
by Peter Stillman
Guideline Publications
Stanford, NY 12167

Grollman EA (ed): *Explaining Death to Children.* Boston, Beacon Press, 1967 (See prologue; explains what *not* to tell children.)

Kushner HS: *When Bad Things Happen to Good People.* New York, Schocken, 1981 (Offers a compassionate and humane approach to dealing with questions of suffering and life and death in a way that affirms humanity and inspires peace of mind.)

For Children

Buscaglia LD: *The Fall of Freddie the Leaf.* New York, Charles B Slack, 1982

Dodge NC: *Thumpy's Story—A Story of Love and Grief* (shared by Thumpy, the Bunny; English and Spanish editions)

Rofes, E (ed): *The Kids Book About Death and Dying.* New York, Little, Brown, 1986 (Researched and written by 11-to-14-year-old students who also recommend other books about death and dying; covers topics such as euthanasia, organ donation, autopsy, emotions, and how children feel about the death of a friend, pet, parent, or their own life-threatening illness. However, section on brain death needs updating.)

Children's Hospice International (CHI)
1101 King Street, Suite 131
Alexandria, VA 22314
(703) 684-0330 or 684-0331

Organizations

The Compassionate Friends
National Headquarters
P.O. Box 3696
Oak Brook, IL 60522
(312) 323-5010

Growth and Development, Altered

Related to **(Specify)**

Definition

Altered growth and development: The state in which an individual has, or is at risk for, impaired ability to perform tasks of his/her age group or impaired growth.

> **Author's Note:** The focus of this category will be children and adolescents. When an adult has not accomplished a developmental task, the nurse should assess for the altered functioning that has resulted from the failure to meet a developmental task, for example, *Impaired Social Interactions* or *Ineffective Individual Coping*.

Defining Characteristics

Major (must be present)

Inability or difficulty performing skills or behaviors typical of his/her age group (*e.g.*, motor, personal/social, language/cognition) (see Table II-8) and/or

Altered physical growth: weight lagging behind height by 2 standard deviations; pattern of height and weight percentiles indicate a drop in pattern

Minor (may be present)

Inability to perform self-care or self-control activities appropriate for age (see Table II-8)

Flat affect, listlessness, decreased responses, slow in social responses, shows limited signs of satisfaction to caregiver, shows limited eye contact, difficulty feeding, decreased appetite, lethargic, irritable, negative mood, regression in self-toileting, regression in self-feeding (see Focus Assessment)

Infants: watchfulness, interrupted sleep pattern

Etiological, Contributing, Risk Factors

Pathophysiological

Circulatory impairment: congenital heart defects, congestive heart failure

Neurological impairment: cerebral damage, congenital defects, cerebral palsy, microencephaly

Gastrointestinal impairment: malabsorption syndrome, gastroesophageal reflux, cystic fibrosis

Endocrine or renal impairment: hormonal disturbance

Musculoskeletal impairment

    Congenital anomalies of extremities   Muscular dystrophy

Acute illness

Prolonged pain

Repeated acute illness, chronic illness

Inadequate caloric, nutritional intake

Treatment-related

Prolonged, painful treatment	Repeated or prolonged hospitalization
Traction or casts	Prolonged bed rest
Isolation	Confinement

Situational (personal and environmental)

Parental knowledge deficit
Stress (acute, transient, or chronic)
Hospitalization or change in usual environment
Separation from significant others (parents, primary caretaker)
Inadequate, inappropriate parental support (neglect, abuse)
Inadequate sensory stimulation (neglect, isolation)
Parent–child conflict
School-related stressors
Parental anxiety
Loss of significant other
Loss of control over environment (established rituals, activities, established hours of contact with family)
Multiple caretakers

Maturational

Infant–Toddler

(birth–3 years)

Lack of Stimulation

Separation from parents/significant others
Change in environment
Restriction of acitivity
Inadequate parental support
Inability to trust significant other
Inability to communicate (deafness)

Preschool Age

(4–6 years)

Restriction of Activity

Loss of ability to communicate
Lack of stimulation
Lack of significant other
Loss of significant other (death, divorce)
Loss of peer group
Loss of independence
Fear of mutilation, pain, abandonment
Removal from home environment

School Age

(6–11 years)

Loss of Individual Control

Loss of significant others
Loss of peer group
Fear of immobility, mutilation, death
Fear of intrusive procedures
Strange environment

Adolescent

(12–18 years)

Loss of independence and autonomy
Disruption of peer relationships
Disruption of body image
Interruption of intellectual achievement
Loss of significant others

Focus Assessment Criteria

See Table II-8 for descriptions of appropriate developmental milestones/behaviors for each age group, as well as information for nursing intervention and parental guidance.

Subjective Data

(Data should be verified with primary caregiver.)
  1. Current nutritional patterns
       Diet recall for past 24 hours (from parent or child, type of food, amounts)
       Diet history
       Height/weight at birth
       Intake pattern
       Child's reaction to eating, feeding
       Parental/child knowledge of nutrition
  2. Physiological alterations
       Presence of nausea, vomiting, diarrhea
       Allergies
       Food intolerances
       Dysphagia
       Fatigue
       Report of other physical symptoms (*e.g.*, rash, URI)
  3. Parental attitudes
       What are the parents' expectations for the child?
       What are the parents' feelings about being parents?
       Did the parents experience poor parenting themselves?
       Parenting approach to care and discipline of child?
       How do the parents feel about home situation?
       How do the parents feel about child's illness, treatments/hospitalization?
       Assess family functioning with appropriate assessment tool.
  4. Stressors in environment
       Illness in family
       Conflict in family
       History of illness or hospitalization of child
       Child's behavior/success in school
       Child's peer/sibling relationships
  5. Developmental level: Behaviors listed under Developmental Tasks (Table II-8) may be assessed through direct observation or report of parent/primary caregiver. The Denver Developmental Screening Tool may be used for children under 6 years of age.

Objective Data

  1. General appearance
       Cleanliness, grooming
       Eye contact
       Facial responses
       Response to stimulation
       Mood (*i.e.*, crying, elated, etc.)
  2. Response/interaction with parent
       Spontaneous, happy when comforted by parent
       Reaction when separated
       Response to procedures, strangers
  3. Nutritional status
       Height/weight (compare to norms in Principles and Rationale for Nursing Care)

Frontal/occipital circumference (also see Focus Assessment Criteria, *Nutrition Altered: Less Than Body Requirements*)
4. Elimination patterns
   Bowel and bladder
   Description, frequency of stool
5. Personal/social
   Language/cognition
   Motor activity: Assess for achievement of developmental skills in appropriate age group (Table II-8)
6. Type of illness, treatments
7. Developmental level (see behaviors described under Developmental Tasks [Table II-8])

Principles and Rationale for Nursing Care

1. Development can be defined as the patterned, orderly, lifelong changes in structure, thought, or behavior that evolve as a result of maturation of physical and mental capacity, experiences, and learning. Development results in the person achieving a new level of maturity and integration. Growth refers to increase in body size, function, complexity of body cell content. For the purposes of this diagnosis, growth and development are synonymous, because any disruption that does not affect development will most likely result in a diagnosis of *Altered Nutrition*.
2. The following assumptions concerning development are relevant:
   - The most rapid growth and development occurs in the early stages of life.
   - Childhood is the foundation period of life and establishes the basis for successful or unsuccessful development throughout life.
   - Growth and development are continuous and occur in spurts, rather than in a straight, upward direction.
   - Development follows a definable, predictable, and sequential pattern.
   - Growth is not necessarily accompanied by a behavioral change.
   - Critical periods exist where development is occurring rapidly and the individual's ability to respond to stressors is limited.
   - Development proceeds in a cephalocaudal, proximodistal direction.
   - Development proceeds from simple to complex.
   - Development occurs in all components of a person (*i.e.,* motor, intellectual, personal, social, language).
   - Development results form biological, maturational, and individual learning.
3. Often development is defined in terms of stages or levels, as is illustrated in Erikson's stages of man, and Piaget's stages of cognition. In addition, development may be defined in terms of tasks that must be accomplished. A developmental task is a growth responsibility that occurs at a particular time in the life of a person. Successful achievement of the task leads to success with later tasks. Development is affected through either an acceleration of the process or a slowing down of the process by a variety of influences. Physiological disruptions, through either genetic malfunction or insult from illness, may potentially alter development, temporarily or permanently. Psychological and social influences may also alter development positively or negatively. The alteration of development in a child is particularly critical because the alteration may establish a basic foundation that then remains faulty for the life of the child. Because of the rapid acceleration of development in childhood, several critical periods exist where influences can easily modify development.
4. Of the range of possible physiological, psychological, and social influences that may

(*Text continues on page 379*)

Table II-8. **Age-related Developmental Needs**

Developmental Tasks/Needs	Parental Guidance	Implications for Nursing
Birth to 1 Year		
PERSONAL/SOCIAL		
Learns to trust and anticipate satisfaction	Encourage parent to respond to cry, meet infants need *consistently.*	Encourage parent to participate in care:
Sends cues to mother/caretaker		Bathing
Begins understanding self as separate from others (body image)	Teach parent not to be afraid they will "spoil" infant with too much attention.	Feeding
		Holding
MOTOR	Talk and sing to child; hold and cuddle often.	Teach parent guidance information.
Responds to sound	Provide variety of stimulation.	Provide ongoing stimulation while confined
Social smile	Allow infant to feed self (cereal, etc.)	through use of toys, mirrors, mobiles, music.
Reaches for objects	Do not prop bottle.	Hold, speak to infant, maintain eye contact.
Begins to sit, creep, pull up and stand with support	*Toys*	Investigate crying.
Attempting to walk	Brightly colored crib toys, mobiles	Do not restrain.
LANGUAGE/COGNITION	Stuffed toys: of varied textures	
Learns to signal wants/needs with sounds, crying	Music boxes	
Begins to vocalize with meaning (two-syllable words: Dada, Mama)	*Safety*	
Comprehends some verbal/nonverbal messages (no, yes, bye-bye)	Be aware of rapidly changing locomotive ability (*i.e.,* childproof kitchen, stairways; small objects within reach; tub safety).	
Learns about words through senses		
FEARS		
Loud noises		
Falling		
1 to 3½ Years		
PERSONAL SOCIAL		
Establishes self-control, decision-making, self-independence (autonomy).	Provide child with peer companionship.	Allow child to take liquids from a cup (including medicines).
Extremely curious, prefers to do things himself.	Allow for brief periods of separation under familiar surroundings.	Allow child to perform some self-care tasks:

(continued)

Demonstrates independence through negativism.

Very egocentric: believes he controls the world.

Learns about words through senses.

MOTOR

Begins to walk and run well.

Drinks from cup, feeds self.

Develops fine-motor control.

Climbs.

Begins self-toileting.

LANGUAGE/COGNITION

Has poor time sense.

Increasingly verbal (4–5 word sentences by age 3½).

Talks to self/others.

Misconceptions about cause/effect.

FEARS

Loss/separation from parents

Darkness

Machines/equipment

Intrusive procedures

Practice safety measures that guard against child's increased motor ability and curiosity (poisoning, falls).

Tell the truth.

Disciplining child for violation of safety rules:

Running in street

Touching electrical wires

Allow child some control over fears:

Favorite toy

Night light

Allow exploration within safe limits.

Explain as simply as possible why things happen.

Allow child to explain why he thinks things are happening.

Correct misconceptions.

Include child in domestic activities when possible:

Dusting

Cleaning spoons

Discuss differences in opinions (between parents) in front of child.

Do not threaten child with what will happen if he does not behave.

Always follow through with punishment.

Toys

Manipulative toys

Puzzles

Bright-colored, simple books

Large-muscle devices (gym sets, etc.)

Music (songs, records)

Wash face and arms

Brush teeth

Expect resistant behavior to treatments; reinforce treatments, not punishments.

Use firm, direct approach and provide child with choices only when possible.

Restrain child when needed.

Explain to parents methods for disciplining child:

Slap hand once (for dangerous touching, e.g., stove)

Sit in chair for 2 minutes (if child gets up, put him back and reset timer)

Explain the need for consistency.

Allow expression of fear, pain, displeasure.

Assign consistent caregiver.

Let child play with simple equipment (stethoscope).

Provide materials for play (favorite toy, night light, etc.).

Be honest about procedure.

Praise child for helping you:

Holding still

Holding the Band-Aid

Give child choices whenever possible.

Tell child he can cry or squeeze your hand, but you expect him to hold still.

Have parents present for procedures when at all possible.

Explore with child his fantasies of the situation:

Use play therapy

Explain the procedure immediately beforehand if short (e.g., injection) and two hours before if longer or intrusive (e.g., x-ray, IV insertion).

Follow home routines when possible.

(continued)

Table II-8. **Age-related Developmental Needs** (continued)

Developmental Tasks/Needs	Parental Guidance	Implications for Nursing
3½ to 5 Years		
PERSONAL/SOCIAL		
Attempts to establish self as like his parents, but independent.	Teach parents to listen to child's fears, feelings.	Encourage expressing of fears.
Explores environment on his own initiative.	Encourage hugs, touch as expressions of acceptance.	Reinforce reality of body image.
Boasts, brags, has feelings of indestructibility.	Provide explanations—simply.	Encourage self-care, decision-making when possible.
Family is primary group.	Limit stimulation from television to avoid intense material.	Involve parents in teaching.
Peers increasingly important.	Focus on positive behaviors.	Provide peer stimulation.
Assumes sex roles.	Allow child to help as much as possible.	Limit physical restraint.
Aggressive.	Provide child with regular contact with other children (e.g., nursery school).	Provide play opportunities for acting out fantasy, story-telling.
MOTOR		
Locomotion skills increase, and coordinates easier.	Explain that television, movies are make-believe.	Explain to child how he can cooperate (e.g., hold still), and expect that he will.
Rides tricycle/bicycle.	Practice definite limit-setting on behavior.	Use play therapy to allow child free expression.
Throws ball, but has difficulty catching.	Offer child choices.	Explain all procedures:
LANGUAGE/COGNITION	Allow child to express anger verbally but limit motor aggression ("You may slam a door but you may not throw a toy").	Use equipment if possible; allow therapeutic play.
Egocentric.	Discipline (examples):	Encourage child to ask questions.
Language skills flourish.	Sit in chair 5 minutes.	Tell child the exact body parts that will be affected.
Generates many questions; how, why, what?	Forbid a favorite pastime (no bicycle riding for 2 hours).	Use models, pictures.
Simple problem-solving; uses fantasy to understand, problem-solve.	Be consistent and firm.	Explain when procedure will occur in relation to daily schedule (e.g., after lunch, after bath).
FEARS	Teach safety precautions about strangers.	
Mutilation	Toys and Games	
Castration	Enjoys "make-believe" play (play house, toy models, etc.)	
Dark	Simple games with others, books, puzzles, coloring	
Unknown		
Inanimate, unfamiliar objects		

(continued)

5 to 11 Years

PERSONAL/SOCIAL

Learns to include values and skills of school, neighborhood, peers.

Peer relationships important.

Focuses more on reality, less on fantasy.

Family is main base of security and identity.

Sensitive to reactions of others.

Seeks approval, recognition.

Enthusiastic, noisy, imaginative, desires to explore.

Likes to complete a task.

Enjoys helping.

MOTOR

Moves constantly.

Physical play prevalent (sports, swimming, skating, etc.).

LANGUAGE/COGNITION

Organized, stable thought.

Concepts more complicated.

Focuses on concrete understanding.

FEARS

Rejections, failure

Immobility

Mutilation

Death

Teach appropriate foods needed each day, provide choices.

Encourage interaction outside home.

Include cooking and cleaning in home activities.

Teach safety (bicycle, street, playground equipment, fire, water, strangers).

Maintain limit-setting and discipline.

Prepare child for bodily changes of pubescence and provide with concrete sex education information (late childhood).

Expect fluctuations between immature and mature behavior.

Respect peer relationships but do not compromise your values (e.g., "But, Mom, all the other girls are wearing makeup!").

Promote responsibility, contribution to family (i.e., duties for helping, etc.).

Promote exploration and development of skills (i.e., joining clubs, sports, hobbies, etc.).

Toys and Games

Group games, board games, art activities, crafts, video games, reading.

Promote family and peer interactions (i.e., visiting, telephone, etc.).

Explain all procedures and impact on body.

Encourage questioning, *active* participation in care.

Be direct about explanation of procedures (i.e., body part involved, use anatomical names, pictures, etc.) step by step.

Be honest.

Reassure child that he is liked.

Provide privacy.

Involve parents but make direction of care the child's decision.

Reason and explain.

Encourage continuance of school work, activities if condition permits (i.e., homework, contact with classmates).

Encourage continuance of hobbies, interests.

11 to 15 Years

PERSONAL/SOCIAL

Family values continue to be significant influence.

Encourage independent problem-solving, decision-making within established values.

Respect privacy.

Accept expression of feelings.

(continued)

Table II-8. **Age-related Developmental Needs** *(continued)*

Developmental Tasks/Needs	Parental Guidance	Implications for Nursing
Peer group values have increasing significance.	Be available.	Direct discussions of care and condition to child.
Early adolescence: outgoing and enthusiastic.	Compliment child's achievements.	Ask for opinions, allow input into decisions.
Emotions are extreme, mood swings, introspection.	Listen to interests, likes, dislikes without passing judgment.	Be flexible with routines, explain all procedures/ treatments.
Sexual identity fully mature.	Respect privacy.	Encourage continuance of peer relationships.
Wants privacy/independence.	Allow independence while maintaining safety limits.	Listen actively.
Develops interests not shared with family.	Provide concrete information about sexuality, function, bodily changes.	Identify impact of illness on body image, future functioning.
Concern with physical self.	Teach about:	Correct misconceptions.
Explores adult roles.	Auto safety	Encourage continuance of school work, hobbies, interests.
MOTOR	Drug abuse	
Well-developed	Alcohol abuse	
Rapid physical growth	Tobacco hazards	
Secondary sex characteristics	Mechanical safety	
LANGUAGE/COGNITION	Sexual abuse	
Plans for future career.	Dating	
Able to abstract solutions and problem-solve in future tense.	Games/Interests	
FEARS	Intellectual games	
Mutilation	Reading	
Disruption in body image	Arts, crafts, hobbies	
Rejection from peers	Video games	
	Problem-solving games	
	Computers	

affect development, many exist within the context of illness and wellness care and are often encountered by nurses as they provide care to children. As a result, nursing interventions should be designed with particular developmental tasks and developmental information as a basis for intervention. As part of the care of the child, the nurse must also consider the impact of the primary caregiver or parent figure on the development of the child. The parent essentially controls most of the psychological and social influences present in the early years of childhood. By virtue of the child's dependence on the parent, these influences can modify development.

5. Illness, hospitalization, separation from parents, conflict, or inadequate support from parents, as well as specific pathophysiological processes that interfere witih growth, may ultimately impact development in a child. The nurse must support the family as well as the child in ensuring continuance of the child's developmental processes throughout the course of his illness if optimal recovery is to be achieved. In addition, the nurse must seek to stimulate as well as maintain the child's unique developmental level to promote optimal recovery. Stimulation of the developmental process may occur through parental support, parental teaching, referral, or direct intervention (see also *Altered Parenting*).

Altered Growth and Development
Related to (Specify)

Assessment
See Defining Characteristics

Outcome Criteria

The child will
- Demonstrate an increase in behaviors in personal/social, language, cognition, motor activities appropriate to age group (specify the behaviors)

Interventions

A. Assess causative or contributing factors
- Lack of knowledge—parental (caregiver)
- Acute or chronic illness
- Stress
- Inadequate stimulation
- Parent–child conflict
- Change in environment

B. Teach parents the age-related developmental tasks and parental guidance information (see Table II-8)

C. Carefully assess child's level of development in all areas of functioning by utilizing specific assessment tools, (*e.g.,* Brazelton Assessment Table, Denver Developmental Screening Tool)

D. Provide opportunities for an ill child to meet age-related developmental tasks

(See Implications for Nursing [Table II-8] to assist with designing interventions)

Birth to 1 year

1. Provide increased stimulation using variety of colored toys in crib (*i.e.,* mobiles, musical toys, stuffed toys of varied textures, frequent periods of holding and speaking to infant).
2. Hold while feeding; feed slowly and in relaxed environment.
3. Provide periods of rest prior to feeding.
4. Observe mother and child during interaction, especially during feeding.
5. Investigate crying promptly and consistently.
6. Assign consistent caregiver.
7. Encourage parental visits/calls and involvement in care, if possible.
8. Provide buccal experience if infant desires (*i.e.,* thumb, pacifier).
9. Allow hands and feet to be free, if possible.

1 to 3¹/₂ years

1. Assign consistent caregiver.
2. Encourage self-care activities (*i.e.,* self-feeding, self-dressing, bathing).
3. Reinforce word development by repeating words child uses, naming objects by saying words, and speaking to child often.
4. Provide frequent periods of play with peers present and with a variety of toys (puzzles, books with pictures, manipulative toys, trucks, cars, blocks, bright colors).
5. Explain all procedures as you do them.
6. Provide safe area where the child can locomote, use walker, creeping area, hold hand while taking steps.
7. Encourage parental visits/calls and involvement in care, if possible.
8. Provide comfort measures after painful procedures.

3¹/₂ to 5 years

1. Encourage self care: self-grooming, self-dressing, mouth care, hair care.
2. Provide frequent play time with others and with variety of toys (*i.e.,* models, musical toys, dolls, puppets, books, mini-slide, wagon, tricycle, etc.).
3. Read stories aloud.
4. Ask for verbal responses and requests.
5. Say words for equipment, objects, and people and ask the child to repeat.
6. Allow time for individual play and exploration of play environment.
7. Encourage parental visits/calls and involvement in care, if possible.
8. Monitor television and utilize television as means to help child understand time ("After Sesame Street, your mother will come").

5 to 11 years

1. Talk with child about care provided.
2. Request input from child (*i.e.,* diet, clothes, routine, etc.).
3. Allow child to dress in clothes instead of pajamas.
4. Provide periods of interaction with other children on unit.
5. Provide craft project that can be completed each day or week.
6. Continue school work at intervals each day.
7. Praise positive behaviors.

8. Read stories, and provide variety of independent games, puzzles, books, video games, painting, etc.
9. Introduce child by name to persons on unit.
10. Encourage visits with and/or telephone calls from parents, sibling, and peers.

11 to 15 years
1. Speak frequently with child about feelings, ideas, concerns over condition or care.
2. Provide opportunity for interaction with others of the same age on unit.
3. Identify interest or hobby that can be supported on unit in some manner and support it daily.
4. Allow hospital routine to be altered to suit child's schedule.
5. Dress in his own clothes if possible.
6. Involve in decisions about his care.
7. Provide opportunity for involvement in variety of activities (*i.e.,* reading, video games, movies, board games, art, trips outside or to other areas).
8. Encourage visits and/or telephone calls from parents, siblings, and peers.

E. Initiate health teaching and referrals when indicated

1. Provide anticipatory guidance for parents regarding constructive handling of developmental problems and support of developmental process (Table II-8) (see *Altered Parenting*).
2. Refer to appropriate agency for counseling or follow-up treatment of abuse, parent–child conflict, chemical dependency, etc. (see *Disabled Family Coping*).
3. Refer to appropriate agency for structured, ongoing stimulation program when functioning is likely to be impaired permanently (*e.g.,* schooling).
4. Refer to community programs specific to contributing factors (*e.g.,* WIC, social services, family services, counseling).
5. Provide list of parent support groups (*i.e.,* ARC, Down Syndrome Awareness, Muscular Dystrophy Association, National Epilepsy).

References/Bibliography

Briggs DC: Your Child's Self Esteem. New York, Doubleday, 1979
Chase RA, Rubin RR: The First Wondrous Year. New York, Macmillan, 1979
Damon W: Social and Personality Development, Essays on the Growth of the Child. New York, WW Norton & Co, 1983
Erikson E: Childhood and Society, 2nd ed. New York, WW Norton & Co, 1963
Garmezy N, Rutter M (eds): Stress, Coping, and Development in Children. St. Louis, McGraw-Hill, 1983
Petrillo M, Sanger S: Emotional Care of Hospitalized Children, 2nd ed. Philadelphia, JB Lippincott, 1980
Piaget J: The Theory of Stages in Cognitive Development. New York, McGraw-Hill, 1969
Poster EC: Stress immunization: Techniques to help children cope with hospitalization. Matern Child Nurs J 12(2):21–24, 1983
Samuels M, Samuels N: The Well Baby Book. New York, Summit Books, 1979
Wong D, Whaley L: Clinical Handbook of Pediatric Nursing, 2nd 3d. St. Louis, CV Mosby, 1986

Health Maintenance, Altered

Related to **Tobacco Use**

Related to **Increased Food Consumption in Response to Stressors and Insufficient Energy Expenditures for Intake**

Related to **Lack of Knowledge (Specify): Potential**

Related to **Lack of Knowledge of Ostomy Care: Potential**

Definition

Altered health maintenance: The state in which an individual or group experiences or is at risk of experiencing a disruption in health because of an unhealthy life-style or lack of knowledge to manage a condition.

Author's Note: *Altered Health Maintenance* is a diagnostic category that can be used to describe a person (or persons) who desires to change an unhealthy life-style (obesity, tobacco use) or who needs teaching for self-management of a disease or condition.

Defining Characteristics (in the absence of disease)

Major (must be present)

Reports or demonstrates an unhealthy practice or life-style, *e.g.:*
  Reckless driving of vehicle
  Substance abuse
  Participation in high-risk activities (*e.g.,* recreational: sky/scuba diving, hang-gliding, occupational: police, firefighter, mining, etc.)
  Presence of obvious behavior disorders (compulsiveness, belligerence)
  Overeating

Minor (may be present)

Reports or demonstrates:
  Skin and nails
    Malodorous   Unusual color, pallor
    Skin lesions (pustules, rashes,   Unexplained scars
      dry or scaly skin)
  Respiratory system
    Frequent infections   Chronic cough   Dyspnea with exertion
  Oral cavity
    Frequent sores (on tongue,   Lesions associated with lack of
      buccal mucosa)   oral care or substance abuse
    Loss of teeth at early age   (leukoplakia, fistulas)
  Gastrointestinal system and nutrition
    Obesity   Chronic bowel irregularity
    Chronic anemia   Chronic dyspepsia

Musculoskeletal system
    Frequent muscle strain, backaches, neck pain
    Diminished flexibility and muscle strength
Genitourinary system
    Frequent venereal lesions and infections
    Frequent use of potentially unhealthful over-the-counter products (chemical douches, vaginal perfumed products, nasal sprays, etc.)
Constitutional
    Chronic fatigue, malaise, apathy
Neurosensory
    Presence of facial tics (nonconvulsant)
    Headaches
Psychoemotional
    Emotional fragility
    Behavior disorders (compulsiveness, belligerence)
    Frequent feelings of being overwhelmed

Etiological, Contributing, Risk Factors

A variety of factors can produce *Altered Health Maintenance*. Some common causes are listed below.

Pathophysiological
New medical condition

Treatment-related
    Lack of previous exposure
    New or complex treatment

Situational (personal, environmental)
    Lack of exposure to the experience
    Language differences
    Information misinterpretation
    Personal characteristics
        Lack of motivation
        Lack of education or
          readiness

Ineffective coping patterns (*e.g.,* anxiety, depression, nonproductive denial of situation, avoidance coping)

    Changes in finances
    Lack of access to adequate health care services
    Inadequate health practice
    External locus of control
    Religious beliefs
    Cultural beliefs

Maturational
Lack of education of age-related factors. Examples include
    Children
        Sexuality and sexual
          development
        Safety hazards

Substance abuse
Nutrition

Adolescents
    Same as children
    Automobile safety
        practices

Substance abuse
    (alcohol, other
    drugs, tobacco)
Health maintenance practices

Adults
    Parenthood
    Sexual function

Safety practices
Health maintenance practices

Elderly
    Effects of aging

Sensory deficits

See Table II-9 for age-related conditions.

Focus Assessment Criteria

This assessment is structured primarily to collect data to determine the person's learning capabilities and limitations.

Subjective Data

1. Does the individual/family report or demonstrate an unhealthy life-style?
2. Does the individual/family report frequent colds, infections, flus, etc.?
3. Determine present knowledge of
    Illness
        Severity   Susceptibility to complications
        Prognosis   Ability to cure it or control its
                                    progression
    Treatment/diagnostic studies
    Preventive measures
4. What is the pattern of adhering to prescribed health behaviors?
    Complete   Not adhering
    Modified
5. Does anything interfere with adherence to the prescribed health behavior?
6. History of disease
    Onset
    Symptoms
    Effects on life-style (relationships, work, leisure activities, finances)
7. Stage of adaptation to disease
    Disbelief   Anger
    Denial   Awareness
    Depression   Acceptance
8. Learning needs (perceived by client, family)
9. Learning ability (client, family)
    Level of education   Language spoken
    Ability to read   Language understood
10. Sociocultural factors
    Traditions   Health care beliefs and practices
    Life-style   Values

Objective Data

1. Ability to perform prescribed procedures
    Competency   Accuracy
2. Level of cognitive and psychomotor development
    Age   Ability to read and write

3. Presence of sensory deficits
    Vision
        Problems in focusing   Partial or total blindness
        Inability to distinguish colors
    Hearing
        Partial or total deafness   Tinnitus
    Sense of smell (altered or lost)
    Sense of taste (altered or lost)
    Sense of touch
        Anesthesia   Paresthesia
4. Physical stability
    a. Circulation/tissue perfusion
        General appearance
        Arterial blood pressure
        Pulse rate and regularity
        Pulse volume (weak, thready, full, bounding)
        Skin (color, temperature, moisture)
        Urine output
        Level of consciousness
    b. Respiratory status
        Rate
        Pattern
        Presence of abnormal breath sounds
        Altered blood gases
        Restlessness
        Irritability
    c. Nutritional/hydration status
        Fluid and electrolyte balance (Na, K, urine specific gravity, skin turgor)
        Intake and output
        Weight change
    d. Activity tolerance (good, fair, poor; see *Activity Intolerance* for additional assessment criteria)

Principles and Rationale for Nursing Care

See *Health-Seeking Behaviors*

Weight Reduction

1. Intake must be reduced to 500 calories per day less than requirement to obtain a one-pound-per-week weight loss.
2. The desirable weight loss rate is 1 to 2 pounds per week.
3. Overeating is a complex multidimensional problem with physical, social, and psychological components.
4. Overweight persons are usually nutritionally deprived.
5. Internal motivation is essential for a successful weight-loss program.
6. An individual's body image and coping patterns influence the weight-loss program's success or failure.
7. Childhood obesity is influenced by genetic factors; cellular structure; general body build; metabolic and endocrine factors (pancreatic insufficiency, hypothyroidism, hypersecretion of adrenal cortex); activity level; infantile obesity; and the psychologi-

(*Text continues on page 390*)

Table II-9. **Primary and Secondary Prevention for Age-Related Conditions**

Developmental Level	Primary Prevention	Secondary Prevention

Infancy (0-1 year)	Parent education
	Infant safety
	Nutrition
	Breast feeding
	Sensory stimulation
	Infant massage and touch
	Visual stimulation
	  Activity
	  Colors
	Auditory stimulation
	  Verbal
	  Music
	Immunizations
	  DPT } at 2, 4, and 6 months
	  TOPV }
	Oral hygiene
	Teething biscuits
	Fluoride
	Avoid sugared food and drink
		Complete physical exam every 2-3 months
		Screening at birth
		  Congenital hip
		  PKU
		  Sickle cell
		  Cystic fibrosis
		  Vision (startle reflex)
		Hearing (response to and localization of sounds)
		TB test at 12 months
		Developmental assessments
		Screen and intervene for high risk
		  Low birth weight
		  Maternal substance abuse during pregnancy
		    Alcohol: fetal alcohol syndrome
		    Cigarettes: SIDS
		    Drugs: addicted neonate, AIDS
		  Maternal infections during pregnancy

Preschool (1-5 years)	Parent education Teething Discipline Nutrition Accident prevention Normal growth and development Child education Dental self-care Dressing Bathing with assistance Feeding self-care	Complete physical exam between 2 and 3 years and preschool (U/A, CBC) TB test at 3 years Development assessments (annual) Speech development Hearing Vision Screen and intervene Lead poisoning Developmental lag Neglect or abuse

(continued)

Strabismus
Hearing deficit
Vision deficit

Immunizations
DPT
TOPV } at 18 months
MMR at 15 months
Hib at 24 mos.
Dental/oral hygiene
Fluoride treatments
Fluoridated water
Dietary counsel

Complete physical exam
TB test every 3 years (at ages 6 and 9)
Developmental assessments
Language
Vision: Snellen charts at school
   6–8 years, use "E" chart
   Over 8 years, use alphabet chart
Hearing: audiogram

School age
(6–11 years)

Health education of child
"Basic 4" nutrition
Accident prevention
Outdoor safety
Substance abuse counsel
Anticipatory guidance for physical changes
   at puberty
Immunizations
Tetanus age 10
DPT
TOPV } boosters between 4 and 6 years
Dental hygiene every 6–12 months
Continue fluoridation
Complete physical exam

Complete physical exam (prepuberty or age 13)
Blood pressure
Cholesterol
TB test at 12 years
VDRL, CBC, U/A
Female: breast self-exam
Male: testicular self-exam
Female, if sexually active: Pap and pelvic exam twice, one year apart
   (cervical gonorrhea culture with pelvic); then every 3 years if both
   are negative

Adolescence
(12–19 years)

Health education
Proper nutrition and healthful diets
Sex education
Sexually transmitted diseases
Safe driving skills
Adult challenges
Seeking employment and career choices
Dating and marriage
Confrontation with substance abuse
Safety in athletics

(continued)

Table II-9.　**Primary and Secondary Prevention for Age-Related Conditions** (continued)

Developmental Level	Primary Prevention	Secondary Prevention
	Skin care	Screening and interventions if high risk
	Dental hygiene every 6–12 months	Depression
	Immunizations	Suicide
	Tetanus without trauma	Substance abuse
	TOPV booster at 12–14 years	Pregnancy
		Family history of alcoholism or domestic violence
Young adult (20–39 years)	Health education	Complete physical exam at about 20 years, then every 5–6 years
	Weight management with good nutrition as BMR changes	Cancer checkup every 3 years
	Life-style counseling	Female: BSE monthly
	Stress management skills	Male: TSE monthly
	Safe driving	All females: baseline mammography between ages 35 and 40
	Family planning	Parents-to-be: high-risk screening for Downs syndrome, Tay-Sachs
	Parenting skills	Female pregnant: screen for VD, rubella titer, Rh factor, amniocentesis for woman 35 years or older (if desired)
	Regular exercise	
	Environmental health choices	Screening and interventions if high risk
	Dental hygiene every 6–12 months	Female with previous breast cancer: annual mammography at 35 years and after
	Immunizations	Female with mother or sister who has had breast cancer, same as above
	Tetanus at 20 years and every 10 years	
	Female: rubella, if serum negative for antibodies	Family history colorectal cancer or high risk: annual stool guaiac, digital rectal, and sigmoidoscopy
	Hepatitis-B for high-risk persons (male homosexuals with multiple partners; occupations at risk—dentist, nurse in dialysis unit, lab technician)	PPD if exposed to TB
Middle-aged adult (40–59 years)	Health education: continue with young adult	Complete physical exam every 5–6 years with complete laboratory evaluation (serum/urine tests, x-ray, EKG)
	Midlife changes, male and female counseling	Cancer checkup every year
	"Empty nest syndrome"	Female: BSE monthly
	Anticipatory guidance for retirement	Male: TSE monthly
	Grandparenting	

(continued)

Dental hygiene every 6–12 months
Immunizations
Tetanus every 10 years
Influenza—annual if high risk (*i.e.* major chronic disease [COPD, CAD])
Pneumococcal—single dose

All females: annual mammography 50 years and over
Schiotz's tonometry (glaucoma) every 3–5 years
Sigmoidoscopy at 50 and 51, then every 4 years if negative
Stool guaiac annually at 50 and thereafter
Screening and intervention if high risk
Endometrial cancer: have endometrial sampling at menopause
Oral cancer: screen more often if substance abuser

Elderly adult (60–74 years)

Health education: continue with previous counseling
Home safety
Retirement
Loss of spouse
Special health needs
Nutritional changes
Changes in hearing or vision
Alterations in bowel or bladder habits
Dental/oral hygiene every 6–12 months
Immunizations
Tetanus every 10 years
Influenza—annual if high risk
Pneumococcal—(one time only)

Complete physical exam every 2 years with laboratory assessments
Annual cancer checkup
Blood pressure annually
Female: BSE monthly
Male: TSE monthly
Female: annual mammogram
Annual stool guaiac
Sigmoidoscopy every 4 years
Schiotz's tonometry every 3–5 years
Podiatric evaluation with foot care PRN
Screen for high risk
Depression
Suicide
Alcohol/Drug Abuse

Old-age adult (75 years and over)

Health education: continue counsel
Anticipatory guidance
Dying and death
Loss of spouse
Increasing dependency upon others
Dental/oral hygiene every 6–12 months
Immunizations
Tetanus every 10 years
Influenza—annual
Pneumococcal—if not already received

Complete physical exam annually
Laboratory assessments
Cancer checkup
Blood pressure
Stool guaiac
Female: mammogram, sigmoidoscopy every 4 years
Schiotz's tonometry every 3–5 years
Podiatrist PRN

cal, social, or cultural use of food for comfort, reward, or solace or as a symbol of affluence.

8. An American's diet currently consists of 42% fat, 12% protein, 22% complex carbohydrates (CHO), and 24% simple carbohydrates. Recommended U.S. Dietary goals are 30% fat, 12% protein, 48% complex carbohydrates (CHO), and 10% simple carbohydrates. (Brody)

9. Any increase in activity will increase energy output and increase caloric deficits of a person following a dietary regimen. (Warwick)

10. Often, obesity is facilitated/aggravated by inappropriate response to external cues, including, most often, stressor. This response sets off an ineffective pattern whereby the individual eats in response to stress cues rather than physiological hunger.

11. The body uses a higher percent of energy (calories) to convert CHO to body fat than it does to convert fat to body fat. The body only needs 135–225 fatty calories to supply daily essential fatty acids.

12. The safest activities for the unconditioned obese person are walking, water aerobics, swimming, and cycling.

13. Fluctuations in body weight are common, especially in females. Daily weights can be misleading and disheartening. Body measurements are a better measurement of losses. Regular exercise will cause lean muscle mass to increase. Since muscle weighs more than fat, this may be reflected on the scale as a weight gain.

Altered Health Maintenance Related to Tobacco Use

Author's Note: This nursing diagnosis can be used in two different situations—for the individual who does not know the hazards of tobacco use and for the individual who desires to quit.

Assessment

Subjective Data
Individual reports
　　History of smoking and/or
　　History of chewing smokeless tobacco

Objective Data
　　Tobacco use behavior (smoking, chewing)
　　Odor of tobacco on breath if smoked
　　Spitting behavior if chewed
　　Staining of teeth, fingernails, and fingertips
　　Cough unrelated to infectious process
　　Frequent respiratory infections (upper and lower tracts)
　　Increased sputum production
　　Presence of oral lesions on mucosal and/or periodontal tissues

Outcome Criteria

The individual will
- Identify short-term and long-term health effects of tobacco use.
- Identify benefits of abstinence from tobacco use.
- Verbalize commitment to personal health and desire to eliminate tobacco use.*
- Devise strategies to assist in smoking/chewing cessation.*
- Significantly decrease amount of tobacco used or stop altogether.*

Interventions

A. Assessment

1. Define tobacco use behavior
   a. Type and quantity
      - Cigarettes
          Filter/nonfilter
          Regular/reduced tar and nicotine
          Pack years
      - Cigars
          Inhaled/not inhaled
          Number per day, number of years
      - Pipe
          Inhaled/not inhaled
          Number of bowls/day
      - Smokeless tobacco (chewing)
          Number of minutes/day
          Number of years
   b. Associated activities
       Job
       Home
       Relaxation
       Stressful events
       Recreation
       Use of alcohol/drugs
   c. Previous attempts to abstain from tobacco use
      - What strategies were used?
      - Why were they not successful?
2. Promote understanding of personal tobacco use behavior
   a. Identify negative aspects of tobacco use with client
      - Physical: exercise intolerance, cough, sputum, frequent respiratory infections, dental disease
      - Environmental: burned clothing/furniture, discolored interiors of home/workplace, malodorous clothing/furniture, dirty ashtrays, house and occupational fires

* These outcome criteria are established only *if* the client desires to quit tobacco use. For the client who does not wish to change tobacco use behaviors, provide information regarding health risks and benefits so that an *informed* choice is made. Avoid being judgmental. Always "keep the door open" should the client later change his mind.

- Social: inability to smoke in public places, offensive nature of tobacco use behaviors to family members, friends, co-workers
- Financial: calculate monetary cost of client's habit with client
- Psychological: unpleasant withdrawal symptoms that occur when tobacco is not available (*e.g.*, midnight "nicotine fits"), decreased self-esteem due to dependency

b. Identify positive aspects of tobacco use with client (use client's own words)

3. Provide information

a. Health risks of tobacco use to self
    Cancer (oral, lung, bladder)
    COPD and respiratory infections
    Arteriosclerosis (coronary and peripheral)
    Hypertension and CVA
    Periodontal disease

b. Health risks of tobacco use to others
    Unborn child
    Infants
    Asthmatics
    Persons with angina
    Persons with allergies

c. Benefits of quitting
    Decreased pulse and blood pressure
    Decreased sputum production
    Pulmonary mucosa regenerates
    Decreased risk of cancer, stroke, MI, COPD
    Improved dental hygiene
    Improved senses of taste/smell

d. Strategies available
    - Individual methods: self-help books and tapes, "cold turkey"
    - Group methods: contact local chapters of American Cancer Society, American Lung Association and private businesses
    - Hypnosis
    - Acupuncture
    - Over-the-counter products: filters, tablet regimens, nontobacco cigarettes*
    - Nicotine-containing chewing gum (prescription only)

e. Discuss strategies to minimize weight gain

f. Discuss symptoms of nicotine withdrawal and assist client to prepare for them.
    Craving for tobacco
    Irritability
    Anxiety
    Difficulty concentrating
    Restlessness
    Headache
    Drowsiness
    Gastrointestinal upsets: diarrhea, cramps
    If client has experienced these symptoms before, suggest he choose a time to quit in which he is experiencing relatively low stress.

4. Provide support and encouragement to promote success

* Caution: risks of the combustion of these products when inhaled are yet undetermined

a. Identify with client significant others who will provide ongoing support of client's abstinence from tobacco use
b. Identify with client persons who may sabotage efforts and devise strategies to minimize their impact
c. Reinforce with client his personal reasons for tobacco use cessation; encourage client to make visible reminders

Altered Health Maintenance
Related to Increased Food Consumption in Response to Stressors and Insufficient Energy Expenditure for Intake

Assessment

Subjective Data
Client states
"I like to eat"
"Eating calms my nerves"
"I don't have time for exercise"
"I don't like sports or exercise"
"I can't exercise"

Objective Data
Weight >10% over ideal for height and frame
Triceps skin fold greater than 15 mm in men and 25 mm in women

---

Outcome Criteria

The individual will
- Identify detrimental patterns of eating
- Identify stressors and effective response patterns
- Describe the relationship among metabolism, intake, and exercise
- Commit to exercise (specify type, amount)

Interventions

A. Assess for causative and contributing factors
1. Lack of knowledge
   - balanced nutritonal intake
   - exercise requirements
2. Inappropriate response to external stressors
3. Lack of initiative, motivation

4. Imbalance in composition of foods (*e.g.,* excess fat or simple carbohydrate intake)
5. Cultural, familial factors
6. Poor eating habits (*e.g.,* eating out, eating on the run, skipping meals)
7. Sedentary life-style, occupation
8. Sabotage by family and significant others

B. Increase awareness of components of intake/activity balance
   1. Multiply female weight by 11 and male weight by 12 to determine calorie intake/day needed to maintain current weight.
   2. One pound of fat is roughly equivalent to 3500 calories. To lose 2 pounds per week, one must cut 7000 calories from weekly intake.
   3. Exercise caloric expenditure charts may be used to determine amount of calories burned per duration increment of activity.
   4. Weight-loss goals may be achieved through a combination of caloric intake reduction and energy expenditure (via exercise) in calories.
   5. Successful weight reduction/maintenance is contingent upon a balance reduced caloric intake and caloric expenditure via exercise.

C. Assist client to identify realistic weight-loss program to fit his or her needs.
   1. Decide on amount of loss desired
   2. Time and duration of program
   3. Cost of various programs
   4. Nutritional soundness
   5. Compatibility with life-style

D. Assist client to anticipate environmental considerations.
   1. Friends, family, co-workers—what are their habits? Would they be supportive?
   2. What types of foods are found in the home? At parties? At work? In the lunch room?
   3. What types of leisure/recreational activities are engaged in? Is person sedentary?
   4. What routes are taken to work? Does client pass by fast-food establishments?
   5. Who does the housework? Gardening? Yard? Errands?
   6. How much television is watched? Do commercials trigger eating?
   7. Has person responded to gimmick advertisements for rapid weight loss (*e.g.,* "sleep away," belts, garments, wraps, lotions, etc.)?

E. Assist client to self-assess present eating/exercise habits by keeping a diary for a week, including usual:
   • Food intake/exercise
   • Location/time of meals
   • Emotions around meal time
   • Who client eats with
   • Skipped meals
   • Snacks

F. Familiarize client with cues that often trigger eating.
   • Eating while doing another activity, *e.g.,* watching TV
   • Eating standing up, *e.g.,* can give illusion of not eating
   • Eating out of boredom or stress because you need a break
   • Eat because everyone else is eating

G. Teach client basics of balanced nutritional intake, including supportive measures.
- Choose a diet plan that encourages high intake of complex carbohydrates (CHO) and limited fat intake.
- Know what you are eating. The "basic four" label is misleading, *e.g.*, a chicken-fried steak is a protein converted to high fat content through its preparation (frying).
- Attempt to obtain fat calories from fruits and vegetables instead of meat and dairy products.
- Eat more chicken and fish because they contain less fat and fewer total calories than beef. Remove fat and skin.
- Be aware of salad toppings and especially dressings with mayonnaise (216–308 calories per 2 oz serving).
- Completely avoid fast foods, because they have high fat and total caloric content.
- Dine in or make special requests in restaurants for food selection/preparations, *e.g.*, salad dressing on side, omit sauce from entree.
- Plan meals in advance.
- If attending a party or restaurants, decide what you will eat ahead of time, and stick to it.
- Adhere to grocery list.
- Involve family in meal planning for better nutrition.
- Buy the highest quality beef. Ground round = 10% fat and hamburger = 25% fat.
- Choose a variety of foods.
- Avoid serving family-style.
- Drink 8–10 8 oz glasses of water daily.
- Measure foods and count calories; keep records.
- Read labels on foods and note food composition and calories per serving.
- Eat slowly.
- Experiment with spices, substitutes, and low-calorie recipes.

H. Discuss benefits of exercise.
- Reduces caloric absorption
- Is an appetite suppressant
- Increases metabolic rate
- Preserves lean muscle mass
- Increases oxygen uptake
- Improves self-esteem
- Decreases depression, anxiety, and stress
- Increases caloric expenditure
- Ups the odds for weight-loss maintenance
- Increases restful sleep
- Improves body posture
- Provides fun, recreation, and diversion
- Increases resistance to degenerative diseases of middle/later years (*e.g.*, heart, blood vessels)

I. Assist client to identify realistic exercise program to fit his or her needs, considering:
- Personality, life-style
- Time factor, time of day

- Season—anticipate and plan
- Sedentary/active occupation
- Safety, *e.g.*, sports injuries, environmental hazards
- Costs—club membership, equipment
- Age, physical size, physical condition

J. Monitor or discuss getting started on the exercise program

- Start slow and easy
- Choose activities using many parts of the body
- Choose an activity that is vigorous enough to cause "healthful fatigue"
- Do reading, consult experts, talk with friends/co-workers who exercise
- Plan a daily walking program and gradually increase rate and length of walk
    1. Start out at 5 to 10 blocks for 0.5 to 1.0 mile/day; increase 1 block or 0.1 mile/week
    2. Remember, progress slowly
    3. Avoid straining or pushing too hard and becoming overly fatigued
    4. Stop immediately if any of the following signs occur:

        Lightness or pain in chest   Dizziness
        Severe breathlessness   Loss of muscle control
        Lightheadedness   Nausea

    5. If pulse is 120 beats per minute (BPM) 5 minutes after stopping exercise, 100 BPM 10 minutes after stopping exercise, or if short of breath 10 minutes after exercise, slow down either the rate of walking or the distance
    6. If unable to walk 5 blocks or 0.5 mile without signs of overexertion appearing, decrease length of walking for one week to point before signs appear and then start to add 1 block/0.1 mile each week
    7. Walk at same rate; time self with stopwatch or second hand on watch; after reaching 10 blocks (1 mile) try to increase speed
    8. Remember, increase only the rate or the length of walk at one time
    9. Establish a regular time of day to exercise, with the goal of 3 to 5 times per week for a duration of 15 to 45 minutes and with a heart rate of 80% of stress test or gross calculation (170 BPM for 20–29 age group; decrease 10 BPM for each additional decade of life, *e.g.*, 160 BPM for ages 30–39, 150 BPM for ages 40–49, etc.)
- Encourage significant others also to engage in walking program
- Add supplemental activity, *e.g.*, park far away, work on garden, walk up stairs, spend weekends at leisure activities such as festivals or art fairs, which require walking
- Work up to one hour of exercise per day at least four days per week
- Avoid lapses of more than two days between exercise days

K. Teach client about the risks of obesity:

- Vascular insufficiency
- Arteriosclerosis, heart disease, hypertension
- Left ventricular hypertrophy
- Diabetes mellitus, gallbladder disease
- Increased risk of complications of surgery
- Respiratory disease
- Joint degeneration
- Increased risk of cancer, *e.g.*, breast
- Increased risk of accident/injury

L. Assist client to increase interest and motivation in weight reduction/exercise program.
- Contract re: realistic short- and long-term goals
- Keep intake/activity records
- Hang an admired photograph on the refrigerator
- Get family involved in project
- Record body measurements and limit weighing to once per week
- Increase knowledge by reading and talking with health-conscious friends and co-workers
- Make new friends who are health-conscious
- Get a friend to go on program too or to be a central support
- Avoid persons who may sabotage attempts
- Reward self on a regular basis
- Remind self that self-image and behavior are learned and can be unlearned
- Build a support system of people who value growth and value you as an individual
- Be aware of rationalization, *e.g.,* a lack of time may be a lack of prioritization
- Keep a list of positive outcomes

M. Reduce inappropriate responses to stressors.
1. Teach to distinguish between urge and hunger
2. Use distraction, relaxation, imagery
3. Use alternative response training:
   - Make a list of external cues/situations that lead to off-target behavior
   - List what you can do constructively instead of indulging in off-target behavior when this occurs (*e.g.,* take a walk)
   - Post the list of alternate behaviors on the refrigerator
   - Reevaluate whether plan is realistic and effective every one to two weeks

N. Assist client to plan for life-long weight maintenance.
- Understand issues of dependency, control and esteem
- Decide on *your* plan for *your* control
- Set realistic short- and long-term goals. Revise as necessary
- Think positive, start slowly
- Give self credit for each achievement, avoid perfectionism
- Build healthy support system

O. Initiate health teaching and referrals as indicated.
- Refer to support groups (*e.g.,* Weight Watchers, Overeater Anonymous, TOPS, trim clubs, The Diet Workshop, Inc.)
- Dietitian for meal planning
- Physician for morbid obesity and evaluation of other health problems

Potential Altered Health Maintenance
Related to Lack of Knowledge of (Specify)

Example: Lack of Knowledge of Dietary Management of Diabetes Mellitus
Lack of Knowledge of Newborn Care

Assessment

Subjective Data

The person states that he
  Is aware of a knowledge deficit
  Is anxious and fearful of unfamiliar situations
  Needs instruction

Objective Data

The person
  Does not participate in his care (when other reasons for noncompliance have been ruled out)
  Exhibits anxious behavior, such as
    Increased verbalization   Restlessness
    Inability to concentrate   Sweating palms
      and retain information   Tremulousness
  Delays seeking medical assistance when it is needed
  Misuses health care system (seeks assistance when he himself could have solved the problem or used a more appropriate resource)

Outcome Criteria

The person will
  • Actively participate in the health behaviors prescribed or desired (such as those behaviors required in preparation for a diagnostic test, surgery, or physical examination, or those behaviors related to recovery from illness and prevention of recurrence of complications)
  • Relate less anxiety, related to fear of the unknown, fear of loss of control, misconceptions, or previously given misinformation
  • Describe disease process, causes, and factors contributing to symptoms, and the procedure(s) for disease or symptom control

---

Interventions

The following interventions represent the teaching/learning activities to deal with a new diagnosis or treatment or the anticipation of an unfamiliar test, procedure, or surgery.

A. Assess the causative and contributing factors (in situations requiring a planned teaching/learning intervention)
  New diagnosis
  Change in existing medical condition/health status
  New or altered treatment regimen

B. Reduce or eliminate barriers to learning
  • Assist person in meeting basic physiological needs, if necessary
  • Support person in progressing through stages of psychosocial adaptation to illness
    1. Stage of disbelief (denial)
      a. Orient person to hospital setting, routines affecting him

     b. Teach with a focus on the present
     c. Provide simple explanations of procedures as they are carried out
     d. Help person feel safe, secure
     e. Concentrate on one-to-one teaching, rather than group teaching
     f. Teach family about the denial that person is having
   2. State of developing awareness (guilt, anger)
     a. Listen carefully to person
     b. Continue teaching with a present-tense focus
     c. Allow hositility to be safely vented
     d. Avoid arguing with person
- Delay teaching until person is ready
- Adapt teaching to person's physical and psychological status
- Allow person to work through and express intense emotions prior to teaching
- Examine person's health beliefs and past experiences related to his illness and assess their impact on his desire to learn

C. Promote person/family learning
- Individualize the teaching approach after a thorough assessment
- Plan and share necessity of learning outcomes with person/family
- Follow the principles of teaching/learning previously listed
- Evaluate person/family behaviors as evidence that learning outcomes have been achieved

D. Promote a positive attitude and active participation of the person and his family
- Solicit expressions of feelings, concerns, and questions from person and family
- Encourage person and family to seek information and become involved in making informed decisions
- Explain person/family responsibilities and how these can be assumed

E. Reduce anxiety
- Encourage verbalization
- Listen attentively
- Meet person's expressed needs prior to giving other information
- Develop trust with frequent, consistent interactions
- Give correct, relevant information
- Give nonthreatening information before more anxiety-producing information
- Explain reason(s) for and intended effect of regimen or surgery, emphasizing the positive
- Explore with person the effects of a new diagnosis, treatment, or surgery on his significant others
- Do not overwhelm person with too much information if anxiety is high or physical condition is unstable
- Allow person to maintain some control over himself and his routines by involving person in care
- Prepare person and family for what to expect concerning his environment, routines, the personnel giving care, sensations experienced, etc.
- Reorient as needed

F. Proceed with health teaching and referrals as indicated

Potential Altered Health Maintenance
Related to Lack of Knowledge of Ostomy Care

Author's Note: Persons undergoing ostomy surgery frequently question whether or not they will be able to lead normal lives. The most commonly expressed fear is that of being offensive to themselves and others. Multiple factors contribute to this fear. During the perioperative period, patients consistently ask the same questions about how the ostomy will affect their life-style: "How will I go to the bathroom? Can I really contain the drainage? Will I have an offensive odor? Will the pouch show through my clothing? How do you empty the pouch? How will I know when to change/empty the pouch? Can I work, travel, swim, play, make love? Can I eat regular food? Can I drink beer? Will my partner still love me? What can I do with the pouch during lovemaking? Can I exercise?"

Satisfactory answers to these questions provide knowledge that will decrease the person's fear and facilitate ostomy self-care. If a person can be taught how to contain the ostomy output in a discreet manner, it may provide the confidence that is necessary to begin working through the emotional issues related to having an ostomy. Because control over elimination is a primary concern, teaching the stoma pouching procedure is used as an example of a nursing intervention to reduce the knowledge deficit of ostomy care. (Maklebust)

Assessment

Subjective Data

The person states that he
  Has a knowledge deficit of ostomy care
  Is anxious and fearful because he does not know about ostomy care
  Needs instruction in ostomy care

Objective Data

The person does not participate in ostomy care.
The person is:
  Unable to state own disease/indications for surgery
  Unable to identify own type of ostomy
  Unable to describe routine ostomy care
  Unable to identify stoma pouching equipment
  Unable to apply, change, or empty stoma pouch
  Unable to maintain peristomal skin integrity

Outcome Criteria

The person will
- Actively participate in the health behaviors prescribed or desired (such as those behaviors required in preparation for a diagnostic test, surgery, or physical examination, or those behaviors related to recovery from illness and prevention of recurrence of complications)
- Relate less anxiety, related to fear of the unknown, fear of loss of control, misconceptions, or previously given misinformation
- Describe disease process, causes, and factors contributing to symptoms, and the procedure(s) for disease or symptom control

Interventions

A. Assess knowledge regarding ostomy and effects on life-style

1. Level of understanding of disease
2. Knowledge of structure and function of affected organs
3. Surgical procedure/stoma location
4. Type of ostomy effluent
5. Knowledge of ostomy care (*e.g.,* diet, activity, hygiene, clothing, sexual function, community resources, employment, travel, odor, skin care, appliances, and irrigation, if applicable)
6. Prior exposure to person with ostomy
7. Familiarity with stoma pouching equipment
8. Emotional status, cognitive ability, and physical limitations (*e.g.,* anxiety, memory, vision, manual dexterity)
9. Life-style/strengths/coping mechanisms
10. Available support systems

See other possible nursing diagnoses for additional interventions, for example:

   a. Anticipatory grief related to perceived loss of adult toileting behavior
   b. Powerlessness related to loss of control over elimination following removal of anal sphincter or urethra
   c. Potential disturbance in self-concept related to sudden change in body structure following ostomy surgery, or
   d. Social isolation related to fear of rejection by others

B. Instruct person on stoma and related information

1. Dispel misinformation/misconceptions regarding ostomy
2. Explain normal anatomical structure and function of GI or GU tract.
3. Explain effects of disease on affected organs.
4. Use diagram/model to show altered route of elimination.
5. Describe appearance and anticipated location of stoma:
   - Stoma will be same color and have same degree of moistness as oral mucous membrane.
   - Stoma has no nerve endings for pain and will not hurt when touched.
   - Stoma will become smaller as the surgical area heals—color will remain the same
   - Stoma size may change depending on illness, hormone levels, weight gain or loss.
6. Discuss need for wearing pouch as a prosthesis or substitute for the removed colon or bladder.
7. Encourage handling of stoma pouching equipment.
8. Teach basic stoma pouching principles:
   a. Peristomal skin should be clean and dry so that appliance will adhere to skin.
   b. A well-fitting appliance should protect all the surrounding skin surface from drainage.
   c. Pouch should be changed when the least amount of drainage is anticipated, usually upon rising.
   d. Pouch should be emptied when one-third to one-half full.
   e. Pouch should be changed routinely before a leak occurs.
   f. Pouch should be changed if burning or itching occurs under the appliance.
   g. Condition of stoma and peristomal skin should be observed during pouch changes.
9. Proceed with teaching necessary procedures. Consistently use same sequence while teaching.
   a. Teach procedure for preparing stoma pouch:
      - Measure stoma.

- Use appliance manufacturer's stoma-measuring card if possible.
- If appliance manufacturer's stoma-measuring card does not accommodate stoma size or shape, teach person to make individual pattern of stoma. Place clear plastic wrap from skin barrier wafer over stoma. Trace stoma with a marking pen. Cut hole in plastic to accommodate stoma.
- Use pattern to trace opening onto the reverse side of a skin barrier wafer.
- Cut opening in center of skin barrier wafer that is slightly larger (approximately 1/8 inch) than stoma
- Secure appropriate odor-proof pouch onto skin barrier wafer (if using two-piece appliance system)
- Remove white paper backing from skin barrier wafer.
- Set pouch aside.

  b. Teach procedure for changing disposable stoma pouch:

- Remove old pouch by gently pushing skin away from paper tape and skin barrier wafer.
- Fold old pouch over on itself and discard in plastic bag.
- Clean peristomal skin with wash cloth and warm tap water.
- Blot or pat skin dry.
- Apply new pouch to abdomen carefully, centering the hole in the skin barrier wafer over the stoma.
- Press on wafer for a few minutes so that heat and pressure of hand will help wafer adhere to skin.
- Secure pouch by "picture framing" wafer with four strips of hypoallergenic paper tape (if wafer does not already have tape attached).

  c. Teach procedure for emptying stoma pouch:

- Sit on toilet.
- Put some toilet paper into toilet bowl so that water does not splash.
- Remove pouch clamp from tail of pouch.
- Empty contents of pouch into toilet.
- Flush toilet.
- Clean inside and outside of pouch tail with toilet paper.
- Squeeze ostomy appliance deodorant into end of pouch.
- Reapply clamp to tail of pouch.

C. Incorporate emotional support into technical self-ostomy care sessions

This allows resolution of emotional issues during acquisition of technical skills. Derricks identified four stages of psychological adjustment that ostomy patients experience.

  a. Narration—Each person recounts his illness experience and reveals his understanding of how and why he finds himself in his current situation.

  b. Visualization and verbalization—The person looks at and expresses feelings about his stoma.

  c. Participation—The person progresses from observer to assistant and then to independent performer of the mechanical aspects of ostomy care.

  d. Exploration—The person begins to explore methods of incorporating the ostomy into his life-style.

Using this adjustment framework helps to establish guidelines for arranging patient experiences in an organized manner.

D. Encourage person to become active in care by gradually increasing his responsibility

Have individual:

- Look at and touch stoma.
- Assumptions cannot be made about a person's reaction to a situation. The reality of the altered body function may overwhelm the person.
- Verbalize feelings about stoma.
- Assure person that his responses are normal and appropriate. Person's perceptions must be validated by the nurse.
- Practice using pouch clamp on empty pouch.
- Beginning with a necessary skill that is apart from the body is less threatening.
- Assist with emptying pouch.
- During ostomy care, person watches health care professionals for signs of revulsion. The nurse's attitude and support are of primary importance.
- Participate in pouch removal.
- Give feedback on progress. Reinforce positive behavior, proper techniques.
- Participate in pouch application. Point out degrees of success achieved toward self-care.
- Demonstrate stoma pouching procedure independently in presence of resource person.
- Evaluate need for further teaching.
- Involve significant other in learning ostomy care principles.
- Assess interactions with significant other.
- Discuss plans to incorporate ostomy into own life-style.
- Suggest a visitor from the United Ostomy Association who can share similar experiences.

E. Initiate health teaching and referrals as indicated:
   1. Relate ostomy care to diet, medications, hygiene, clothing, sexual function, community resources, employment, travel, odor, skin care, appliances, and irrigation, if applicable. Review follow-up care and signs/symptoms to report to enterostomal (ET) nurse or physician.
   2. Discuss community resources/self-help groups:
      - Visting nurse
      - United Ostomy Association
      - Foundation for Ileitis and Colitis
      - Recovery of male potency—help for the impotent male
      - American Cancer Foundation
      - Community suppliers of ostomy equipment
      - Financial reimbursement for ostomy equipment

References/Bibliography

Albert M: Health screening to promote health for the elderly. Nurse Pract 12(5):42, 1987

American Cancer Society: The Cancer-Related Health Checkup. New York, American Cancer Society, 1980

Bartlett EE: Behavioral diagnosis: A practical approach to patient education. Patient Counsel Health Educ 4(1):29–35, 1982

Beloc N, Breslow L: The relation of physical health status and health practice. Prev Med 1:409–421, 1972

Bille D (ed): Practical Approaches to Patient Teaching. Little, Brown Co, Boston, 1981

Breslow L, Somers A: The lifetime health-monitoring program. N Engl J Med 296:601–608, 1977

Carlson CE, Blackwell B: Behavioral Concepts and Nursing Intervention, 2nd ed. Philadelphia, JB Lippincott, 1978

Chestnut CH: Treatment of postmenopausal osteoporosis. Compr Ther 10(7):41–47, 1984

Chow MP, Durand BA, Feldman MN et al: Handbook of Primary Care. New York, John Wiley & Sons, 1979

Christman NJ, Kirchhoff KT: Preparatory sensory information. In Bulechek G, McCloskey J (eds): Nursing Interventions: Treatments for Nursing Diagnoses. Philadelphia, WB Saunders, 1985

Cohen N: Three steps to better patient teaching. Nursing 10(2):72–74, 1980

Coralli C et al: Osteoporosis: Significance, risk factors and treatment. Nurse Pract 11(9):25, 1986

Czerwinski B: Manual of Patient Education for Cardiopulmonary Dysfunctions. St. Louis, CV Mosby, 1980

Doak CC, Doak LG, Root JH: Teaching Patients with Low Literacy Skills, Philadelphia, JB Lippincott, 1985

Duvall EM: Marriage and Family Development, 5th ed. Philadelphia, JB Lippincott, 1977

Eisenberg A, Eisenberg H: Alive and Well: Decision in Health. New York, McGraw-Hill, 1979

Falvo DR: Effective Patient Education. Rockville, MD, Aspen Systems Corp, 1985

Flynn PA: Holistic Health: The Art and Science of Care. Bowie, MD, Robert J. Brady, 1980

Frank T et al: Pertussis immunizations? Pediatr Nurs 10(5):360, 1984

Hill L, Smith N: Self-Care Nursing. Englewood Cliffs, NJ, Prentice-Hall, 1985

Hymovich DP, Barnard MV: Family Health Care, 2nd ed. New York, McGraw-Hill, 1979

Implementing Patient Education in the Hospital. Chicago, American Hospital Association, 1979

Jensen DP: Patient contracting. In Bulechek G, McCloskey J (eds): Nursing Interventions: Treatments for Nursing Diagnoses. Philadelphia, WB Saunders, 1985

Kandzari J, Howard J: The Well Family: A Developmental Approach to Assessment. Boston, Little, Brown & Co, 1981

Kelly K, McClelland E: Discharge planning. In Bulechek G, McCloskey J (eds): Nursing Interventions: Treatments for Nursing Diagnoses. Philadelphia, WB Saunders, 1985

Lieberman MA, Borman LD: Self-Help Groups for Coping with Crisis. San Francisco, Jossey-Bass, 1979

Montag M, Swenson P: Fundamentals of Nursing Care, 5th ed. Philadelphia, WB Saunders, 1959

Ouslander JC, Beck JC: Defining the health problems of the elderly. Annu Rev Public Health 3:55–83, 1982

Pajares KF et al: Rubella vaccination. Pediatr Nurs 10(1):72, 1984

Pender NJ: Self-modification. In Bulechek G, McCloskey J (eds): Nursing Interventions: Treatments for Nursing Diagnoses. Philadelphia, WB Saunders, 1985

Periodic health exam: A guide for designing individualized preventive health care in the asymptomatic adult. Ann Intern Med 95:729–732, 1981

Pritchett S: Patient, Family and Community Health Education. Atlanta, Pritchett and Hull Associates, 1977

Rankin SH, Duffy KL: Patient Education: Issues, Principles, & Guidelines. Philadelphia, JB Lippincott, 1983

Redman B: Curriculum in patient education. Am J Nurs 78:1363, 1366, 1978

Redman BK: The Process of Patient Education, 5th ed. St. Louis, CV Mosby, 1984

Redman BK, Thomas SA: Patient teaching. In Bulechek G, McCloskey J (eds): Nursing Interventions: Treatments for Nursing Diagnoses. Philadelphia, WB Saunders, 1985

Rimar JM: Haemophilus Influenzae Type b Polysaccharide Vaccine. MCN 11:57, 1986

Smitherman C: Nursing Actions for Health Promotion. Philadelphia, FA Davis, 1981

Spitzer WO: Report of the task force on the periodic health examination. Can Med Assoc J 121:193–254, 1979

Storlie F: Patient Teaching in Critical Care. New York, Appleton-Century-Crofts, 1975

Todd B: Preventing influenza and pneumonia. Geriatr Nurs pp 399-401, Nov–Dec 1984

Wilberding JZ: Values Clarification. In Bulechek G, McCloskey J (eds): Nursing Interventions: Treatments for Nursing Diagnoses. Philadelphia, WB Saunders, 1985

Wilson-Barnett J, Osborne J: Studies evaluating patient teaching: Implications for practice. Int J Nurs Stud 20(1):33–44, 1983

Woldum KM, Bower KA, Ryan-Morrell V: Patient education: Tools for Practice. Rockville, MD, Aspen System Corp, 1985

Woldum KM, Ryan-Morrell V, Towson MC: Patient Education: Foundations of Practice. Rockville, MD, Aspen Systems Corp, 1985

Zander K, Bower K, Foster S et al: Practical Manual for Patient Teaching. St. Louis, CV Mosby, 1978

Tobacco Use

Hughes JR, Miller SA: Nicotine gum to help stop smoking. JAMA 252(20):2855–2858, 1984
Lefcoe NM, Ashley MJ, Pederson LL, Keays JJ: The health risks of passive smoking. Chest 84(1):90–95, 1983
Mennies JH: Smoking: The physiologic effects. Am J Nurs 83(8):1143–1146, 1983
Squier CA: Smokeless tobacco and oral cancer: A cause for concern? CA 34(5):242–247, 1984

Ostomy Care

Alterescu V: The ostomy: What do you teach the patient? Am J Nurs 85(11):1250–1253, 1985
Boarini J: The ostomy, what can go wrong? Am J Nurs 85(12):1361, 1985
Bollinger B: A Teenager's Ostomy Guide. Available from Hollister, Inc., 2000 Hollister Drive, Libertyville, IL 60048
Borden N: Outcome standards for the ostomy client. J Enterostomal Therapy 10:128–131, 1983
Broadwell DC, Jackson B: Principles of Ostomy Care. St. Louis, CV Mosby, 1982
Broadwell DC, Sorrells, SL:
   Summary of Your Ileostomy Care
   Summary of Your Colostomy Care
   Summary of Your Urinary Diversion Care
   Ostomy Care for Children
Available from Bard Home Health Division, C.R. Bard, Inc., P.O. Box 18, Berkeley Heights, NJ 07922
Brogna L: Self-concept and rehabilitation of the person with an ostomy. J Enterostomal Therapy 12(6):205–209, 1985
Derricks V: Nursing practices that affect the dynamics of rehabilitation for patients with an ostomy. ANA Clinical Sessions. Kansas City, ANA, 1974
Given BA, Simmons SJ: Gastroenterology in Clinical Nursing, 4th ed. St Louis, CV Mosby, 1984
Jacobs M. Geels W: Signs and Symptoms in Nursing: Interpretation and Management. Philadelphia, JB Lippincott, 1985
Jeter KF: "Help For Incontinent People" Report. Available from HIP, PO Box 544, Union, SC 29373
Jeter KF: These Special Children. Available from Bull Publishing Co., PO Box 208, Palo Alto, CA 94302
Lee D: Standards of Enterostomal Therapy Practice. Newport Beach, CA, IAET, 1981
Maklebust J: United Ostomy Association visits and adjustment following ostomy surgery. J Enterostomal Therapy 12(3):84–92, 1985
Moss RC: Overcoming fear, a review of research on patient, family instruction. AORN J 43(5):1107–1114, 1986
Mullen BD, McGinn K: The Ostomy Book. Available from Bull Publishing Co., PO Box 208, Palo Alto, CA 94302
Smith DB: Patient teaching. In Smith DB, Johnson DE (eds): Ostomy Care and the Cancer Patient: Surgical and Clinical Considerations, pp 85–92. Orlando, FL, Grune & Stratton, 1986
Smith DB, Johnson DE: Preoperative preparation. In Smith DB, Johnson DE (eds): Ostomy Care and the Cancer Patient: Surgical and Clinical Considerations, pp 4–5. Orlando, FL, Grune & Stratton, 1986
Watson PG: Meeting the needs of patients undergoing ostomy surgery. J Enterostomal Therapy 12(4):121–124, 1985
Watt RC: The ostomy, why is it created? Am J Nurs 85(1):1242–1245, 1985

Obesity

See *Altered Nutrition: Less Than Body Requirements* for additional sources of information.
Brody J: Jane Brody's Nutrition Book. New York, W Norton & Co, 1981
Brownell KD, Stunkard AJ: Exercise in the development and control of obesity. In Stunkard AJ (ed): Obesity. Philadelphia, WB Saunders, 1980
Danforth E: Diet and obesity. Am J Clin Nutr 41:1132–1145, 1985
Fernstein AR: The treatment of obesity: An analysis of methods, results, and factors that influence success. J Chronic Dis 11:349–393, 1960

Fox SM III, Naughton JP, Haskell WL: Physical activity in prevention of coronary heart disease. Ann Clin Res 3:404–432, 1971

Franklin BA, Rubenfire M: Losing weight through exercise. JAMA 244:377–379, 1980

Hoepfel HJ: Improving compliance with an exercise program. Am J Nurs 81:560–563, 1981

Holmes N, Ardito EA, Stevenson D, Lucas CP: In Storlie J, Jordan HA (eds): Behavioral Management of Obesity, pp 137–150. New York, Spectrum Publications, Inc, 1984

Jacobson P: Help for fat teenagers. Pediatr Nurs 5(2):49–50, 1979

Kaufmann NA: Eating habits and opinions of teenagers on nutrition and obesity. J Am Diet Assoc 66:264–268, 1975

Overeaters Anonymous: A self-help group. Am J Nurs 81:560–563, 1981

Pavlou KN, Steffee NP, Lerman RH, Burrows BA: Effects of dieting and exercise on lean body mass, oxygen uptake and strength. Med Sci Sports Exer 17:466–469, 1985

Pitta P, Alpert M, Perelle A: Cognitive stimulus-control program for obesity with emphasis on anxiety and depression reduction. Int J Obes 4:227–233, 1980

Schroeder MA (ed): Symposium on obesity. Nurs Clin North Am 17(2), 1982

Smith GS, Delprato DJ: Stimulus control of covert behaviors (urges). Psychol Record, 26:461–466, 1976

Stunkard AJ: Biological and psychological factors in obesity. In Goodstern RK (ed): Eating and Weight Disorders, pp 1–31. New York, Springer Publishing Co, 1983

Wadden TA, Stunkard AJ, Brownell KD: Very low calorie diets: Their efficacy, safety and future. Ann Intern Med 99:675–684, 1983

Warwick M, Garrow JS: The effect of addition of exercise to a regime of dietary restriction on weight loss, nitrogen balance, resting metabolic rate and spontaneous physical activity in three obese women in a metabolic ward. Int J Obes 5:25–32, 1981

Wilson GT, Brownell KD: Behavior therapy for obesity: Including family members in the treatment process. Behav Ther 9:943–945, 1978

Wooley SC, Wooley OW, Dyrenforth SR: Theoretical, practical, and social issues in behavioral treatments of obesity. J Appl Behav Anal 12:3–25, 1979

Stress Management

Alberti RE, Emmons ML: Your Perfect Right: A Guide to Assertive Behavior. San Luis Obispo, CA, Impact Publishers, 1974

Bloom L, Coburn K, Pearlman J: The New Assertive Woman. New York, Dell Publishers, 1976

Girdano DD, Everly GS: Controlling Stress and Tension. Englewood Cliffs, NJ, Prentice-Hall.

Girdano DD, Everly GS: The Stress-Mess Solution. Bowie, MD, Robert J. Brady, 1980

Martin RA, Poland EY: Learning to Change: A Self-Management Approach to Adjustment. New York, McGraw-Hill, 1980

Exercise

Cantu RC: Toward Fitness: Guided Exercise for Those with Health Problems. New York, Human Sciences Press, 1980

Ellfeldt L, Lowman CL: Exercises for the Mature Adult. Springfield, IL, Charles C Thomas, 1973

Getchell L: Physical Fitness: A Way of Life, 2nd ed. New York, John Wiley & Sons, 1979, 1973

Kuntzelman CT: The Complete Book of Walking. New York, Simon and Schuster, 1979

Nutrition/Dental

Beal VA: Nutrition in the Life Span. New York, John Wiley & Sons, 1980

Diet and Dental Health. Chicago, IL, American Dental Association, 1975

A Healthier Mouth: It's Up to You. Jersey City, NJ, Block Drug Company, 1975

McGill M, Pye O: The No-Nonsense Guide to Food and Nutrition. New York, Butterick Publishing, 1978

Safety

See *Potential for Injury* References/Bibliography

Resources for the Consumer

National Self-Health Clearinghouse, Graduate School and University Center of the City University of New York (CUNY), 33 West 42nd Street, Room 1227, New York, NY 10036, (212)840-7606. Publishers of *Self-Help Reporter*.

Community Wellness Resource Centers

The Center for Health Promotion, 601 Brookdale Towers, 2810 Fifty-seventh Avenue N, Minneapolis, MN 55430

Good Health Program, Skokie Valley Community Hospital, 9600 Gross Point Road, Skokie, Illinois 60076

Organizations

American Cancer Society
American Dental Association
American Heart Association

Health-Seeking Behaviors

Related to **(Specify)**

Definition

Health-seeking behaviors: The state in which an individual in stable health actively seeks ways to alter personal health habits and/or the environment in order to move toward a higher level of wellness.*

Author's Note: This diagnostic category can be used to describe the individual/family that desires health teaching related to the promotion and maintenance of health (preventive behavior, age-related screening, optimal nutrition, etc). This diagnostic category should be used to describe an asymptomatic person. However, it can be used for a person with a chronic disease to help that person attain a higher level of wellness. For example, a woman with lupus erythematosus can have the diagnosis.

Defining Characteristics

Major (must be present)

Expressed or observed desire to seek information for health promotion

Minor (may be present)

Expressed or observed desire for increased control of health practice
Expression of concern about current environmental conditions on health status
Stated or observed unfamiliarity with wellness community resources
Demonstrated or observed lack of knowledge in health-promotion behaviors

Etiological, Contributing, Risk Factors

Situational (personal, environmental)

Role changes
    Marriage   "Empty-nest" syndrome
    Parenthood   Retirement
Lack of knowledge of need for:
    Preventive behavior (disease)   Regular exercise program
    Screening practices for age and risk   Constructive stress management
    Optimal nutrition and weight con-   Supportive social networks
       trol   Responsible role participation

Maturational

See Table II-9 for age-related situations.

* Stable health status is defined as age-appropriate illness prevention measures achieved, client reports good or excellent health, and signs and symptoms of disease, if present, are controlled.

Focus Assessment Criteria

Subjective
Does the individual/family practice primary prevention? (Refer to Table II-9 for age-related prevention behaviors.)

Does the individual/family report a recent change in role responsibilities because of:

Marriage	Parenthood
Death	"Empty-nest" syndrome
Divorce	Retirement

Principles and Rationale for Nursing Care

General
1. Montag and Swenson wrote that healthy individuals are able to
   - Perform their chosen work without excessive stressor strain
   - Exert themselves physically without exhaustion
   - Feel refreshed after rest and relaxation
   - Set and attain realistic goals
   - Enjoy the company of other people
   - Enjoy periods of solitude
2. Many members of the population view health as absence of disease. Rather, health can be viewed as a return (or recovery) to a previous state or to a heightened awareness of the individual's full potential and life meaning. (Flynn)
3. The control of major health problems in the U.S. depends directly on modification of individual behavior and habits of living. (Flynn)
4. Forty percent of the population is more than 20 pounds overweight. (Knowles)
5. Seventy percent to eighty percent of accidents at home are related to parental drinking. (Flynn)
6. Belloc and Breslow correlated well-being and increased life span to the following seven practices:
   - Sleeping 7–8 hours nightly
   - Eating three meals at regular times
   - Eating breakfast daily
   - Maintaining desirable body weight
   - Avoiding excessive alcohol consumption
   - Participating in regular exercise
   - Abstaining from smoking
7. In addition to addressing life-styles to promote wellness, total health depends on (Flynn)
   - Eradication of poverty and ignorance
   - Availability of jobs
   - Adequate housing, transportation, and recreation
   - Public safety
   - Aesthetically pleasing and beneficial environment

Screening
1. Screening is the administration of a specific procedure to an asymptomatic person for the purpose of early detection of disease.
2. Assumptions concerning screening are that
   The procedure is acceptable to the at-risk population, is relatively simple and not

time-consuming, and is available at a reasonable cost

The disease would not ordinarily be suspected because of lack of symptoms

Detection of the disease during this period will improve morbidity/mortality from that condition

The disease is significantly prevalent

Adequate treatment for the disease is available

Treatment for the disease will improve the quality of life, and this outcome outweighs any adverse effects of the screening procedure

3. The tasks of screening are to

Identify major disabling conditions

Investigate the personal and social benefits of early detection and intervention for asymptomatic persons with the condition (*e.g.,* facilitate family coping, minimize disability and cost, prevent premature death, improve productivity of affected persons, decrease overall morbidity and mortality)

Identify persons at high risk for specific conditions through *personal medical history* (*e.g.,* concurrent disease such as diabetes mellitus involves greater risk for hypertension), *family medical history* (*e.g.,* breast cancer, diabetes, hypertension), and *social history* (*e.g.,* substance abuse–cancer, heart disease; sexual patterns—veneral disease; domestic violence—person abuse)

Identify tests and procedures that accurately detect the condition (who will do them? how often are they done? who bears the cost?)

Plan a strategy for disseminating screening information to health care professionals and the public

Plan evaluation of screening effectiveness

4. Screening must be individualized based upon personal health risk profile, developmental level and age, and the right to self-determination and protection of dignity.

5. Screening is directed toward two populations: those identified as at high risk and the general population.

6. Types of screening measures include

Physical findings (periodic exams by health care professionals and self-exams of breast, testicles, and skin)

Survey of risk factors (smoking, alcohol abuse)

Laboratory tests (serum–*e.g.,* sickle-cell in blacks, PKU in newborns; urine—*e.g.,* renal disease in the elderly; x-ray—*e.g.,* dental caries, chest TB)

7. Nurses are in an especially effective position to screen because they

Permeate every segment of society

Are knowledgeable about health and physical examination

Believe in a holistic philosophy of care

Consider client teaching a vital aspect of the nursing role

Interface with multiple health professions

Prevention

1. The goals of prevention are
   - Avoidance of disease by choosing a healthy life-style
   - Decrease in mortality due to disease by early detection and intervention
   - Improvement of quality of life
2. The three levels of prevention are primary, secondary, and tertiary.
3. The primary level of prevention involves actions that prevent disease and accidents and promote well-being. Key concepts are as follows:

Concept	*Examples*
Wellness A life-style that incorporates the principles of health promotion and is directed by self-responsibility	Diet low in salt, sugar, and fat Regular exercise and stress management Elimination of smoking Minimal alcohol intake
Self-help Mutual sharing with others who have similar needs	La Leche League Childbirth Education Assertiveness training Specific written resources (books, pamphlets, magazines) Public media (radio, television)
Safety	Adherence to speed limits Use of seat belts and car seats Proper storage of household poisons
Immunizations	Children: DPT Nonpregnant women of childbearing age: Rubella vaccine if antibody titer is negative Elderly: influenza, pneumonia

4. The secondary level of prevention concerns actions that promote early detection of disease and subsequent intervention (see screening principles), both routine physical examination by a health professional at regular intervals and self-examination. Self-examination is a twofold process
   (1) A general awareness of changes of body parts, functions, and sensations, and the possible implications of these changes.

   Cancer warning signs

   Change in bowel or bladder habits
   Sore that does not heal
   Unusual bleeding or discharge
   Thickening or lump in breast or elsewhere
   Indigestion or difficulty in swallowing
   Obvious change in wart or mole
   Nagging cough or hoarseness

   Arthritis warning signs

   Stiffness on arising
   Persistent pain
   Pain or tenderness in one or more joints
   Swelling in one or more joints
   Recurrence of these symptoms, especially when they involve one or more joints

   Heart attack signals

   Chest pain, usually behind sternum
   Pain in jaw, neck, or arm
   Pressure or tight sensation in chest, possibly associated with sweating, nausea, shortness of breath, and feeling weak
   (2) Specific and purposeful examination of one's own body parts for abnormality (*e.g.*, breast, testicles, skin)
5. The tertiary level of screening involves actions that restore and rehabilitate in the presence of illness. For example, for a person with coronary artery disease, these would be

Restorative (surgery, such as coronary artery bypass, angioplasty and medications)

Rehabilitative (stress management, exercise program, stop smoking, "zipper club" [self-help group])

6. Potential barriers to prevention are found both in the health care system and in the individual. The system may be

Disease-oriented rather than health-oriented

Composed of health care professionals who are taught to focus on fragment systems of the human body rather than take a holistic approach

Functioning on a financial system that rewards treatment of illness, not prevention

Difficult to reach or may have previously proved unsatisfactory

The client may:

Believe that the health/illness state is determined by forces (fate, luck) outside himself (external locus of control)

Perceive the behavior needed as unacceptable or uncomfortable

Practice sociocultural behaviors that are not healthful (*e.g.,* obesity is considered desirable, salt is prevalent in diet)

Experience psychological disturbances that impede incentive to practice healthy behaviors

Lack financial resources

Teaching/Learning Process

1. Patient/health education is the teaching-learning process of influencing client and family behavior through changes in knowledge, attitudes, and beliefs and through the acquisition of psychomotor skills. The goal of patient teaching is to help the client assume responsibility for self-care.

   The teaching-learning process consists of "steps," which are actually the components of the nursing process: assessment, planning, implementing, and evaluating. Patient education is a constellation of interventions, including self-modification (Pender), patient contracting (Jensen), values clarification (Wilberding), and preparatory sensory information (Christman and Kirchoff). It may be appropriate to use one of these interventions in the assessment phase (*i.e.,* values clarification) in order to determine the optimal combination of educational interventions for a particular client.

2. Each person should be assessed for the knowledge and skill needed to monitor health status (*e.g.,* home blood glucose monitoring in diabetes), control or cure disease, or prevent disease (*e.g.,* diet, medication therapy, life-style changes), and prevent recurrence or complications (*e.g.,* postoperative leg exercises).

3. Inaccurate perceptions of health status usually involve misunderstanding of the nature and seriousness of the illness, susceptibility to complications, and the need for procedures for cure or control of illness.

4. Psychological manifestations of anxiety and denial may have resulted from misconceptions, not knowing what to do, or not knowing how to carry out prescribed behaviors.

5. Teaching should be routinely incorporated as an integral part of nursing care whenever a new diagnosis or change in regimen is made or when the client faces an unfamiliar situation.

A. Assessment of Learning Needs, Readiness to Learn, and Factors That Will Influence Learning

1. An assessment prior to teaching will facilitate the meaningfulness, efficacy, and overall success of the teaching-learning process by defining *what* content should be present, *how* the content should be given, *when* the client is ready to learn, and *who* should be included in the process.
2. Each person learns in his own unique way.
3. Learning is dependent on physical and emotional readiness. The client needs to be relatively free of pain and extreme anxiety to learn.
4. High anxiety decreases learning, while slight anxiety may increase learning.
5. Client motivation is one of the most important variables affecting the amount of learning that takes place.

B. Planning for the Attainment of Realistic Goals by Client and Family

1. Planning goals and teaching strategies must be started only after a thorough assessment.
2. Planning should include the involvement of the client and family in goal-setting.
3. Goals must be written in the format of behavioral objectives, which are specific and observable behaviors to be accomplished by client and family at the completion of the learning experience.
4. Planning should also include a determination of teaching strategies to be employed to enable the client and family to achieve the goals set.
5. The best combination of educational methods, content, and learning materials for some clients is not necessarily the best combination for others.

C. Implementing the Teaching Plan

1. Teaching is planned, structured, and sequenced communication to produce learning.
2. Teaching can be formal with the use of audiovisual aids, or it can be informal, occurring in conjunction with other forms of nursing care.
3. Active participation on the part of the client and family enhances learning and retention and is essential if learning is to occur.
4. Learning is increased when roles are clearly defined (*i.e.,* who is the learner and who is the teacher)
5. Learning requires energy. More information is learned with the least amount of energy when the nurse presents the information at a level consistent with the client's ability, when there is an association between the content presented and something the client already knows or has experienced, and when information is given in response to an expressed need of the client and family.
6. Use of audiovisual aids enhances learning.
7. Retention of information is increased when the teaching-learning process involves a variety of senses.
8. Repetition stengthens learning. Retention is increased when facts or skills are repeated. Overlearning increases retention.
9. Retention is better when the information learned is put into immediate use than when its application is delayed.
10. No single educational input, by itself, should expect to have a lasting effect on behavior, unless it is reinforced by other educational efforts.
11. Teaching is most effective in changing behavior if it is in response to a newly diagnosed illness or new treatment for the client.

12. Learning is made easier when the learner is aware of his progress.
13. Reward is a stronger inducement to learning than punishment.
14. Learning is enhanced in an environment free of distractions and other obstacles.
15. Learning is increased when the nurse communicates the necessity of learning and her own enjoyment and expertise as a facilitator in the teaching-learning process.

D. Evaluating the Teaching-learning Process

1. Evaluation involves determining whether or not the planned goals are able to be achieved by client and family.
2. Evaluation methods include observing client and family behaviors, skill performance, etc., and asking questions related to the behavioral objectives that were mutually planned with client and family.
3. If learning cannot be demonstrated, further assessments and revisions in the teaching plan are necessary.

E. Factors Affecting Learning/Factors Affecting the Learner

Physical factors that affect learning include
    Presence of acute illness
    Fluid and electrolyte imbalance
    Nutritional status
    Illness or treatments that interfere with mental alertness (pain, medications)
    Illness or treatments that interfere with motor abilities (fatigue, equipment)
    Activity tolerance (endurance)
Personal factors that affect learning include
    Age
    Intelligence
    Level of motivation
    Level of anxiety
    Denial of disease process
    Depression
    Stage of adaptation to illness
    Past experiences or knowledge
    Locus of control
    Perception of
        Seriousness of condition
        Susceptibility to complications
        Prognosis
        Ability to control progression or to cure condition
Socioeconomic factors that affect learning include
    Language
    Life-style
    Support system
    Financial status
    Past experiences with health care
    Cultural background
    Transportation
        Health care facility
        Drugstore

F. Factors Resulting in Ineffective Teaching

Inadequate or no assessment prior to teaching
Assessment data were not communicated or not considered when teaching (the most

influential assessment factors are psychological status, physical stability, educational level, cultural background, socioeconomic status)

Teaching was not individualized

Information not presented at a level consistent with the client's ability

Tendency to talk down to client

Use of misunderstood terms

Fragmented presentation of information

Too much information given, with important information hidden or lost among irrelevant information

No repetition of information

No feedback given in relation to process (or client is punished for not learning)

No evaluation of client learning made

G. Factors Reflecting Ineffective Interaction

Client and family not involved with planning learning goals—which may be unrealistic

Cultural differences between nurse and client may create stereotyping, thus interfering with teaching

Discouragement of questions, hindering learner involvement

No opportunity to practic psychomotor skills or put learned information into practice

Distractions in environment

Smoking

1. Smoking has immediate and long-term effects on the respiratory system.
2. Immediate effects are paralysis of the ciliary cleansing mechanism of the lungs (which should keep breathing passages free of inhaled irritants and bacteria); irritation of the lining of the lungs, causing an inflammatory response; increased production of mucus; and decreased oxygenation.
3. Long-term effects are *permanent* disabling of the ciliary cleansing mechanism; reduction of the number of macrophages in the airways; a *permanent* decrease in the lung's ability to fight infection; increased production of mucus cells; a significant increase in the risk of developing pulmonary disease (a history of 15 to 20 "pack years" indicates a high risk); possible enlargement of the distal air passages; and chronic CO_2 retention, which results in hypoxia's becoming the drive to breathe, rather than hypercarbia (increased CO_2).
4. Smoking has immediate and long-term effects on the cardiovascular system.
5. Immediate effects are vasoconstriction and decreased oxygenation of the blood, elevated blood pressure, increased heart rate and possible dysrhythmias, and an increase in the work of the heart.
6. Long-term effects include an increased risk for coronary artery disease and myocardial infarction. Smoking also contributes to hypertension, to peripheral vascular disease (*e.g.*, leg ulcers), and to chronically abnormal arterial blood gases (low oxygen, or pO_2, and high carbon dioxide, or pCO_2).

Nutrition

See Principles and Rationale for Nursing Care for *Altered Nutrition*

Exercise

1. A regular exercise program should
   Be enjoyable
   Utilize a minimum of 400 calories in each session
   Sustain a heart rate of approximately 120 to 150 beats per minute

Involve rhythmical alternate contracting and relaxing of muscles

Be integrated into the person's life-style 4 to 5 days per week (at least 30 to 60 minutes)

2. Regular exercise can provide the person with increased

Cardiovascular-respiratory endurance

Muscle strength

Muscle endurance

Flexibility

Ability to deliver nutrients to tissue

Ability to tolerate psychological stress

Ability to reduce body fat content

3. An exercise program should include

A warm-up session (10 minutes of stretching exercises)

Endurance exercises

A cool-down session (5 to 10 minutes)

4. Before beginning an exercise program, the person must consider

Physical limitations (consult nurse or physician)

Personal preferences

Life-style

Community resources

What clothing is needed (shoes)

How to monitor pulse before, during, and after exercise

5. The person is taught to monitor his pulse before, during, and after exercise to assist him to achieve his target heart rate and not to exceed his maximum advisable heart rate for his age (Kuntzelman).

Age	Maximum Heart Rate	Target Heart Rate
30	190	133–162
40	180	126–153
50	170	119–145
60	160	112–136

Osteoporosis

1. "Twenty-five percent of all white women over age 60 suffer from some sign or symptom of osteoporosis, *e.g.,* fracture of hip, wrist or spine, back pain following spinal fracture or height loss." (Chestnut)

2. Factors that contribute to a woman's risk of osteoporosis are loss of female hormones after menopause, low calcium intake, insufficient exercise, small stature, fair skin, family history, cigarette smoking, excessive alcohol consumption, excessive caffeine intake, and excessive protein consumption. (Chestnut)

High-Risk Elderly

1. The elderly represent 11% of the population but consume 30% of the money spent on health care and 50% of the federal health budget. (Ouslander)

2. Albert proposes that one way to reduce cost is to schedule cost-effective health screening techniques rather than annual comprehensive health exams.

3. Conservative, nonpharmacological treatments should be tried first with the elderly. If medications are ordered, low doses should be used and titrated up if needed. (Albert)

4. The elderly tolerate caffeine poorly. It contributes to insomnia, anxiety, tremors, cardiac dysrhythmias, calcium wasting, and urinary incontinence. (Albert)

Health-Seeking Behaviors
Related to (Specify)

Assessment
Refer to Defining Characteristics

Outcome Criteria

The person will
- Describe screening that is appropriate for age and risk factors
- Perform self-screening for cancer
- Participate in a regular physical exercise program
- State an intent to use positive coping mechanisms and constructive stress management
- Agree with self-responsibility for wellness (physical, dental, safety, nutritional, family)

Interventions

A. Assess for factors that contribute to the promotion and the maintenance of health

Knowledge of disease and preventive behavior
Appropriate screening practices for age and risk
Good nutrition and weight control
Regular exercise program
Constructive stress management
Supportive social networks

B. Promote health behaviors in the person and the family
1. Determine the person's or family's knowledge or perception of
   a. Specific diseases (*e.g.,* heart disease, cancer, respiratory disease, childhood diseases, infections, dental disease)
   b. Susceptibility (*e.g.,* presence of risk factors, family history)
   c. Seriousness
   d. Value of early detection
2. Determine the person's or family's past patterns of health care
   a. Expectations
   b. Interactions with health care system or providers
   c. Influences of family, cultural group, peer group, mass media
3. Provide specific information concerning screening for age-related conditions (refer to Table II-9)
4. Discuss the role of nutrition in health maintenance and the prevention of illness (see Principles and Rationale for Nursing Care for *Altered Nutrition* for specific explanations)
   a. Basic four food groups
   b. Nutrient needs related to age, level of physical activity, pregnancy, and lactation

   c. The prudent use of
        Salt (see *Fluid Volume Excess* for foods high in sodium)
        Canned vegetables
        Fried foods
        Red meats
        Fats (butter, margarines)
        High-calorie desserts
        Snack foods (potato chips, candy, soda)
        Refined sugar
        Foods containing nitrosamines (smoked meats, preservatives)
   d. The generous use of health-promoting foods
      (1) Cruciferous vegetables (broccoli, cabbage, cauliflower, Brussels sprouts)—protect against colorectal cancer
      (2) High-fiber foods—protect against colorectal cancer
      (3) Calcium-containing foods (dairy, dark leafy vegetables, etc.)—protect against osteoporosis
   e. See *Altered Health Maintenance* for specific information concerning weight control

5. Discuss the benefits of a regular exercise program
   • See Principles and Rationale for Nursing Care for the positive effects of a regular exercise program
   • Determine the optimal exercise for the individual, considering physical limitations, preferences, and life-style
        Walking briskly
        Jogging
        Running
        Aerobic exercises
        Aerobic dancing
        Swimming
        Bicycling
        Skipping rope
   • Stress the importance of beginning any physical activity slowly

6. Discuss the elements of constructive stress management
        Assertiveness training
        Problem-solving
        Relaxation techniques
        See Appendix X for relaxation techniques and Appendix VII for guidelines for problem-solving
        See Pertinent Literature for the Consumer on assertiveness and problem-solving self-help books

7. Discuss strategies for developing positive social networks
   a. Relate the functions of a support system
      • Provide love and affection
      • Share common social concerns
      • Serve as buffers for life's stressors
      • Prevent isolation
      • Respect mutual pursuits of members
      • Cooperate for the purpose
      • Provide dependable assistance (emotional and economic, if appropriate)
   b. Suggest methods for strengthening this system
      • Be supportive of others

- Practice active listening by allowing yourself to listen attentively to the other person, such as:
  - Don't interrupt the person
  - Allow a few seconds to lapse between dialogue to provide time to gather thoughts and to reduce the "rush to speak"
c. Provide others with opportunities to share their concerns without judgment. Refrain from giving solutions to problems of others; rather, a discussion of options may be indicated (*e.g.,* "You have several options: You can quit your job, request a transfer, discuss the problem with your boss or do nothing")
d. When confronted with a relationship problem, review the situation
     What is the problem?
     Who/what is responsible for the problem?
     What are the options?
     What are the advantages and disadvantages of each option?
     (See Appendix VII for guidelines for problem-solving)
e. Provide warmth and affection to significant others
  - Praise a child's accomplishments
  - Praise all attempts at accomplishments
  - Practice open shows of affection (*e.g.,* with children [boys and girls], with spouse, and with others)
f. Practice mutual goal-setting to direct common efforts and reevaluate them periodically
g. Offer sincere assistance to individuals to promote trust
h. Build relationships with individuals and families who share common interests and values
i. Recognize when additional assistance is needed
     Marital counseling
     Self-help groups
     Health professional
     Religious affiliation
j. Allow oneself and each member of the family—children, spouse, parents—to enhance personal identity by pursuing individual interests (refer to **Altered Growth and Development** for age-related needs of children)

C. Initiate health teaching and referrals as indicated

1. Review the daily health practices of the individual (adults, children)
     Dental care
     Food intake
     Fluid intake
     Exercise regime
     Leisure activities
     Responsibilities in the family
   Use of
     Tobacco
     Salt, sugar, fat products
     Alcohol
     Drugs (over-the-counter, prescribed)
   Knowledge of safety practices
     Fire prevention
     Water safety
     Automobile (maintenance, seat belts)

Bicycle

Poison control

2. Suggest selective disease-preventing behaviors when **appropriate**
   a. Skin cancers

      Avoid frequent sun exposure

      Avoid tanning salons

      Wear effective sunscreens and protective clothing
   b. Venereal diseases

      Use barrier contraceptive methods
   c. AIDS

      Use condoms

      Avoid high-risk sexual practices
   d. Hepatitis B

      Hepatitis vaccine, if high risk
   e. Hearing loss

      Use ear protection routinely (*e.g.,* mowing lawn, around machinery)

      Avoid loud music (headphones, etc.)

      Avoid prolonged exposure to loud noises
   f. Congential deformities

      Avoid the use of alcohol and drugs during pregnancy
   g. Oral cancers

      Avoid tobacco chewing

      Avoid concurrent heavy use of alcohol and tobacco
   h. Lung cancers, COPD

      Avoid tobacco smoking

      Avoid chronic exposure to known inhalable carcinogens (*e.g.,* asbestos)
   i. Coronary artery disease

      Avoid obesity

      Avoid cholesterol

      Avoid tobacco use

      Practice stress management

      Exercise regularly
   j. Stroke

      Avoid tobacco use, especially if taking oral contraceptives
   k. Reye syndrome

      Avoid aspirin products in children with viruses
   l. Osteoarthritis

      Avoid obesity

      Avoid repeated trauma to joints
   m. Osteoporosis for high-risk women (refer to Principles for high-risk characteristics
      • Vitamin D supplement
      • Calcium supplement
      • Regular exercise
      • Reduction of or abstinence from caffeine, alcohol

3. Refer to selected nursing diagnoses for additional information on and assessment of

   Safety needs: see *Potential for Injury*

   Activity needs: see *Diversional Activity Deficit*

   Affiliative needs: see *Social Isolation*

   Parenting needs: see *Altered Parenting*

   Family needs: see *Altered Family Processes*

   Spiritual needs: see *Spiritual Distress*

Sexual needs: see *Altered Sexuality Patterns*

Self-care needs: see *Impaired Home Maintenance Management; Knowledge Deficit*

Emotional needs: see *Ineffective Individual Coping; Anxiety; Fear; Grieving; Disturbance in Self-Concept;* and *Powerlessness*

References/Bibliography

Bruhn JG, Cordova FG, William JA, Fuentes RG Jr: The wellness process. J Community Health, 2(3):209–221, 1977

Dunn HL: High Level Wellness. Thorofare, NJ, Charles B Slack, 1977

Hall BA, Allan JD: Sharpening nursing's focus by focusing on health. Nurs Health Care, 7(6): 315–320, 1986

Laffrey SC, Loveland-Cherry CJ, Winkler SJ: Health behavior: Evolution of two paradigms. Public Health Nurs 3(2): 92–100, 1986

Pender NJ: Health Promotion in Nursing Practice. Norwalk, CT, Appleton-Century-Crofts, 1982

Travis JW: Wellness Workbook for Helping Professionals. Mill Valley, CA, Wellness Associates, 1981

See also References/Bibliography for *Altered Health Maintenance*

Home Maintenance Management, Impaired

Related to **(Specify)**

Definition

Impaired home maintenance management: The state in which an individual or family experiences or is at risk to experience a difficulty in maintaining self or family in a home environment.

> **Author's Note:** This diagnostic category can describe situations in which the individual and/or family needs specific instructions in order to manage home care of a family member and/or activities of daily living.

Defining Characteristics

Major (must be present)

> Outward expressions of difficulty by individual or family
> > In maintaining the home (cleaning, repairs, financial needs) or
> > In caring for self or family member at home

Minor (may be present)

> Poor hygienic practices
> > Infections
> > Infestations
> > Accumulated wastes
> > Unwashed cooking and eating
> > > equipment
> > Offensive odors
> Impaired caregiver
> > Overtaxed
> > Anxious
> > Lack of knowledge
> > Negative response to ill member
> Unavailable support system

Etiological, Contributing, Risk Factors

Pathophysiological

> Chronic debilitating disease
> > Diabetes mellitus
> > Chronic obstructive
> > > pulmonary disease
> > Congestive heart failure
> > Cerebral vascular acci-
> > > dent
> > Cancer
> > Arthritis
> > Multiple sclerosis
> > Muscular dystrophy
> > Parkinson's disease

Situational (personal, environmental)

> Injury to individual or family member (fractured limb, spinal cord injury)
> Surgery (amputation, ostomy)
> Impaired mental status (memory lapses, depression, anxiety—severe panic)
> Substance abuse (alcohol, drugs)
> Unavailable support system

Loss of family member
Addition of family member (newborn, aged parent)
Lack of knowledge
Insufficient finances

Maturational

Infant: Newborn care, high risk for sudden infant death syndrome
Elderly: Family member with deficits (cognitive, motor, sensory)

Focus Assessment Criteria

Owing to the variability and complexity of this diagnostic category, the nurse must determine whether the entire assessment must be performed or just selected areas. For example, if an elderly man lives alone, delete the assessment of the family. If a family is in crisis (financial or emotional), delete assessment of the functional status of the individual.

If a member is ill or disabled, the entire assessment may be indicated.

Subjective Data

Assessment of Individual Function
Vision
    Adequate
    Corrected (date of last prescription)
    Complaints of
        Blurriness   Difficulty in focusing
        Loss of side vision   Inability to adjust to darkness
Hearing
    Adequate
    Use of hearing aid (condition, batteries)
    Need to lip-read
Thermal/tactile
    Adequate
    Altered sense of cold/hot
Mental status
    Alert
    Drowsy
    Confused
    Oriented to time, place, events
    Complaints of
        Vertigo   Orthostatic hypotension
        Altered sense of balance
Mobility
    Ability to ambulate
        Around room   Around house
        Up and down stairs   Outside house
    Ability to travel
        Drive car (date of last   Use public transportation
            reevaluation)   Get in and out of vehicles
    Devices
        Cane   Prosthesis
        Wheelchair   Condition of devices
        Walker   Competence in their use

Shoes/slippers
    Proper fit   Nonskid soles
    Condition
Self-care activities: ability to
    Dress and undress   Use the toilet
    Groom self   Eat
    Bathe
Housekeeping activities: ability to
    Clean   Shop
    Launder clothes   Prepare food
Miscellaneous
    Drug therapy
        Type, dosage   Storage
        Labeling   Ability to self-medicate safely
    Communication: ability to
        Write   Contact emergency assistance
        Use phone
    Support system
        Help available from relatives, Club or religious contacts
            friends, neighbors   Emergency help available
    Community resources (*e.g.,* public health nurses, homemaker service, Meals on
        Wheels)
    Public transportation

Objective Data

Assessment of Individual Function
Physical appearance (groomed, unkempt)
Gait (steady, unsteady, use of aids)
Cognitive processes
    Ability to communicate needs
    Ability to interact
    History of wandering (witnessed, reported by others)
    Assess for presence of
        Anger   Withdrawal
        Depression   Faulty judgment
Treatment-related activities
    Presence of barriers to performance
        Lack of knowledge   Sensory deficits (visual, tactile)
        Lack of resources (support   Cognitive deficits
            system, equipment, financial) Emotional deficits
        Motor deficits (weakness,   Environmental (bathroom/water
            paralysis, amputation)   not accessible)

Assessment of Family Function. (The following focuses on the assessment of the ability of
the family to care for family member at home. For an assessment of the family unit, refer
to assessment criteria for *Altered Family Processes.*)
Knowledge and skills
    Assess the family or caretaker for ability to perform the following safely and correctly
        Treatments   Emergency treatment if
        Bathing   appropriate (*e.g.,* cardiac
        Medication administration   arrest, seizures)

Emotional response
  Assess the family or caretaker for the presence of
    Overprotecting the person
    Neglect of other family members
    Neglect of other responsibilities
    Resentment of responsibilities
    Inability to ask for or accept
      relief from responsibilities
    Unrealistic expectations of
      future recovery
  Assess the disabled or ill individual for the presence of
    Impossible demands upon time of
      caretaker
    Resentment when caretaker is
      away
    Lack of diversional activities
    Lack of vocational or educational
      pursuits
Resources
  Assess knowledge of family or caretaker of resources available for
    Emergency care
    Equipment
      Purchase
      Maintenance
      Repair
    Financial support
    Relief from caretaking
      responsibilities
        Close relative or neighbor
        Church group
        Community agency
    Medical follow-up care

Assessment of Home Environment of Children
Presence of/Report of:
  Provisions for play
    Appropriate play materials
    Safe play area (indoors, outdoors)
    Special place designated for child's possessions
  Stimulating environment
    Selected use of television (amount, type)
    Activities for age-related development (see *Altered Growth and Development*)
    Family time (meal, joint activities)
    Family outings
  Affectionate environment
    Touching, holding
    Speaks with pride about child
    Conversations convey positive feelings

Assessment of Housing
Type (rent, own)
    Apartment   Duplex   Single family house
Appearance: presence of
    Insects (flies, roaches)
    Rodents/vermin
    Offensive odors
    Unwashed cooking equipment
    Accumulation of dirt, food
      wastes, or hygiene wastes
Physical facilities
    Number of rooms for family
      members
    Toilet facilities (accessibility)
    Heating
    Ventilation
    Handrails (stairs)
    Lighting
    Water supply
    Sewage disposal
    Garbage disposal
    Screens
Safety
  Are there any adaptations that need to be made in the home for the individual?
    Better communication (telephone)

Access (in and out of home, to rooms)

Bathroom (*e.g.*, grab bar, bath bench, nonskid floors)

Refer to Focus Assessment Criteria for *Potential for Injury* for an assessment of hazards in the home.

Principles and Rationale for Nursing Care

1. Home care by professionals should be preventive, supportive, and therapeutic.

   Preventive measures include health education, home safety, and stress management.

   Supportive care can be legal, financial, nutritional, social, religious, and homemaking.

   Therapeutic care involves nursing care, therapists (occupational, speech), dental, and medical.

2. Discharge planning begins at admission, with the nurse determining the anticipated needs of the person and family after discharge: the individual's self-care ability, the availability of support, homemaker services, equipment needs, community nursing services, and therapy (physical, speech, occupational).

3. The home environment must be assessed for safety prior to discharge: location of bathroom, access to water, cooking facilities, and environmental barriers (stairs, narrow doorways).

4. Community agencies can provide the opportunity for home care and allow for the person to remain at home.

5. In determining an individual's ability to care for himself at home, assess his ability to function and protect self. Consider such things as: motor deficits, sensory deficits, and mental status.

6. To assess, teach, and evaluate the individual or the family's ability to perform learned skills after discharge, use on-unit situations, whereby the person(s) takes responsibility for care, and day, overnight, or weekend leave to home. A home visit may be indicated by a nurse or a community health nurse.

7. Some families are unable to meet the home needs of ill members and require assistance. Families who are able to meet the needs of ill members should also be provided with periodic assistance or relief.

8. The effects on the life of a caretaker of a chronically ill person depend on (Goldstein):

   The ill person's level of disability and dependence

   The health and functional mobility of the caretaker

   The availability of assistance (type and frequency)

   The other responsibilities the caretaker has

9. The time and energy demands of caretaking may compete with other role responsibilities (*e.g.*, spouse, mothering, occupational).

10. Role fatigue describes the situation where the caregiver must devote the majority of time to caregiving, thus requiring that all other roles and responsibilities be subordinated to the demands of caretaking.

11. Persons and families with cancer have certain ongoing needs that may necessitate interventions at home:

    Teaching needs (disease, treatment, diagnostic studies)

    Surgery (recovery, wound care)

    Coping with the diagnosis

    Fear of the future

    Treatment effects and side-effects (radiotherapy, chemotherapy)

    Inability to perform role responsibilities

    Biologic needs (disease- or treatment-related; *e.g.*, nutrition, elimination, comfort)

12. Stetz reported that spouse caregivers of individuals with cancer described the following caregiving demands (in priority):
    - Physical care treatment regimen, coping with the changes
    - Household responsibilities, finances
    - Witnessing the experience
    - Fatigue, illness, change in pattern of living (*e.g.,* social life)
    - Constant vigilance
    - Unsatisfactory information exchange with health care provider or institution
    - The meaning of cancer
    - Unknown future
    - Changes in relationship with ill spouse
13. Male caregivers experienced greater difficulty in managing the household, while female caregivers experienced greater difficulty with observing their ill mate's suffering. (Stetz)

Impaired Home Maintenance Management
Related to (Specify)

Statement Examples: **Inability to Perform Household Activities Post-Myocardial Infarction**
Inability to Perform Home Activities Secondary to Impaired Vision

Assessment
Refer to Defining Characteristics

Outcome Criteria

The person or caretaker will
- Identify factors that restrict self-care and home management
- Demonstrate the ability to perform skills necessary for the care of the individual or home
- Express satisfaction with home situation

Interventions
The following interventions apply to many individuals with impaired home management, regardless of etiology.

A. Assess for causative or contributing factors
Lack of knowledge
Insufficient funds
Lack of necessary equipment or aids
Inability to perform household activities (illness, sensory deficits, motor deficits)

Impaired cognitive functioning
Impaired emotional functioning

B. Reduce or eliminate causative or contributing factors if possible

1. Lack of knowledge for home care
   - Determine with the person and family the information needed to be taught and learned
   - Initiate the teaching
   - Refer to a community nursing agency for follow-up
   - Refer to *Health-Seeking Behaviors* for additional interventions on teaching
2. Lack of necessary equipment or aids
   - Determine the type of equipment needed, considering availability, cost, and durability
   - Seek assistance from agencies that rent or loan supplies
     a. Teach the care and maintenance of supplies that increase length of use
     b. Consider adapting equipment to reduce cost
3. Insufficient funds
   - Consult with social service department for assistance
   - Consult with service organizations for assistance
     - American Heart Association
     - The Lung Association
     - American Cancer Society
4. Inability to perform household activities
   Determine the type of assistance needed (*e.g.*, meals, housework, transportation) and assist the individual to obtain them.
   a. Meals
      - Discuss with relatives the possibility of freezing complete meals that require only heating (*e.g.*, small containers of soup, stew, casseroles)
      - Determine the availability of meal services for ill persons (Meals on Wheels, church groups)
      - Teach persons about foods that are easily prepared and nutritious (*e.g.*, hard-boiled eggs)
   b. Housework
      - Contract with an adolescent for light housekeeping
      - Refer to community agency for assistance
   c. Transportation
      - Determine the availability of transportation for shopping and health care
      - Request rides with neighbors to places they drive routinely
5. Impaired mental processes
   - Assess the ability of the individual to safely maintain a household
   - Refer to *Potential for Injury* related to lack of awareness of hazards
6. Impaired emotional functioning
   - Assess the severity of the dysfunction
   - Refer to *Ineffective Individual Coping* for additional assessment and interventions.

C. Initiate health teaching and referrals as indicated

1. Discuss the implications of caring for a chronically ill family member
   Amount of time
   Effects on other role responsibilities (spouse, children, job)
   Physical requirements (lifting)

2. Share alternatives to reduce strain and fatigue of caretaking responsibilities
   - Acquire relief from responsibilities at least twice a week for at least 3 hours (sitter, neighbors, relatives)
   - Enlist the aid of others to meet some of the needs of the ill person (hairdresser, transporting to physician's office)
   - Plan to utilize at least one hour a day as leisure time (*e.g.,* after ill person is asleep)
   - Maintain contacts with friends and relatives even if only by phone; let friends know that you do use sitters so they can include you in some social activities
   - Allow the caretaker opportunities to share problems and feelings
3. Commend caregivers for their concern, diligence, and perseverance in caring for the loved one at home

References/Bibliography

Archbold P: Impact of parent caring on middle-aged offspring. Gerontol Nurs 6:60, 1980

Craven R: The effects of illness on family function. Nurs Forum 2:191–193, 1972

Coyle N: A cancer centers outreach . . . maintain these patients at home, Sloan-Kettering. Am J Nurs 85(5):590, 594, 1985

Davis AJ: Disability, home care, and the caretaking role in family life. J Adv Nurs 5:475–484, 1980

Edstrom S, Miller MW: Preparing the family to care for the cancer patient at home: A home care course. Cancer Nursing 4:49–52, 1981

Eggert GM, Granger CV, Morris R et al: Caring for the patient with long-term disability. Geriatrics 32(6):102–106, 1977

Ellmyer P, Thomas N: A guide to your patient's safe home use of oxygen. Nursing 12(1):55–57, 1982

Fitting M, Rabins P, Lucas MJ, Eastham J: Caregivers for dementia patients: A comparison of husbands and wives. Gerontologist 26:248–252, 1986

Ford M, Wasilewicz C: Bridging the gap between hospital and home. Canadian Nurse 77(1):44–47, 1981

Fortinsky R, Granger CV, Seltzer GB: The use of functional assessment in understanding home care needs. Med Care 19:489–497, 1981

Goldstein V: Caretaker Role Fatigue. Nurs Outlook 29:23–30, 1981

Googe M, Varricchio C: A pilot investigation of home health care needs of cancer patients and their families. Oncology Nursing Forum 8(3):24–28, 1981

Harvey BL: Your patient's discharge plan: Does it include home care referral? Nursing 11(7):48–51, 1981

Heller BR, Walsh FJ, Wilson KM: Seniors helping seniors: Training older adults as new personnel resources in home health care. J Gerontol Nurs 7:552–555, 1981

Hunter G, Johnson SH: Physical support systems for the homebound oncology patient. Oncology Nursing Forum 7(3):21–23, 1980

Jelneck LJ: The special needs of the adolescent with chronic illness. Matern Child Nurs J 2:57–61, 1977

Klopovich P, Suenram D, Cairns N: A common sense approach to caring for children with cancer: The community health care nurse. Cancer Nursing 3:201–208, 1980

MacVicar M, Archoid PA: A framework for family assessment in chronic illness. Nurs Forum 15:180–194, 1976

Mailick M: The impact of severe illness of the individual and family: An overview. Soc Work Health Care 5:117–128, 1979

McCorkle R et al: What nurses need to know about home care. Oncol Nurs Forum 11(6):63–69, 1984

Pappas JP: Strategic planning for home health care. Caring 4(10):24–25, 27–29, 1983

Pigg J: Fifty helpful hints for active arthritis patients. Nursing 4(4):39–41, 1974

Rathlev M, McNamara M: Teaching families to give trach care at home. Nursing 12(6):70–71, 1982

Schmidt MD: Meet the health care needs of older adults by using a chronic care model in the home setting. J Gerontol Nurs 11(9), 1983

Stetz KM: Caregiving demands during advanced cancer—The spouse's needs. Cancer Nurs 10(5):260–268, 1987

Symposium on community health/home care. Nurs Clin North Am 15:321–428, 1980

White HA, Briggs AM: Home care of persons with respiratory problems. Topics in Clinical Nursing 2(4):69–77, 1980

Hopelessness

Related to **(Specify)**

Definition

Hopelessness: A sustained subjective emotional state in which an individual sees no alternatives or personal choices available to solve problems or to achieve what is desired and cannot mobilize energy on own behalf to establish goals.

> **Author's Note:** Hopelessness differs from powerlessness in that a hopeless person sees no solution to his problem and/or way to achieve what is desired, even if he has control of his life. A powerless person may see an alternative or answer to the problem, yet be unable to do anything about it because of lack of control and resources.

Defining Characteristics

Major (must be present)

Expresses profound, overwhelming, sustained apathy in response to a situation perceived as impossible with no solutions (overt or covert).

Examples of expressions are:
- "I might as well give up because I can't make things better"
- "My future seems awful to me"
- "I can't imagine what my life will be like in 10 years"
- "I've never been given a break, so why should I in the future"
- "Life looks unpleasant when I think ahead"
- "I know I'll never get what I really want"
- "Things never work out how I want them to"
- "It's foolish to want or get anything because I never do"
- "It's unlikely I'll get satisfaction in the future"
- "The future seems vague and uncertain"

Physiological
- Slowed responses to stimuli

Emotional

The hopeless person often has difficulty experiencing feelings, but may feel:
- Unable to seek good fortune, luck, or God's favor
- He has no meaning or purpose in life
- "Empty or drained"
- A sense of loss and deprivation

Person exhibits
- Passiveness
- Decreased verbalization
- Lack of ambition, initiative, and interest

Cognitive
- Decreased problem-solving and decision-making capabilities

- Deals with past and future, not here and now
- Decreased flexibility in thought processes
- Lacks imagination and wishing capabilities
- Unable to identify and/or accomplish desired objectives and goals
- Unable to plan, organize, or make decisions
- Unable to recognize sources of hope

Minor (may be present)

Physiological
- Anorexia
- Weight loss
- Decreased exercise
- Increased sleep

Emotional

Person feels:
- Incompetent
- "A lump in his throat"
- Discouraged with self and others
- "At the end of his rope"
- Tense
- Helpless
- Overwhelmed (feels he just "can't . . . ")
- Loss of gratification from roles and relationships
- Vulnerable

Person exhibits
- Poor eye contact; turns away from speaker; shrugs in response to speaker
- Apathy (decreased response to internal and external stimuli)
- Decreased affect
- Decreased motivation
- Despondency
- Sighing
- Social withdrawal
- Lack of involvement in self-care (may be cooperative in nursing care but offers little help to self)
- Passively allows care
- Regression
- Resignation
- Depression
- Anger
- Destructiveness

Cognitive
- Conveys negative and/or slowed thought processes
- Decreased ability to integrate information received
- Loss of time perception for past, present, and future
- Decreased ability to recall from the past
- Confusion
- Decreased ability to communicate effectively
- Distorted thought perceptions and associations
- Unreasonable judgment
- Suicidal thoughts
- Has unrealistic perceptions in relation to hope

Etiological, Contributing, Risk Factors

Pathophysiological:

Any chronic and/or terminal illness can cause or contribute to hopelessness (*e.g.,* heart disease, kidney disease, cancer, AIDS).

Associated factors include:
- Failing or deteriorating physiologic condition
- Impaired body image
- New and unexpected signs or symptoms of previous disease process
- Prolonged pain, discomfort, weakness
- Impaired functional abilities (walking, elimination, eating)

Treatment-related

Prolonged treatments (*e.g.,* chemotherapy, radiation) that cause discomfort
Prolonged treatments with no positive results
Treatments that alter body image (*e.g.,* surgery, chemotherapy)
Prolonged diagnostic studies that yield no significant results
Prolonged dependence on equipment for life support (*e.g.,* dialysis, respirator)
Prolonged dependence on equipment for monitoring bodily functions (*e.g.,* telemetry)

Situational

Prolonged activity restriction (*e.g.,* fractures, spinal cord injury)
Prolonged isolation due to disease processes (*e.g.,* infectious diseases, reverse isolation for suppressed immune system)
Separation from significant others (parents, spouse, children, others)
Inability to achieve goals in life that one values (marriage, education, children)
Inability to participate in activities one desires (walking, sports)
Loss of something or someone valued (spouse, children, friend, financial resources)
Prolonged caretaking responsibilities (spouse, child, parent)
Exposure to long-term physiological or psychological stress
Loss of belief in transcendent values/God

Maturational

Child

Loss of caregiver
Loss of trust in significant other (parents, sibling)
Abandonment by caregivers
Loss of autonomy related to illness (*e.g.,* fracture)
Loss of bodily functions
Inability to achieve developmental tasks (trust, autonomy, initiative, industry)

Adolescent

Loss of significant other (peer, family)
Loss of bodily functions
Change in body image
Inability to achieve developmental task (role identity)

Adult

Impaired bodily functions, loss of body part
Impaired relationships (separation, divorce)
Loss of job, career

Loss of significant others (death of children, spouse)
Inability to achieve developmental tasks (intimacy, commitment, productiveness)
Elderly
  Sensory deficits
  Motor deficits
  Loss of independence
  Loss of significant others, things
  Inability to achieve developmental tasks (integrity)

Focus Assessment Criteria

Hopelessness is a subjective emotional state in which the nurse must validate with the individual. Emotional and cognitive areas must be assessed carefully by the nurse to make the inference that the person is experiencing hopelessness. Some of these same cues may be seen in persons with diagnoses of *Social Isolation, Powerlessness, Self-Concept Disturbance,* and/or *Spiritual Distress.*

Subjective Data

1. Presence of illness and/or treatment
     Chronic, prolonged, deteriorating, exhausting
2. Activities of daily living
   - Exercise: amount, type
   - Sleep: time, amount, quality
   - Hobbies: self-interest activities
   - Self-care participation
   - Appetite: eating habits
3. Energy and motivation
   - Does the person feel exhausted, tired?
   - Does the person have any goals or desires?
   - What are these goals and desires? Are they realistic?
   - Does this person feel he can achieve them?
   - Does this person feel overwhelmed?
   - What does he feel he can achieve?
   - Does he express an interest in self-care?
   - Does he express an interest in social activities?
   - Does he express an interest in any activities?
4. Meaning and purpose in life
   - What does this person value most in life? Why?
   - Is he able to achieve this value?
   - What does this person describe as his purpose and/or role in life?
   - Is this purpose/role fulfilled?
   - What in life has the most meaning to this person?
   - Is this available to this person at this time?
   - Are his perceptions of his meaning and purpose realistic and/or achievable?
   - What kind of relationship does he have with God?
   - Does this relationship give meaning or purpose to his life?
5. Choice and/or control in situations
   - What does he perceive as his most difficult problem? Why?
   - What does he feel the solution to the problem is? Is this solution realistic?

- What kind of problem-solving and/or decision-making skills does this person have? Planning skills? Organizing skills?
- Is his perception of the problem distorted? If so, how?
- Have other alternatives to his problem been considered and/or tried?
- Does this person feel he has any controlling influence in the situation?
- How flexible or rigid are this person's thought processes?

6. Future options
   - What does the person believe the future will bring? Negative or positive things?
   - Does this person look forward to the future? What does he say about his past?
   - What does he see as worth living for?
   - How does the future look to this person?
   - How does this person perceive his present illness? Its effect on his life? Its effect on his relationships?
   - How does this person perceive his current treatments for his illness? Promising, or stressful and useless?
   - Does this person recognize any sources of hope?
   - Does this person have any wishes or dreams?
   - What does he want most in life?
   - Does this person have suicidal thoughts? If so, explore why.

7. Significant relationships
   - Who does this person perceive as the most significant other in his life?
   - What is this person's current relationship with this significant other person?
   - What are this person's feelings toward this significant other now?
   - Is this relationship currently pleasing and/or helpful to this person?
   - Does this person have contact with this significant other now?
   - Has divorce or death of spouse, or death of child, sibling, friend, pet, occurred recently?
   - Has this person moved away from significant others recently?

Objective Data

General appearance
- Grooming
- Posture
- Eye contact
- Speed of activities

Principles and Rationale for Nursing Care

Hope

1. Hope is an unconscious cognitive behavior that energizes and allows one to act, achieve, and utilize crisis as an opportunity for growth. It activates the motivational system.
2. Hope is closely related to confidence, wishing, faith, inspiration, determination, choice, and autonomy.
3. Although wishing and hoping are related, a person may or may not be committed to his wishes, but he is committed to his hoped-for events. Therefore, giving up hope is more harmful than giving up a wish. Hope is more rational and logical than wishing.
4. A hoping person has realistic desires that he feels will in some way improve his life when they occur.

5. Hope is future and reality oriented. A hopeful person wants a desired change in his current life. He feels that change is possible and that there is a way out of his difficulties.
6. Early childhood experiences influence a person's ability to hope. A person learns to hope if a trusting environment is promoted.
7. Hope is related to faith because many people experience hope by recognizing their reliance on higher powers to restore meaning and purpose in their lives.
8. Hope is related to help from others, in that a person feels his external resources may be supportive to him when his internal resources and strengths seem insufficient to cope with a situation (*e.g.*, a family and/or significant other is often a source of hope).
9. Watson (1979) has identified hope as both a curative and a "carative" factor in nursing. Hope, along with faith and trust, provides psychic energy to draw upon to aid in the curative process.
10. It has been observed that hope prolongs life in critical survival conditions, while a loss of hope often results in death (Korner, 1970).
11. A hoping person feels autonomous in making decisions about choices open to him.
12. Hope can be shared, but this involves close human relationships, trust, and understanding.
13. Kübler-Ross observed that those who expressed hope coped more effectively during their difficult dying periods. She also noted that death occurred soon after these individuals stopped expressing hope.
14. Hope helps a person to feel whole.

Hopelessness

1. Hopelessness is an emotional state in which a person feels that life is too much to handle—that it is impossible. A person who lacks hope sees no possibility that his life will improve and no solution to problems. He believes that neither he nor others can do anything to help.
2. Hopelessness is related to despair, helplessness, doubt, grief, apathy, sadness, depression, and suicide.
3. A hospitalized person is often depressed but not necessarily hopeless.
4. It has been observed that hope reflected in clients' drawings has a direct relationship to the clients' improvement, whereas a lack of hope is related to recurrence of disease. Therefore, a nurse can be helpful to clients in finding their resources of hope. The presence of cancer has been significantly predicted in individuals on the basis of identifying the presence of hopelessness in the person's life prior to the diagnosis of cancer. Therefore, terminal illness may result in hopelessness, and a life state of hopelessness may result in terminal illness (Schmale and Iher, 1966).
5. Hopelessness results in three basic categories of feelings:
   a. Sense of the impossible; what the person feels he must do, he cannot; he feels trapped
   b. Overwhelmed; tasks and others are perceived as too big and difficult to handle and the self is perceived as small
   c. Apathy; the person has no goals; no sense of purpose
6. A person experiencing hopelessness cannot imagine anything that can be done or is worth doing, nor can he imagine beyond what is currently occurring.
7. Hopeless persons lack internal resources or strengths (*e.g.*, autonomy, self-esteem, integrity) to draw upon. Regardless of age, they reach outside themselves for help because their internal resources may be depleted.

8. Some degree of hopelessness is involved in everyone's life. It occurs in various forms and is a more common and usual feeling than reported (*e.g.,* we all must die; it is hopeless to hope for anything else).

9. Hopelessness is most often observed in those who are rigid and inflexible in their thoughts, feelings, and actions.

10. Often people have ideals that are hopeless in reality (*e.g.,* not to die, we can trust everyone, all people should always act appropriately).

11. If hopelessness is recognized and dealt with imaginatively, it can result in movement, growth, and resourcefulness. Rigidity never overcomes hopelessness.

12. A person can cope with a part of his life he views as hopeless if he is able to realize that there are other factors in his life that are hopeful. For example, a person may realize he may never walk again, yet he will be able to go home and be in the company of his grandchildren and move around. Therefore, hopelessness can lead to the discovery of alternatives that provide meaning and purpose in life. It is essential to keep hopelessness out of the way of hope.

13. Motivation is essential in the recovery process of hopelessness. The client must determine a goal even if he has low expectations of achieving it. The nurse is the catalyst to encourage the client to take the first step to identify a goal. After this is accomplished, another goal must be created.

14. The health care team must be hopeful if the client is to be hopeful; otherwise, the client views all efforts of the team as a waste of time.

15. The more the client believes he can attain a goal, the more important that goal becomes in providing hope for the client.

16. The nurse mobilizes the client's internal and external resources to strengthen his hope, motivation, and will to live.

17. Often when a person's internal and external resources are exhausted, he relies on his relationship with God for hope. He may feel more secure in placing hope in God than in other people or himself. Hoping in God may not mean an abrupt end to crisis, but gives the person a sense of God's control of circumstances and ability to support a person during this time. Meaning and purpose for life and suffering may be found in a client's relationship with God and the knowledge of His control. Hope for a client's future may depend on his perception of a promise of eternal fellowship with God that continues after this present life on earth ends. With this eternal relationship with God comes the belief in God's promise to end all suffering and restore harmonious relationships—man with God, himself, and others.

Hopelessness
Related to (Specify)

Assessment
See Defining Characteristics

Outcome Criteria

Short Term

The person will
- Share suffering openly and constructively with others
- Reminisce and review his life positively
- Consider his values and the meaning of life
- Express feelings of optimism about the present
- Express feelings of positive relationships with significant others
- Express confidence in a desired outcome
- Express confidence in self and others
- Verbalize realistic goals

Long Term
- The person will demonstrate an increase in energy level as evidenced by activities (*i.e.,* self-care, exercise, hobbies, etc.)
- Express positive expectations about the future
- Demonstrate initiative, self-direction, and autonomy in decision-making and activities
- Make statements similar to the following:
  "I am looking forward to . . . "
  "When things are not so good, it helps me to think of . . . "
  "I have enough time to do what I want."
  "There are more good times ahead."
  "I expect to succeed in . . . "
  "I expect to get more out of the good things in life."
  "My past experiences have helped me be prepared for my future."
  "In the future, I'll be happier."
  "I have faith in the future."

Interventions

A. Assist the person to identify and express feelings

1. Listen to and treat the person as an individual
2. Convey empathy to promote verbalization of doubts, fears, and concerns
3. Validate and reflect impressions with the person
4. Accept the person's feelings (*i.e.,* trust his will to live if it exists, accept his anger)
5. Encourage the person to verbalize why and how hope is significant in his life
6. Encourage expressions of how hope is uncertain in his life and areas in which hope has failed him
7. Assist the person to recognize that hopelessness is a part of everyone's life that demands recognition. It can be utilized as a source of energy, imagination, and freedom that encourages a person to consider alternate choices. It leads to self-discovery.
8. Assist the person to understand that he can deal with the hopeless aspects of his life by separating them from the hopeful aspects. Help the person identify areas of hopelessness in his life and acknowledge them. Help him to distinguish between the

possible and the impossible. The nurse mobilizes a client's internal and external resources in order to promote hope as follows.

B. Assess and mobilize the person's internal resources (autonomy, independence, rationale, cognitive thinking, flexibility, spirituality)

1. Emphasize the client's strengths, not weaknesses
2. Compliment the client on appearance and/or efforts when appropriate
3. Promote motivation by:
   a. Identifying client's values and interests
   b. Identifying client's areas of success and usefulness; emphasize his past accomplishments
   c. Utilize this information to develop goals with the client
   d. Assist the client to identify sources of hope (*i.e.,* relationships, faith, things to accomplish)
   e. Assist the client to develop realistic short-term and long-term goals (progress from simple to more complex; may use a "goals poster" to indicate type and time for achieving specific goals)
   f. Teach the client to monitor specific signs of progress to use as self-reinforcement
   g. Encourage "means—end" thinking in positive terms (*i.e.,* If I do this and . . . , then I'll be able to . . .)
4. Assist the client with problem-solving and decision-making (See Appendix VII)
   a. Respect the client as a competent decision-maker; treat his decisions and desires with respect
   b. Encourage verbalization to determine the client's perception of choices
   c. Clarify and modify the client's perceptions of reality
   d. Correct misinformation
   e. Assist the client to identify those problems he cannot resolve in order to advance to problems he can resolve. In other words, assist the client to move away from dwelling on the impossible and hopeless and to begin to deal with matters that are realistic and hopeful.
   f. Assess the client's perceptions of self and others in relation to size. (This person often perceives others in the world as large and difficult to deal with and perceives himself as small.) If his perceptions are unrealistic, assist him to reassess them in order to restore proper size to his world.
   g. Promote flexibility. Encourage the client to try alternatives and take risks.
   h. Teach and support the client to use rational inquiry (to seek more information).
5. Assist the client to learn effective coping skills
   a. Teach the client the importance of mutuality in sharing concerns.
   b. Explain the benefits of distraction from negative events.
   c. Teach the client the value of confronting issues.
   d. Teach and assist patient relaxation techniques (see Appendix X) prior to anticipated stressful events.
   e. Encourage mental imagery to promote positive thought processes (see Appendix X).
   f. Allow the client time to reminisce to gain insight into past experiences.
   g. Teach the client to "hope to be" the best person possible today and to appreciate the fullness of each moment.
   h. Teach the client to maximize esthetic experiences (*e.g.,* smell of coffee, back rub, or feeling the warmth of the sun or a breeze)

    i. Teach the client to anticipate experiences he takes delight in each day (*e.g.,* walking, reading favorite book, writing letter)

C. Assess and mobilize person's external resources (significant others, health care team, support groups, God and/or higher powers)

  1. Family and/or significant others
    a. Involve family and/or significant others in plan of care
    b. Encourage family to express their love and need for the person
    c. Emphasize the importance of sustaining and supportive positive relationships
    d. Foster and encourage the client to spend increased time and/or thoughts with loved ones in healthy relationships
    e. Teach the family their role in sustaining hope
    f. Convey hope, information, and confidence to family as their feelings will be conveyed to the client
    g. Discuss the client's meaningful goals with family
    h. Utilize touch and closeness with the client to demonstrate to the family that this is acceptable (provide privacy)
    i. Help the client to recognize that he is loved, cared about, and important to the lives of others regardless of his failing health
    j. Utilize and emphasize family strengths of endurance, courage, and patience
  2. Health Care Team
    a. Develop positive-trusting nurse-client relationship by:
        Answering questions
        Respecting client's feelings
        Providing consistent care
        Following through on requests
        Touch
        Providing comfort
        Honesty
    b. Convey attitude of "We care too much about you to let you just give up" and/or "I can help you"
    c. Hold conferences and share client's goals with staff
    d. Provide staff support groups, utilize team care conferences
    e. Encourage the client to utilize and work with the health care team to cope with problems
    f. Share advances in technology and research for treatment of diseases
  3. Support Groups
    a. Encourage person to share concerns with others who have had similar problem and/or disease and have had positive experiences from coping effectively with it
    b. Provide information on self-help groups (*i.e.,* "Make today count"—40 chapters in US and Canada; "I can cope"—series for cancer patients; "We Can Weekend"—for families of cancer patients)
    c. Initiate referrals when indicated
  4. God and/or higher powers
    a. Assess belief support system (value, past experiences with, religious activities, relationship with God, meaning and purpose of prayer; refer to *Spiritual Distress*)
    b. Create environment in which client feels free to express self spiritually
    c. Acknowledge the client's belief system
    d. Allow the client time and opportunities to reflect on the meaning of suffering, death, and dying
    e. Accept, respect, and support the patient's hope in God

D. Identify the individual at risk for self-harm (Refer to *Potential for Self-harm*)

Initiate referrals as indicated
- Counseling
  - Spiritual
  - Family
- Crisis hot line

References/Bibliography

Beck AT, Weissman A: The measurement of pessimism: The hopelessness scale. J Consult Clin Psychol 42(6):861–865, 1972

Beck MB, Rawlins RP, Williams SR: Mental Health Psychiatric Nursing, A Holistic Life-Cycle Approach, pp 499-536. CV Mosby, St Louis, 1984

Buehler JA: What contributes to hope in the cancer patient? Am J Nurs 75:1353–1356, 1975

Dubree M, Vogelpohl R: When hope dies—so might the patient. Am J Nurs 80:2046—2049, 1980

Fish S, Shelly JA: Spiritual Care: The Nurse's Role, 2nd ed, pp 40–45. Downers Grove, IL, Intervarsity Press, 1983

Gottschalk LA: A hope scale applicable to verbal samples. Arch Gen Psychiatry 30:779–787, 1974

Hinds PS: Inducing a definition of "hope" through the use of grounded theory methodology. J Adv Nurs 9:357–362, 1984

Korner IN: Hope as a method of coping. J Consult Clin Psychol 34(2):134–139, 1970

Kubler–Ross E: Death: The Final Stage of Growth. Englewood Cliffs, NJ, Prentice-Hall, 1975

Lynch WF: Image of Hope; Imagination as a Healer of the Hopeless, pp 47–62. Baltimore, Helicon, 1965

Limandri BJ, Boyle DW: Instilling hope. Am J Nurs 78:79–80, 1978

Martocchio BC, Dufault K: In hospice compassionate care and the dying experience. Nurs Clin North Am 20(2):380–391, 1985

Miller JF: Inspiring hope. Am J Nurs 85:22–25, 1985

Peck ML: The therapeutic effect of faith. Nurs Forum 20(2):154–167, 1981

Schmale AH, Iher HP: The affect of hopelessness and the development of cancer. Psychosom Med 28(5):714–721, 1966

Schnieder JS: Hopelessness and helplessness. JPN and Mental Health Services, pp 12–16, March 1980

Taylor PB, Gideon MD: Holding out hope to your dying patient; paradoxical but possible. Nursing 12:42–45, 1982

Watson J: Nursing: The Philosophy and Science of Caring. Boston, Little, Brown & Co, 1979

Infection, Potential for

Related to **(Specify Risk Factors)**

Definition

Potential for infection: The state in which an individual is at risk to be invaded by an opportunistic or pathogenic agent (virus, fungus, bacteria, protozoa or other parasite) from external sources.

Author's Note: *Potential for Infection* describes a situation when host defenses are compromised, thus becoming more susceptible to environmental pathogens.

Defining Characteristics

Evidence of risk factors such as:
    Altered production of leukocytes
    Altered immune response
    Altered circulation (lymph, blood)
    Presence of favorable conditions for infection (see Etiological, Contributing, Risk Factors)
    History of infection

Etiological, Contributing, Risk Factors

A variety of health problems and situations can create favorable conditions that would encourage the development of infections.
Some common factors are:

Pathophysiological

Chronic diseases
    Cancer   Hematologic   Respiratory disorders
    Renal failure   disorders   Collagen diseases
    Arthritis   Diabetes mellitus   Heritable disorders
          Hepatic disorders

Alcoholism
Immunosuppression
Immunodeficiency
Altered or insufficient leukocytes
Blood dyscrasias
Impaired oxygen transport
Altered integumentary system
Periodontal disease
Obesity
Loss of consciousness
Hormonal factors

Treatment-related

Medications
Antibiotics
Steroids
Antiviral agents
Insulin

Antifungal agents
Tranquilizers

Immunosuppressants

Surgery
Radiation therapy
Dialysis
Total parenteral nutrition
Chemotherapy
Presence of invasive lines (*e.g.,* IVs, Foley catheter, enteral feedings)
Tracheostomy

Situational (personal, environmental)

Prolonged immobility
Trauma (accidental, intentional)
Postpartum period
Contact with contagious agents (nosocomial or community acquired)
Postoperative period
Increased length of hospital stay

Malnutrition
Stress
Bites (animal, insect, human)
Thermal injuries
Warm, moist, dark environment (skin folds, casts)
Inadequate personal hygiene
Lack of immunizations
Smoking

Maturational

Newborns
Lack of maternal antibodies (dependent on maternal exposures)
Lack of normal flora
Open wounds (umbilical, circumcision)
Immature immune system
Infant/childhood
Lack of immunization
Elderly
Debilitated
Immune response decreased
Chronic diseases

Focus Assessment Criteria

Subjective Data

1. Does the person complain of:
Continuous fevers
Intermittent fevers
Previous infections
• Urinary tract

- Respiratory
- Wound
- Cutaneous
- GI

Pain or swelling
- Generalized
- Localized

2. History of recent travel
   Within US
   Outside US
3. History of exposure to infectious diseases*
   Airborne (most childhood infections, chickenpox, tuberculosis)
   Vector-borne and other vector-associated infections (malaria, plague)
   Vehicle-borne and other food- and water-borne infections (hepatitis A, Salmonellas)
   Contact-spread (most common type of exposure)
   - Direct (person to person)
   - Indirect (instruments, clothing, etc., to person)
   - Contact droplet (pneumonias, colds, etc.)
4. History of risk factors associated with infections (See Etiological, Contributing, Risk Factors)

Objective Data

1. Presence of wounds
   Surgical
   Burns
   Invasive devices (trach, IV, drains)
2. White blood cell count (WBC)
3. Temperature
4. Cultures

Principles and Rationale for Nursing Care

General

1. There are two parameters that can assist to identify individuals at risk for infection—predictive factors and confounding factors. (Owen)
2. Predictors are controllable factors that have been identified as increasing the risk of infection by interfering or compromising the host defenses. Intervention can be implemented to control or influence the degree of risk associated with these factors. (Owen)
3. Confounding factors are factors that augment the risk of infection. They are not singularly controllable during hospitalization but can enhance one's predictive risk for infection significantly. (Owen)
4. The following are confounding factors:
   - Age
   - Anatomic determinants
   - Metabolic determinants
   - Decreased numbers of neutrophils
   - Diminished or defective immunoglobulin synthesis or rapid loss of immunoglobulin

* See *Potential for Infection Transmission:* Principles and Rationale for Nursing Care

- Defective cell-mediated immune mechanisms
- Antimicrobial therapy
5. Resistance to infection is dependent on the host's immune response (susceptibility), the dose of the infecting agent, and the virulence of the organism. Factors influencing the host's immune response include:
   - Anatomic barriers—each system has specific lines of defenses.
   - Therapies—pose a threat to normal lines of defense by either invasiveness or alteration of body function.
   - Developmental and heritable factors—factors that have negative impact on the individual's immune system function (e.g., newborn status); agammaglobulinemia.
   - Hormonal factors—the male is more vulnerable to infection than the female; pregnancy increases the female's vulnerability; steroid therapy increases vulnerability in both sexes.
   - Age—includes both extremes of age (immaturity or degeneration of the immune system).
   - Nutrition influences protein synthesis and phagocytosis, decreasing the body's vulnerability to infection.
   - Fever—hyperthermia may inhibit the growth of organisms; hypothermia may decrease the effects of the fever.
   - Secretions such as mucus, saliva, and skin secretions contain substances that are bactericidal, decreasing the risk of infection and colonization.
   - Endotoxins, a product of some gram-negative bacteria, have a limited ability to kill other bacteria or increase an individual's resistance to some infections.
   - Interference—the interaction between two distinct organisms that are parasitizing the host leads to interference, in which one remains dominant and the other is suppressed.
   - The inflammatory response consists of the following: (1) activation of leukocytes, (2) plasma proteins, which localize and phagocytize the infectious process, and (3) increased blood and lymph flow that dilutes and flushes out toxic materials; this process causes a local increase in temperature.
   - Phagocytosis is the process by which parasites are removed by means of engulfment and digestion.
6. "Any person can be infected with HIV (the AIDS virus) even with no symptoms. It takes 6 weeks to 6 months after exposure for a person to develop HIV antibodies. Therefore, nurses must use precautions with blood and body fluids from all patients to protect themselves from exposure to HIV. These precautions also protect against other infectious organisms."
   - Wash hands before and after all patient or specimen contact.
   - Handle the blood of all patients as potentially infectious.
   - Wear gloves for potential contact with blood and body fluids.
   - Place used syringes immediately in nearby impermeable container; do not recap or manipulate needle in any way!!
   - Wear protective eyewear and mask if splatter with blood or body fluids is possible (e.g., bronchoscopy, oral surgery).
   - Wear gowns when splash with blood or body fluids is anticipated (e.g., L & D).
   - Handle all linen soiled with blood and/or body secretions as potentially infectious.
   - Process all laboratory specimens as potentially infectious.
   - Wear mask for TB and other respiratory organisms (HIV is not airborne).
   - Place resuscitation equipment where respiratory arrest is predictable. (California Nurses Association. Used with permission.)

Host Defenses
Specific host defenses of each system that influence the immune response include:

Central Nervous System
> Because the most common route for both bacterial and viral infections of the central nervous system is the hematogenous route, blood host defenses play an important primary role.

Cutaneous
1. Skin provides a first line of defense against organisms, both anatomically and chemically.
2. Sweat glands and sebaceous glands do not allow overgrowth of bacteria.
3. The acid pH of the skin does not allow pathogenic organisms to grow or survive on the skin for any length of time.
4. Eye infections are controlled by the flushing and lysozyme action of tears. Organisms are flushed through the lacrimal duct and deposited in the nasopharynx.

Blood
1. The circulating blood is the major vehicle for transporting internal defense mechanisms.
2. The febrile response is associated with circulating pyrogens to the hypothalamus.

Genitourinary Tract
1. Anatomical structure eliminates easy ascent of perineal microorganisms into the bladder.
2. Mucous layer allows entrapment of organisms and engulfment by bladder cells.
3. The pH and osmolality of urine prevent bacterial multiplication.
4. The ability to empty the bladder completely eliminates stasis of invading organisms and allows for continual flushing.

Respiratory Tract
1. The nares entrap the majority of foreign matter on the mucus membranes as a result of turbulence caused by the turbinates and hairs.
2. The mucociliary transport system consists of cilia and mucus, which remove additional matter passing to the upper and lower bronchi.
3. Lysozymes and IgA, a secretion of phagocytes, are found in nasal secretions and assist in the prevention of colonization.
4. Particles reaching as far as the alveoli can be removed through the expulsive action of sneezing and coughing, and the gag reflex.
5. Phagocytosis occurs in the alveoli, with the macrophages utilized as a major defense mechanism.

GI Tract
1. A mucous layer traps ingested microbes in the epithelium of the GI tract.
2. Gastric acids kill most organisms.
3. Peristalsis aids in the removal of organisms.
4. Intestinal secretions contain antibody (IgA), bile salts, lysozyme, glycolipids, and glycoproteins that prevent proliferation and adherence.
5. Normal gut flora interact to restrict overproliferation.

Wounds
1. Skin provides a first line of defense; the opening of the skin, either surgically or traumatically, potentiates infection.
2. A wound essentially closes within 24 hours, eliminating the risk of direct inoculations of organisms.

3. Wound infections rely on the capabilities of other host defenses to assist in the healing process.
4. Risk factors associated with wound infections depend on (1) endogenous factors such as presence of confounding factors, skin preparation, the use of prophylactic antibiotics; and (2) exogenous factors such as the preoperative scrub, barrier techniques, airborne contamination, environmental disinfection, wound care, and the condition of the wound at the time of closure.

Potential for Infection
Related to (Specify)

Assessment
See Etiological, Contributing, Risk Factors

Outcome Criteria

The person will:
- Demonstrate meticulous handwashing technique by the time of discharge.
- Be free from nosocomial infectious processes during hospitalization.
- Demonstrate knowledge of risk factors associated with potential for infection and will practice appropriate precautions to prevent infection.

Interventions

A. Identify individuals at high risk for nosocomial infections

1. Assess for predictors
- Infection (preoperatively)
- Abdominal or thoracic surgery
- Surgery longer than two hours
- G.U. procedure
- Instrumentation (ventilator, suction, catheters, nebulizers, tracheostomy, invasive monitoring)
- Anesthesia
2. Assess for confounding factors
- Age less than 1 year or greater than 65 years
- Obesity
- Underlying disease conditions (COPD, diabetes, cardiovascular blood dyscrasias)
- Substance abuse
- Medications (steroids, chemotherapy, antibiotic therapy)
- Nutritional status (intake less than minimum daily requirements)
- Smoker
3. Label individual who has one or more confounding factors and one or more predictors with *Potential for Infection* on their care plan. (Owen M, Grier M: Infection Risk Assessment Guide, 1987. Unpublished, used with permission)

B. Reduce the entry of organisms into individuals

1. Meticulous hand-washing to prevent the spread of infection.
2. Maintain aseptic technique for all invasive devices
3. Implement isolation measures dependent on the causative organism (see *Potential for Infection Transmission*)
4. Limit unnecessary diagnostic or therapeutic procedures
5. Change opened containers on a regular basis
6. Reduce presence of airborne microorganisms
7. Ensure proper ventilation and proper surface cleaning (damp dust)

Cutaneous
1. Maintain dry skin surface and acidic *p*H
2. Avoid damage to skin surface
3. Follow procedures for care of sites (Foley catheter, IV)

Genitourinary tract
1. Assess the need for catheterization daily
2. Keep urinary drainage devices below bladder or clamp during transport
3. Maintain acidic *p*H of urine
4. Investigate possibility of incomplete bladder emptying

C. Protect the immune-deficient individual from infection

1. Place in private room
2. Instruct individual to ask all visitors and personnel to wash their hands before approaching individual
3. Limit visitors when appropriate
4. Screen all visitors for known infections or exposure to infections
5. Restrict invasive devices (IV, lab specimens) to those that are absolutely necessary
6. Teach individual and family members signs and symptoms of infection
7. Evaluate individual's personal hygiene habits
8. Provide immune globulin to individuals exposed to specific diseases that might be life threatening (*i.e.,* chickenpox, hepatitis)

D. Reduce individual's susceptibility to infection

1. Encourage and maintain caloric and protein intake in diet (see *Altered Nutrition*)
2. Assess the client for adequate immunizations against childhood diseases, bacterial infections (*e.g.,* pneumococcal and *Haemophilus influenzae* vaccines), and other viral infections (flu virus vaccines)
3. Monitor use or overuse of antimicrobial therapy
4. Administer prescribed antimicrobial therapy within 15 minutes of scheduled time to ensure adequate maintenance of therapeutic levels (prevention of resistant strains or organisms)
5. Observe for clinical manifestations of infection in individuals at high risk
6. Minimize length of stay in hospital to prevent colonization with nosocomial organisms
7. Observe for superinfection development in individuals currently receiving antimicrobial therapy

E. Initiate health teaching and referrals as indicated

1. Instruct individual and family regarding the causes, risks and communicability of the infection
2. Report communicable diseases as appropriate to public health department

References/Bibliography

Axnick K, Yardbrough M: Infection Control: An Integrated Approach. St Louis, CV Mosby, 1984

Bennett JV, Brachman PS: Hospital Infections. Boston, Little, Brown & Co, 1979

Brunner LS, Suddarth DS: The Lippincott Manual of Nursing Practice, 4th ed. Philadelphia, JB Lippincott, 1986

California Nurses Association: AIDS Education and Training. San Francisco, CNA, 1988

Haley RW: Managing Hospital Infection Control for Cost-Effectiveness: A Strategy for Reducing Infectious Complications. Chicago, American Hospital Association, 1986

Hoeprich PD: Infectious Diseases. Philadelphia, Harper & Row, 1983

Larson E: Clinical Microbiology and Infection Control. Boston, Blackwell Scientific Publications, 1984

Owen M, Grier M: Infection Risk Assessment Guide. Unpublished, 1987

Wenzel RP: CRC Handbook of Hospital Acquired Infections. Boca Raton, FL, CRC Press, 1981

Guidelines for the Prevention and Control of Nosocomial Infections. U.S. Department of Health & Human Services, Centers for Disease Control, Atlanta, 1981–1986

Infection Transmission, Potential for *

Related to **(Specify)**

Related to **Lack of Knowledge of Reducing the Risk of Transmitting the AIDS Virus**

Definition

Potential for infection transmission: The state in which an individual is at risk for transferring an opportunistic or pathogenic agent to others.

Defining Characteristics

Presence of risk factors (See Etiological, Contributing, Risk Factors)

Etiological, Contributing, Risk Factors

Pathophysiological

Colonization with highly antibiotic-resistant organism.
Airborne transmission exposure
Contact transmission exposure (direct, indirect, contact droplet)
Vehicle transmission exposure
Vector-borne transmission exposure

Treatment-related

Contaminated or dirty surgeries (I&D, traumatic wound)
Drainage devices (urinary, chest tubes)
Suction equipment
Invasive devices (endotracheal tubes)

Situational (personal, environmental)

Disaster with hazardous infectious material
Unsanitary living conditions (sewage, personal hygiene)
Areas considered high risk for vector-borne diseases (malaria, rabies, bubonic plague)
Areas considered high risk for vehicle-borne disease (hepatitis A, *Shigella, Salmonella*)
Lack of knowledge
Intravenous drug use
Multiple sex partners

---

* This diagnostic category is not currently on the NANDA list but has been included for clarity or usefulness.

Maturational

Newborn
> Birth outside hospital setting in uncontrolled environment
> Exposure during prenatal or perinatal period to communicable disease via maternal source.

Focus Assessment Criteria

(Refer also to *Potential for Infection*)

Subjective Data
> History of infection
> Onset of symptoms
> Exposure to communicable disease
> Sexual practices

Objective Data
> Extent of infection—amount of coughing, bleeding, drainage
> Hygienic practices of patient
> Mode of transmission
>> Blood/body fluids
>> Purulent drainage
>> Respiratory secretions
>> Oral–fecal
>> Vector

Principles and Rationale for Nursing Care

General

In order to spread an infection, three elements are required (refer to Figure II-2):
- A source of infecting organisms
- A susceptible host
- A means of transmission for the organism

1. Sources of infecting organisms include:
   a. Clients, personnel, and visitors with acute disease, incubating infection, or colonized organisms without apparent disease
   b. Person's own endogenous flora (autogenous infection)
   c. Inanimate environment, including equipment and medications
2. Susceptibility of the host varies according to
   a. Immune status of the host
   b. Ability to develop a commensal relationship with the infecting organism and become an asymptomatic carrier
   c. Preexisting diseases affecting the client
3. Means of transmission for the organism include one or more of the following:
   a. Contact transmission, the most frequent method of transferring organisms. It can be divided into three subgroups:
      1. Direct contact—involves direct physical transfer between a susceptible host and an infected or colonized person.
      2. Indirect contact—involves the exchange of organisms between a host and contaminated objects, usually inanimate.

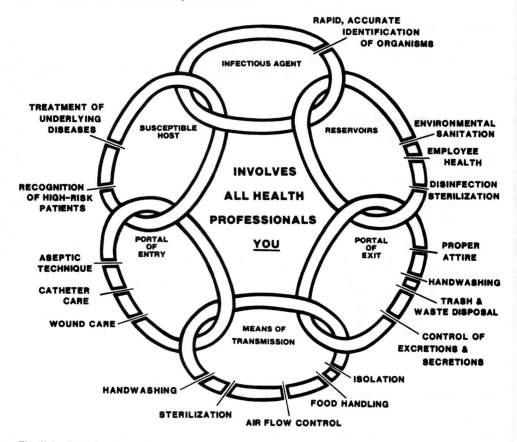

Fig. II-2 Breaking the chain of infection. (Adapted from the APIC Starter Kit with permission from the Association for Practitioners in Infection Control, Mundelein, Illinois, copyright APIC, 1978)

      3. Droplet contact—involves the transfer of organisms from coughing, sneezing, or talking by an infected person into the conjunctivae, nose, or mouth of a susceptible host. Droplets travel no more than 3 feet.
  b. Vehicle route transmission infections are spread through a means such as:
      1. Food (*e.g.*, hepatitis A, *Salmonella*)
      2. Water (*e.g.*, *Legionella*)
      3. Drugs (*e.g.*, IV-contaminated products)
      4. Blood (*e.g.*, hepatitis B, AIDS)
  c. Airborne transmission infections are disseminated via droplet nuclei (residue of evaporated droplets that may remain suspended in the air for long periods of time) or dust particles in the air containing the infectious agent.
  d. Vector-borne transmission infections are spread through vectors such as animals or insects.
4. The practice of Universal Precautions requires that precautions be taken with all blood and body fluids. However, those patients with suspected or confirmed medical

diagnosis indicative of an infectious disease process need to be documented with a comprehensive plan of care for that infection or potential infection. That can be done most expeditiously through the nursing diagnosis *Potential for Infection Transmission.*

5. "Any person can be infected with HIV (the AIDS virus) even with no symptoms. It takes 6 weeks to 6 months after exposure for a person to develop HIV antibodies. Therefore, nurses must use precautions with blood and body fluids from all patients to protect themselves from exposure to HIV. These precautions also protect against other infectious organisms."
   - Wash hands before and after all patient or specimen contact.
   - Handle the blood of all patients as potentially infectious.
   - Wear gloves for potential contact with blood and body fluids.
   - Place used syringes immediately in nearby impermeable container; do not recap or manipulate needle in any way!!
   - Wear protective eyewear and mask if splatter with blood or body fluids is possible (*e.g.,* bronchoscopy, oral surgery).
   - Wear gowns when splash with blood or body fluids is anticipated (*e.g.,* L & D).
   - Handle all linen soiled with blood and/or body secretions as potentially infectious.
   - Process all laboratory specimens as potentially infectious.
   - Wear mask for TB and other respiratory organisms (HIV is not airborne).
   - Place resuscitation equipment where respiratory arrest is predictable. (California Nurses Association)

Acquired Immunodeficiency Syndrome (AIDS)

1. AIDS is caused by a retrovirus labeled human immunodeficiency virus (HIV). Transmission is made by contaminated semen, vaginal fluids, or blood.
2. The reported cases nationally according to risk groups are:
   73% homosexuals
   17% intravenous drug users
   10% babies of infected mothers, recipients of infected blood transfusions
3. AIDS has a latency or incubation period of 18 months to 5 years. During this period the individual is transmitting disease through sexual activity or contaminated blood.
4. Human immunodeficiency virus (HIV) destroys the body's T and B lymphocytes, thus making the host susceptible to a select group of diseases (refer to Table II-10).
5. AIDS is a terminal disease with a mortality rate of greater than 95% at 2 years.

Potential for Infection Transmission
Related to (Specify)

Assessment
See Defining Characteristics

Table II-10. **List of Most Frequent Infections and Neoplasms in Acquired Immunodeficiency Syndrome (AIDS)**

Problem	Site
AIDS-Related Complex	
Candida albicans	Mouth (thrush)
Herpes simplex	Mucocutaneous; may be severe
Herpes zoster	Disseminated; may be severe
Lymphadenopathy	Generalized (always more than one lymph node)
Fevers	Usually greater than 100°F; persistent over months
Diarrhea	No organism recovered, or conventional organisms recovered
Weight loss	Progressive and sustained
Night sweats	Characteristically severe and drenching; persistent and sustained over months
Thrombocytopenia	Often accompanied by petechia; may be severe and life-threatening
Infections	
Candida albicans	Mouth (thrush); throat
Cryptococcus neoformans	Central nervous system (CNS); pulmonary; disseminated
Pneumocystis carinii	Pneumonia
Toxoplasma gondii	CNS
Histoplasma gondii	CNS
Cryptosporidium	Intestine; diarrhea
Cytomegalovirus (CMV)	Retinas; intestine; pulmonary; disseminated
Herpes simplex	Mucocutaneous; severe
Herpes zoster	Disseminated; severe
Human immunodeficiency virus (HIV)	CNS, disseminated
Progressive multifocal leukoencephalopathy	CNS
Mycobacterium avium-intracellulare (MAI)	Disseminated
Mycobacterium tuberculosis	Pulmonary (TB)
Neoplasms	
Kaposi's sarcoma	Skin; disseminated
Burkitt's lymphoma	Lymphatic system
Non-Hodgkin's lymphoma	Lymphatic system
Mycosis fungoides	Skin (dermal lymphoma)

(Source: Keating SB, Kelman GB: Home Health Care Nursing Concepts and Practice, p 251. Philadelphia, JB Lippincott, 1988

Outcome Criteria

The person will
- Relate the need to be isolated until noninfectious
- Describe the mode of transmission of disease by the time of discharge
- Demonstrate meticulous hand washing during hospitalization

Interventions

A. Identify susceptible host individuals based on focus assessment for potential for infection and history of exposure

B. Identify the mode of transmission based on infecting agent
   1. Airborne
   2. Contact
      - Direct
      - Indirect
      - Contact droplet
   3. Vehicle-borne
   4. Vector-borne

C. Reduce the transfer of pathogens
   1. Initiate appropriate isolation precautions (see Table II-11)
   2. Secure appropriate room assignment dependent on the type of infection and hygienic practices of the infected person.
   3. Adhere to the Universal Infection Precautions
      - Wash hands before and after all patient or specimen contact.
      - Handle the blood of all patients as potentially infectious.
      - Wear gloves for potential contact with blood and body fluids.
      - Place used syringes immediately in nearby impermeable container; do not recap or manipulate needle in any way!!
      - Wear protective eyewear and mask if splatter with blood or body fluids is possible (*e.g.,* bronchoscopy, oral surgery).
      - Wear gowns when splash with blood or body fluids is anticipated (*e.g.,* L & D)
      - Handle all linen soiled with blood and/or body secretions as potentially infectious.
      - Process all laboratory specimens as potentially infectious.
      - Wear mask for TB and other respiratory organisms (HIV is not airborne).
      - Place resuscitation equipment where respiratory arrest is predictable. (California Nurses Association)

D. Initiate health teaching and referrals as indicated
   1. Referral to infection control practitioner for follow-up with the Health Department regarding family exposure and cause of exposure, and to assist in appropriate isolation of the patient
   2. Patient education regarding hand-washing as the single most important measure to prevent the spread of infection.
   3. Patient education regarding the chain of infection and patient responsibility in both the hospital and at home

(*Text continues on page 469*)

Table II-11. **Disease-specific Isolation Precautions***

	Precautions Indicated						
Disease	Private Room?	Masks?	Gowns?	Gloves?	Infective Material	Apply Precautions How Long?	Comments
Acquired immunodeficiency syndrome (AIDS)	Yes if patient hygiene is poor	No	Yes if soiling is likely	Yes for touching infective material	Blood and body fluids	Duration of illness	Use caution when handling blood and blood-soiled articles. Take special care to avoid needlestick injuries. If gastrointestinal bleeding is likely, wear gloves if touching feces.
Gastroenteritis							
Campylobacter species	Yes if patient hygiene is poor	No	Yes if soiling is likely	Yes for touching infective material	Feces	Duration of illness	
Clostridium difficile	Yes if patient hygiene is poor	No	Yes if soiling is likely	Yes for touching infective material	Feces	Duration of illness	
Cryptosporidium species	Yes if patient hygiene is poor	No	Yes if soiling is likely	Yes for touching infective material	Feces	Duration of illness	
Escherichia coli (enteropathogenic, enterotoxic, or enteroinvasive)	Yes if patient hygiene is poor	No	Yes if soiling is likely	Yes for touching infective material	Feces	Duration of illness	
Giardia lamblia	Yes if patient hygiene is poor	No	Yes if soiling is likely	Yes for touching infective material	Feces	Duration of illness	

(continued)

Rotavirus	Yes if patient hygiene is poor	No	Yes if soiling is likely	Yes for touching infective material	Feces	Duration of illness or 7 days after onset, whichever is less
Salmonella species	Yes if patient hygiene is poor	No	Yes if soiling is likely	Yes for touching infective material	Feces	Duration of illness
Shigella species	Yes if patient hygiene is poor	No	Yes if soiling is likely	Yes for touching infective material	Feces	Until 3 consecutive cultures of feces taken after ending antimicrobial therapy are negative for infecting strain
Unknown etiology	Yes if patient hygiene is poor	No	Yes if soiling is likely	Yes for touching infective material	Feces	Duration of illness
Viral	Yes if patient hygiene is poor	No	Yes if soiling is likely	Yes for touching infective material	Feces	Duration of illness
Yersinia enterocolitica	Yes if patient hygiene is poor	No	Yes if soiling is likely	Yes for touching infective material	Feces	Duration of illness
Gonorrhea	No	No	No	No	Discharge may be

(continued)

Table II-11. **Disease-specific Isolation Precautions*** (continued)

Disease	Precautions Indicated					Infective Material	Apply Precautions How Long?	Comments
	Private Room?	Masks?	Gowns?	Gloves?				
Hepatitis, viral Type A (infectious)	Yes if patient hygiene is poor	No	Yes if soiling is likely	Yes for touching infective material		Feces may be	For 7 days after onset of jaundice	Hepatitis A is most contagious before symptoms and jaundice appear; once these appear, small, inapparent amounts of feces, which may contaminate the hands of personnel during patient care, do not appear to be infective. Thus, gowns and gloves are most useful when gross soiling with feces is anticipated or possible.
Type B ("serum hepatitis"), including hepatitis B antigen (HBsAg) carrier	No	No	Yes if soiling is likely	Yes if touching infective material		Blood and body fluids	Until patient is HBsAg-negative	Use caution when handling blood and blood-soiled articles. Take special care to avoid needlestick injuries. Gowns are indicated when clothing may become contaminated with body fluids or blood (for example, when blood splattering is anticipated). If gastrointestinal bleeding is likely, wear gloves if touching feces. A private room may be indicated if profuse bleeding is likely to cause environmental contamination.

(continued)

Disease					Blood and body fluids		Comments
Non-A, Non-B	No	No	Yes if soiling is likely	Yes for touching infective material		Duration of illness	Currently, the period of infectivity cannot be determined.
Herpes simplex *(Herpesvirus hominis)* Encephalitis	No	No	No	No			
Mucocutaneous, disseminated or primary, severe (skin, oral, and genital)	Yes if patient hygiene is poor	No	Yes if soiling is likely	Yes for touching infective material	Lesion secretions from infected site	Duration of illness	
Mucocutaneous, recurrent (skin, oral, and genital)	No	No	No	Yes for touching infective material	Lesion secretions from infected site	Until all lesions are crusted	
Neonatal (see comments for newborn with perinatal exposure)	Yes	No	Yes if soiling is likely	Yes for touching infective material	Lesion secretions	Duration of illness	The same isolation precautions are indicated for infants delivered (either vaginally or by cesarean section if membranes have been ruptured for more than 4–6 hours) to women with active genital herpes simplex infections. Infants delivered by cesarean section to women with active genital herpes simplex infections before and probably within 4–6 hours after membrane rupture are at minimal risk of developing herpes simplex infection; *(continued)*

Table II-11. **Disease-specific Isolation Precautions*** *(continued)*

Disease	Private Room?	Precautions Indicated			Infective Material	Apply Precautions How Long?	Comments
		Masks?	Gowns?	Gloves?			
							the same isolation precautions may still be indicated, however. (American Academy of Pediatrics Committee on Fetus and Newborn. Perinatal herpes simplex virus infections. Pediatrics 1980; 66:147–149. Also: Kibrick S, Herpes simplex infection at term. JAMA 1980; 243:157–160.)
Herpes zoster (varicella-zoster), Localized in immunocompromised patient, or disseminated	Yes	Yes	Yes	Yes for touching infective material	Lesion secretions and possibly respiratory secretions	Duration of illness	Localized lesions in immunocompromised patients frequently become disseminated. Because such dissemination is unpredictable, use the same isolation precautions as for disseminated disease. Persons who are not susceptible do not need to wear a mask. Persons susceptible to varicella-zoster

(continued)

Condition	Private Room	Gowns	Masks	Gloves	Infective Material	Duration	Comments
							(chickenpox) should, if possible, stay out of room. Special ventilation for the room, if available, may be advantageous, especially for outbreak control. Exposed susceptible patients should be placed on isolation precautions beginning at 10 days after exposure and continuing until 21 days after last exposure.
Localized in normal patient	Yes if patient hygiene is poor	No	No	Yes for touching infective material	Lesion secretions	Until all lesions are crusted	Persons susceptible to varicella-zoster (chickenpox) should, if possible, stay out of room. Roommates should not be susceptible to chickenpox.
Meningitis Aseptic (nonbacterial or viral meningitis) (also see specific etiologies)	Yes, if patient hygiene is poor	No	Yes if soiling is likely	Yes for touching infective material	Feces	For 7 days after onset	Enteroviruses are the most common cause of aseptic meningitis.
Bacterial, gram-negative enteric, in neonates	No	No	No	No	Feces may be		During a nursery outbreak, cohort ill and colonized infants, and use gowns if soiling is likely and gloves if touching feces.
Fungal	No	No	No	No			

(continued)

Table II-11. **Disease-specific Isolation Precautions*** (continued)

Disease	Precautions Indicated				Infective Material	Apply Precautions How Long?	Comments
	Private Room?	Masks?	Gowns?	Gloves?			
Haemophilus influenzae, known or suspected	Yes	Yes for those close to patient	No	No	Respiratory secretions	For 24 hours after start of effective therapy	
Listeria monocytogenes	No	No	No	No			
Neisseria meningitidis (meningococcal), known or suspected	Yes	Yes for those close to patient	No	No	Respiratory secretions	For 24 hours after start of effective therapy	
Pneumococcal	No	No	No	No			
Tuberculous	No	No	No	No			Patient should be examined for evidence of current (active) pulmonary tuberculosis. If present, precautions are necessary (see tuberculosis).
Other diagnosed bacterial	No	No	No	No			
Meningococcemia (meningococcal sepsis)	Yes	Yes for those close to patient	No	No	Respiratory secretions	For 24 hours after start of effective therapy	
Multiply-resistant organisms† infection or colonization‡							

(continued)

Infection	Private Room	Masks	Gowns	Gloves	Infective Material	Duration of Precautions	Comments
Gastrointestinal	Yes	No	Yes if soiling is likely	Yes for touching infective material	Feces	Until off antimicrobials and culture-negative	In outbreaks, cohorting of infected and colonized patients may be indicated if private rooms are not available.
Respiratory	Yes	Yes for those close to patient	Yes if soiling is likely	Yes for touching infective material	Respiratory secretions and possibly feces	Until off antimicrobials and culture-negative	In outbreaks, cohorting of infected and colonized patients may be indicated if private rooms are not available.
Skin, Wound, or Burn	Yes	No	Yes if soiling is likely	Yes for touching infective material	Pus and possibly feces	Until off antimicrobials and culture-negative	In outbreaks, cohorting of infected and colonized patients may be indicated if private rooms are not available.
Urinary	Yes	No	No	No	Urine and possibly feces	Until off antimicrobials and culture-negative	Urine and urine-measuring devices are sources of infection, especially if the patient (or any nearby patients) has indwelling urinary catheter. In outbreaks, cohorting of inpatients and colonized patients may be indicated if private rooms are not available.
Pneumonia Bacterial not listed elsewhere (including gram-negative bacterial)	No	No	No	No	Respiratory secretions may be		

(continued)

Table II-11. **Disease-specific Isolation Precautions** * (continued)

Disease	Private Room?	Precautions Indicated Masks?	Precautions Indicated Gowns?	Precautions Indicated Gloves?	Infective Material	Apply Precautions How Long?	Comments
Chlamydia	No	No	No	Yes for touching infective material	Respiratory secretions	Duration of illness	
Viral (see also specific etiologic agents) Adults	No	No	No	No	Respiratory secretions may be		
Viral Infants and young children	Yes	No	Yes if soiling is likely	No	Respiratory secretions	Duration of illness	Viral pneumonia may be caused by various eitologic agents, such as parainfluenza viruses, influenza viruses, and, particularly, respiratory syncytial virus, in children less than 5 years old (Committee on Infectious Diseases, American Academy of Pediatrics, 1982 Red Book); therefore, precautions to prevent their spread are generally indicated. Maintain precautions indicated for the etiology that is most likely.
Etiology unknown							
Fungal	No	No	No	No			

(continued)

Haemophilus influenzae							
Adults	No	No	No	No	Respiratory secretions may be		
Infants and children (any age)	Yes	Yes for those close to patient	No	No	Respiratory secretions	For 24 hours after start of effective therapy	
Legionella	No	No	No	No	Respiratory secretions may be		
Meningococcal	Yes	Yes for those close to patient	No	No	Respiratory secretions	For 24 hours after start of effective therapy	
Mycoplasma (primary atypical pneumonia, Eaton agent pneumonia)	No	No	No	No	Respiratory secretions may be		A private room may be useful for children
Pneumococcal	No	No	No	No	Respiratory secretions may be for 24 hours after start of effective therapy		
Pneumocystis carinii	No	No	No	No	Respiratory secretions		
Staphylococcus aureus	Yes	Yes for those close to patient	Yes if soiling is likely	Yes for touching infective material	Respiratory secretions	For 48 hours after start of effective therapy	

(continued)

Table II-11. **Disease-specific Isolation Precautions*** (continued)

Disease	Precautions Indicated						Apply Precautions How Long?	Comments
	Private Room?	Masks?	Gowns?	Gloves?	Infective Material			
Streptococcus, group A	Yes	Yes for those close to patient	Yes if soiling is likely	Yes for touching infective material	Respiratory secretions		For 24 hours after start of effective therapy	A private room is especially important for children.
Tuberculosis								
Extrapulmonary, draining lesion (including scrofula)	No	No	Yes if soiling is likely	Yes for touching infective material	Pus		Duration of drainage	
Extrapulmonary, meningitis	No	No	No	No				
Pulmonary, confirmed or suspected (sputum smear is positive or chest x-ray appearance strongly suggests current [active] TB, for example, a cavitary lesion	Yes with special ventilation	Yes if patient is coughing and does not reliably cover mouth	Yes if gross contamination of clothing is likely	No	Airborne droplet nuclei		In most instances the duration of isolation precautions can be guided by clinical response and a reduction in numbers of TB or-	Prompt use of effective antituberculous drugs is the most effective means of limiting transmission. Gowns are not important because TB is rarely spread by fomites, although gowns are indicated to prevent gross contamination of clothing. For more detailed guidelines refer to

(continued)

is found), or laryngeal disease.							ganisms on sputum smear. Usually this occurs within 2–3 weeks after chemotherapy is begun. When the patient is likely to be infected with isoniazid-resistant organisms, apply precautions until patient is improving and sputum smear is negative for TB organisms.	"Guidelines for Prevention of TB Transmission in Hospitals" (1982), Tuberculosis Control Division, Center for Prevention Services, Centers for Disease Control, Atlanta, GA (HHS Publication No. [CDC] 82-8371) and CDC Guideline for Infection Control in Hospital Personnel. In general, infants and young children do not require isolation precautions because they rarely cough and their bronchial secretions contain few TB organisms compared to adults with pulmonary TB.
Wound infections Major	Yes	No	Yes if soiling is likely	Yes for touching infective material	Pus	Duration of illness	Major = draining and not covered by dressing or dressing does not adequately contain the pus.

(continued)

Table II-11. **Disease-specific Isolation Precautions*** *(continued)*

Disease	Precautions Indicated				Infective Material	Apply Precautions How Long?	Comments
	Private Room?	Masks?	Gowns?	Gloves?			
Minor or limited	No	No	Yes if soiling is likely	Yes for touching infective material	Pus	Duration of illness	Minor or limited = dressing covers and adequately contains the pus, or infected area is very small, such as a stitch abscess.

(Source: U.S. Public Health Service, Centers for Disease Control)

*Universal Infection Precautions must be utilized with blood and body fluids from all patients. The above table summarizes the specific precautions for diagnosed infections.

†The following multiply-resistant organisms are included:
Gram-negative bacilli resistant to all aminoglycosides that are tested. (In general, such organisms should be resistant to gentamicin, tobramycin, and amikacin for these special precautions to be indicated.)
Staphylococcus aureus resistant to methicillin (or nafcillin or oxacillin if they are used instead of methicillin for testing).
Pneumococcus resistant to penicillin.
Haemophilus influenzae resistant to ampicillin (beta-lactamase positive) and chloramphenicol.
Other resistant bacteria may be included if they are judged by the infection control team to be of special clinical and epidemiologic significance.

‡Colonization may involve more than 1 site.

Potential for Infection Transmission Related to **Lack of Knowledge of Reducing the Risk of Transmitting the AIDS Virus**

Focus Assessment Criteria

Subjective Data

Individual states that he is fearful of contracting AIDS

Objective Data

1. The person reports
   - Not using preventive methods
   - High-risk sexual behaviors
2. The person is a member of a high-risk group (homosexual, bisexual, prostitute, intravenous drug user, multiple sexual partners, or other)

Outcome Criteria

- The person will describe the causes of AIDS and situations/factors contributing to its transmission.
- The person will relate practices that reduce the transmission of the AIDS virus sexually.
- The person will describe how to disinfect equipment.

Interventions

A. Identify susceptible host individual

   Homosexuals
   Bisexuals
   Intravenous drug users
   Prostitutes
   Hemophiliacs
   Human immunodeficiency virus (HIV)–positive individuals
   Multiple sexual partners

B. Counsel susceptible host individuals to be tested for AIDS

C. Discuss the mode of transmission of the virus in semen or vaginal fluids and blood (Source: Understanding AIDS)

   Vaginal, anal, or oral sex with susceptible host individuals
   Unprotected sex with infected person
   Sharing drug needles and syringes

D. Prevent the transfer of virus
  1. Abstain from sexual activity
  2. Engage in sexual activity with one mutually, faithful, uninfected partner
  3. Avoidance of intravenous drug (street) use

E. Reduce the risk of transmission of AIDS with susceptible host individuals
  1. Explain low-risk sexual behaviors
      Mutual masturbation
      Massage
      Vaginal intercourse with condom
  2. Explain the risk of ejaculate contact with broken skin or mucous membranes (oral, anal)
  3. Teach to use condoms of latex rubber, not "natural membrane" condoms; teach appropriate storage to preserve latex
  4. Explain the need to use water-based lubricants to reduce prophylactic breaks. Avoid petroleum-based lubricants, which dissolve latex
  5. Explain that a condom with a spermicide may provide additional protection by decreasing the number of viable HIV particles

F. Teach how to disinfect equipment possibly contaminated with the AIDS virus at home (needles, syringes, sex toys)
  1. Wash under running water
  2. Fill or wash with household bleach
  3. Rinse well with water

G. Provide facts to dispel the myths regarding AIDS transmission
  1. The AIDS virus is not transmitted by mosquitoes, swimming pools, clothes, eating utensils, telephones, toilet seats, or close contact (at work, school, etc.)
  2. Saliva, sweat, tears, urine, and feces do not transmit the AIDS virus
  3. Donating blood cannot transmit the AIDS virus.
  4. Blood for transfusions is tested to substantially reduce the risk of contracting the AIDS virus.

H. Initiate health teaching and referrals as indicated
  1. Refer to infection control practitioners
  2. Provide with AIDS hot line (1-800-342-AIDS) for more information
  3. Emphasize the need to be careful about the person you become sexually involved with (past sexual partners, experimented with drugs)
  4. Provide the community and schools with the facts regarding the transmission of AIDS and dispel myths

References/Bibliography

Books and Articles

Axnick K, Yarbrough M (eds): Infection Control: An Integrated Approach. St Louis, CV Mosby, 1984

Barrick B: The homosexual client with AIDS and the intravenous drug user with AIDS. In Keating S, Kelman G: Home Health Care Nursing, pp 249–269. Philadelphia, JB Lippincott, 1988

Bennett JV, Brachman PS (eds): Hospital Infections. Boston, Little, Brown & Co, 1979

Centers for Disease Control. Human immunodeficiency virus infection in the United States: A review of current knowledge. MMWR 36(Suppl 5–6), 1987

Garner JS, Simmons BP: Guidelines for isolation precautions in hospitals, CDC Guidelines. Infect Control 4(4):245–375, 1983

Resources for the Consumer

Literature
Available through county health departments (all major communicable diseases)
Understanding AIDS. HHS Publication No. (CDC) HHS-88-8404
Surgeon General
Association for Practitioners in Infection Control (APIC, Mundelein, Illinois)

Organizations
American Lung Association

Injury, Potential for

Related to **Sensory or Motor Deficits**
Related to **Lack of Awareness of Environmental Hazards**
Related to **Maturational Age of Hospitalized Child**
Related to **Vertigo Secondary to Orthostatic Hypotension**

Aspiration, Potential for

Related to **(Specify)**

Poisoning, Potential for

Suffocation, Potential for

Trauma, Potential for

Definitions

Potential for injury: The state in which an individual is at risk for harm because of a perceptual or physiological deficit, a lack of awareness of hazards, or maturational age.

Potential for aspiration: The state in which an individual is at risk for entry of secretions, solids, or fluids into the tracheobronchial passages.

472

Potential for poisoning: The state in which an individual is at high risk of accidental exposure to or ingestion of drugs or dangerous substances.

Potential for suffocation: The state in which an individual is at risk for smothering and asphyxiation.

Potential for trauma: The state in which an individual is at high risk of accidental tissue injury (*e.g.,* wound, burns, fracture)

> **Author's Note:** This diagnostic category has four subcategories—Potential for Aspiration, Poisoning, Suffocation, and Trauma. The interventions to prevent poisoning, suffocation, and trauma are included under the general category *Potential for Injury.* Should the nurse choose to isolate interventions only for prevention of poisoning, suffocation, or trauma, then the diagnostic category *Potential for Poisoning, Potential for Suffocation,* or *Potential for Trauma* would be useful.

Defining Characteristics

Presence of risk factor (*e.g.*)

Evidence of environmental hazards*	History of accidents
Lack of knowledge of environmental hazards	Impaired mobility
	Sensory deficits
Lack of knowledge of safety precautions	

Etiological, Contributing, Risk Factors

Pathophysiological

Altered cerebral function
  Tissue hypoxia
  Post trauma
  Vertigo

Syncope
Confusion

Altered mobility
  Unsteady gait

Loss of limb

Impaired sensory function
  Vision
  Hearing

Thermal/touch
Smell

Pain
Fatigue
Orthostatic hypotension
Vertebrobasilar insufficiency
Cervical spondylosis
Subclavian steal
Vestibular disorders
Carotid sinus syncope
Seizures
Hypoglycemia
Electrolyte imbalance
Amputation

* See Etiological, Contributing, Risk Factors, and Focus Assessment Criteria for specific hazards.

Arthritis
Cerebral vascular accident
Parkinsonism
Congestive heart failure
Dysrhythmias
Depression

Treatment-related

Medications
    Sedatives
    Vasodilators
    Antihypertensives
Casts/crutches, canes, walkers

Hypoglycemics
Diuretics
Phenothiazines

Situational (personal, environmental)

Decrease or loss of short-term memory
Dehydration (*e.g.,* in summer)
Prolonged bed rest
Stress
Vasovagal reflex
Faulty judgment
Alcohol
Poisons (plants, toxic chemicals)
Household hazards
    Unsafe walkways
    Unsafe toys
Automotive hazards
    Lack of use of seat belts
        or child seats
Fire hazards
    Smoking in bed
    Gas leaks

Faulty electric wires
Improperly stored poisons

Mechanically unsafe vehicle

Improperly stored petroleum
    products

Unfamiliar setting (hospital, nursing home)
Improper footwear
Inattentive caretaker
Improper use of aids (crutches, canes, walkers, wheelchairs)
Environmental hazards (home, school, hospital)
History of accidents

Maturational

Infant/child
    High risk for maturational age
    Suffocation hazards (improper crib, pillow in crib, plastic bags, unattended in
        water—bath, pool, choking on toys, food)
    Improper use of bicycles, kitchen utensils/appliances, sports equipment, lawn equip-
        ment
    Poison (plants, cleaning agents, medications)
    Fire (matches, fireplace, stove)
    Falls
Adolescent: Automobile, bicycle, alcohol, drugs
Adult: Drugs, automobile, alcohol
Elderly: Motor and sensory deficits, medication (accidental overdose), cognitive deficits

Focus Assessment Criteria

This entire assessment is indicated only when the individual is at high risk for injury because of personal deficits, alterations (*e.g.,* mobility problems), or maturational age. In households without such a family member, the functional assessment of the individual can be deleted.

Subjective Data

Physical Capabilities of the individual (as reported by person or caretaker)

1. Vision
   - Adequate
   - Corrected (date of last prescription)
   - Complaints of
     - Blurriness
     - Loss of side vision
     - Difficulty in focusing
     - Inability to adjust to darkness
2. Hearing
   - Adequate
   - Use of hearing aid (condition, batteries)
   - Need to read lips
   - Inadequate
3. Thermal/tactile
   - Adequate
   - Altered sense of hot/cold
4. Mental status
   - Alert
   - Drowsy
   - Confused
   - Oriented to time, place, events
   - Cognitive stage (immature reasoning/judgment)
   - Complaints of
     - Vertigo
     - Altered sense of balance
     - Orthostatic hypotension
5. Mobility
   - Ability to ambulate
     - Around room
     - Up and down stairs
     - Around house
     - Outside house
   - Ability to travel
     - Drive car (date of last reevaluation)
     - Use public transportation
   - Devices
     - Cane
     - Wheelchair
     - Walker
     - Prosthesis
     - Condition of devices
     - Competence in their use
   - Shoes/slippers
     - Condition
     - Fit
     - Nonskid soles
   - Abilities related to developmental milestones
     - Turning over
     - Sitting
     - Standing
     - Climbing
     - Crawling
     - Walking
6. Self-care activities: ability to
   - Dress and undress
   - Groom self
   - Reach the toilet
   - Bathe self
   - Eat
7. Housekeeping activities: ability to
   - Clean
   - Launder clothes
   - Shop
   - Prepare food

8. Miscellaneous
    Drug therapy
        Type, dosage
        Labeling
    Communication
        Can write
        Use phone
    Support system/primary caregiver
        Help available from relatives,
            friends, neighbors
        History of "blackouts"

Storage
Ability to self-medicate safely

Contact emergency assistance
Can make needs known

Club and church contacts

Objective Data

Physical Capabilities of the Individual
Gait/mobility
    Steady   Unsteady   Requires aids
Cognitive processes
  Ability to communicate needs
  Ability to interact
  History of wandering (witnessed and reported by others)
  Ability to understand cause and effect
Assess for presence of
    Anger   Withdrawal
    Depression   Faulty judgment
Self-care activities: ability to
    Dress and undress   Bathe
    Groom self   Eat
    Reach toilet

Housing Assessment
Rent or own
Type (apartment, duplex, single family house)
Physical amenities
    Number of rooms for family   Lighting
        members   Water supply
    Toilet facilities   Sewage
    Heating   Garbage disposal
    Ventilation
Safety
  Adaptations that may need to be made
    Replace nonsturdy furniture
    Gates for stairs
    Better communication facilities (telephone)
    Easier passage from room to room and into and out of house
    Bathroom safety (grab bar, bath bench, nonskid floors)
  Walkways (inside and outside)
    Sidewalks (uneven, broken)
    Stairs (inside and outside)
        Broken steps   Lighting
        No hand rails   Protection for children
    Halls
        Cluttered   Poor lighting

Electrical considerations
    Absence of outlet covers
    Cords frayed and unanchored
    Outlets overloaded; accessible to children; near water
    Switches too far from bedside
Lighting
    Adequate or inadequate
    At night; and outdoors
    To bathroom at night
Floors
    Even or uneven
    Highly polished
    Rugs not anchored
Kitchen
    Pot handles not turned inward
    Stove (grease or flammable objects on stove)
    Refrigerator (improperly stored food; inadequate temperatures)
Toxic substances
    Stored in food containers, not properly labeled and accessible to children
    Medications kept beyond date of expiration
    Poisonous household plants
Fire protection
    Matches/lighters accessible to children
    No fire extinguishers
    Improper storage of corrosives, combustibles
    Lack of furnace maintenance
    No fire escape plan, no fire extinguishers
    Emergency telephone numbers not accessible (firehouse, police)
Hazards for children in nursery
    Cribs near drapery cords
    Cribs with wide slat openings
    Plastic bags
    Pillows in crib
    Space between mattress and crib rails
    Unattended without crib rails up
    Unattended on changing table
    Pacifier hung around infant's neck
    A propped bottle placed in infant's crib
    Toys with pointed edges, removable parts
Hazards for children in household
    Accessible purses with medications, lighters, matches
    Objects with lead paint
    Poisonous plants (see Table II-12 for specific plants)
    Open windows without screens or loose screens
    Plastic bags
    Furniture with glass or sharp corners
    Open doorways, stairways
Outdoor hazards for children
    Porches without rails
    Play area without fence
    Backyard pools

Table II-12. **Poisonous Substances Around the House**

Drugs

Aspirin	Cough medicines	Laxatives
Tranquilizers	Vitamins	Oral contraceptives
Barbiturates		

Petroleum Products

Cleaning Agents

Soaps and polishes	Disinfectants	Drain cleaners

Poisonous Plants

Amaryllis	Holly	Oleander
Azalea	Iris	Poinsettia
Baneberry	Jack-in-the-pulpit	Poison hemlock
Belladonna	Jerusalem cherry	Poison ivy
Bittersweet	Jimsonweed	Pokeweed
Bloodroot	Lily of the valley	Potato leaves
Castor-bean plant	Marijuana	Rhododendron
Climbing nightshade	Mistletoe	Rhubarb leaves
Daffodil	Morning glory	Tomato leaves
Dieffenbachia	Mountain laurel	Wisteria
Foxglove	Mushrooms	Yew

Miscellaneous

Baby powder	Cosmetics	Lead paint

Domestic/wild animals
Poisonous plants
Fall assessment
See Figure II-3.

Principles and Rationale for Nursing Care

General

1. There is an increased incidence of injuries in the confused elderly. Confusion in the aged can result from
   Toxic effects of drugs
   Sensory overload (too many details in a new situation)
   Physiological states such as fatigue or elimination problems (*e.g.*, constipation or a full bladder) or pain
   Sensoriperceptual problems
   Hypoxia
2. Dangerous drugs and products that are accessible to children and confused persons can result in accidental poisoning.
3. Accidents occur more frequently
   During the initial period of hospitalization and between the hours of 6 and 9 PM
   During peak activity periods (mealtime, playtime)
   In unfamiliar surroundings
   With inadequate lighting
   At holidays
   On vacations
   During home repairs

1. Name: 2. D.O.B.:   3. Sex:
4. Date: 5. Day of week: 6. Time of day:
7. Diagnoses:
8. Witnessed by staff: ( ) yes   ( ) no
9. Location of fall: ( ) Room   ( ) BR   ( ) DR   ( ) Lounge
                ( ) outdoors   ( ) shower   ( ) hallway   ( ) other
10. Vital signs: BP _____   P _____   R _____   T _____
             Orthostatic BP: lying _____,   standing _____
11. Description of fall (if applicable):
     ( ) from bed, side rails ( ) up, ( ) down
     ( ) getting in and out of bed
     ( ) from wheelchair
     ( ) ambulatory: ( ) assisted, ( ) unassisted
     ( ) tub, shower
     ( ) found on floor, wet floor ( ) yes, ( ) no
     ( ) restraints ordered: ( ) yes, ( ) no
         In place? ( ) yes, ( ) no
     ( ) from stretcher
     ( ) assistive devices: ( ) yes, ( ) no
         ( ) wheelchair, ( ) walker, ( ) cane
     ( ) environmental hazard identified? Describe:
12. Patient's account of fall:
13. Nurse's account of fall:
14. Patient's mental status prior to fall (baseline):
15. Patient's mental status at time of fall: ( ) alert, ( ) disoriented, ( ) confused,
         ( ) sedated, ( ) other _____
16. Type of injury: ( ) laceration, ( ) hematoma, ( ) burn, ( ) abrasion, ( ) sprain,
         ( ) fracture, ( ) other _____
17. Was the patient experiencing any of the following at the time of the fall:
     ( ) acute confusion
     ( ) difficulty with ambulation
     ( ) bowel or bladder urgency
     ( ) emotional upset, anger, or agitation
     ( ) medically unstable at time of fall
     ( ) lightheadedness
     ( ) palpitations
     ( ) chest pain
     ( ) shortness of breath
     ( ) one-side weakness
18. After the fall, did the patient:
     Lose consciousness ( ) yes, ( ) no
     Lose bladder/bowel control ( ) yes, ( ) no
19. Previous falls: ( ) yes, ( ) no
     No. during past 6 months _____
     No. resulting in injury _____
20. Number of different medications patient has taken during the last 24 hours, including
     prns: _____.
21. Medication categories:
     ( ) cardiac meds
     ( ) diuretic or antihypertensive
     ( ) neuroleptic (sedative, hypnotic, antidepressant, psychotropic, antianxiety)
     ( ) analgesic
     ( ) laxative or stool softener
22. What measures can be taken to prevent recurrence:
23. Postinjury care given:
24. Treatment plan:

Fig. II-3 Fall assessment. (Data from Hernandez and Miller, 1986; Barbieri, 1983; Tideiksaar, 1984; Schulman and Acquaviva, 1987)

4. Seventy percent of all fatal falls occur in people 65 years of age and over (National Safety Council).
5. The highest risk for falls occurs in people who are confused or agitated.
6. Persons over 60 usually need twice as much light to perform a task as a 20-year-old.
7. Visual difficulty because of glare is often responsible for falls in the aged, who have an increased susceptibility to glare. Incandescent (nonfluorescent) lighting produces less glare and therefore provides better illumination for the aged.
8. Color contrast between the object and the background increases visualization (*e.g.*, white against black).
9. Fasting for diagnostic tests causes dehydration and weakness that contribute to accidents.
10. Falls can result when urinary urgency and frequency cause a person to rush to the bathroom.
11. Some common drugs contributing to postural hypotension are:

Diuretics	Antihistamines
Pheothiazines	Alcohol
Antidepressants	Levodopa
Barbiturates	Diazepam

12. Table II-12 lists common sources of poisoning in the home.

Children

1. Accidents rank number one as the cause of death and injury for children under the age of 19.
2. Mechanical suffocation is the most frequent accident for infants under 1 year of age.
3. Accidental poisoning is the major cause of death in children 1 to 5 years old (see Table II-12).
4. In each stage of development, a child is prone to a specific type of accident.
    Neonatal: motor vehicle accidents (lack of infant seat)
    1 month: falls (from rolling)
    2 months: burns from high water temperature   ⎫ motor vehicle
    4 to 6 months: walking injuries, electrical burns   ⎬ accidents
    9 to 12 months: house injuries (sharp objects, poisons, unsafe toys)
    1 to 3 years: playground injuries, tricycles, burns and poisoning   ⎭ mechanical suffocation
    3 to 5 years: motor vehicles, falls
    School age: fire, water, motor vehicles, bicycles, playground equipment, animal bites
    Adolescent: motor bikes, bicycles (risk-taking), substance abuse
5. Traditional lap belts should be worn only by children over 40 or 50 pounds, and the shoulder belt should not be used for children weighing less than 55 pounds because of the danger of strangulation.
6. Children should be taught early (when 2 years old) and constantly reminded about rules regarding streets, playground equipment, fires, water (pools, bathtubs), animals, strangers.
7. Seven hundred thirty-eight children drowned in 1982 and 3,000 children experienced near-drowning, with one third left with neurologic deficits; 68,000 persons had nonsubmersion accidents in and around swimming pools. (Baxter)
8. Sixty-eight percent of the near-drowning accidents take place while a parent is supervising the child, resulting from a momentary lapse of attention. (Baxter)
9. Effective swimming depends on intellectual as well as physical maturity. Organized

swimming lessons may give parents a false sense of security that their child "can swim." (Baxter)

10. Swimming programs that use total submersion put an infant at risk for water intoxication, hypothermia, and bacterial infections. In addition, they may learn to fear the water. (Brill)

Blood Pressure

1. Blood pressure (necessary for tissue perfusion) is dependent upon two factors: the force of the flow of blood (cardiac output), and the diameter of the blood vessel.
2. Blood pressure is affected by the sympathetic and parasympathetic nervous systems. The *sympathetic nervous system increases blood pressure* by increasing heart rate and ventricular contraction (thereby increasing cardiac output and increasing the force of blood flow) and by controlling the diameter of the arterioles and resistance of blood vessels (*i.e.,* blood vessel constriction). The *parasympathetic nervous system decreases blood pressure* by relaxation of the vessel walls and by vagal stimulation, causing a decreased heart rate (thereby decreasing cardiac output and decreasing the force of blood flow).
3. Blood pressure is dependent upon adequate circulating blood volume (*i.e.,* dehydration predisposes one to hypotension).
4. Constricted vessels cause a rise in blood pressure, while dilated vessels cause a drop in blood pressure.
5. *Systolic blood pressure* is dependent upon cardiac stroke volume (pressure within the vessels while the heart is contracting).
6. *Diastolic blood pressure* is dependent upon the condition of the vessels while the heart is at rest (vessel resistance).
7. *Arterial* blood flow is enhanced by a *dependent* position and inhibited by an *elevated* position (gravity pulls blood downward, away from the heart).
8. *Venous* blood flow is enhanced by an *elevated* position and inhibited by a *dependent* position (gravity pulls blood downward, toward the heart).

Hypotension

1. Hypotension causes impaired tissue perfusion of all body organs.
2. The length of time that tissue can survive without adequate blood supply (perfusion) is determined by the tissue type and the metabolic needs of the cell: the heart, brain, lungs, and kidneys may suffer the most catastrophic results, while extremities may tolerate hypotension for quite a long time without problems.
3. Metabolic needs are reduced by hypothermia and increased by hyperthermia (fever).
4. Decreased tissue perfusion (hypotension) causes cellular hypoxia, resulting in ischemia, cellular swelling, and eventually cellular death.
5. Orthostatic hypotension (a sudden drop in blood pressure of 22 mm Hg or more when going from a lying or sitting position to a standing position) is frequently seen associated with
   Decreased blood volume or dehydration
   Prolonged immobility or bedrest
   Aging
   Impaired skeletal muscle function
   Severe varicose veins
   Medications (diuretics, antihypertensives, vasodilators, antipsychotics, and anti-Parkinsonian drugs)
6. Prolonged bed rest causes skeletal muscle weakness and decreased venous tone, predisposing the individual to orthostatic hypotension.

7. Orthostatic drop may be greater in the morning because blood volume tends to decrease during the night.

High-risk Elderly

1. Falls occur with greater frequency in the elderly, and the mortality, dysfunction, disability, and need for medical services that result are greater than in younger age groups. Unintentional injury, a category including falls, motor vehicle accidents, and burns, is the seventh leading cause of death in the elderly, and the incidence of falls represents over 60% of that category.
2. Goals for prevention and management of falls focus on reducing the likelihood of falls by reducing environmental hazards, strengthening individual competence to resist falls and fall-related injury, and providing postfall injury care. Although determining the cause of falls in the elderly is often difficult, falls are believed to be associated with a breakdown in neurological, visual, and vestibular mechanisms, decreasing the individual's ability to maintain an upright posture when balance is threatened. Certain factors such as medications and disease patterns further compromise homeostatic mechanisms. In addition, certain variables may increase the likelihood of sustaining injury as a result of a fall, such as osteoporosis and debilitating disease conditions.
3. A fall-free existence is not always possible for some individuals. Increased independence and mobility may be an important and valuable trade-off for an increased risk of falling. Collaboration among the individual, family, and team members helps arrive at the decision of a less restricted environment.

Potential for Injury
Related to Sensory or Motor Deficits

Assessment

Subjective Data

The person reports
　　Past history of falls and injuries
　　　　Decreased or absent vision
　　　　Decreased or absent hearing
　　　　Decreased or absent thermal
　　　　　perception

Limited movement
Pain
Vertigo

Objective Data

　　Inflamed joints
　　Contractures
　　Skeletal deformities
　　Unsteady gait
　　Paralysis
　　Weakness

Muscle spasms
Crutches
Walker, cane
Prosthesis
Evidence of past injuries
　(bruises, burn marks)

Outcome Criteria

The person will
- Identify factors that increase the potential for injury
- Relate an intent to utilize safety measures to prevent injury (*e.g.,* remove throw rugs or anchor them)
- Relate an intent to practice selected prevention measures (*e.g.,* wear sunglasses to reduce glare)
- Increase his daily activity, if feasible

Interventions

A. Assess for the presence of causative or contributing factors

Unfamiliar surroundings
Impaired vision
 Altered spatial judgment
 Blurred vision
 Diplopia
 Blind spots
 Cataracts
 Altered peripheral vision
 Hemianopia (loss of half the visual field)
 Increased susceptibility to visual glare
 Decreased ability to distinguish object from background
Decreased hearing acuity
Decreased tactile sensitivity (touch)
Orthostatic hypotension
Hypoglycemia
 Unstable gait
 Pain
 Fatigue
 Improper shoes or slippers
 Improper use of crutches, canes, walkers
 Joint immobility
 Side-effects of medication (*e.g.,* tranquilizers, diuretics)
 Hazardous environmental factors

B. Reduce or eliminate causative or contributing factors if possible

1. Unfamiliar surroundings
   - Orient each new admission to surroundings, explain the call system, and assess the person's ability to use it
   - Closely supervise the person during the first few nights to assess safety
   - Utilize night light
   - Encourage the person to request assistance during the night
   - Teach the person about side-effects of certain drugs (*e.g.,* dizziness, fatigue)
   - Keep bed at lowest level during the night
2. Impaired vision
   a. Provide safe illumination or teach person to
      - Provide adequate lighting in all rooms, with soft light at night

- Have light switch easily accessible, next to bed
- Provide background light that is soft

   b. Teach person to reduce glare
- Avoid all glossy surfaces (*e.g.,* glass, highly polished floors)
- Use diffuse light rather than direct light; use shades that darken the room
- Turn head away when switching on a bright light
- Wear sunglasses or hats with brims, or carry umbrellas, to reduce glare outside
- Avoid looking directly at bright lights (*e.g.,* headlights)

   c. Teach person or family to provide sufficient color contrast for visual discrimination
- Color-code edges of steps (*e.g.,* with colored tape)
- Avoid white walls, dishes, counters
- Avoid clear glasses (*i.e.,* use smoked glass)
- Choose objects colored black on white (*e.g.,* black phone)
- Avoid colors that merge (*e.g.,* beige switches on beige walls)
- Paint doorknobs bright colors

3. Decreased tactile sensitivity

   a. Teach preventive measures
- Assess temperature of bath water and heating pads prior to use
- Use bath thermometers
- Assess extremities daily for undetected injuries
- Keep feet warm and dry and skin softened with emollient lotion (lanolin, mineral oil)

   b. See *Altered Tissue Perfusion: Peripheral* for additional interventions

4. Decreased hearing acuity
- Determine if the person has had his hearing evaluated professionally
- Assist him in making a decision regarding the use or type of hearing aid if indicated
- Teach him, when driving, to leave car window partially open to allow warning signals to be heard (*e.g.,* sirens) and set air conditioner, heater, or radio low so outside noises can be heard

5. Orthostatic hypotension
- See *Potential for Injury Related to Vertigo Secondary to Orthostatic Hypotension* for additional interventions

6. Unstable gait

   a. Crutches
- Teach exercises to strengthen arm and shoulder muscles to facilitate use of crutches; use weights and parallel bars
- Measure and fit crutches to each person (2 to 3 inches between top of crutch and armpit); improper length of crutches may cause nerve damage or falls
- Instruct person to wear shoes that fit properly and have nonskid soles
- Assess ability to walk and climb up and down stairs
- Consult with physical therapist for proper gait training

   b. Canes
- Teach person to hold cane in hand opposite affected leg and move cane and impaired limb together
- Cane should be proper length to allow person to extend elbow and bear weight on hand
- Cane should be fitted with rubber tip
- Consult with physical therapist for proper gait training

   c. Walkers
- Teach person exercises to strengthen triceps muscles used in proper crutch walking
- See that floors are clean and dry and free of obstacles and that rugs are anchored
- Instruct person to wear properly fitted shoes with nonslip soles
- Consult with physical therapist for proper gait training

   d. Prosthesis
- Teach person to bathe and inspect stump daily
- Instruct person to put on prosthesis soon after rising to minimize stump swelling
- Prepare person for crutch walking with triceps exercises using weights and parallel bars
- Consult with physical therapist for proper gait training

7. Side-effects of medications
- Assess for the presence of side-effects of drugs that may cause vertigo

Hypotension	Vasodilation
Sedation	Vasoconstriction
Hypokalemia	

8. Hazardous environmental factors

   a. Teach person to
- Eliminate throw rugs, litter, and highly polished floors
- Provide nonslip surfaces in bathtub or shower by applying commercially available traction tapes
- Provide hand grips in bathroom
- Provide railings in hallways and on stairs
- Remove protruding objects (*e.g.,* coat hooks, shelves, light fixtures) from stairway walls

   b. Instruct staff to
- Keep side rails on bed in place and bed at the lowest position when person is left unattended
- Keep bed at lowest position with wheels locked when stationary
- Teach person in wheelchair to lock and unlock wheels
- Ensure that persons' shoes or slippers have nonskid soles

C. Describe and document falls

1. Refer to Focus Assessment (Fig. II-3) for fall assessment
2. Document the results of the assessment.

D. Initiate health teaching and referrals as indicated

1. Teach measures to prevent auto accidents
- Frequently reevaluate ability to drive vehicles
- Wear good-quality sunglasses (gray or green) to reduce glare
- Keep windshields clean and wipers in good condition
- Place mirrors on both sides of car
- Stop periodically to stretch and rest eyes
- Know the effects of medications on driving ability
- Do not smoke while driving or drive after drinking

2. Teach measures to prevent pedestrian accidents
- Allow enough time to cross streets
- Wear garments that reflect light (beige, white) at night

- Wait to cross on the sidewalk, not the street
- Look both ways
- Do not rely solely on green traffic lights to provide safe crossing (right turn on red light may be legal, or driver may disobey traffic regulations)

3. Teach measures to prevent burns
- Equip home with smoke alarm system and check its function each month
- Have a hand fire extinguisher
- Set thermostats for water heater to provide warm but not scalding water
- Use baking soda or a lid cover to smother a kitchen grease fire
- Do not wear loose-fitting clothing (*e.g.,* robes, nightgowns) when cooking
- Do not smoke when sleepy
- Ensure that portable heaters are safely used
- See *Potential for Injury Related to Lack of Awareness of Environmental Hazards* for additional safety measures

4. Refer individuals with motor or sensory deficits for assistance in identifying environmental hazards
- Local fire company
- Community nursing agency
- Accident-prevention information (see References/Bibliography)

5. Discuss the benefits of a walking program to increase circulation if permissible; instruct to
- Rest 10 to 15 minutes before walking
- Start slowly (10 minutes)
- Increase time gradually
- Refrain from drinking caffeine products (coffee, tea, chocolate, cola) 2 to 3 hours before walking
- Wait 2 hours after meals to walk
- Expect some muscle soreness; reduce activity if pain or breathlessness occur

6. Assist person and family to evaluate environmental hazards
7. Refer person to public health or visiting nurse for home visit
8. Refer person to physical therapist for evaluation of gait

Potential for Injury
Related to Lack of Awareness of Environmental Hazards

Assessment

Subjective Data
The person reports
    Past history of accidents

Objective Data
Presence of hazards (see Focus Assessment Criteria)

Outcome Criteria

The person or family will
- Identify potentially hazardous factors in the environment
- Report safe practices in the home
- Teach children safety habits

Interventions

A. Identify situations that contribute to accidents

Unfamiliar setting (homes of others, hotels)
Children
Peak activity periods (during meal preparation, holidays)
New equipment (bicycle, chain saw, lawn mower, snow blower)
Lack of awareness of or disregard for environmental hazards

1. Unfamiliar setting
   - Instruct to leave a light on for access to bathroom during night
   - With small children, instruct parents to
     a. Inspect the area (inside and outside) for hazards before allowing child to play
     b. Expect the child to explore hidden areas
     c. Have infants sleep on floor on padding rather than in beds without rails
2. Children
   - Teach parents to expect frequent changes in infants' and children's ability and to take precautions (*e.g.*, infant who suddenly rolls over for the first time might be on a changing table unattended)
   - Discuss with parents the necessity of constant monitoring of small children
   - Provide parents with information to assist them in selecting a babysitter
     a. Determine previous experiences and knowledge of emergency measures
     b. Observe the interaction of the sitter with the child (*e.g.*, pick up the sitter one-half hour before you are ready to leave)
   - Teach parents to expect children to mimic them, and to teach children what they can do with or without supervision
     a. Tell the child to ask you before attempting a new task
     b. Don't take pills in front of children
   - Explain and expect compliance with certain rules (depending on age) regarding

Streets	Fire
Playground equipment	Animals
Water (pools, bathtubs)	Strangers
Bicycles	

   - Role-play with children to assess understanding of the problem

     "You are walking home from school and a strange man pulls up in a car near you. What do you do?"

     "While walking past a barbecue, your dress catches on fire. What do you do?"
3. Peak activity periods
   - Provide the child with a special distraction (*e.g.*, clay) while preparing meal
   - Place the child in a playpen to provide a safe place that does not require close supervision
   - Assess the safety of holiday decorations prior to use

     Christmas trees

Fire or electrical hazard   Lighted candles
Poorly anchored   Ceramic pieces

4. New equipment
   - Teach to read directions completely before using a new appliance or a piece of equipment
   - Determine the limitations of the equipment
   - Unplug and turn off any appliance that is not functioning before examining (*e.g.,* lawn mower, snow blower, electric mixer)
   - Determine that a new bicycle is the correct size for the child before allowing unrestricted riding
   - Examine new toys for removable parts and chemical and electrical hazards before allowing child to play
5. Lack of awareness of environmental hazards
   - Teach to avoid unsafe practices and prevent injury
     a. Automobiles
        Driving a mechanically unsafe vehicle
        Not using or misusing seat restraints
        Driving after partaking of alcohol or drugs
        Driving with unrestrained babies and children in the car
        Driving at excessive speeds
        Driving without necessary visual aids
        Driving with unsafe road or road crossing conditions
        Nonuse or misuse of necessary headgear for motorcyclist
        Children riding in front seat of car
        Backing up without checking location of small children
        Warming a car in a closed garage
     b. Bicycles, wagons, skateboards, and skates carrying passengers
        No reflectors or lights
        Not in single file
        Riding a too-large bicycle
        Lack of knowledge of rules of the road
        Use of skateboards or skates in heavily traveled areas
     c. Flammables
        Igniting gas leaks
        Delayed lighting of gas burner or oven
        Experimenting with chemicals or gasoline
           Unscreened fires, fireplaces, heaters
           Inadequately stored combustibles, matches, or oily rags
           Smoking in bed or near oxygen
           Highly flammable children's toys or clothing
           Playing with fireworks or gunpowder
           Playing with matches, candles, cigarettes, lighters
           Wearing of plastic aprons or flowing clothing around open flame
     d. Household
        Kitchen
           Grease waste collected on stoves
           Wearing of plastic aprons or flowing clothing around open flame
           Use of cracked glasses or dishware
           Use of improper canning, freezing, or preserving methods
           Knives stored in an uncovered fashion
           Pot handles facing front of stove

Use of thin or worn potholders or oven mitts
Stove controls on front
Bathroom
  Unlocked medicine cabinet
  Lack of grab rails in bathtub
  Lack of nonskid mats or emory strips in bathtub
  Poor lighting in bathroom and hallways
  Improper placement of electrical outlets
Chemicals and irritants
  Improperly labeled medication containers
  Medications kept in containers other than original ones
  Poor illumination at the medicine cabinet
  Improperly labeled containers of poisons and corrosive substances
  Expired medications that dangerously decompose
  Toxic substances stored in accessible areas (*e.g.,* under sink)
  Inadequately stored corrosives (*e.g.,* lye)
  Contact with intense cold
  Overexposure to sun, sunlamps, heating pads
Lighting and electrical
  Uncovered outlets
  Unanchored electrical wires
  Overloaded electrical outlets
  Overloaded fuse boxes
  Faulty electrical plugs, frayed wires, or defective electrical appliances
  Inadequate lighting over landings and stairs
  Inaccessible light switches (*e.g.,* bedside)
  Use of machinery or appliances without prior instruction
Water and pools
  Discourage use of flotation or swim aids (water wings, tubs) with
    children who can't swim
  Teach safe water behavior
    No running, pushing
    No jumping on others
    No swimming alone
    No playful screaming for help
    No diving in water less than 8 feet deep
    No swimming after meals
    No swimming during electrical storms
    Avoid excessive alcohol use
  Enclose pool
    Use a 5–5 1/2 foot fence
    Use a fence that children can't climb
    Use self-locking gates
  Remove pool cover completely
  Avoid free-floating pool covers
  Teach safe diving and sliding techniques
    Allow diving only from diving boards
    Discourage running dives
    Teach to steer upward with hands and head
    Descend pool slide sitting with feet first
  Have life-saving equipment at pool side (life preserver, rope, or hook)

Learn CPR and how to respond to accidental submersion
  - Remove from water
  - If spinal injury is suspected, immobilize on a board and apply a cervical collar
  - Clear airway of debris
  - If person is unresponsive, place on side if vomiting occurs
  - Remove wet clothes, dry and cover with blankets (including head)
  - Begin CPR and continue until help arrives

Miscellaneous

Unsupervised contact with animals and poisons in environment (plants, pool chemicals, pills)

Obstructed passageways

Unsafe window protection in home with young children

Guns or ammunition stored in unlocked fashion

Large icicles hanging from roof

Icy walkways

Glass sliding doors that look open when closed

Low-strung clothesline

Discarded or unused refrigerators or freezers without removed doors

e. Infants and children

Household

Pillows in crib

Staircases without stair gates

Crib mattresses that do not fit snugly

Cribs with slat opening to allow child's body to fall through, catching the head

Glass or sharp-edged tables

Porches and decks without railings

Poisonous plants (see Table II-12)

Furniture painted with lead paint

Unsupervised bathing

Open windows

Propped bottle in crib

Toys

Sharp edges

Easily breakable parts

Removable small pieces

Balloons

Lollipops

Pacifier around neck

Miscellaneous

Unattended in shopping cart

Unattended in car

Cribs, walkers, high chairs with movable parts that trap child (*e.g.*, springs)

B. Initiate health teaching and referrals as indicated

- Instruct parents how to "child proof" the home
- Instruct parents to keep poisons and corrosive substances in tightly closed, carefully marked containers in locked closets
- Parents should discard unused supplies of medications and keep needed medications in locked, inaccessible medicine closet

- Parents should be taught how to administer antidotes for specific toxic substances
- Parents should also have the phone number of the Poison Control Center in a convenient place
- Refer individuals to local poison control center for "Mr. Yuk" poison warning stickers and advice on emergency procedures; teach the child what a Mr. Yuk sticker means
- Instruct parents on the use of ipecac and its availability
- Assist family to evaluate environmental hazards in home; consult public health agency
- Install specially designed locks to prevent children from opening closets where combustible, corrosive, or flammable materials or medications are stored
- Instruct parents to use socket covers to prevent accidental electrical shocks to children
- Teach parents about hazards of lead paint ingestion and how to identify "pica" in a child
- Refer parents to public health department if lead paint screening is necessary
- Encourage use of child-proof caps
- Advise parents to avoid storing dangerous substances in containers ordinarily used for foods
- Refer parents to automobile club for information regarding safety car seats for children
- Refer parents to local fire department for assistance in staging home fire drills

Potential for Injury
Related to Maturational Age of Hospitalized Child

Assessment

Subjective Data

The parent (primary caregiver) reports child's unique cognitive and motor abilities
Developmental milestones the child has achieved

Objective Data

Presence of hazards (see Focus Assessment Criteria)
Evidence that child/adolescent's abilities are changing (*e.g.*, the infant may turn over for the first time in the hospital)

Outcome Criteria

The child/adolescent will be
- Free from injury from potentially hazardous factors that are identified in the hospital environment

The family will
- Reinforce and demonstrate safe practices in the hospital

Interventions

A. Protect the infant/child from injury in the hospital by controlling hazards that are age-related

Infant (1–12 months)

Ensure that the infant can be identified by an identification band and a tag on his crib.

Keep unsafe toys out of reach (*e.g.,* buttons, beads, balloons, broken toys, sharp-edged toys, other small toys).

Use restraints to prevent infant from removing catheters, eye patches, IV infusions, dressings, and feeding tubes, as needed.

Keep siderails up in locked position when child is in crib.

Fasten safety straps on infant seats, swings, highchairs, and strollers.

Do not allow bottles to be propped. The infant should be held with his head in an upright position.

Do not place pillows in crib.

Place one hand over the child while weighing, changing diapers, etc., to keep infant safe.

Do not allow infant to wear pacifier on a string around the neck.

Check bath water to make sure that the temperature is appropriate. Never leave infant alone while bathing! Support the small infant's head out of the water.

Check the temperature of formula, especially if it is heated in the microwave.

Position crib away from bedside stand, infusion pumps, etc., to prevent child from reaching unsafe objects (*i.e.,* dials on infusion pump, suction machine, electrical outlets).

Do not allow parents to smoke or drink hot beverages in infant's room.

Foods that must be chewed or are small enough to occlude the airway should not be offered (*i.e.,* nuts, popcorn, hard candy, whole hot dogs). Forks and knives are not appropriate utensils for infants.

Discard syringes, needles, med packets, plastic bags safely.

Protect with shoes or slippers the feet of the infant who is able to walk.

Transport the infant safely to other areas of the hospital (*i.e.,* x-ray, laboratory).

Remind parents to have approved car seat in their automobile to transport the child home.

Assess each unique situation for potential for injury to the infant.

Early Childhood (13 months–5 years)

Ensure that the young child is identifiable by name band and name tag on crib.

Keep siderails up in locked position when child is in crib—top and bottom compartments; use siderails on youth beds.

Monitor child at all times when eating, bathing, playing, and toileting.

Keep cleaning agents, sharp items, and plastic bags out of reach.

Secure thermometer while taking temperature (use rectal or axillary method with toddler and oral method when child is old enough not to bite down on thermometer).

Assess for loose teeth, and document on records.

Check the temperature of bath water before immersing child.

Use electric beds with extreme caution. For example, children may get their fingers caught or get under the bed and be at risk for a crushing injury.

Position crib/bed away from bedside stand, infusion pumps, etc., to prevent child from reaching unsafe objects.

Keep child safe when mobile:
> Protect child's feet with shoes or slippers when ambulating.
> Keep bathroom and closet doors firmly shut.
> Check any tubing attached to child to prevent kinking or dislodgement.
> Apply safety straps when child is in highchair, stroller or on a cart.
> Transport safely to other areas of the hospital (*i.e.*, x-ray).
> Use restraints to prevent child from removing catheters, eye patches, IV infusion, dressings, and feeding tubes, as needed.
> Place one hand over child when weighing, changing diapers, etc., to prevent falls.

Do not call medications "candy."

Do not permit the child to chew gum, eat hard candy, nuts, whole hot dogs, or fish with bones.

Set limits: Enforce and repeat to child what he can do in the hospital and to which areas he may go.

Provide with age-appropriate, safe toys (see manufacturer's guidelines.)

Do not allow parents to smoke or drink hot beverages in the child's room.

Feed the child in a quiet environment; ensure that the child is seated while eating to prevent choking.

Remind parents to have approved car seat in automobile to transport child home.

Assess each unique situation for potential for injury to the young child.

Schoolager/adolescent (6–12 years/13–18 years)

Ensure that the schoolager/adolescent can be identified by a name band and a tag on his bed. Schoolagers may claim to be someone else to joke with the nurse, not realizing the danger of this.

Assess for loose teeth and document on records.

Assess for self-care deficits and activity intolerance because the schoolager/adolescent may not ask for help when ambulating, bathing, toileting, and so forth.

Apply safety straps when transporting via cart or wheelchair.

Set limits: Enforce and reiterate to the child what he can do and to what areas he may go in the hospital.

Provide with age-appropriate activities. Supervise therapeutic play closely and do not allow child to use syringes as squirt guns.

Do not allow parents to smoke or drink hot beverages in the child's room.

Encourage child/adolescent to wear Medic Alert necklace or bracelet, if appropriate. Encourage to carry I.D. in wallet/purse.

Remind to wear seat belt in auto when discharged.

Assess each unique situation for potential for injury to the schoolager/adolescent.

Potential for Injury Related to Vertigo
Secondary to Orthostatic Hypotension

Assessment

Subjective Data

Individual reports:
- Dizziness

- Blurred vision
- Vertigo
- History of "blackouts"

Objective Data

Bracheal systolic blood pressure decreases 20 mm Hg when moving from lying to standing position

---

Outcome Criteria

The individual will
- Relate methods of preventing sudden decreases in cerebral blood flow due to orthostatism
- Demonstrate maneuvers to change position and avoid sudden drop in cerebral pressure
- Relate fewer episodes of dizziness or vertigo

Interventions

A. Identify contributing factors
- Medications
- Cardiac dysrhythmias
- Arterial stenosis or occlusion
- Hypertension or rotation of the neck
- Prolonged recumbent position
- Sudden change in position (from lying to sitting or standing)

B. Assess for orthostatic hypotension
- Take bilateral bracheal pressures with the person supine
- If the bracheal pressures are different, use the arm with the higher reading and take the blood pressure immediately after the individual stands up quickly; report differences to the physician
- Ask the individual to describe sensations

C. Discuss physiology of orthostatic hypotension with individual
- Age-related changes in vessel
- Volume of blood in lower extremities
- Sympathetic nervous system response
- Effects of prolonged bed rest

D. Teach techniques to avoid orthostatic hypotension
- Change positions slowly
- Move from lying to an upright position in stages:
  Sit up in bed
    Dangle first one leg, then the other over the side of the bed
  Allow a few minutes before going on to each step
  Gradually pull oneself from a sitting to a standing position
  Place a chair, walker, cane, or other assistive device nearby to use to steady oneself when getting out of bed

- Avoid stooping to pick something from the floor; use an assistive device available from an orthotics department or a self-help store to pick up items from the floor
- Use waist-high elastic stockings
    Place stockings on in A.M. before getting out of bed
    Avoid sitting for long periods of time
    Remove stockings when supine

E. Encourage person to increase daily activity if permissible

- Discuss the value of daily exercise (increases circulation, decreases the process of osteoporosis, increases energy levels, reduces stress, and contributes to an overall state of well-being)
    Establish an exercise program

F. Teach person precautions to avoid injury

- Discuss the potential hazards of hypotension (drinking, smoking, cooking)
- Teach person to increase fluid intake during periods of excess fluid loss (diaphoresis, exercise)
- Discuss factors that increase vasodilation (alcohol—initially followed by vaso-constriction; extreme warmth)

Potential for Aspiration

Related to **(Specify)**

Definition

Potential for aspiration: The state in which an individual is at risk for entry of secretions, solids, or fluids into the tracheobronchial passages.

Defining Characteristics

Presence of favorable conditions for aspiration (see Etiological, Contributing, and Risk Factors)

Etiological, Contributing, Risk Factors (related to's)

Pathophysiological

Reduced level of consciousness/unconsciousness
Dementias anesthesia
Seizures
Alcohol/drug-induced
Depressed cough/gag reflexes
Cerebral vascular accident
Parkinsonism
Head injury
Debilitating conditions
Paralysis
Increased intragastric pressure (decreased gastrointestinal motility, delayed gastric
emptying)
   Autonomic dysfunction
   Pregnancy
   Obesity
   Electrolyte imbalance
   Ileus
   Intestinal obstruction
   Gastro outlet syndrome
Impaired swallowing
   Achalasia   Myasthenia gravis
   Scleraderma   Guillain-Barré syndrome
   Hiatal hernia   Multiple sclerosis
   Esophageal strictures   Muscular dystrophy
Tracheoesophageal fistula
Catatonic

Treatment-related

Facial/oral surgery/trauma
Neck surgery/trauma
Wired jaws

Gastrointestinal tubes
Tracheostomy or endotracheal tubes
Enteral feedings
Anesthesia

Situational

Inability/impaired ability to elevate upper body
Alcohol use during meals

Maturational

Newborns
Premature
Cleft palate
Children (high-risk age 1–3)
Elderly
Poor dentition

Focus Assessment Criteria

Subjective Data

History of a problem with swallowing or aspiration
History of: (see pathophysiological etiologies)

Objective Data

Height and weight
Ability to swallow, chew, feed self
Neuromuscular impairment
Decreased/absent gag reflex
Decreased strength on excursion of muscles involved in mastication
Perceptual impairment
Facial paralysis
Mechanical obstruction
Edema
Tracheostomy tube
Tumor
Perceptual patterns/awareness
Level of consciousness
Condition of oropharyngeal cavity
Nasal regurgitation
Hoarseness
Aspiration
Coughing a second or two after swallowing
Dehydration
Apraxia

Principles and Rationale for Nursing Care

1. Swallowing is a complicated mechanism with three stages: voluntary, pharyngeal and esophageal.
2. The voluntary stage is the moving of the food from the palate to the pharynx.
3. The pharyngeal stage is automatic as follows:
   • soft palate is pulled up to close the posterior nares

- palatopharyngeal folds on the sides of the pharynx constrict to permit passage of properly masticated food
- epiglottis swings backward over larynx opening to prevent aspiration into the trachea
- relaxation of hypopharyngeal sphincter stretches the opening of the esophagus
- rapid peristaltic wave forces food into the upper esophagus

4. The esophageal stage moves the food from the pharynx to the stomach by peristaltic movements controlled by vagal reflexes.
5. Central nervous system depression interferes with the protective mechanism of the sphincters.
6. Nasogastric and endotracheal tubes cause incomplete closure of the esophageal sphincters.
7. Individuals with debilitating conditions who aspirate are at high risk for aspiration pneumonia.
8. The volume and characteristics of the aspirated contents influence morbidity and mortality. Food particles can cause mechanical blockage. Gastric juice erodes alveoli and capillaries and causes chemical pneumonitis.
9. Regurgitation is often silent in persons with decreased sensorium or depressed mental states.
10. Tracheostomy tubes interfere with the synchrony of the glottic closure. Inadequate cuff inflation provides a path for aspirate.
11. Increased intragastric pressure can contribute to regurgitation and aspiration. Situations that increase intragastric pressure are bolus tube feedings, obstructions,. obesity, pregnancy, and autonomic dysfunction.
12. Individuals undergoing caesarean sections are high risk for aspiration because of increased intragastric pressure.

Potential for Aspiration
Related to (Specify)

Assessment
See Defining Characteristics

Outcome Criteria

The person will
- not experience aspiration
- relate measures to prevent aspiration

Interventions

A. Assess causative or contributing factors

1. Susceptible individual
   - Reduced level of consciousness
   - Autonomic disorders

- Debilitated
- Newborns
2. Tracheostomy/endotracheal tubes
3. Gastrointestinal tubes/feedings

B. Reduces the risk of aspiration in:

1. Individuals with decreased strength, decreased sensorium, or autonomic disorders
   - Maintain a side-lying position if not contraindicated by injury
   - If the person cannot be positioned on his side, open oropharyngeal airway by lifting the mandible up and forward, with the head tilted backward (for a small infant, hyperextension of the neck may not be effective)
   - Assess for position of the tongue, assuring that it has not dropped backward, occluding the airway
   - Keep the head of the bed elevated, if not contraindicated by hypertension or injury
   - Maintain good oral hygiene: Clean teeth and use mouthwash on cotton swab; apply petroleum jelly to lips, removing encrustations gently
   - Clear secretions from mouth and throat with a tissue or gentle suction
   - Reassess frequently for presence of obstructive material in mouth and throat
   - Reevaluate frequently for good anatomic positioning
   - Maintain side-lying position after feedings
2. With tracheostomies or endotracheal tubes
   a. Inflate cuff:
      - during continuous mechanical ventilation
      - during and after eating
      - during and 1 hour after tube feedings
      - during IPPB treatments
   b. Suction q1–2 hours and p.r.n.
3. With gastrointestinal tubes and feedings
   a. Verify placement of feeding tube with air auscultation for tubes positioned via the nasogastric or nasojejunal route
   b. Aspirate for residual contents before each feeding for tubes positioned gastrically
   c. Elevate head of bed 30–45 minutes during feeding periods, and one (1) hour after to prevent reflux by use of reverse gravity
   d. Administer feeding if residual contents are less than 150 ml (intermittent)
      or
      Administer feeding if residual is not greater than 150 ml at 10–20% of hourly rate (continuous)
   e. Regulate gastric feedings using an intermittent schedule allowing periods for stomach emptying between feeding intervals
4. With newborns and premature infants with cleft lip and/or palate
   a. Position infant's head in an upright position
   b. Utilize a large soft nipple with large hole or Lamb's nipple (long, soft)
   c. The nipple hole should be large enough for the feeding to be under 30 minutes
   d. Do not position the nipple through the cleft
   e. Apply gentle counter pressure on the base of the bottle to assist the infant with tongue and palate control of the milk flow
   f. Burp frequently because of excessive air swallowing
   g. If nipple feeding is unsuccessful, use a rubber-tipped syringe to deposit the formula on the back of the tongue
5. With an elderly person with difficulties chewing and swallowing (see *Impaired Swallowing*)

C. Initiate health teaching and referrals as indicated

- Instruct person and/or family on causes and prevention of aspiration
- Have family demonstrate tube feeding technique
- Refer to community nursing agency for assistance at home
- Teach about the danger of eating when under the influence of alcohol
- Teach the Heimlich or abdominal thrust manuever to remove aspirated foreign bodies

Potential for Poisoning

Definition
Potential for poisoning: The state in which an individual is at high risk of accidental exposure to or ingestion of drugs or dangerous substances.

> **Author's Note:** This diagnostic category has four subcategories—Potential for Aspiration, Poisoning, Suffocation, and Trauma. The interventions to prevent poisoning, suffocation, and trauma are included under the general category *Potential for Injury*. Should the nurse choose to isolate interventions only for prevention of poisoning, suffocation, or trauma, then the diagnostic category *Potential for Poisoning, Potential for Suffocation,* or *Potential for Trauma* would be useful.

Defining Characteristics
Presence of risk factors (See Etiological, Contributing, Risk Factors for *Potential for Injury*)

Potential for Suffocation

Definition

Potential for suffocation: The state in which an individual is at risk for smothering and asphyxiation.

> **Author's Note:** This diagnostic category has four subcategories—Potential for Aspiration, Poisoning, Suffocation, and Trauma. The interventions to prevent poisoning, suffocation, and trauma are included under the general category *Potential for Injury*. Should the nurse choose to isolate interventions only for prevention of poisoning, suffocation, or trauma, then the diagnostic category *Potential for Poisoning, Potential for Suffocation,* or *Potential for Trauma* would be useful.

Defining Characteristics

Presence of risk factors (See Etiological, Contributing, Risk Factors for *Potential for Injury*)

Potential for Trauma

Definition

Potential for trauma: The state in which an individual is at high risk of accidental tissue injury (*e.g.,* wound, burns, fracture)

Author's Note: This diagnostic category has four subcategories—Potential for Aspiration, Poisoning, Suffocation, and Trauma. The interventions to prevent poisoning, suffocation, and trauma are included under the general category *Potential for Injury.* Should the nurse choose to isolate interventions only for prevention of poisoning, suffocation, or trauma, then the diagnostic category *Potential for Poisoning, Potential for Suffocation,* or *Potential for Trauma* would be useful.

Defining Characteristics

Presence of risk factors (See Etiological, Contributing, Risk Factors for *Potential for Injury*)

References/Bibliography

Articles

Barbiere E: Patient falls are not patient accidents. J Gerontol Nurs 9(3):164–173, 1983
Cooper S: Accidents and older adults. Geriatr Nurs 2:287–290, 1981
Hernandez M, Miller J: How to reduce falls. Geriatr Nurs 7(2):97–102, 1986
Kulikowski E: A study of accidents in a hospital. Supervisor Nurse 8(3):64–68, 1979
Lynn FH: Incidents—need they be accidents? Am J Nurs 80:1098–1101, 1980
Rauckhorst LM: Community and home assessment. J Gerontol Nurs 6:319–327, 1980
Riffle K: Falls: Kinds, causes, and prevention. Geriatr Nurs 3:165–169, 1982
Schulman B, Acquaviva T: Falls in the elderly. Nurse Pract 12(11):30, 1987
Simons RS: The occupational health nurse: Safety's overlooked resource. Occupational Health Nurse 28(2):7–12, 1980
Spellbring A et al: Improving safety for hospitalized elderly. J Gerontol Nurs 14(2):31–37, 1988
Symposium on Injuries and Injury Prevention. Pediat Clin North Am 32(1), 1985
Tideiksaar R: Fall assessment record. J Am Geriatr Soc 32(7):539, 1984
Witte N: Why the elderly fall. Am J Nurs 79:1154–1160, 1979

Child Safety

Brill J: Dispelling the myth of the drown proof child. Contemp Pediatr 4(6):30, 1987
Karp S: A 10 point program for bicycle safety. Contemp Pediatr 4(6):16, 1987
McIntire M, Angle CR: Poison control: A model for childhood safety. Pediatrician 5:180–184, 1976
Newest guidelines on pediatric CPR and first aid. Contemp Pediatr 4(6):47, 1987
Wheatley G: Introduction: Childhood accidents. Pediatr Ann 6(11):12–26, 1977

Orthostatic Hypotension

Adelman EM: When the patient's blood pressure falls: What does it mean? What do you do? Nursing 10(2):26, 1980

Alfaro R: Pneumatic antishock trousers, how and when to use them. Dimens Crit Care Nurs 1(1):7–16, 1982

Berne RM, Levy MN: Cardiovascular Physiology. St Louis, CV Mosby, 1981

Rubenstein LZ, Robbins AS: Falls in the elderly: A clinical perspective. Geriatrics 39(4):67–78, 1984

Wade DW: Teaching patients to live with chronic orthostatic hypotension. Nurs 12(7):64–65, 1982

West CM: Ischemia in pathophysiological phenomena. In Carrieri VK, Lindsey AM, West CM (eds): Nursing: Human Responses to Illness. Philadelphia, WB Saunders, 1986

Resources for the Consumer

Literature

Making Products Safer (Pamphlet no. 524)

What Should Parents Expect from Children? (Pamphlet no. 357)

Request the above and a list of other publications from Public Affairs Pamphlets, 381 Park Avenue South, New York, NY 10016 (50 cents for each pamphlet)

Fontana VJ: A Parent's Guide to Child Safety. New York, TY Crowell, 1973

Poison Prevention Packaging available free from the Consumer Product Safety Commission, Washington, DC 20207

Kids Aren't Drownproof, The Kids Aren't Drownproof Coloring Book, Is Your Pool Safe? and What Every Parent Should Know About Water Safety. The Community Association for the Retarded, 3864 Middlefield Road, Palo Alto, CA 94303

Never Leave a Child Alone. Accident Prevention Committee, American Academy of Pediatrics, PO Box 2134, Inglewood, CA 90305

Safe Swimming for Your Boy or Girl. The Injury Prevention Program (TIPP), American Academy of Pediatrics, Publications Department, 141 Northwest Point, PO Box 927, Elk Grove Village, IL 60007.

Knowledge Deficit

Definition

Knowledge deficit: The state in which an individual or group experiences a deficiency in cognitive knowledge or psychomotor skills regarding the condition or treatment plan.

Author's Note: Knowledge deficit does not represent a human response, alteration, or a pattern of dysfunction but rather an etiological or contributing factor.* Lack of knowledge can contribute to a variety of responses, *e.g.,* anxiety, self-care deficits, noncompliance. All nursing diagnostic categories have related patient/ family teaching as a part of nursing interventions, *e.g., Altered Bowel Elimination, Impaired Verbal Communication.* When the teaching directly relates to a specific nursing diagnosis, incorporate the teaching in the plan. When lack of or insufficient knowledge is the primary cause of a diagnosis or a risk factor for a potential diagnosis, list lack of knowledge as a "Related to." For example when specific teaching is indicated prior to a procedure, *Anxiety Related to Unfamiliar Environment* procedure can be used. When information giving is directed to assist a person or family with a decision, *Decisional Conflict* may be indicated. Other examples of diagnostic statements with lack of knowledge as the "Related to" are
- *Potential Altered Health Maintenance* related to lack of knowledge of diabetes mellitus, management and signs/symptoms of complications
- *Potential Impaired Home Maintenance Management* related to lack of knowledge of home care and community resources
- *Potential for Injury* related to lack of knowledge of bicycle safety

Defining Characteristics

Major (must be present)

Verbalizes a deficiency in knowledge or skill/request for information
Expresses "inaccurate" perception of health status
Does not perform correctly a desired or prescribed health behavior

Minor (may be present)

Lack of integration of treatment plan into daily activities
Exhibits or expresses psychological alteration (*e.g.,* anxiety, depression) resulting from misinformation or lack of information

---

* Jenny J: Knowledge Deficit: Not a Nursing Diagnosis. Image 19(4):184–185, 1987

Mobility, Impaired Physical

Related to **Limited Use of Lower Limbs**

Related to **Limited Use of Upper Limbs**

Definition

Impaired physical mobility: A state in which the individual experiences or is at risk of experiencing limitation of physical movement.

> **Author's Note:** This diagnostic category describes an individual with limited use of arm(s) or leg(s). Nursing interventions would focus on strengthening and restoring function and preventing deterioration. Frequently, the impaired mobility becomes the etiology for other nursing diagnoses such as *Self-Care Deficit, Potential for Injury* or *Potential for Disuse Syndrome.*

Defining Characteristics

Major (must be present)

Inability to move purposefully within the environment, including bed mobility, transfers, ambulation

Minor (may be present)

Range-of-motion limitations
Limited muscle strength or control
Impaired coordination

Etiological, Contributing, Risk Factors

Pathophysiological

Neuromuscular impairment
   Autoimmune alterations (multiple sclerosis, arthritis)
   Nervous system diseases (Parkinsonism, myasthenia gravis)
   Muscular dystrophy
   Partial or total paralysis (spinal cord injury, stroke)
   Central nervous system (CNS) tumor
   Increased intracranial pressure
   Sensory deficits
Musculoskeletal impairment
   Spasms
   Flaccidity, atrophy, weakness
   Connective tissue disease (systemic lupus erythematosus)
   Edema (increased synovial fluid)

Treatment-related

External devices (casts or splints, braces, IV tubing)
Surgical procedures (amputation)

Situational (personal, environmental)

Trauma
Depression
Pain

Maturational

Elderly: Decreased motor agility, muscle weakness

Focus Assessment Criteria

Subjective Data

1. History of systemic disorders
    Neurologic
        CVA, head trauma, increased intracranial pressure
        Multiple sclerosis, polio, Guillain-Barré, myasthenia gravis
        Spinal cord injury, tumor, birth defect
    Cardiovascular
        Myocardial infarction   Congenital heart anomaly
        Congestive heart failure
    Musculoskeletal
        Osteoporosis   Fractures
        Arthritis
    Respiratory
        Chronic obstructive pulmonary   Orthopnea
            disease (COPD)   Pneumonia
        Dyspnea on exertion
    Debilitating diseases
        Cancer   Endocrine disease
        Renal disease
2. History of symptoms that interfere with mobility
        Onset   Frequency
        Duration   Precipitated by what?
        Location   Relieved by what?
        Description   Aggravated by what?
3. History of symptoms (complaints of)
    Pain
    Muscle weakness
    Fatigue
        Attributed to?   Amount of time out of bed
        Induced by?   Amount of time sleeping or
                                                 resting
4. History of recent trauma or surgery
        Fractures   Head injury   Abdominal surgery or
                                                         injury
5. Current drug therapy
        Sedatives, hypnotics, CNS depressants   Laxatives   Other

Objective Data

1. Dominant hand

   Right   Left   Ambidextrous

2. Motor function

Right arm	Strong	Weak	Absent	Spastic
Left arm	Strong	Weak	Absent	Spastic
Right leg	Strong	Weak	Absent	Spastic
Left leg	Strong	Weak	Absent	Spastic

3. Mobility

Ability to turn self	Yes	No	Assistance needed (specify)
Ability to sit	Yes	No	Assistance needed (specify)
Ability to stand	Yes	No	Assistance needed (specify)
Ability to transfer	Yes	No	Assistance needed (specify)
Ability to ambulate	Yes	No	Assistance needed (specify)

   Weight-bearing (assess both right and left sides)

   Full   As tolerated

   Partial   Non–weight bearing

   Gait

   Stable   Unstable

   Assistive devices

   Crutches   Walker   Prosthesis

   Cane   Wheelchair   Other

   Braces

   Restrictive devices

   Cast or splint   Ventilator   IV

   Traction   Drain   Monitor

   Braces   Foley   Dialysis

   Range of motion (shoulders, elbows, arms, hips, legs)

   Full   Limited (specify)   None

4. Endurance (see *Activity Intolerance* for additional information)

   a. Assess

   Resting pulse, blood pressure, respirations

   BP, respirations, and pulse immediately after activity

   Pulse every 2 minutes until pulse returns to within 10 beats of resting pulse

   b. After activity, assess for presence of indicators of hypoxia (showing intensity, frequency, or duration of activity must be decreased or discontinued) as follows

   Blood pressure

   Failure of systolic rate to   Increase in diastolic of 155 mmHg
   increase

   Respirations

   Excessive rate increases   Dyspnea

   Decrease in rate   Irregular rhythm

   Cerebral and other changes

   Confusion   Weakness

   Uncoordination   Pallor

   Change in equilibrium   Cyanosis

5. Peripheral circulation

   Capillary refill time (normal less than 3 seconds)

   Skin color, temperature, and turgor

Peripheral pulses (rate, quality)

Brachial	Popliteal
Radial	Posterior tibial
Femoral	Pedal

6. Motivation (as perceived by nurse and stated by person)

Excellent	Satisfactory	Poor

Principles and Rationale for Nursing Care

Guidelines for Range of Motion (ROM)

1. There are three ROM categories—passive, active, and functional.

   Passive ROM keeps muscles and joints limber. One person passively moves another person's muscles (*e.g.,* the helper lifts and moves the person's legs).

   Active ROM exercise limbers and strengthens muscles and joints. The person actively uses his muscles, (*e.g.,* while lying down, the person moves his legs).

   Functional ROM strengthens muscles and joints while performing necessary activity (*e.g.,* walking). Performed by individual himself.

2. Never do range of motion passively if the individual can do it actively.

3. Once the individual can perform active ROM, progress to functional activities.

4. During ROM, the individual's legs and arms should be moved gently to within his pain tolerance; perform ROM slowly to allow the muscles time to relax.

5. Support the extremity above and below the joint.

6. For passive ROM, the supine position is the most effective. The individual who performs ROM himself can use a supine or sitting position.

7. Do range of motion daily with bed bath, 3 to 4 times daily if there are specific problem areas. Try to incorporate into activities of daily living.

Transfers

1. Before transferring anyone, the nurse should assess the number of personnel needed for assistance.

2. The individual should be positioned on the side of the bed. His feet should be touching the floor, and he should be wearing stable shoes or slippers with nonskid soles.

3. For getting in and out of bed, weight-bearing on the uninvolved or stronger side should be encouraged.

4. Wheelchair should be locked before transfer. If using a regular chair, be sure it will not move.

5. The person should be instructed to use the arm of the chair closer to him for support while standing.

6. The nurse should have her arms around the person's rib cage, and her back should be straight, with knees slightly bent.

7. The person should be told to place his arms around the nurse's waist or rib cage, *not her neck.*

8. The nurse should support the person's legs by bracing his with hers. (While facing the person, she should lock his knees with her knees.)

9. Hemiplegic individuals should be instructed to pivot on the uninvolved foot.

10. For individuals with lower limb weakness or paralysis, a sliding board transfer may be used.

    The person should wear pajamas so he will not stick to the board.

    The person needs good upper extremity strength to be able to slide his buttocks from the bed to the chair or wheelchair. (Wheelchairs should have removable arms.)

When the person's arms are strong enough, he should progress to a sitting transfer without the board, if he can lift buttocks enough to clear bed and chair seat.

11. If the person's legs give out, the nurse should guide him gently to the floor and *seek additional assistance.*

Positioning

1. The nurse should assess how frequently position needs to be changed (every 15 minutes to 2 hours), depending on individual's status—*e.g.,* person with spinal cord injury may need his position changed every 15 minutes).
2. People should be positioned with the goal of ambulation in mind (*e.g.,* knees slightly flexed.
3. The nurse should assess problem areas: head, joints, extremities.

   If possible, only one pillow should be used under the *head* to prevent flexion contractions of the neck. Shoulder position should be changed throughout the day (adduction, abduction, overhead extension).

   Arms should be abducted with elbows in slight flexion. The wrist should be in neutral position with the fingers slightly flexed and the thumb slightly abducted and flexed. Arms and hands should be elevated to prevent dependent edema.

   Prolonged periods of hip flexion (*e.g.,* when head of bed is elevated) should be avoided. The prone position should be encouraged if tolerated by the individual.

   External leg rotation should be prevented by placing a small towel lateral to the leg. Pillows should not be placed under knees. If the lower extremity is to be elevated, pillows should be placed under the calf. (Knee flexion contractures can prevent ambulation.)

   Ankles should be in the position of 90°. A footboard may be required to prevent prolonged plantar flexion and shortening of the Achilles tendon. Active movement of the ankle during the day is essential.

4. Pillows or soft towel or blanket rolls may be used to protect specific areas from pressure (*e.g.,* bridging by use of rolled blanket under an ankle, preventing weight on heel).
5. Shearing forces should be minimized when changing the person's position. During transfers, the person's buttocks should be lifted, rather than dragged, whenever possible. A turning sheet should be used to assist the individual to change positions.
6. See Principles and Rationale for Nursing Care under *Activity Intolerance* and *Impaired Skin Integrity* for additional information.

High-risk Elderly Persons

1. About one-tenth of noninstitutionalized elderly persons report some limitation in mobility, and of the institutionalized elderly, over 90% are dependent in at least one activity of daily living (Brody and Foley, 1985). Problems with mobility are often the reason for nursing home admission or extensive in-home care. Assessment of mobility determines the extent of functional impairment as a result of disease or disability.
2. The effects of immobility in the elderly are particularly dangerous. Muscle weakness, atrophy, and decreased endurance are quick to occur, and the biochemical and physiological effects such as nitrogen loss and hypercalciuria are important to consider (Hogue, 1985). Permanent functional loss is more likely with prolonged

immobility, and in addition, elderly persons are vulnerable to new morbidity such as pneumonia, pressure sores, falls and fracture, osteoporosis, incontinence, confusion, and depression. Every effort toward prevention and mobilization should be made.

3. Pain and depression are linked in the elderly; effective management of both is sometimes necessary. Inadequate pain relief may be a primary factor leading to depression in some individuals, but depression should not be discounted as a secondary feature of pain. Depression may require aggressive management including drugs and other therapies (Kwentus et al., 1985).

Impaired Physical Mobility
Related to Limited Use of Lower Limbs

Assessment

Subjective Data

Pain

Fatigue

Numbness and tingling

Weakness

Objective Data

Inability to move or coordinate one or both lower limits

Limitations in range of motion of lower limbs

Mechanical devices restricting mobility (*e.g.,* cast, traction)

Refusal to acknowledge existence of limbs (*e.g.,* post-CVA)

Impaired ability to transfer with or without adaptive devices (bed-chair, chair-commode)

Impaired ability to perform activities of daily living

Impaired sitting or standing balance

Impaired ability to ambulate with or without assistive devices

Alterations in gait patterns

Partial or total loss of one or both lower limbs

Impaired ability to move within physical environment (*e.g.,* curbs, stairs)

Outcome Criteria

The person will

- Demonstrate the use of adaptive devices to increase mobility
- Utilize safety measures to minimize potential for injury
- Describe rationale for interventions
- Demonstrate measures to increase mobility
- Report an increase in strength and endurance of upper limbs

Interventions

A. Assess causative factors

Trauma (*e.g.,* cartilage tears, fractures, amputations)

Surgical procedure (*e.g.,* joint replacement, reduction of fractures, vascular surgery)

Debilitating disease (*e.g.,* diabetes, cancer, rheumatoid arthritis, multiple sclerosis, stroke)

B. Reduce or eliminate contributing factors

1. Increase limb mobility
   - Perform range-of-motion exercises (frequency to be determined by condition of the individual)
   - Support extremity with pillows to prevent or reduce swelling
   - Medicate for pain as needed, especially before activity* (see *Altered Comfort*)
   - Apply heat or cold to reduce pain, inflammation, and hematoma*
   - Apply cold to reduce swelling post-injury (usually first 48 hours)*
   - Encourage the person to perform exercise regimens for specific joints as prescribed by physician or physical therapist
2. Position the person in alignment to prevent complications
   - Avoid pillows under knee; support calf instead
   - Point toes and knees toward ceiling when the client is in a supine position
   - Use footboard to prevent foot drop
   - Avoid prolonged periods of hip flexion (*i.e.,* sitting position)
   - To position hips, place rolled towel lateral to hip to prevent external rotation
   - Change position every 15 minutes to 2 hours depending on individual's skin tolerance to pressure
3. Maintain good body alignment when mechanical devices are used
   a. Traction devices
      - Assess for correct position of traction and alignment of bones
      - Observe for correct amount and position of weights
      - Allow weights to hang freely, with no blankets or sheets on ropes
      - Assess for changes in circulation; check pulse quality, skin temperature, color of extremities, and capillary refill (should be <2 sec)
      - Assess for changes in circulation (numbness, tingling, pain)
      - Assess for changes in mobility (ability to flex/extend unaffected joints)
      - Assess for signs of skin irritation (redness, ulceration, blanching)
      - Assess skeletal traction pin sites for loosening, inflammation, ulceration, and drainage; clean pin insertion sites (procedure may vary with type of pin and physician's order)
      - Encourage isometrics* and prescribed exercise program.
   b. Casts
      - Assess for proper fit of casts (they should not be too loose or too tight)
      - Assess circulation to the encasted area every 2 hours (color and temperature of skin, pulse quality, capillary refill <2 sec)
      - Assess for changes in sensation of extremities every two hours (numbness, tingling, pain)
      - Assess motion of uninvolved joints (ability to flex and extend)

---

* May require a physician's order.

- Assess for skin irritation (redness, ulceration, or complaints of pain under the cast)
- Keep cast clean and dry; do not allow sharp objects to be inserted under cast; petal rough edges with adhesive tape; place soft cotton under edges that seem to be causing pressure points
- Allow cast to air dry while resting on pillows to prevent dents
- Observe cast for areas of softening or indentation
- Exercise joints above and below cast if allowed (*e.g.,* wiggle fingers and toes every two hours)
- Assist with prescribed exercise regimens and isometrics of muscles enclosed in casts*
- Keep extremities elevated after cast application to reduce swelling

c. Braces
- Assess for correct positioning of braces
- Observe for signs of skin irritation (redness, ulceration, blanching, itching, pain)
- Assist with exercises as prescribed for specific joints
- Have the person demonstrate correct application of the brace

d. Prosthetic devices
- Observe for signs of skin irritation of the stump before applying prosthetic device (stump should be clean and dry; Ace bandage should be rewrapped and securely in place)
- Have the person demonstrate the correct application of the prosthesis
- Assess the person for gait alterations or improper walking technique
- Proceed with health teaching if indicated

e. Ace bandages
- Assess for correct position of Ace bandage
- Apply Ace bandage with even pressure, wrapping from distal to proximal portions, and making sure that the bandage is not too tight or too loose
- Observe for "bunching" of the bandage
- Observe for signs of irritation of skin (redness, ulceration, excessive tightness)
- Rewrap Ace bandage b.i.d. or as needed, unless contraindicated (*e.g.,* if the bandage is a postoperative compression dressing, it should be left in place)
- When wrapping lower extremity, leave the heel exposed, using figure-8 technique

Note: Some mechanical devices may be removed for exercises, depending on nature of injury or type and purpose of device. Consult with the physician to ascertain when the person may remove the device.

4. Provide progressive mobilization*
- Assist the person slowly to sitting position
- Allow the person to dangle his legs over the side of the bed for a few minutes before he stands up
- Limit time to 15 minutes, three times a day, the first few times out of bed
- Increase the person's time out of bed, as tolerated by 15-minute increments
- Progress to ambulation with or without assistive devices
- If unable to walk, assist the person out of bed to a wheelchair or chair

* May require a physician's order

- Encourage ambulating for short frequent walks (at least 3 times daily), with assistance if unsteady
- Increase lengths of walks progressively each day

C. Provide health teaching as indicated

1. Teach the person methods of transfer from bed to chair or commode and to standing position
2. Teach how to ambulate with adaptive equipment (*e.g.*, crutches, walkers, canes)
   a. Instruct the individual in weight-bearing status
   b. Observe and teach the use of
      (1) Crutches
         - No pressure should be exerted on axilla; hand strength should be used
         - Type of gait varies with individual's diagnosis
         - Measure crutches 2 to 3 inches below axilla, and tips 6 inches away from feet
      (2) Walkers
         - Use arm strength to support weakness in lower limbs
         - Gait varies with individual's problems
      (3) Wheelchairs
         - Practice transfers
         - Practice maneuvering around barriers
      (4) Prostheses (teach about the following)
         - Stump wrapping prior to application of the prosthesis
         - Application of the prosthesis
         - Principles of stump care
         - Importance of cleaning the stump, keeping it dry, and applying the prosthesis only when the stump is dry
   c. Teach the individual safety precautions
      - Protect areas of decreased sensation from extremes of heat and cold
      - Practice falling and how to recover from falls while transferring or ambulating
      - For decreased perception of lower extremity (post-CVA "neglect"), instruct the individual to check where limb is placed when changing positions or going through doorways; and check to make sure both shoes are tied, that affected leg is dressed with trousers, and that pants are not dragging
      - Instruct individuals who are confined to wheelchair to shift position and lift up buttocks every 15 minutes to relieve pressure; maneuver curbs, ramps, inclines, and around obstacles; and lock wheelchairs prior to transferring
   d. Practice proper positioning, range of motion (active or passive), and prescribed exercises
   e. Practice stair-climbing if individual's condition permits
   f. Observe for complications of immobility
      Phlebitis (*i.e.*, redness, tenderness, swelling of calves)
      Pressure ulcer (*i.e.*, blanching of skin, redness, itching, pain)
      Infection after limb surgery (*i.e.*, pain, swelling, redness)
      Neurovascular compromise (*i.e.*, numbness, tingling, pain, blanching, decreased pulse quality, coolness of skin)

Impaired Physical Mobility
Related to Limited Use of Upper Limbs

Assessment

Subjective Data

The person reports

Pain	Fatigue
Loss of sensation (numbness, tingling	Weakness

Objective Data

Inability to move one or both upper extremities
Impaired grasp
Limited range of motion of one or more upper limbs
Mechanical devices preventing full range of motion (*e.g.,* traction, cast)
Inability to perform self-care activities
Neglect of one or both upper limbs
Partial or total loss of upper limb(s)
Impaired coordination of upper limb(s)

Outcome Criteria

The person will
- Demonstrate modes of adaptation to disability, *e.g.,* use of adaptive equipment such as universal cuff
- Relate rationale for interventions
- Report on increase in strength and endurance of upper limbs

---

Interventions

A. Assess causative factors

Trauma (*e.g.,* fractures, crushing injuries, lacerations, amputations)
Surgical procedure (*e.g.,* joint replacement, reduction of fractures, removal of tumors, mastectomy)
Systemic disease (*e.g.,* multiple sclerosis, CVA, Guillain-Barré, rheumatoid arthritis, Parkinson's, lupus)

B. Reduce or eliminate contributing factors

1. Increase limb mobility if possible
   - Assist with range of motion exercises*
   - Elevate extremity with pillows or sling above level of the heart to prevent or reduce swelling (may be contradindicated in CHF)
   - Medicate for pain as needed, especially before activity* (see *Altered Comfort*)

---

* May require a physician's order

- Apply cold to reduce swelling post-injury (usually first 48 hours)*
- Assist with exercise regimens for specific joints as prescribed by physician or physical therapist (*e.g.,* for joint replacements)*

2. Position the person in alignment to prevent complications
   - Arms abducted from the body with pillows
   - Elbows in slight flexion
   - Wrist in a neutral position, with fingers slightly flexed, and thumb abducted and slightly flexed
   - Position of shoulder joints changed during the day (*e.g.,* abduction, adduction, range of circular motion)

3. Prevent injury when mechanical devices are used
   a. Traction devices
      - Assess for correct alignment of bones and position of weights
      - Allow weights to hang freely with no blankets or sheets on ropes
      - Assess for changes in circulation; check pulse quality, skin temperature, color of extremities, and capillary refill (should be <2 sec)
      - Assess for changes in sensation (numbness, tingling, pain)
      - Assess for changes in mobility (ability to flex/extend unaffected joints)
      - Assess for signs of skin irritation (redness, ulceration, flaking)
      - Assess skeletal traction, pin sites for loosening, inflammation, or skin ulceration; clean pin insertion sites b.i.d. (procedure may vary with type of pin and physician's order)
      - Encourage isometrics and prescribed exercise program*
   b. Casts
      - Assess for tightness of cast
        - Circulation: temperature, color, check pulses, capillary refill should be <2 seconds
        - Sensation: numbness, tingling, increased pain
        - Motion: ability to flex, extend
      - Assess for skin irritation: redness ulceration, complaints of pain under cast
      - Keep cast clean and dry; petal edges with adhesive tape if necessary; no sharp objects down into cast
      - Allow cast to air dry; observe for areas of softening
      - Exercise joints above and below cast; prescribed exercise regimens and isometrics of muscles enclosed in casts
      - After application, elevate extremity on pillows to prevent or reduce swelling
   c. Slings
      - Assess for correct application; sling should be loose around neck and should support elbow and wrist above level of the heart
      - Remove slings for range of motion*
   d. Ace bandages (care as for lower limbs' bandages)
      - Observe for correct position
      - Apply with even pressure, wrapping distally to proximally
      - Observe for "bunching"
      - Observe for signs of skin irritation (redness, ulceration) or tightness (compression)
      - Rewrap Ace bandages b.i.d. or as needed, unless contraindicated (*e.g.,* if bandage is postoperative compression dressing, check physician's orders)

* May require a physician's order

4. Encourage use of affected arm when possible
   - Encourage the person to use affected arm for self-care activities (*e.g.,* feeding himself, dressing, brushing hair)
   - For post-CVA neglect of upper limb (see also *Unilateral Neglect*)
     a. Place objects to affected side to encourage use of "forgotten" limb
     b. Stand to the person's side and encourage him to use all fields of vision
        Note: Some mechanical devices may be removed for exercises, depending on nature of injury or type and purpose of device. Physician's orders should be consulted.
   - Instruct the person to utilize unaffected arm to exercise the affected arm.
   - Use appropriate adaptive equipment to enhance the use of arms
     - Universal cuff for feeding in individuals who have poor control in both arms, hands
     - Large-handled or padded silverware to assist individuals with poor fine motor skills
     - Dishware with high edges to prevent food from slipping
     - Suction-cup aids to hold dishes in place to prevent sliding of plate
   - Use a warm bath to alleviate early morning stiffness and improve mobility
   - Encourage the individual to practice handwriting skills, if able
   - Allow time for the individual to practice using affected limb.

C. Proceed with health teaching as indicated
   - Have the person demonstrate range of motion and prescribed exercises
   - Have the person demonstrate the care of adaptive and mechanical devices
   - Teach the person safety precautions
   - Practice difficult maneuvers (*e.g.,* cooking with one hand)
   - For areas of decreased sensation, instruct the person to take precautions with heat, cold, and sharp objects
   - For neglect of upper extremity, instruct the person to observe and check for positioning, exposure to irritants, or sharp objects
   - Teach person methods of performing self-care activities (see self-care deficits)
   - Teach individual when to alternate rest and activity of joints

References/Bibliography

Banwell BF: Exercise and mobility in arthritis. Nurs Clin North Am 19(4):605–616, 1984

Brody J, Foley E: Epidemiologic considerations. In Schneider E (ed): The Teaching Nursing Home: A New Approach to Geriatric Research, Education, and Clinical Practice, pp 9–25. New York, Raven Press, 1985

Farrell J: Illustrated guide to Orthopedic Nursing, 2nd ed. Philadelphia, JB Lippincott, 1982

Gartland J: Fundamentals of Orthopedics. Philadelphia, WB Saunders, 1965

Hogue C: Mobility. In Schneider E (ed): The Teaching Nursing Home: A New Approach to Geriatric Research, Education, and Clinical Care, pp 231–244. New York, Raven Press, 1985

Krusen FH, Kottke FJ, Elwood P Jr (eds): Handbook of Physical Medicine and Rehabilitation. Philadelphia, WB Saunders, 1971

Kwentus J, Harkins S, Lignon N et al: Current concepts of geriatric pain and its treatment. Geriatrics 40(4):48–57, 1985

Lieberson S, Mendes DG: Walking in bed: Strength and mobility of the lower extremities of bedridden patients. Phys Ther 59:1112–1115, 1979

Meissner JE: Elevate your patient's level of independence. Nursing 10(9):72–73, 1980

Milazzo V: Exercise class for patients in traction. Am J Nurs 81:1843–1844, 1981

Olson EV (ed): The hazards of immobility. Am J Nurs 67:780–797, 1967

Sine R (ed): Basic Rehabilitation Techniques, 2nd ed. Rockville, MD, Aspen Systems Corporation, 1981

Noncompliance

Related to **Anxiety**

Related to **Negative Side-Effects of Prescribed Treatment**

Related to **Reported Unsatisfactory Relationship with Caregiving Environment or Caregivers**

Definition

Noncompliance: The state in which an individual or group desires to comply but is prevented from doing so by factors that deter adherence to health-related advice given by health professionals.

Author's Note: The use of the nursing diagnosis *Noncompliance* describes the individual who desires to comply but is prevented from doing so by the presence of certain factors. The nurse must attempt to reduce or eliminate these factors for the interventions to be successful. However, the nurse is cautioned against using the diagnosis of noncompliance to describe an individual who has made an informed autonomous decision not to comply.

Defining Characteristics

Major (must be present)

Verbalization of noncompliance or nonparticipation or confusion about therapy and/or
Direct observation of behavior indicating noncompliance

Minor (may be present)

Missed appointments
Partially used or unused medications
Persistence of symptoms*
Progression of disease process*
Occurrence of undesired outcomes* (postoperative morbidity, pregnancy, obesity, addiction, regression during rehabilitation)

Etiological, Contributing, Risk Factors

Pathophysiologial

Impaired ability to perform tasks because of disability (*e.g.,* poor memory, motor and sensory deficits)
Chronic nature of illness

---

* When these characteristics are considered to be the result of noncompliance, one is assuming that the therapy prescribed has been proved to be effective and is appropriate.

Increasing amount of disease-related symptoms despite adherence to advised regimen.

Treatment-related

Side-effects of therapy
Previous unsuccessful experiences with advised regimen
Impersonal aspects of referral process
Nontherapeutic environment
Complex, unsupervised, or prolonged therapy
Financial cost of therapy
Nontherapeutic relationship between client and nurse

Situational (personal, environmental)

Concurrent illness of family member
Inclement weather preventing client from keeping appointment
Nonsupportive family, peers, community
Knowledge deficit
Lack of autonomy in health-seeking behavior
Health beliefs run counter to professional advice
Poor self-esteem
Disturbance in body image

Maturational

Developmental maturity of client is incompatible with his/her age

Focus Assessment Criteria

Subjective Data

What is the person's general health motivation?
  Does client seek help when needed?
  Does client accept the diagnosis as valid?
  Does client intend to make the advised life-style alterations?
What is the person's perception of his present state of health?
  Does client consider himself to be generally well?
  Is there fear of a specific illness?
  Does client believe his illness is severe?
How does the person view the advised treatment regimen?
Does the person report
  Unacceptable side-effects of therapy?

Unpleasant taste	Pain	Time-consuming or
Difficulty swallowing	Heavy expenses	inconvenient

  Inability to repeat or demonstrate the prescribed behavior?

Exercise program	Drug names and	Treatment procedure
Next appointment date	schedule	

  Situations that interfere with prescribed behavior?

Family demands	Occupations	Travel (hotels, restau-
Stress	Lack of transportation	rants)

  Does family member report any of the above problems?

Objective Data

Assess for the presence of
  Missed appointments

Obstacles to self-care
>   Inability to read   Musculoskeletal deficits
>   Immaturity   Cognitive deficits
>   Memory lags   Pain

Evidence of obstacles in caregiving environment
>   Long waiting period   Hurried atmosphere

Evidence of noncompliance
>   Persistence of symptoms   With medications (pill count, serum
>   Progression of disease   drug levels

Principles and Rationale for Nursing Care

1. Since the diagnosis of noncompliance has a high subjective component, the nurse is cautioned not to utilize the diagnosis as a reflection of the nurse's value judgment but, rather, to seek to identify causative and contributing factors.
2. Both clients and health care professionals share the responsibility for noncompliance and must work together to correct it.
3. There is a gray area between noncompliance and making an informed decision not to adhere to health-related advice. For example, the individual who does not take his medication because he is unable to swallow pills is different from the person who refuses chemotherapy because he is exhausted from previous treatments and is ready to die. In both cases, the nurse intervenes to elicit reasons for this behavior. However, only in the first circumstance are attempts made to change the situation.
4. When evaluating noncompliance related to medication, the nurse must consider the following factors that may affect drug absorption, metabolism, effectiveness, side-effects, and excretion: body weight, age, time of administration, route of administration, genetic factors, basal metabolic rate, interactions with other drugs and foods, presence of organ disease (*e.g.,* liver and kidneys), altered body chemistry (*e.g.,* hypokalemia), and infection.
5. When a client reports symptomatic side-effects from a new drug, consider the many manifestations of the human allergic response: hives and the entire spectrum of rashes, respiratory discomfort and distress, pruritus, watery eyes, swelling of mucous membranes, and gastrointestinal discomforts.

Noncompliance
Related to Anxiety

Assessment

Subjective Data

The person states
>   He is anxious or fearful
>   He has not followed advice of health care professional

Objective Data

The person exhibits nonverbal signs of anxiety
>   Tachycardia   Chest pain
>   Perspiration   Dyspnea

Headache   Cold extremities
GI discomfort   Tachypnea
Insomnia

Outcome Criteria

The person will
• Verbalize fears related to health needs
• Identify factors that are contributing to anxiety
• Identify alternatives to present coping patterns

Interventions

A. Assess causative or contributing factors

Negative experiences with disease or with health care system (either personally or
    through others)
Stressors

B. Reduce or eliminate causative or contributing factors if possible

1. Negative experiences with health care system.
   • Using open-ended questions, encourage person to talk about previous experiences
     with health care (*e.g.,* hospitalizations, family deaths, diagnostic tests, blood
     tests, x-rays)
   • Ask client directly, "What are your concerns about
     . . . taking this drug?"
     . . . following this diet?"
     . . . having a blood test?"
     . . . going through the cystoscopy?"
     . . . having your gallbladder removed?"
     . . . using a diaphragm?"
     . . . paying for the operation?"
   • Encourage client to talk about how the diagnosis and treatment might affect him
     and/or significant others
   • Acknowledge appropriateness of being fearful
   • Correct any misconceptions
   • Give appropriate instructions
   • Discuss the effects of anxiety on pain, breathing, healing, and general comfort
     (see also *Anxiety; Fear*)
2. Stressors
   • Assess person for recent changes in life-style (personal, work, family, health,
     financial)
   • Facilitate recognition by person of how those factors are affecting his health
   • Assist person to manage his stressors; see the appropriate diagnosis that reflects
     the stressor

     Fear   Spiritual Distress
     Anxiety   Altered Thought Process
     Grieving   Ineffective Individual Coping
     Altered Nutrition   Altered Family Process
     Self-Care Deficit

C. Initiate referrals if indicated

Dietician
Nutrition support
Home health
Social service
Other community agencies

Noncompliance
Related to Negative Side-Effects of Prescribed Treatment

Assessment

Subjective Data

The person states that he has altered the prescribed health behavior because of discomforts related to treatment(s)

"Medications make me sick"
"Medications make me tired"

The person describes symptoms such as

Dizziness	Indigestion
Headache	Drowsiness
Dry mouth	Sexual difficulties
Pain	Depression
Diarrhea	

The person states that treatments are inconvenient

Objective Data

Any lab test indicative of treatment effects (*e.g.,* toxic drug levels, hypokalemia due to diuretics)

Physical findings

Rashes	Hyperpigmentation
Hives	Dehydration
Loss or growth of hair	Drowsiness
Fat deposits	

Outcome Criteria

The person will
- Describe experiences that cause him to alter prescribed behavior
- Describe appropriate treatment of side effects, if necessary
- Demonstrate appropriate alternatives to the previous plan

Interventions

A. Assess causative or contributing factors of prescribed therapy

Requires prolonged period of time
Is unsupervised
Is complex, with numerous medications, or special equipment is needed
Is very costly
Involves changes in lifelong habits
Is inconvenient in terms of time, place, or side-effects
Is culturally unacceptable

B. Assess the person's complaints

Onset and duration?
Associated with activity? food? stress?

C. Review present medication therapy (prescribed and over-the-counter)

- Identify present therapy (names, dosages, time taken)
- Identify possible adverse interactions among drugs (consult pharmacist)
- Establish whether toxicity is present (blood level of drug)*

D. Assist person to reduce causative factors

- For gastric irritation, suggest that drug be taken with milk or food; may be advisable to eat yogurt (unless contraindicated)
- For drowsiness, take medication at bedtime or late in afternoon; consult physician for dose reduction
- For leg cramps (hypokalemia), increase intake of foods high in potassium (oranges, raisins, tomatoes, bananas)
- For other side-effects, consult pertinent references
- Use long-acting intramuscular preparations whenever possible; this includes some antibiotics and antipsychotic medications
- Suggest that physicians use combination pills if available (*e.g.,* Aldoril [methyldopa and hydrochlorothiazide] and Triavil [perphenazine and amitriptyline])
- When appropriate, be sure client is taking the fewest number of pills possible (check dosages to provide the largest dose available in the fewest number of pills)*
- Instruct client to take pills twice rather than four times per day whenever appropriate*
- Encourage prescription of generic drugs for persons with financial concerns
- When treatments require more than one set of hands, evaluate home help situation (see *Impaired Home Maintenance Management*)
- When expensive equipment is involved for treatments at home, make appropriate referrals to social workers and local agencies

E. Initiate health teaching and referrals as indicated

- Teach importance of adhering to prescribed regime
- Teach what to expect (effects of drug or treatment; side-effects)

---

* May require a physician's order

Noncompliance
Related to Reported Unsatisfactory Relationship with Caregiving Environment or Caregivers

Assessment

Subjective Data

Verbalizes dissatisfaction with setting, caregivers, or treatment regime

Objective Data

Clients seen in waiting areas for long periods of time
Schedules are overbooked
There is a shortage of caregiving personnel
Clients and caregivers are culturally unrelated
Client is seen by a different caregiver at each visit
Physical setting lacks privacy
Setting is located in dangerous or inaccessible area
Prescribed therapies are not provided by caregiving setting
Treatments prescribed are complex or costly

Outcome Crisis

The person will
- Express anger, frustrations, confusion related to aspects of the clinical setting to nurse
- Identify sources of dissatisfaction
- Offer suggestions of what would be more satisfactory

Interventions

A. Assess causative or contributing factors

1. Referral process
   Prolonged period between referral and scheduled appointment
   Referral to a clinic rather than to a specific caregiver
   Referral by person other than self
2. Method of scheduling
   Block scheduling, or "first come, first serve," rather than individual appointments
   Overbooked schedule preventing reasonable amount of time for visit
3. Communication barriers
   Presence of language barrier
   Teaching center in which a variety of students see clients and disturb continuity
   Goals of personnel and clients differ
   Personnel lack interest or expertise necessary to develop trust of clients
   Personnel make decisions *for* client, rather than *with* him
   Conflicting messages from variety of health professionals to client

4. Physical setting
    Crowded, impersonal seating in waiting areas
    Clients seen in curtained booths rather than individual rooms
    Location is not on public transportation lines
    Location is in a neighborhood different from client's

B. Eliminate or reduce contributing factors if possible

1. Referral process
   - Whenever possible, allow client to make own appointments
   - Shorten referral waiting time
   - Personnel handling referral appointments should inquire about transportation and child care, suggesting help available if needed
   - Send reminder postcard to client before appointment
   - Personnel initiating referral should give client adequate explanations as to why it is indicated and what is expected from the visit

2. Method of scheduling
   - If possible, give individual appointments
   - Do not schedule unreasonable number of clients for a given time period

3. Communication barriers
   - Allow person an opportunity to make the decisions about his own health care; assume an advisory approach when counseling, rather than one that is dictatorial
   - Consider the use of contracting when behavior modification is indicated; include caregiver in the contract as well as the client
   - Schedule interpreters whenever non–English speaking clients are anticipated (consult "language banks" in larger institutions)
   - For the caregiver who knows small amounts of a language (Spanish, for example), make note cards inscribed with key words appropriate to the clinical setting
   - In teaching centers where clients may see different students at each visit, schedule primary nurses to stop in to see each patient
   - Plan patient care conferences, including members of all involved health professions, at regular intervals to promote seeing clients as individuals

4. Physical setting
   - Utilize waiting time for teaching (*e.g.,* group classes)
   - Use as many resources as possible to make waiting and caregiving areas pleasant, welcoming, and nonclinical
   - Utilize blank wall space for health education materials, pictorial progress of client, holiday decorations, original artwork by clients, etc.
   - Ensure privacy during interviews, examinations, and procedures
   - Causative factors related to the location of the clinical setting, safety, and transportation are difficult problems to correct; nurses may make proposals for
         Special buses
         Enhanced security
         Ramps for wheelchairs
         Improved lighting in parking areas and walkways
         More nearby parking facilities
   - Arrange for home visit if appropriate
   - Utilize community resources (*e.g.,* transportation for disabled or senior citizens)

C. Encourage person to verbalize frustrations with the clinical setting in the context of a therapeutic nursing relationship

References/Bibliography

Books and Articles

Becker H (ed): The Health Belief Model and Personal Health Behavior. Thorofare, NJ, Charles B. Slack, 1974

Edel MK: Noncompliance: An appropriate nursing diagnosis? Nurs Outlook 33(4):183–185, 1985

Haynes R, Taylor D, Sackett D: Compliance in Health Care. Baltimore, Johns Hopkins Press, 1979

Kinnaird LS, Yoham MA, Kieval YM: Patient compliance in rehabilitating programs. Nurs Clin North Am 17(3):523–532, 1982

Komaroff L: The practitioner and the compliant patient. Am J Public Health 66(9):833–835, 1976

Marston MV: Compliance with medical regimes: A review of the literature. Nursing Res 19(4):312–323, 1970

Ryan P, Falco SM: A pilot study to validate the etiologies and defining characteristics of the nursing diagnosis of noncompliance. Nurs Clin North Am 20(4):685–695, 1985

Scherwitz L, Leventhal H: Strategies for increasing patient compliance. Health Values 2(6):301–306, 1978

Steckel SB: Predicting, measuring, implementing and following-up on patient compliance. Nurs Clin North Am 17(3):491–497, 1982

Thomson PS, Willis JC: Compliance changes in a black lung clinic. Nurs Clin North Am 17(3):513–521, 1982

Resources for the Consumer

Literature

Food-drug interactions: Can what you eat affect your medication? Elizabeth, NJ, Wakefern Food Corporation

Nutrition, Altered
Less Than Body Requirements

Related to **Chewing or Swallowing Difficulties**

Related to **Anorexia**

Related to **Difficulty or Inability to Procure Food**

Impaired Swallowing

Related to **(Specify)**

Altered Nutrition:
Less Than Body Requirements

Definitions

Altered nutrition: Less than body requirements: The state in which an individual who is not NPO experiences or is at risk of experiencing reduced weight related to inadequate intake or metabolism of nutrients.

> **Author's Note:** This diagnostic category describes individuals who can ingest food but have difficulty. This category should not be used to describe individuals who are NPO or cannot ingest food. Those situations should be described by the collaborative problem of:
>
> Potential Complication: electrolyte imbalances
> negative nitrogen balance
>
> Nurses monitor to detect complications of an NPO state and confer with medicine for parenteral therapy. Some nursing diagnoses that may relate to an individual who is NPO are *Potential Altered Oral Mucous Membrane* and *Altered Comfort*.

Defining Characteristics

Major (must be present)

One who is not NPO reports or has: inadequate food intake less than recommended daily allowance (RDA) with or without weight loss and/or

Actual or potential metabolic needs in excess of intake with or without weight loss

Minor (may be present)

Weight 10% to 20% + below ideal for height and frame

Triceps skin fold, mid-arm circumference, and mid-arm muscle circumference less than 60% standard measurement

Tachycardia on minimal exercise and bradycardia at rest

Muscle weakness and tenderness

Mental irritability or confusion

Decreased serum albumin

Decreased serum transferrin or iron-binding capacity

Etiological, Contributing, Risk Factors

Pathophysiological

Hyperanabolic/catabolic states

    Burns (post-acute phase)   Cancer

    Infection   Trauma

Chemical dependence

Faulty metabolism

    Cirrhosis   Gastric resection

Dysphagia
  Cerebrovascular accident
  Amyotrophic lateral sclerosis
  Cerebral palsy
Absorptive disorders
  Crohn's disease
  Cystic fibrosis
  Diverticulosis
Stomatitis
Trauma
Altered level of consciousness

Muscular dystrophy
Parkinson's disease
Neuromuscular disorders

Treatment-related
Surgery
Medications (chemotherapy)
Surgical reconstruction of mouth
Wired jaw
Radiation therapy
Inadequate absorption as a side effect
  Colchicine
  Pyrimethamine
  Antacid

Neomycin
Para-aminosalicyclic acid

Situational (personal, environmental)
Fear of choking
Anorexia
Depression
Stress
Social isolation
Nausea and vomiting
Allergy
Parasites
Inability to procure food (physical limitations; financial or transportation problems)
Lack of knowledge of adequate nutrition
Crash or fad diet
Inability to chew (wired jaw, damaged or missing teeth, ill-fitting dentures)
Diarrhea
Lactose intolerance
Ethnic/religious eating patterns

Maturational
Infants/children: Congenital anomalies, growth spurts, developmental eating disorders
Adolescent: Anorexia nervosa (post-acute phase)
Elderly: Altered sense of taste

Focus Assessment Criteria

Subjective Data
History of problem (childhood, sociocultural influences)
Diet recall for past 24 hours
  Is that the usual intake pattern?

Diet history
Past diets
Amount weight lost
Weight gained back (how soon? how much?)

Present Dietary Patterns

Diet diary (for overweight person)
Instruct person to record for one week
What, when, where, and why eaten
Whether doing anything else (*e.g.,* television, reading)
Emotions just before eating
Others present
Food source and preparation
Living arrangements
Financial status

Activity Level

Occupation
Exercise (what? how often?)

Coping Pattern

Response to stress (eat or not eat?)
Perceptions of problem
Perceptions of causation
Desire to change
Support system available (strengths/limitations)

Knowledge of Nutrition

Basic food groups
Foods high and low in calories
Relationship of activity vs. metabolism
Portion size

Physiological Alterations

Medication history
Medical/surgical history
Presence of

Allergies	Fatigue
Nausea	Dysphagia
Vomiting	Pain
Anorexia	Stomatitis

See *Nausea/Vomiting, Impaired Swallowing, Pain* for additional interventions.

Objective Data

Height and weight
Compare to standardized chart according to sex (see tables under Principles and
Rationale for Nursing Care)
Anthropometric measurements (refer to Principles and Rationale for Nursing Care
for standard charts)
Triceps skin fold
Mid-arm circumference

Mid-arm muscle circumference
Condition of hair, skin, nails, mouth, and teeth (see *Altered Oral Mucous Membrane*)
Ability to chew, swallow, feed self

Diagnostic Studies

Hemoglobin
Serum albumin
Serum transferrin or iron-binding capacity
Total Lymphocytes count
Thyroid function
Triglycerides
Cholesterol
Calcium
Iron
Vitamin B_{12}
Folic acid
Urinary creatinine height
Lipoproteins
Potassium
Serum uric acid

Principles and Rationale for Nursing Care

General

1. Food habits are influenced by personal preferences, culture and religion, economic factors, family eating patterns, and knowledge of nutrition.
2. The body requires a minimum level of nutrients for health and growth. During the life span, the nutritional needs of individuals vary, as indicated in Table II-13.
3. Inability to meet metabolic requirements results in loss of weight, poor health, and decreased ability of the body to grow or repair itself.
4. Metabolic needs are increased in the presence of trauma, sepsis, infection, and cancer.
5. To obtain a one-pound weight gain, 3500 calories above metabolic requirements must be acquired.
6. Anorexia is a complex multidimensional problem involving physical, social, and psychological components.
7. Nutritional deficiencies in the elderly can result from chronic disease, anemia, anorexia, dental status, financial problems, loneliness, the inability to procure or prepare foods, and fluid imbalance.
8. The person with cancer experiences nutritional problems that are disease-related and treatment-related, as indicated below.

Disease-Related

Malabsorption
Diarrhea
Constipation
Anemia
Protein deficits
Fatigue

Treatment-Related

Stomatitis
Diarrhea
Nausea and vomiting
Anorexia
Fatigue

9. Tables II-14 and II-15 can be used to compare the individual's weight for height and anthropometric measurements.

Table II-13.   **Age-Related Daily Nutritional Requirements**

Age	Daily Nutritional Requirements
Infants	
Newborn	12–18 oz milk
2–3 months	20–30 oz milk
4–5 months	25–35 oz milk; strained vegetables and fruits; egg yolks
6–7 months	28–40 oz milk; above solids, plus meat
8–11 months	24 oz milk; 3 regular meals
1–2 years	24 oz milk; 1000 calories
Children	
Preschool (3–5 years)	1500 calories; 40 gm protein

	Basic 4 food groups
	    4–6 servings fruits and vegetables
	    2 or more servings meat/protein (2 oz portions)
	    4 servings bread or cereal
	    4 servings dairy

School (6–12 years)	80 calories/kg; 1.2 (gm/kg) protein

	Basic 4 food groups (as preschool)
	    1.5–2 gm calcium
	    400 units vitamin D
	    1.5–3 liters water

Adolescent (13–17 years)	2200–2400 calories for females 3000 calories for males

	Basic 4 food groups (as preschool)
	    50–60 gm protein
	    3 gm calcium
	    400 units vitamin D

Adults	
	1600–3000 calorie range (based on physical activity, emotional state, body size, age, and individual metabolism)

	Basic 4 food groups
	    2 servings dairy
	    at least 2 servings meat/protein
	    4–6 servings fruits/vegetables
	    4 servings bread or cereal

	Males need increased protein, ascorbic acid, riboflavin, and vitamins E and B_6
	Females need the above and also increased iron and vitamins A and B_{12}

Pregnant women
(2nd and 3rd trimesters)
	Daily calorie requirement
	    11–15 yr 2500
	    16–22 yr 2400
	    23–50 yr 2300

	Increase protein 10 gm or 1 serving meat 1.2–3.5 gm calcium Increase vitamins A, B, and C 30–60 mg iron

(continued)

Table II-13. **Age-Related Daily Nutritional Requirements** (continued)

Age	Daily Nutritional Requirements
Lactating women	2500–3000 calories (500 over regular diet)
	Basic 4 food groups 4 servings meat/protein 5 servings dairy 4+ servings grain 5+ servings vegetables 2+ servings Vitamin C-rich 1+ green leafy 2+ others
	Fluids 2–3 quarts (1 qt milk) Increase in Vitamin A, C, niacin
Over 65	Basic 4 food groups (same as adult)
	Caloric requirements decrease with age (1600–1800 for female, 2000–2400 for male) but are dependent on activity, climate, and metabolic needs
	Ensure intake of essential amino acids, fatty acids, vitamins, elements, fiber, and water
	60 mg ascorbic acid
	40–60 mg protein
	800 mg calcium (1500 mg for females)
	10 mg iron

High-risk Elderly

1. In general, the elderly need the same kind of balanced diet as any other age group but with fewer calories. However, diets of elderly clients tend to be insufficient in iron, calcium, and vitamins (Drugay, 1986). The combination of long-established eating patterns, income, transportation, housing, social interaction, and the effects of chronic or acute disease influence the person's nutritional intake and health.
2. Several problems that affect the elderly can be managed effectively when nutritional considerations are given priority in planning (e.g., constipation, osteoporosis, lactose intolerance, anemia).
3. Several situations that affect the elderly client's ability to procure or ingest foods are:
   - Anorexia due to medications, grief, depression, illness
   - Impaired mental status leading to inattention to hunger or selecting insufficient kinds/amounts of food
   - Impaired mobility or manual dexterity (paresis, tremors, weakness, joint pain, or deformity)
   - Voluntary fluid restriction for fear of urinary incontinence
   - Small frame or history of undernutrition
   - Inadequate income to purchase food
   - Lack of transportation to buy food or facility to cook
   - New dentures or poor dentition
   - Dislike of cooking and eating alone
   - Refusal to eat related to death wish or depression
4. Constipation, a frequent geriatric complaint, has been shown to be well managed without laxatives when fluids and fiber (e.g., bran) are increased in the diet and

Table II-14. **Weight for Height and Body Frame***

Men

Height Feet	Inches	Small Frame	Medium Frame	Large Frame
5	2	128–134	131–141	138–150
5	3	130–136	133–143	140–153
5	4	132–138	135–145	142–156
5	5	134–140	137–148	144–160
5	6	136–142	139–151	146–164
5	7	138–145	142–154	149–168
5	8	140–148	145–157	152–172
5	9	142–151	148–160	155–176
5	10	144–154	151–163	158–180
5	11	146–157	154–166	161–184
6	0	149–160	157–170	164–188
6	1	152–164	160–174	168–192
6	2	155–168	164–178	172–197
6	3	158–172	167–182	176–202
6	4	162–176	171–187	181–207

Women

Height Feet	Inches	Small Frame	Medium Frame	Large Frame
4	10	102–111	109–121	118–131
4	11	103–113	111–123	120–134
5	0	104–115	113–126	122–137
5	1	106–118	115–129	125–140
5	2	108–121	118–132	128–143
5	3	111–124	121–135	131–147
5	4	114–127	124–138	134–151
5	5	117–130	127–141	137–155
5	6	120–133	130–144	140–159
5	7	123–136	133–147	143–163
5	8	126–139	136–150	146–167
5	9	129–142	139–153	149–170
5	10	132–145	142–156	152–173
5	11	135–148	145–159	155–176
6	0	138–151	148–162	158–179

To Make an Approximation of Your Frame Size . . .

Extend your arm and bend the forearm upward at a 90 degree angle. Keep fingers straight and turn the inside of your wrist toward your body. If you have a caliper, use it to measure the space between the two prominent bones on *either side* of your elbow. Without a caliper, place thumb and index finger of your other hand on these two bones. Measure the space between your fingers against a ruler or tape measure. Compare it with these tables that list elbow measurements for *medium-framed* men and women. Measurements lower than those listed indicate you have a small frame. Higher measurements indicate a large frame.

Men

Height in 1" Heels	Elbow Breadth
5'2"–5'3"	2½"–2⅞"
5'4"–5'7"	2⅝"–2⅞"
5'8"–5'11"	2¾"–3"
6'0"–6'3"	2¾"–3⅛"
6'4"	2⅞"–3¼"

Women

Height in 1" Heels	Elbow Breadth
4'10"–4'11"	2¼"–2½"
5'0"–5'3"	2¼"–2½"
5'4"–5'7"	2⅜"–2⅝"
5'8"–5'11"	2⅜"–2⅝"
6'0"	2½"–2¾"

*Weights at ages 25–59 based on lowest mortality. Weight in pounds according to frame (in indoor clothing weighing 5 lb for men and 3 lb for women; shoes with 1" heels).
(Revised Height–Weight Tables derived from life-insurance statistics prepared by the Metropolitan Life Insurance Company: men and women. Copyright 1983, Metropolitan Life Insurance Company)

Table II-15. **Anthropometric Measurements (adult)***

Test	Sex	Reference	>90% Reference	90%–60% Reference	<60% Reference
Mid-Arm Circumference (MAC)(in cm)					
	Male	29.3	>26.3	26.3–17.6	<17.6
	Female	28.5	>25.7	25.7–17.1	<17.1
Mid-Arm Muscle Circumference (MAMC)(in cm)					
	Male	25.3	>22.8	22.8–15.2	<15.2
	Female	23.2	>20.9	20.9–13.9	<13.9
Triceps Skin Fold (TSF)(in mm)					
	Male	12.5	>11.3	11.3–7.5	< 7.5
	Female	16.5	>14.9	14.9–9.9	< 9.9

* If measurements are below 90% reference, nutritional support program may be indicated. (Jelliffe DB: The Assessment of the Nutritional Status of the Community. World Health Organization Monograph No. 53. Geneva, WHO, 1966)

activity is increased or abdominal exercises initiated. Clients with diverticulosis also benefit from a high-fiber diet.

5. Adequate intake of calcium and vitamin D can maintain bone strength and calcium stores, a most important consideration in osteoporosis.
6. Persons receiving diuretics must be closely observed for adequate hydration (intake and output) and electrolyte balance, especially sodium and potassium. Potassium-rich foods should be regularly included in the diet.
7. Anorexia or dry mouth due to medication can be attenuated by altering the time of medication administration or offering fluids shortly before mealtime to stimulate the appetite and moisten the oral mucosa.
8. Persons who are impaired either physically or cognitively should receive the necessary support and supervision in selecting foods and in self-feeding.
9. Persons with lactose intolerance should try foods such as yogurt and ice cream, which seem to cause less flatulence and cramping, to meet their calcium needs.
10. Anemia due to iron deficiency usually occurs over a period of time and may be affected by chronic diseases and insufficient dietary iron intake. Increasing the intake of foods rich in vitamin C, folic acid, and dietary iron can improve the conditions necessary for optimal absorption of iron. Iron supplementation is often necessary.

Altered Nutrition: Less Than Body Requirements
Related to Chewing or Swallowing Difficulties

Assessment

Subjective Data

The person reports
    Dry mouth
    Sores in mouth
    "Can't chew (swallow)"

Objective Data

    Wired jaw
    Paresis involving muscles required for chewing or swallowing
    Impaired or broken teeth, missing teeth, ill-fitting dentures
    Stomatitis
    Decreased/absent gag reflex

Outcome Criteria

The person will
- Describe causative factors when known
- Describe rationale and procedure for treatment
- Experience adequate nutrition through oral intake
- Increase oral intake as evidenced by (specify)

Interventions

A. Assess causative factors

    Mechanical obstruction (wired jaw)
    Neurologic condition causing muscle weakness, slowness, uncoordination, paralysis, or a combination of these (CVA, amyotrophic lateral sclerosis, parkinsonian syndrome) (see *Impaired Swallowing*)
    Decreased salivation (radiation therapy)
    Dental disorders
    Stomatitis (see *Altered Oral Mucous Membrane*)

B. Reduce or eliminate causative and contributing factors if possible

1. Mechanical obstruction
    a. Instruct or assist person to
      - Keep a record of intake
      - Perform oral hygiene immediately after eating (*e.g.*, Water Pik-type cleansing [preferred])

        Swishing low-calories carbonated beverage around mouth

        Swishing solution of 1/2 or 1/4 hydrogen peroxide and 1/2 or 3/4 water around mouth (solution can be flavored with mouthwash)

  b. Teach techniques to maintain adequate nutritional intake and stimulate appetite

- Vary liquids to allow for different textures and tastes (*e.g.,* juices, cream soups)
- Use commercially prepared or home-made high-protein/calorie supplements (*e.g.,* enrich milk [mix 1 quart fresh milk with 1 cup instant nonfat milk] and blenderize with various flavorings—ripe banana, ice cream, syrups, fresh or frozen fruit)

2. Decreased salivation

  a. Instruct or assist person to

- Increase liquid intake with meals
- "Wet" food to make up for lack of saliva
- Use artificial saliva
- Papain tablets, 10 minutes before eating
- Meat tenderizer made from papaya enzyme applied to oral cavity with lemon glycerin swab 10 minutes before eating
- Suck on lemon immediately before eating to stimulate salivation (overuse can damage tooth enamel)
- Avoid consuming only milk and milk products because they tend to form a tenacious mucus

  b. Check medications person is on for side-effects of dry mouth/decreased salivation

  c. Teach person to rinse mouth whenever needed to remove debris, stimulate gums, or lubricate and refresh mouth

3. Swallowing difficulties

  a. Before beginning feeding, assess that person is adequately alert and responsive, is able to control mouth, has cough/gag reflex, and can swallow own saliva

  b. Have suction equipment available and functioning properly

  c. Position person correctly

- Have individual sit upright (60°–90°) in chair or dangle feet at side of bed if possible (prop pillows if necessary)
- Have individual assume position 10 to 15 minutes before and after eating
- Have individual flex head forward on the midline about 45° to keep esophagus patent

  d. Start with small amounts and progress slowly as person learns to handle each step

        Part of eyedropper filled with water

        Whole eyedropper

        Use juice in place of water

        1/4 teaspoon semi-solid (applesauce)

        1/2 teaspoon semi-solid

        1 teaspoon semi-solid

        pureed food or commercially prepared baby foods

        1/2 cracker

        Soft diet

        Regular diet

- For person who has had a CVA, place food at back of tongue and on side of face he can control
- Feed slowly, making certain previous bite has been swallowed

   e. Reduce noxious stimuli
- Minimize distractions by turning off television or radio and secluding individual for the feeding session
- Keep patient focused on task by giving directions until he has finished swallowing each mouthful

      "Move food to middle of tongue"

      "Raise tongue to roof of mouth"

      "Think about swallowing"

      "Swallow"

      "Cough to clear airway"

   f. Check that mouth is empty before continuing
- Make sure food has not collected in the cheek pouches

   g. Instruct or assist person to
- Administer good oral hygiene before and after feedings
- Avoid spicy, acid, or salty foods
- Avoid rough foods (raw vegetables, bran)
- Soak "dry" foods (toast) to soften
- If cold foods are soothing to individual, add ice or ice cream to gain extra coldness
- Avoid smoking and alcohol (they may irritate mouth or throat)

C. Initiate health teaching and referrals as indicated

- Consult with speech pathologist for assistance with persons with swallowing difficulties
- Consult with dietician for assistance with diet plan
- Explain to individual and significant others rationale of treatment and how to proceed with it
- See *Altered Oral Mucous Membrane Related to Stomatitis* if indicated
- See *Impaired Swallowing* if indicated

Altered Nutrition: Less Than Body Requirements
Related to Anorexia

Anorexia is a lack of appetite for food or fluids.

Assessment

Subjective Data

The person reports

   He is not hungry

   Nausea

   Cannot concentrate on food

Objective Data

Weight loss

Intake less than recommended daily allowance (RDA)

Outcome Criteria

The person will
- Increase oral intake as evidenced by (specify)
- Describe causative factors when known
- Describe rationale and procedure for treatments

Interventions

A. Assess causative factors

Alteration in sense of taste or smell

Social isolation

Radiation therapy or chemotherapy

Alteration in body image or self-concept

Early satiety

Noxious stimuli (pain or painful or unpleasant procedures, fatigue, odors, nausea and vomiting)

B. Reduce or eliminate contributing factors if possible

1. Altered sense of taste or smell
   - Explain to person the importance of consuming adequate amounts of nutrients
   - Teach person to use spices to help improve the taste and aroma of food (lemon juice, mint, cloves, basil, thyme, cinnamon, rosemary, bacon bits)
   - Teach protein sources he may find more acceptable than red meat
        Eggs and dairy products
        Chicken and turkey
        Fish (if not strong-smelling)
        Marinated meat (in wine, vinegar)
        Soy products (tofu)
   - Chopped or ground meats/protein sources may be more acceptable
   - Mixing protein and vegetables may be more acceptable
   - Refer to meals as "snacks" to make them sound smaller
2. Social isolation
   - Encourage individual to eat with others (meals served in dining room or group area, at local meeting place such as community center, by church groups)
   - Provide daily contact through phone calls by support system
   - See *Social Isolation* for additional interventions
3. Noxious stimuli (pain, fatigue, odors, nausea, and vomiting)
   a. Pain
      - Plan care so that unpleasant or painful procedures do not take place before meals
      - Medicate individual for pain ½ hour before meals according to physician's orders

- Provide pleasant, relaxed atmosphere for eating (no bedpans in sight; don't rush); try a "surprise" (*e.g.,* flowers with meal)
- Arrange plan of care to decrease or eliminate nauseating odors or procedures near mealtimes

b. Fatigue
- Teach or assist individual to rest before meals
- Teach individual to spend minimal energy in food preparation (cook large quantities and freeze several meals at a time; request assistance from others)

c. Odor of food
- Teach him to avoid cooking odors—frying foods, brewing coffee—if possible (take a walk; select foods that can be eaten cold)
- Suggest using foods that require little cooking during periods of anorexia

d. Nausea and vomiting
- Encourage frequent small amounts of ice chips or cool clear liquids (dilute tea, Jell-O water, flat ginger ale or cola) unless vomiting continues (adults 30 to 60 ml q ½–1 hour; children 15 to 30 ml q ½–1 hour)
- Consider giving medications by suppository rather than by mouth
- Decrease the stimulation of the vomiting center

  Reduce unpleasant sights and odors

  Provide good mouth care after vomiting

  Teach person to practice deep breathing and voluntary swallowing to suppress the vomiting reflex

  Instruct him to sit down after eating but not to lie down

  Encourage him to eat smaller meals and eat slowly
- Restrict liquids with meals to avoid overdistending the stomach; also avoid fluids 1 hour before and after meals
- If possible, avoid the smell of food preparation
- Try eating cold foods, which have less odor
- Loosen clothing
- Sit in fresh air
- Avoid lying down flat for at least 2 hours after eating (an individual who must rest should sit or recline so head is at least 4 inches higher than feet)

See *Impaired Swallowing* for additional interventions

C. Promote foods that stimulate eating and increase protein consumption

1. Maintain good oral hygiene (brush teeth, rinse mouth) before and after ingestion of food
2. Offer frequent small feedings (six per day plus snacks) to reduce the feeling of a distended stomach
3. Allow individual to choose food items as close to actual eating time as possible
4. Arrange to have highest protein/calorie nutrients served at the time individual feels most like eating (*e.g.,* if chemotherapy is in early morning, serve in late afternoon)
5. Encourage significant others to bring in favorite home foods
6. Instruct person to
   - Eat dry foods (toast, crackers) upon arising
   - Eat salty foods if permissible
   - Avoid overly sweet, rich, greasy, or fried foods
   - Try clear cool beverages
   - Sip slowly through straw
   - Take whatever he feels he can tolerate
   - Eat small portions low in fat and eat more frequently

7. Try commercial supplements available in many forms (liquids, powder, pudding); keep switching brands until some are found that are acceptable to individual in taste and consistency
8. Teach techniques to individual and family for home food preparation
   - Add powdered milk or egg to milkshakes, gravies, sauces, puddings, cereals, meatballs, or milk to increase protein calorie content
   - Add blenderized or baby foods to meat juices or soups
   - Use fortified milk (*i.e.,* 1 cup instant nonfat milk to 1 quart fresh milk)
   - Use milk or half-and-half instead of water when making soups and sauces; soy formulas can also be used
   - Add cheese or diced meat whenever able
   - Add cream cheese or peanut butter to toast, crackers, celery sticks
   - Add extra butter or margarine to soups, sauces, vegetables
   - Spread toast while hot
   - Use mayonnaise (100 cal/T) instead of salad dressing
   - Add sour cream or yogurt to vegetables or as dip
   - Use whipped cream (60 cal/T)
   - Add raisins, dates, nuts, and brown sugar to hot or cold cereals
   - Have extra food (snacks) easily available
9. Review high calorie vs. low calorie foods
10. If lactose-intolerant, explore alternate dairy source to drinking milk (*i.e.,* cheese, yogurt, acidophilus milk)

D. Initiate health teaching and referrals as indicated
   1. Dietitian for meal planning
   2. Psychiatric therapy when indicated
   3. Community meal centers
   4. Support groups for anorexics

Altered Nutrition: Less Than Body Requirements
Related to Difficulty or Inability to Procure Food

Altered ability to procure food is the inability to acquire food because of physical, economic, or sociocultural barriers.

Assessment

Subjective Data
The person reports
"Can't afford to buy food"
"Don't know how to fix foods"
"Too much bother to fix meals for one person"

Objective Data
> Inability to speak or understand English
> Activity restriction

Outcome Criteria

The person will
- Describe causative factors when known
- Identify a method to acquire food on a regular schedule

Interventions

A. Assess causative factors

> Inadequate economic resources to obtain adequate nutrition
> Sociocultural barrier
> Physical inability to procure food, related to health problem such as COPD, cardiac condition, CVA, or quadriplegia

B. Eliminate or reduce contributing factors if possible

1. Inadequate economic resources
   - Assess eligibility for food stamps, or other government-funded programs for low-income groups; consult with social service
   - Suggest co-operatives or local farmers' markets for shopping
   - Buy foods and meats on sale and freeze; utilize cheaper cuts and tenderize
   - Suggest foods that are low in cost and nutritionally high; decrease use of prepackaged or prepared items
     > Beans and legumes as protein source
     > Powdered milk (alone or mixed half-and-half with whole milk)
     > Seasonal foods when plentiful
   - Encourage growing a small garden or participating in a community plot
   - Freeze or can fruits and vegetables in season (refer to county agricultural agent for information on canning and freezing)
2. Sociocultural barrier
   - Introduce individual to locally available foodstuffs and instruct in their preparation
   - Suggest substitutions of locally available foodstuffs for those to which individual is accustomed
   - Refer to adult education home economics classes for food preparation
   - Assist individual in recognizing and using additional outlets and sources of food (grocery stores, meat and fruit markets)
   - Encourage peer-group meetings among people of similar backgrounds to allow learning and exchange of ideas
   - Acquaint with ethnic food store locations if available
3. Physical deficits
   - Promote alternate methods of food procurement and preparation
     a. Assess support systems for someone willing to purchase or prepare food for individual or take him to store
        > Supermarkets that deliver
        > Meals on Wheels or similar service

Homemaker

Group housing

Door-to-store bus service

  b. Teach the individual or others to cook enough for six meals at one time and freeze; make own complete "frozen dinners"

- Aid person in planning daily activities to account for energy need in shopping for food and preparing meals

Rest periods before and after activity

Rest periods during activity if needed

C. Initiate health teaching and referrals as indicated

1. Social worker, occupational therapist, or visiting nurse, as needed
2. Adult education programs
3. Local extension office for information on vegetable gardening, community gardens, and techniques of freezing and canning foods
4. Dietician for meal planning

References/Bibliography

Books and Articles

Buckley JE, Addicks CL, Maniglia J: Feeding patients with dysphagia. Nurs Forum 15(1):69–85, 1976

Cooper KH: The New Aerobics. New York, Bantam Books, 1979

Cockram D, Kaminski M: Current concepts in nutritional assessment. Nutritional Support Services 6(5):14–15, 1986

Dansky KM: Assessing children's nutrition. Am J Nurs 77:1610–1611, 1977

Drugay M: Nutritional evaluation: Who needs it. J Gerontol Nurs 12(4):14–18, 1986

Ewald EB: Recipes for a Small Planet. New York, Ballantine Books, 1973

Forlaw L, Bayu L (eds): Symposium on Nutrition. Nurs Clin North Am 18(1), 1983

Glucroft J: Slim test update. Nutritional Support Services 6(5):16, 1986

Griffin KM, Stubbert J, Breckenridge K: Teaching the dysphagic patient to swallow. RN 37(9):60–63, 1974

Kaminski MV Jr, Jeejeebhoy KN: Modern clinical nutritional assessment—diagnosis of malnutrition and selection of therapy. American Journal of Intravenous Therapy and Clinical Nutrition 6(3):31–50, 1979

Kornguth ML: Nursing management—when your client has a weight problem. Am J Nurs 81:553–554, 1981

Mitchell HS, Rynbergen HJ, Anderson L et al (eds): Cooper's Nutrition in Health and Disease, 16th ed. Philadelphia, JB Lippincott, 1976

Molleson A: New Dimensions in Nutrition. Columbus, Ohio, Ross Laboratories, 1980

Rang ML: Bibliography for nutrition in pregnancy. J Obstet Gynecol Neonatal Nurs 9:55–58, 1980

Rouedu JR: Dysphagia: An Assessment and Management Program for the Adult. Minneapolis, Sister Kenny Institute-Abbott-Northwestern Hospital, 1980

Sine R, Liss S, Roush R et al: Basic Rehabilitation Techniques. Germantown, MD, Aspen Systems Corp, 1977

Sussman A, Goode R: Walking for Pleasure, for Health and Serenity. New York, Famolau, 1977

Worthington B (ed): Symposium on nutrition. Nurs Clin North Am 14(2), 1979

Resources for the Consumer

Literature

Chamberlain AS: The Soft Foods Cookbook. Garden City, NY, Doubleday

Chemotherapy and You (N.I.H. Pub. No. 81-1136). These three pamphlets available from U.S. Department of Health, Office of Cancer Communications, National Cancer Institute, Building 31, Room 108A18, Bethesda, Maryland 20205

Diet and Nutrition (N.I.H. Pub. No. 81-2038). A resource for parents of children with cancer.

Eating Hints (N.I.H. Pub. No. 81-2079). Recipes and tips for better nutrition during cancer treatment

Goldbeck N: As you Eat So Your Baby Grows: A Guide to Nutrition in Pregnancy. Available from Ceres Press, Box 87, Dept D, Woodstock, NY 12498 ($1.75)

McGill M, Pye O: The No-Nonsense Guide to Food and Nutrition. Piscataway, NJ, New Century, 1982

List of publications. Society for Nutrition Education, 2140 Shattuck Avenue, Suite 1110, Berkeley, CA 94704

Impaired Swallowing

Related to
(Specify)

Definition

Impaired swallowing: The state in which an individual has decreased ability to voluntarily pass fluids and/or solid foods from the mouth to the stomach.

Defining Characteristics

Major (must be present)

Observed evidence of difficulty in swallowing and/or
Evidence of aspiration
Stasis of food in oral cavity

Minor (may be present)

Coughing
Choking
Apraxia (ideational, constructional, or visual)

Etiological, Contributing, Risk Factors

Pathophysiological

Cleft lip/palate
Neuromuscular disorders (*e.g.,* cerebral palsy, muscular dystrophy, myasthenia gravis, Guillain-Barré, botulism, poliomyelitis, Parkinson's disease)
Neoplastic disease (disease affecting brain and/or brain stem)
Cerebrovascular accident
Right or left hemispheric damage to brain
Damage to 5th, 7th, 9th, 10th, or 11th cranial nerve
Tracheoesophageal fistula
Tracheoesophageal tumors, edema

Treatment-related

Surgical reconstruction of the mouth and/or throat
Anesthesia
Mechanical obstruction (tracheostomy tube)

Situational (personal, environmental)

Altered level of consciousness
Fatigue
Limited awareness
Altered sense of taste
Irritated oropharyngeal cavity

Maturational
>   Infant/children: congenital anomalies, developmental disorders

Focal Assessment Criteria

Subjective Data

>   History of problem with swallowing
>   Diet recall for past 24 hours
>>   Is that the usual intake pattern?
>   History of problem foods
>   Diet history
>   Weight change
>   Present dietary pattern
>>   Diet diary
>>   Food source and preparation
>>   Living arrangements
>>   Financial status
>   Coping pattern
>>   Perception of problem
>>   Perception of causation
>   Knowledge of nutrition
>>   Basic food groups
>>   Foods high and low in calories
>   Physiological alterations
>>   Medical history
>>   Presence of:
>>>   Allergies
>>>   Vomiting
>>>   Fatigue
>>>   Dysphagia
>>>   Pain
>>>   Stomatitis

Objective Data

>   Height and weight
>   Ability to swallow, chew, feed self
>   Neuromuscular impairment
>>   Decreased/absent gag reflex
>>   Decreased strength on excursion of muscles involved in mastication
>>   Perceptual impairment
>>   Facial paralysis
>   Mechanical obstruction
>>   Edema
>>   Tracheostomy tube
>>   Tumor
>   Perceptual patterns/awareness
>   Level of consciousness
>   Condition of oropharyngeal cavity
>   Nasal regurgitation
>   Hoarseness
>   Aspiration

Cough a second or two after swallowing
Dehydration
Apraxia

Principles and Rationale for Nursing Care

1. Swallowing has an intellectual component as well as a physical one.
2. Swallowing (deglutition) can be divided into three phases:
   a. voluntary
   b. pharyngeal
   c. esophageal
3. The 5th, 7th, 9th, 10th, and 11th cranial nerves are involved in deglutition.
4. Swallowing is a complex activity.
5. A cough reflex is essential for rehabilitation, but a gag reflex is not.
6. Do not confuse the ability to chew with the ability to swallow. See also *Altered Nutrition: Less Than Body Requirements*.
7. An individual may have more than one type of swallowing impairment.

Swallowing, Impaired
Related to (Specify)

Some statement examples are:
- Related to mechanical impairment of mouth
- Related to muscle paralysis or paresis
- Related to inability to participate in automatic eating behavior secondary to decreased cognition

Assessment

See Defining Characteristics

Outcome Criteria

The person will
- Report improved ability to swallow

The person and/or family will
- Describe causative factors when known
- Describe rationale and procedures for treatment

Interventions

A. Assess for causative or contributing factors

1. Mechanical impairment of oropharyngeal structures
   a. Congenital anomalies

      b. Cleft lip/palate
      c. Cranial nerve damage (5th, 7th, 9th, 10th, and/or 11th)
      d. Surgical reconstruction of mouth
      e. Cerebrovascular accident
      f. Altered level of consciousness
      g. Fatigue
      h. Reddened, irritated oropharyngeal cavity
      i. Decreased/absent gag reflex
  2. Muscle paralysis or paresis
      a. Post-CVA
      b. Cranial nerve damage
      c. Decreased/absent gag reflex (*e.g.* postradiation)
  3. Impaired cognition or awareness
      a. Cortical damage
      b. Apraxia
      c. Aphasia

B. Reduce or eliminate causative/contributing factors in individuals with:

  1. Mechanical impairment of mouth—Assist the individual with moving the bolus of food from the anterior to the posterior of mouth
      a. Place food in the posterior mouth where swallowing can be assured, using
        • A syringe with a short piece of tubing attached
        • A glossectomy spoon
        • Soft food of a consistency that can be manipulated by the tongue against the pharynx, such as gelatin, custard, or mashed potatoes
      b. Prevent/decrease thick secretions
        • Artifical saliva
        • Papain tablets dissolved in mouth 10 minutes before eating
        • Meat tenderizer made from papaya enzyme applied to oral cavity 10 minutes before eating
        • Frequent mouth care
        • Increase fluid intake
        • Check medications for potential side-effects of dry mouth/decreased salivation
  2. Muscle paralysis or paresis
    Strengthen muscles by the following measures:
    • Pass a #14 or #16 feeding tube several times a day while verbally encouraging person to swallow
    • Talk the person through the process of swallowing a feeding tube
    • Instruct/guide person through swallowing tube himself
    • Increase size of feeding tube to #18 tube if further strengthening is required
    • Encourage person to think about swallowing while doing it
    • Progress to ice chips, water, and then food when danger of aspiration is decreased
  3. Impaired cognition or awareness
      a. General
        • Remove feeding tube during training if increased gag reflex is present
        • Concentrate on solids rather than liquids, since liquids are generally less well tolerated
        • Keep extraneous stimuli at minimum while eating (*e.g.,* no television or radio, no verbal stimuli unless directed at task)
        • Have person concentrate on task of swallowing

- Have person sit up in chair with neck slightly flexed
- Instruct person to hold breath while swallowing
- Observe for swallowing and check mouth for emptying
- Avoid overloading mouth, because this decreases swallowing effectiveness
- Give solids and liquids separately

b. Person with aphasia, or left hemispheric damage
- Demonstrate expected behavior
- Reinforce behaviors with simple one-word commands

c. Person with apraxia, or right hemispheric damage
- Divide task into smallest units possible
- Assist person through each task with verbal commands
- Allow person to complete one unit fully before giving next command
- Continue verbal assistance at each eating session until no longer needed
- Incorporate written checklist as a reminder to person

Note: Person may have both left and right hemispheric damage and require a combination of the above techniques.

C. Reduce the possibility of aspiration

1. Before beginning feeding, assess that person is adequately alert and responsive, is able to control mouth, has cough/gag reflex, and can swallow own saliva
2. Have suction equipment available and functioning properly
3. Position person correctly
   - Have individual sit upright (60°–90°) in chair or dangle feet at side of bed if possible (prop pillows if necessary)
   - Have individual assume position 10 to 15 minutes before eating and maintain position for 10 to 15 minutes after finishing eating
   - Have individual flex head forward on the midline about 45° to keep esophagus patent
4. Keep individual focused on task by giving directions until he has finished swallowing each mouthful
   - "Take a breath"
   - "Move food to middle of tongue"
   - "Raise tongue to roof of mouth"
   - "Think about swallowing"
   - "Swallow"
   - "Cough to clear airway"
   - Reinforce voluntary action
5. Start with small amounts and progress slowly as person learns to handle each step
   - Ice chips
   - Part of eyedropper filled with water
   - Whole eyedropper
   - Use juice in place of water
   - 1/4 teaspoon semi-solid
   - 1/2 teaspoon semi-solid
   - 1 teaspoon semi-solid
   - Pureed food or commercial baby foods
   - One-half cracker
   - Soft diet
   - Regular diet
   - For person who has had a CVA, place food at back of tongue and on side of face he can control

- Feed slowly, making certain previous bite has been swallowed
- Some individuals do better with foods that hold together, such as soft-boiled eggs or ground meat and gravy

D. Initiate health teaching and referrals as indicated

- Consult with speech pathologist
- Consult with dietician for meal planning
- Explain to individual and significant others rationale of treatment and how to proceed with it
- See *Altered Oral Mucous Membrane Related to Stomatitis* if indicated
- See *Nutrition, Altered: Less Than Body Requirements*

Note: If the above strategies are unsuccessful, consultation with physician may be necessary for alternative feeding techniques such as tube feedings or parenteral nutrition.

References/Bibliography

Forlaw L: The critically ill patient: Nutritional implications. Nurs Clin North Am 18:111–117, 1983

Gettrust KV, Ryan SC, Engleman DS: Applied Nursing Diagnosis: Guides for Comprehensive Care Planning, pp 15–16. New York, John Wiley & Sons, 1984

Iverson T, Carpenter M, Haskin D, Maas M et al: Fulfilling nutritional requirements. J Gerontol Nurs 14(4):16–24, 1988

Lang C, Cooning S, Newman S: Nutritional support: A foundation for critical care. Critical Care Quarterly 5(2):45–47, 1982

Larsen GL: Chewing and swallowing. In Martin N, Holt NB, Hicks DB (eds): Comprehensive Rehabiliation Nursing, pp 173–185. New York, McGraw-Hill, 1981

McNally J, Stair J, Somerville E (eds): Guidelines for Cancer Nursing Practice. Orlando FL, Grune & Stratton, 1985

Salmond S: How to assess the nutritional status of acutely ill patients. Am J Nurs 80:922–924, 1980

Tilton CN, Maloof M: Diagnosing the problem in stroke. Am J Nurs 82:596–601, 1982

Welnetz K: Maintaining adequate nutrition and hydration in the dysphagic ALS patient. Can Nurse 79(3):30–34, 1983

Worthington-Roberts B, Karkeck JM: Nutrition. In Carnevali D, Patrick M (eds): Nursing Management for the Elderly, 2nd ed, pp 189–218. Philadelphia, JB Lippincott, 1986

Nutrition, Altered: More Than Body Requirements

Related to **Imbalance of Intake vs. Activity Expenditures**

Definition

Altered nutrition: More than body requirements: The state in which the individual experiences or is at risk of experiencing weight gain related to an intake in excess of metabolic requirements

> **Author's Note:** Obesity is a complex condition with sociocultural, psychological, and metabolic implications. This diagnostic category, when used to describe obesity or overweight conditions, focuses on them as a nutritional problem. The focus of treatment is behavioral modification and life-style changes. It is recommended that *Altered Health Maintenance Related to Intake in Excess of Metabolic Requirements* be used in place of this diagnostic category. When weight gain is the result of physiological conditions (*e.g.,* altered taste) or pharmacological interventions (*e.g.,* corticosteroid), this diagnostic category can be clinically useful.

Defining Characteristics

Major (must be present)

Overweight (weight 10% over ideal for height and frame), or
Obese (weight 20% or more over ideal for height and frame)
Triceps skin fold greater than 15 mm in men and 25 mm in women

Minor (may be present)

Reported undesirable eating patterns
Intake in excess of metabolic requirements
Sedentary activity patterns

Etiological, Contributing, Risk Factors

Pathophysiological

Altered satiety patterns
Decreased sense of taste and smell

Treatment-related

Medications (corticosteriods)
Radiation (decreased sense of taste and smell)

Situational (personal, environmental)

Pregnancy (at risk to gain more than 25–30 pounds)

Maturational

Adult/elderly: Decreased activity patterns; decreased metabolic needs

Focus Assessment Criteria

See *Altered Nutrition: Less Than Body Requirements*

Principles and Rationale for Nursing Care

Obesity

1. Intake must be reduced to 500 calories per day less than requirement to obtain a one-pound-per-week weight loss.
2. The desirable weight loss rate is 1 to 2 pounds per week.
3. Overeating is a complex multidimensional problem with physical, social, and psychological components.
4. Overweight persons are usually nutritionally deprived.
5. Exercise produces weight loss by increasing the caloric utilization by the body. Exercise does not have to occur in one time period to lose weight but may be spread out over a period of days and still be successful.
6. Internal motivation is essential for a successful weight-loss program.
7. An individual's body image and coping patterns influence the weight-loss program's success or failure.
8. Childhood obesity is influenced by genetic factors; cellular structure; general body build; metabolic and endocrine factors (pancreatic insufficiency, hypothyroidism, hypersecretion of adrenal cortex); activity level; infantile obesity; and the psychological, social, or cultural use of food for comfort, reward, or solace or as a symbol of affluence.
9. See *Altered Nutrition: Less Than Body Requirements* for additional principles.

Altered Nutrition: More Than Body Requirements
Related to Imbalance of Intake vs. Activity Expenditures*

Assessment

Subjective Data

Client states
"I like to eat"
"Eating calms my nerves"
"I don't have time for exercise"
"I don't like sports or exercise"
"I can't exercise"

Objective Data

Weight >10% over ideal for height and frame
Triceps skin fold greater than 15 mm in men and 25 mm in women

---

* This specific diagnosis describes the individual who ingests calories in excess of metabolic need.

Outcome Criteria

The person will
- Experience increased activity expenditure with weight loss
- Describe relationship between activity level and weight
- Identify eating patterns that contribute to weight gain
- Lose weight

Interventions

A. Assess causative factors

Stress response (increased oral intake)
Lack of basic nutritional knowledge
Low body image or self-concept (see *Ineffective Individual Coping Related to Depression*)
Ethnic or cultural values
Boredom
Sedentary life-style or work

B. Increase individual's awareness of those actions that contribute to excessive oral intake
- Request him to write down all the food he has eaten for the past 24 hours
- Instruct him to keep a diet diary for one week
  What, when, where, and why eaten?
  Whether doing anything else (*e.g.,* watching television, preparing dinner)
  Emotions just before eating
  Others present (snacking with spouse, children)
- Review diet diary with individual to point out patterns (*i.e.,* time, place, persons, emotions, foods) that affect intake
- Review high- and low-calorie food items

C. Assist person to set realistic goals (*i.e.,* decreasing oral intake by 500 calories will result in a 1-to-2-lb loss each week)
- Calculate requirements for actual weight minus 15 pounds and recalculate every two months or as necessary (actual weight in pounds $- 15 \times 10 =$ maximum daily calories allowed if there is to be a weight loss)
- Plan balanced acceptable diet (remember cultural and personal preferences and use exchange lists; diet should provide choices)
- Plan for extra calories on weekends or as a special treat
- Select non-food rewards such as new clothes or a night out

D. Alter identified patterns of eating

For example, if Friday night is the time when excess eating occurs, plan to be out on Friday night; if the person eats while watching television, keep hands occupied in another manner such as knitting or crocheting, limit television watching, or eat low-calorie snacks such as unbuttered popcorn, raw celery, and carrots.

E. Teach behavior modification techniques
- Eat only at a specific spot at home (*i.e.,* kitchen table)
- Do not eat while doing other activities such as reading or watching television; eat only when sitting
- Drink 8-oz glass of water immediately before eating
- Decrease second helpings, fat and fatty foods, sweets and sugar and alcohol
- Use small plates (portions look bigger)
- Prepare small portions, just enough for a meal, and discard leftovers
- Never eat from another person's plate
- Eat slowly and chew thoroughly
- Put down utensils and wait 15 seconds between bites
- Eat low-calorie snacks that need to be chewed to satisfy oral need (carrots, celery, apples)
- Decrease liquid calories; drink diet sodas or water
- Plan eating splurges (save a number of calories a day and have a treat once a week) but eat only a small amount of splurge foods

F. Increase activity level*
- Use stairs instead of elevator
- Park at outer edge of parking lot
- Plan a daily walking program and gradually increase rate and length of walk
  1. Start out at 5 to 10 blocks for 0.5 to 1.0 mile/day; increase 1 block or 0.1 mile/week
  2. Remember, progress slowly
  3. Avoid straining or pushing too hard and becoming overly fatigued
  4. Stop immediately if any of the following signs occur:

Lightness or pain in chest	Dizziness
Severe breathlessness	Loss of muscle control
Lightheadedness	Nausea

  5. If pulse is 120 beats per minute (BPM) 5 minutes after stopping exercise, or if pulse is 100 BPM 10 minutes after stopping exercise, or if short of breath 10 minutes after exercise, slow down either the rate of walking or the distance
  6. If unable to walk 5 blocks or 0.5 mile without signs of overexertion appearing, decrease length of walking for one week to before signs appear and then start to add 1 block/0.1 mile each week
  7. Walk at same rate; time self with stopwatch or second hand on watch; after reaching 10 blocks (1 mile) try to increase speed
  8. Remember, increase only the rate *or* the length of walk at one time
  9. Establish a regular time of day to exercise, with the goal of 3 to 5 times per week for a duration of 15 to 45 minutes and with a heart rate of 80% of stress test or gross calculation (170 BPM for 20–29 age group; decrease 10 BPM for each additional decade of life—*e.g.,* 160 BPM for ages 30–39, 150 BPM for ages 40–49, etc.)
- Encourage significant others to engage in walking program also

G. Add additional exercise as tolerated

Television or tape cassette exercise program	Dancing
Exercycle	Swimming
Spa/gym/YMCA	Bicycling

* **Caution:** If health problem exists, consult physician before increasing activity.

H. Initiate health teaching and referrals as indicated

- Explain basic nutritional knowledge
- Explain health hazards of overweight
- Explain the benefits of exercise (*e.g.,* consumes calories, reduces stress)
- Refer to support groups (*e.g.,* Weight Watchers, Overeaters Anonymous, TOPS, trim clubs, The Diet Workshop, Inc.)
- Dietician for meal planning
- Physician for morbid obesity and evaluation of other health problems

Bibliography

See *Altered Nutrition: Less Than Body Requirements* for additional sources of information.
Hoepfel HJ: Improving compliance with an exercise program. Am J Nurs 80:449–450, 1980
Jacobsen P: Help for fat teenagers. Pediatr Nurs 5(2):49–50, 1979
Kaufmann NA: Eating habits and opinions of teenagers on nutrition and obesity. J Am Diet Assoc 66:264–268, 1975
Overeaters anonymous: A self-help group. Am J Nurs 81:560–563, 1981
Schroeder MA (ed): Symposium on Obesity. Nurs Clin North Am 17(2), 1982

Nutrition, Altered: Potential For More Than Body Requirements

Definition

Altered nutrition: Potential for more than body requirements: The state in which an individual is at risk of experiencing an intake of nutrients that exceeds metabolic needs.

Author's Note: This diagnostic category is similar to *Potential Altered Nutrition: More Than Body Requirements*. It describes an individual who has a family history of obesity, is demonstrating a pattern of higher weight, and/or has had a history of excessive weight gain. (*e.g.,* previous pregnancy). Until clinical research differentiates this category from other presently accepted categories, use *Altered Health Maintenance* (*Actual* or *Potential*) or *Potential Altered Nutrition: More Than Body Requirements* to direct teaching to assist families and individuals to identify unhealthy dietary patterns.

Defining Characteristics

Reported or observed obesity in one or both parents
Rapid transition across growth percentiles in infants or children
Reported use of solid food as major food source before 5 months of age
Observed use of food as reward or comfort measure
Report of observed higher baseline weight at beginning of each pregnancy
Dysfunctional eating patterns

Parenting, Altered

Related to **Impaired Parental–Infant Attachment (Bonding)**

Parental Role Conflict

Related to **The Illness and/or Hospitalization of a Child**

Parenting, Altered

Related to **Impaired Parental–Infant Attachment (Bonding)**

Definition
Altered parenting: The state in which one or more caregivers experiences a real or potential inability to provide a constructive environment that nurtures the growth and development of his/her/their child (children).

> **Author's Note:** A family's ability to function is at a high risk of developing problems when the child or parent has a condition that increases the stress of the family unit. The term *parent* refers to any individual(s) defined as the primary caregiver(s) for a child.

Defining Characteristics

Major (must be present)

Inappropriate parenting behaviors, and/or
Lack of parental attachment behavior

Minor (may be present)

Frequent verbalization of dissatisfaction or disappointment with infant/child
Verbalization of frustration of role
Verbalization of perceived or actual inadequacy
Diminished or inappropriate visual, tactile, or auditory stimulation of infant
Evidence of abuse or neglect of child
Growth and development lag in infant/child

Etiological, Contributing, Risk Factors
Individuals or families who may be at high risk for developing or experiencing parenting difficulties:

Parent(s)

Single	Emotionally disturbed	Terminally ill
Adolescent	Alcoholic	Acutely disabled
Abusive	Addicted to drugs	Accident victim

Child

Of unwanted pregnancy	Physically handicapped	Terminally ill
Of undesired sex	Mentally handicapped	Rebellious
With undesired characteristics	Hyperactive	

Situational (personal, environmental)

Separation from nuclear family
Lack of extended family

Lack of knowledge
Economic problems
    Inflation   Unemployment
Relationship problems
    Marital discord   Stepparents
    Divorce   Live-in boy/girl friend
    Separation   Relocation
Change in family unit
    New child   Relative moves in

Other

History of ineffective relationships with own parents
Parental history of abusive relationship with parents
Unrealistic expectations of child by parent
Unrealistic expectations of self by parent
Unrealistic expectations of parent by child
Unmet psychosocial needs of child by parent
Unmet psychosocial needs of parent by child

Focus Assessment Criteria

Applies to each individual (mother and father) and to family unit
1. Attachment behavior
    Pregnancy
        Planned?   Was an abortion considered?
        Desired?   If yes, why was decision
                                    changed?

    Prenatal
        Verbalizes anticipation   Seeks prenatal care
        Selects name   Follows the regimen
        Plans layette   Decides about infant feeding
                                    (breast or bottle)
    Intrapartum
        Participates in the decision and the birthing process
        Verbalizes positive feelings
        Attempts to see infant as soon as delivered
        Responds positively (happy) or negatively (sad, apathetic, disappointed, an-
            gry, ambivalent)
        Holds and talks to infant
        Uses baby's name
        Talks to baby's father
    Postpartum
        Verbalizes positive feelings
        Seeks proximity by holding infant closely; touches and hugs
        Smiles and gazes at infant; seeks eye-to-eye contact
        Seeks family resemblance (*i.e.,* "has my eyes," "sleeps like his father")
        Refers to infant by name and sex
        Expresses interest in learning infant care
        Performs nurturing behavior (*i.e.,* feeding, changing)
2. Family structure/roles
    Characteristics of the family: age and sex of family members, cultural and
        religious backgrounds, occupations of parent(s).

Roles of parent(s) within and outside of family structure; identify potential for role conflicts

Demands of daily living (employment, financial)

Social support systems of parent(s)

Location of most relatives

Frequency of visits with relatives

Length of time lived at present residence

Patterns of parental socialization with friends and relatives

Interrelationship between parents

3. Parenting knowledge/experience

Parents' recall of their relationship with their parent or caretakers and types of discipline and punishment used

Experiences with previous pregnancies

Knowledge of developmental needs and demands

Parental expectations of child

Parent or parents' understanding of the child's reaction to hospitalization and/or illness

4. Parent/child relationship

Subjective

Parental level of satisfaction with child

Amount of play activities between mother and child

Amount of play activities between father and child

Amount of caretaking activities between mother and child

Amount of caretaking activities between father and child

Provisions for child development (toys, verbal stimulation)

Reasons for disciplining

Methods of discipline or punishment

5. Individuals (parent, child) at high risk for parenting problems

Assess for presence of at-risk factors in parent and child (see Etiological, Contributing, Risk Factors)

Objective

Child's affect (animated, warm, apathetic, cold, withdrawn)

Presence of touching/holding behavior

Presence of injuries

Explanation by child and parent

Correlation of explanation to injury

History of injuries (type, causes)

Observe

Parent–child interactions

Parental participation in caretaking activities

Parental comforting of child

Parental gathering and assimilation of information related to their child and themselves

Parental ability to interpret hospital/illness-related events for their child

Family communication patterns

Visiting patterns and changes in visiting patterns

Principles and Rationale for Nursing Care

In the past, because of living in extended families, young children observed and frequently assisted in the birth and care of infants. Today in the United States, because of our mobile society and the more isolated nuclear family life-style, young men and women often approach parenthood with only a vague recollection of their own childhood, no knowledge of the birthing process, and limited, if any, experience in infant and child care.

General

1. Parenting is a learned behavior, and in general people parent as they were parented.
2. Support groups partially replacing the extended family have become very popular and useful in providing knowledge regarding the birth process and in developing parenting skills.
3. Parents need confidence, as well as skill, in order to be comfortable in their new role. The nurse is in the enviable position of being able to assist families by providing them with information on parenting.
4. Situations that contribute to potential or actual alteration in parenting are often related to ineffective individual or family coping.
5. See *Altered Growth and Development* for age-related developmental tasks with related interventions.

Bonding/Attachment

1. Research indicates that there is a "sensitive period" during the newborn's first minutes and hours of life during which the child is beautifully equipped to meet and interact with the parents. Close contact at this time and in the days to follow is most beneficial to the bonding process.
2. The process of bonding begins before conception by planning the pregnancy and its conception as described by the following steps (Josten): planning the pregnancy, confirming the pregnancy, accepting the pregnancy, feeling fetal movement, accepting the fetus as an individual, giving birth, hearing and seeing the baby, touching and holding the baby, and caring for the baby.
3. The period from birth to three days is an important period for father–child bonding.
4. Bonding is promoted by seeing, touching, and caring for the infant.
5. Participation of the father in caregiving activities in American society has increased. Fathers who choose the traditional role (allowing the mother to be totally responsible for caretaking activities) must be assessed in their sociocultural context.
6. Attachment during the postpartum period is influenced by three factors: the characteristics of the baby—its appearance (attractive) and behavior (alert); the characteristics of each parent (satisfaction with baby, beliefs about ability to care for baby, ability to console and comfort baby, frequency of interactions with baby); and support—the availability of a positive resource person (relative, neighbor) and the availability of follow-up for high-risk families.
7. The bonding process is impeded when the parent(s) and child are separated because of the condition of the infant or a parent.
8. Parents are reluctant to form attachments to a sick infant because of their fear of loss. This reluctance creates tremendous guilt.
9. Parents must be given the opportunity for grief work in the case of an ill or defective infant before attachment can begin.
10. No single behavior during pregnancy or in the postpartum period can be a conclusive sign of attachment difficulty. The presence of several characteristic signs should direct the nurse to gather more data.
11. The use of birthing rooms enhances the bonding process because of the decrease in interruptions.

General Guidelines for Nurses and Parents

1. Practice open, honest dialogues. Never threaten (*e.g.*, "If you are bad I will not take you to the movies").
2. Do not lecture. Tell the child he was wrong and let it go. Spend time talking about pleasant experiences.
3. Compliment children on their achievements. Make each child feel important and special. Especially tell a child when he has been good; try not to focus on negative behavior.
4. Do not be afraid to hold and hug (boys as well as girls).
5. Set limits and keep them. Expect cooperation. Encourage the child to participate in activities that conform to your values. Do not be trapped by, "But everybody else can."
6. Let the child help you as much as possible.
7. Discipline the child by restricting his activity. For a younger child, sit him in a chair for 3 to 5 minutes. If the child gets up, spank him once and put him back. Continue until the child sits for the prescribed time. For an older child, restrict bicycle riding or movie-going (pick an activity that is important to him).
8. Make sure the discipline corresponds to the unacceptable behavior. Children should be allowed opportunities to make mistakes and to verbally express anger.
9. Spank only once (the first spank is for the child, the rest are for you). Stay in control. Try not to discipline when you are irritated.
10. Remember to examine what you are doing when you are not disciplining your child (*e.g.*, enjoying each other, loving each other).
11. Never reprimand a child in front of another human being (child or adult). Take the child aside and talk.
12. Never decide you cannot control a child's destructive behavior. Examine your present response. Are you threatening? Do you follow through with the punishment or do you give in? Has the child learned you do not mean what you say?
13. Be a good model (the child learns from you whether you intend it or not). Never lie to a child even when you think it is better; the child must learn that you will not lie to him, no matter what.
14. Children learn to be responsible adults by having responsibilities as children. Give each child a responsibility suited to his age, such as picking up toys, making beds, or drying dishes. Expect the child to complete the task.
15. Share your feelings with children (happiness, sadness, anger). Respect and be considerate of the child's feelings and of his right to be human.

Altered Parenting
Related to Impaired Parental–Infant Attachment (Bonding)

Bonding is the strong attachment formed between parent and child.

Assessment

Subjective Data
The parent verbalizes
    Feelings of inadequacy
    Disgust at infant's bodily functions
    Resentment toward infant
    Disappointment in sex of physical characteristics of infant

Objective Data
    Does not hold infant close
    Does not seek eye-to-eye contact
    Does not talk to infant or call infant by name
    Inattentive to infant's needs
    Asks no questions about care
    Cries, appears sad
    Is hostile to father

Outcome Criteria

The parent will
  • Demonstrate increased attachment behaviors, such as holding infant close, smiling and talking to infant, and seeking eye contact with infant
  • Request to be involved in infant's care
  • Begin to verbalize positive feelings regarding the infant

---

Interventions

A. Assess causative or contributing factors
  1. Maternal
        Unwanted pregnancy
        Prolonged or difficult labor and delivery
        Postpartum pain or fatigue
        Lack of positive support system (mother, spouse, friends)
        Lack of positive role model (mother, relative, neighbor)
  2. Parental inadequate coping patterns (one or both parents)
        Alcoholic
        Drug addict
        Marital difficulties (separation, divorce, violence)

Change in life-style related to new role
Adolescent parent
Career change (*e.g.,* working woman to mother)
Illness in family
3. Infant
Premature, defective, ill
Multiple birth

B. Eliminate or reduce contributing factors if possible

1. Illness, pain, fatigue
   - Establish with mother what infant-care activities are feasible
   - Provide mother with uninterrupted sleep periods of at least 2 hours during the day and 4 hours during the night
   - Provide relief for discomforts
     a. Episiotomy
        - Evaluate degree of pain
        - Assess for hematomas and abscesses
        - Provide with comfort measures (ice, warm compresses, analgesics*)
     b. Hemorrhoids
        - Prevent and treat constipation
        - Provide comfort measures (compresses with witch hazel, suppositories,* analgesics*)
     c. Breast engorgement of nursing mother
        - Nurse as frequently as possible
        - Apply warm compresses (shower) before nursing
        - Apply cold compresses following nursing
        - Try hand massage, hand expressing, or breast pump between nursing
        - Offer mild analgesics
        - See *Ineffective Breastfeeding*
     d. Breast engorgement of non-nursing mother
        - Offer analgesics as ordered
        - Apply ice packs
        - Encourage use of a good supporting brassiere that covers the entire breast
2. Lack of experience or lack of positive mothering role model
   - Explore with mother her feelings and attitudes concerning her own mother
   - Assist her to identify someone who is a positive mother and encourage her to seek that person's aid
   - Outline the teaching program available to her during hospitalization
   - Determine who will assist her at home initially
   - Identify community programs and reference material that can increase her learning about child care after discharge (see References/Bibliography)
3. Lack of positive support system
   a. Identify mother's support system and assess its strengths and weaknesses
   b. Assess the need for counseling
      - Encourage the parent(s) to express feelings about the experience and about the future
      - Be an active listener to the parent(s)
      - Observe the parent(s) interacting with the infant
      - Assess for resources (financial, emotional) already available to the family

* May require a physician's order.

- Be aware of resources available both within the hospital and in the community
- Counsel the parent(s) on assessed needs
- Refer to hospital or community services

C. Provide opportunities for the bonding process

1. Promote bonding in the immediate postdelivery phase
   - Encourage mother to hold infant following birth (may need a short recovery period)
   - Provide skin-to-skin contact if desired; keep room warm (72° to 76°) or use a heat panel over the infant
   - Provide mother with an opportunity to breast-feed if desired
   - Delay the administration of silver nitrate to allow for eye contact
   - Give family as much time as they need together with minimum interruption from the staff (the "sensitive period" lasts from 30 to 90 minutes)
   - Encourage father to hold infant
2. Facilitate the bonding process during the postpartum phase
   - Check mother regularly for signs of fatigue, especially if she had anesthesia
   - Offer flexible rooming-in to the mother; establish with her the amount of care she will assume initially and support her requests for assistance
   - Discuss the future involvement of the father in the infant's care (if desired, plan opportunities for father to participate in his child's care during visits)
3. Provide support to the parent(s)
   - Listen to the mother's replay of her labor and delivery experience
   - Allow for verbalization of feelings
   - Indicate acceptance of feelings
   - Point out the infant's strengths and individual characteristics to the parent(s)
   - Demonstrate the infant's responses to the parents
   - Have a system of follow-up following discharge, especially for families considered at risk (*e.g.,* phone call or a home visit by the community health nurse)
   - Be aware of resources and support groups available within the hospital and the community and refer the family as needed
4. Assess the need for teaching
   - Observe the parent(s) interacting with the infant
   - Support each parent's strengths
   - Assist each parent in those areas where they are uncomfortable (role modeling)
   - Offer classes in infant care
   - Have handouts and audiovisual aids available for parent(s) to view at odd hours
   - Assess for level of knowledge in the area of growth and development and provide information as needed
   - See References/Bibliography for recommended printed material on parenting and child care

D. Initiate referrrals as needed

- Consult with community agencies for follow-up visits if indicated
- Refer parents to pertinent organizations (see References/Bibliography)

Parental Role Conflict*

Related to **Illness and/or Hospitalization of a Child**

Definition

Parental role conflict: The state in which a parent or primary caregiver experiences or perceives a change in role in response to external factors (*e.g.,* illness, hospitalization, divorce, separation).

> **Author's Note:** This diagnostic category describes a parent or parents whose previously effective functioning ability is challenged by external factors. In certain situations, such as illness, role confusion and conflict are expected. This category differs from *Altered Parenting*, which describes a parent (or parents) who demonstrates or is at high risk to demonstrate inappropriate parenting behaviors and/or lack of parental attachment. If parents are not assisted in adapting their role to external factors *Parental Role Conflict* can lead to *Altered Parenting*.

Defining Characteristics

Major (must be present)

Parent(s) express(es) concerns about changes in parental role
Demonstrated disruption in care and/or taking routines

Minor (may be present)

Parent(s) express(es) concerns/feelings of inadequacy to provide for child's physical and emotional needs during hospitalization or in the home
Parent(s) express(es) concerns about effect of child's illness on family
Parent(s) express(es) concerns about care of siblings at home
Parent(s) express(es) guilt about contributing to the child's illness through lack of knowledge, judgment, etc.
Parent(s) express(es) concern about perceived loss of control over decisions relating to the child
Parent(s) is (are) reluctant, unable, or unwilling to participate in normal caretaking activities, even with encouragement and support
Parent(s) verbalize(s), demonstrate(s) feelings of guilt, anger, fear, anxiety, and/or frustration

Etiological, Contributing, Risk Factors

Situational (personal, environmental)

Illness of child

* This diagnostic category was developed by the Nursing Diagnosis Discussion Group, Rainbow Babies' and Children's Hospital, University Hospitals of Cleveland. The interventions were written by this Group and Susan Kitchell.

Birth of a child with a congenital defect and/or chronic illness
Hospitalization of a child with an acute or chronic illness
Change in acuity, prognosis, or environment of care (*e.g.,* transfer to or from an ICU)
Invasive or restrictive treatment modalities (*e.g.,* isolation, intubation, etc.)
Home care of a child with special needs (*e.g.,* apnea monitoring, postural drainage, hyperalimentation)
Interruptions of family life due to treatment regimen

Separation
   Divorce   Death
   Remarriage   Illness of caretaker

Change in family membership
   Birth, adoption
   Addition of relatives (*e.g.,* grandparent, siblings)

Focus Assessment Criteria

See *Altered Parenting*

Principles and Rationale for Nursing Care

See *Altered Parenting*

Parental Role Conflict
Related to Illness and/or Hospitalization of a Child

Assessment

Subjective/Objective Data
See Defining Characteristics

Outcome Criteria

Parent(s) will
- Demonstrate control over decision-making regarding the child, collaborate with health professionals in making decisions about the health/illness care of the child
- Relate information about the child's health status and treatment plan
- Participate in caring for the child in the home/hospital setting to the degree he/she/they desire
- Verbalize feelings about the child's illness and the hospitalization

---

Interventions

1. Help parent(s) adapt parenting behaviors to allow for continuation of parenting role during hospitalization and/or illness

- Use role-supplementation strategies to help parents adapt parenting role to meet the needs of the child
- Use role model parenting behaviors appropriate to child's developmental stage and medical condition
    Instruct parents to continue limit-setting strategies and demonstrations of caring behaviors (*e.g.*, touching, hugging despite hospitalization and equipment)
- Provide information to empower parent(s) to adapt parenting role to the situation of hospitalization and/or the event of chronic illness of the child
- Provide information about hospital routines and policies such as visiting hours, mealtimes, division routines, medical and nursing routines, rooming-in, etc.
- Introduce self and other health care workers involved in the child's care and explain the role of each member of the team
- Explain procedures and tests to parent(s); help them interpret these activities to the child; discuss child's age-appropriate range of responses
- Assess usual parenting role or interpretation of real or perceived parental role
- Assess parental knowledge about child's normal growth and development, safety issues, etc., and offer supplemental information as appropriate (see *Altered Growth and Development*))
- Teach parent(s) special skills needed to provide for the physical and health care needs of the child

2. Facilitate parent(s) receiving information about the child's health status and treatment plan
   - Foster open communication between self and parent(s), allowing time for questions, frequent repetition of information; provide direct and honest answers
   - Facilitate open communication between parents and other members of the health care team
   - Approach parents with new information, do not make them assume the responsibility for seeking out the information
   - When parents cannot be with their child, facilitate information-sharing through telephone calls; allow parents to call primary nurse or nurse caring for child
   - Facilitate interdisciplinary communication so that all members of the health care team will have congruent and consistent information to share with the family
   - Assess parental understanding of the child's illness
   - Explain and intepret medical terminology to parent(s) to aid in their understanding of the child's condition
   - Interpret hospital environment and events to parent(s)
   - Use role model interpretations of events to child, help parents interpret to child and other family members
   - Respect confidentiality of information, share information about child with parent(s) only, instruct other family members to obtain information from parent(s)

3. Support continued decision-making of parent(s) regarding the child's care
   - Provide parent(s) opportunity to help formulate plan of care for their child
   - Use parent(s) as source of information about the child, his/her usual behaviors, reactions, and preferences
   - Recognize parent(s) as "expert(s)" about their child
   - Allow parent(s) the choice to be present during treatments and procedures
   - Involve parent(s) in decisions about the child's care, giving them choices whenever possible
   - Encourage both parents to share responsibility in decision-making as appropriate to their usual pattern

4. Allow parents to participate in caring for their child to the degree they desire
   - Provide for 24-hour rooming-in for at least one parent and extended visiting for other family members
   - Collaborate and negotiate with parent(s) about parental tasks they wish to continue to do, tasks they wish others to assume, tasks they wish to share, and task they want to learn to do, continually assess changes in their desired involvement in care
   - Assess parental ability to comfort the child, use comfort strategies that parent(s) have indicated for the child
   - Allow parent(s) to have uninterrupted time with the child
   - Provide consistent caregivers for the family through primary nursing; explain the primary nurse's role, responsibilities, and commitment to the parent and child
   - Explore with parent(s) their personal responsibilities (*i.e.,* work schedule, sibling care, household responsibilities, responsibilities to extended family); assist them in establishing a schedule that allows for sufficient caretaking time for the child and/or visiting time with the hospitalized child without frustration in meeting other role responsibilities (*e.g.,* if visiting is not possible until evening hours, delay child's bath time and allow parent to bathe child then)
5. Support parental ability to normalize the hospital/home environment for themselves and the child
   - Orient parent(s) and child to hospital setting prior to admission, if possible, through prehospitalization or pretransfer tour
   - Orient parent(s) to the hospital environment: kitchen, playroom, tub room, treatment room, parent's lounge
   - Orient parent(s) on how to obtain needed supplies for self and child
   - Orient parent(s) to other hospital area: cafeteria, chapel, gift shop, library, Ronald McDonald house
   - Encourage parent(s) to bring clothing and toys from home
   - Allow parent(s) to prepare home-cooked food or bring food from home if desired
   - Encourage opportunities for families to eat meals together
   - Construct daily routine around home routine as indicated by parent(s)
   - Provide privacy for parent–child interactions (*i.e.,* privacy for breastfeeding of infants, family time for teens and parents)
   - Provide parent(s) with comfortable visiting and sleeping accommodations at the bedside, if possible, for easy access to the child
   - Attempt to minimize stressors of the unit/division (*i.e.,* noise level, overaccess by hospital personnel, unplanned patient care) that disrupt quiet/rest periods
   - Provide age-appropriate developmental (school) and diversional activities for the child to provide for parenting opportunities
   - Assist parent(s) in understanding the effects of illness and or hospitalization of the child; explain and clarify as necessary
   - Encourage opportunities for parent(s) to take the child on leaves from the hospital, including visits home, as possible
   - Use an interdisciplinary approach to care-planning to minimize the length of hospitalization
6. Help parent(s) verbalize feelings about the child's illness and/or hospitalization and adaptation of the parenting role to the situation
   - Encourage parent(s) to express feelings and concerns about the child's illness and/or hospitalization and about the perceived need for parental role change
   - Provide opportunities for parent(s) to be alone, not in the presence of the child, so they may feel free to express feelings, frustrations, fears

- Indicate acceptance of parental feelings
- Provide supportive climate in which parents feel comfortable sharing their concerns
- Identify members of the staff who have established a therapeutic relationship with the parent(s)
- Provide opportunities for parent(s) to talk about themselves, events related to hospitalization/illness, and real/perceived conflicts and changes in their role, whether temporary or permanent
- Facilitate process of adjustment to the diagnosis/prognosis and planning for future care

7. Provide for physical and emotional needs of parent(s) so that they have the energy and support to continue parenting during illness/hospitalization
   - Assess and facilitate parental ability to meet self-care needs (*i.e.,* rest, nutrition, activity, privacy, etc.)
   - Allow parent(s) an opportunity to determine the care-giving schedule to correspond with a schedule to meet their own needs
   - Assess support systems: parent to parent, family, friends, minister, etc.
   - Assess, acknowledge, and facilitate family strengths
   - Facilitate and reinforce effective coping strategies employed by parent(s)
   - Continue to listen to parental concerns regarding the child and parental role
   - Continue to assess additional stressors in the family setting

8. Initiate referrals if indicated: chaplain, social service, community agencies (respite care), parent self-help groups

References/Bibliography

General

Admire G, Byer L: Counseling the pregnant teenager. Nursing 11(4):62–63, 1981

Algren C: Role perception of mothers who have hospitalized children. Children's Health Care, 14(1), 1985

Aguilera, DC, Messick JM: Crisis Intervention: Theory and Methodology. St. Louis, CV Mosby, 1974

Anderson J, Chung J: Culture and illness: Parents' perceptions of their child's long term illness. Nursing Papers 19(4):40–52, 1982

Anthony C, Koupernik C: The Child in His Family: The Impact of Disease and Death. New York, John O. Wiley & Sons, 1973

Ayer A: Is partnership with parents really possible? MCN 3(2):107, 1978

Bishop B: A guide to assessing parenting capabilities. Am J Nurs 75:1784–1787, 1975

Brink R: How serious is the child's behavioral problem? Matern Child Nurs J 7(1):33–36, 1982

Cameron J: Year-long classes for couples becoming parents. Matern Child Nurs J 4(5):358–362, 1979

Carter M, Miles M, Bufford T, Massanein R: Parent environmental stress in pediatric intensive care units. Dimen Crit Care Nurs 4(3):180–188, 1985

Chan J, Leff P: Parenting the chronically ill child in the hospital: Issues and concerns. Children's Health Care, 11(1):9–16, 1982

Dressen S: The young adult: Adjusting to single parenting. Am J Nurs 76:1286–1289, 1976

Ferraro A, Longo D: Nursing care of the family with a chronically ill, hospitalized child: An alternative approach. Image 16(3):77–81, 1985

Fife B, Huhman M, Keck J: Development of a clinical assessment scale: Evalution of the psychosocial impact of childhood illness on the family. Issues Compr Pediatr Nurs 9(1):11–31

Freiberg K: How parents react when their child is hospitalized. Am J Nurs 72:1270–1272, 1972

Hawkins-Walsh E: Diminishing anxiety in parents of sick newborns. Matern Chil Nurs J 5(1):30–34, 1980

Hayes V, Knox J: The experience of stress in parents of children hospitalized with long term disabilities. J Adv Nurs 9:333–341, 1984

Hill R: Generic features of families under stress. In Paral HJ (ed): Crisis Intervention: Selected Readings, New York, Family Service Association of America, 1966

Hobbs N, Perrin J: Issues in the Care of Children with Chronic Illness. San Francisco, Jossey-Bass, 1985

Hymovich D: Parents of sick children, their needs and tasks. Pediatr Nurs 2(6):9–13, 1976

Hymovich D: Assessing the impact of chronic childhood illness on the family and parent coping. Image 13:71–74, 1981

Jackson P, Braadham R, Burwel, H: Child care in the hospital: A parent/staff partnership. MCN 3(2):104–107, 1978

Jay SS: Pediatric intensive care: Involving parents in the care of their child. Matern Child Nurs J 6:195–204, 1977

Johnson SH: Nursing Assessment and Strategies for the Family at Risk: High-Risk Parenting, 2nd ed. Phildelphia, JB Lippincott, 1986

Johnston M: Cultural variations in professional and parenting patterns. J Obstet Gynecol Neonatal Nurs 8(4):9–15, 1980

Malinowski JS: Answering a child's questions about sex and a new baby. Am J Nurs 79:1956–1968, 1979

McKeever P: Fathering the chronically ill child. Matern Child Nurs J 6(2):124–128, 1981

Meleis A: Role insufficiency and role supplementation: A conceptual framework. Nurs Res 24(4):264–271, 1975

Melichar M: Using crisis theory to help parents cope with a child's temper tantrums. Matern Child Nurs J 5(3):181–185, 1980

Mercer RT: Teenage motherhood: The first year. J Obstet Gynecol Neonatal Nurs 9(1):16–29, 1980

Miezio P: Parenting Children with Disabilities: A Professional Source for Physicians and a Guide for Parents. New York, Dekkar, 1983

Mishel M: Parents' perception of uncertainty concerning their hospitalized child. Nurs Res 32(6):324–330, 1983

Moore ML: Newborn, Family, and Nurse. Philadelphia, WB Saunders, 1981

Morrow N, Johnson R: Coping strategies used by parents during their child's hospitalization in an intensive care unit. Children's Health Care, 14(1):14–21, 1985

Nelms B: What is a normal adolescent? Matern Child Nurs J 6(6):402–406, 1981

Petrillo M, Sangay S: Emotional Care of the Hospitalized Child. Philadelphia, JB Lippincott, 1980

Rapoff M: Helping parents to help their children comply with treatment regimens for chronic disease. Issues Compr Pediat Nurs 9(3):147–156, 1986

Roy M Sr: Role cues and mothers of hospitalized children. Nurs Res 16(2):178–182, 1967

Stranik JK, Hogberg BL: Transition into parenthood. Am J Nurs 79:90–93, 1979

Trahd GE: Sibling of chronically ill children: Helping them cope. Pediatr Nurs 12(3):191–193, 1986

Waley L, Wong D: Nursing Care of Infants and Children. St. Louis, CV Mosby, 1979

Woolery L, Barkley N: Enhancing couple's relationship during prenatal and postnatal classes. Matern Chil Nurs J 6(3):184–188, 1981

Abuse

Helfer RE, Kempe CH: Helping the Battered Child and His Family. Philadelphia, JB Lippincott, 1972

Olson RJ: Index of suspicion: Screening for child abusers. Am J Nurs 76:108–110, 1976

Symposium on child abuse and neglect. Nurs Clin North Am 16(2), 1981

Tagg PI: Nursing interventions for the abused child and his family. Pediatr Nurs 2(5):36–39, 1976

Wegmann M, Lancaster J: Child neglect and abuse. Family and Community Health 11(2):11–17, 1981

Bonding

Dean P, Morgan P, Towle JM et al: Making baby's acquaintance a unique attachment. Strategy 7(1):37–41, 1982

Jenkins R, Westhus NK: The nurse role in parent-infant bonding: Overview, assessment, intervention. J Obstet Gynecol Neonatal Nurs 10(2):114–118, 1981

Josten L: Prenatal assessment guide for illuminating possible problems with parenting. Matern Child Nurs J 6(2):113–117, 1981

Klaus MH, Kennell JH: Maternal/Infant Bonding. St. Louis, CV Mosby, 1976
Mercer R: Nursing Care for Parents at Risk. Thorofare, NJ, Charles B Slack, 1977

Resources for Parents

Literature

Adams DW, DeVeau EJ: Coping With Childhood Cancer, Virginia, Reston, 1984
Child Care Manual. ROCOM Press, P.O. Box 1577, Newark, New Jersey 07101
Christophersen ER: Little People: Guidelines for Common Sense Childrearing. Lawrence, KS, H & H Enterprises, 1977
Mash EJ: Behavior Modification Approaches to Parenting. New York, Brunner/Mazel Publishers, 1976
Salk L, Kramer R: How to Raise a Human Being. New York, Warner Books, 1973
Your Child From 1 to 6, U.S Department of Health, Education, and Welfare, Children's Bureau, Publication No. 30, Washington, DC 20014

Organizations

Parents Without Partners, 7910 Woodmount Avenue, 1000 Washington, DC 20014; also local chapters
LaLeche League International, 9616 Minneapolis Avenue, Franklin Park, Illinois 60131; also local chapters
Parent Effectiveness Training, 531 Stevens Avenue, Solana Beach, California 92075
Parents for Parents, Inc., 125 Northmore Drive, Yorktown Heights, NY 10598
Federation for Children with Special Needs, 312 Stuart Street, Boston, MA 02116

Local Counseling Services

Catholic Charities, Jewish Family Services, Christian Family Services, community agencies, and mental health centers

Post-Trauma Response

Related to **The Subjective Experience of (an) Overwhelming Traumatic Event(s)**

Rape Trauma Syndrome

Post-Trauma Response*

Related to **The Subjective Experience of (an) Overwhelming Traumatic Event(s)**

Definition

Post-trauma response: A state in which the individual experiences a sustained painful response to (an) overwhelming traumatic event(s), which has not been assimilated.

Defining Characteristics

Major (must be present)

Reexperience of the traumatic event, which may be identified in cognitive, affective, and/or sensory motor activities such as:

Flashbacks, intrusive thoughts
Repetitive dreams/nightmares
Excessive verbalization of the traumatic events
Survival guilt or guilt about behavior required for survival
Painful emotion, self-blame, shame, or sadness
Vulnerability or helplessness, anxiety, or panic
Fear of repetition, death, or loss of bodily control
Angry outburst/rage, startle reaction
Hyperalertness or hypervigilance

Minor (may be present)

Psychic/emotional numbness
Impaired interpretation of reality, impaired memory
Confusion, dissociation, or amnesia
Vagueness about traumatic event
Narrowed attention, or inattention/daze
Feeling of numbness, constricted affect
Feeling detached/alienated
Reduced interest in significant activities
Rigid role-adherence or stereotyped behavior
Altered life-style
Submissiveness, passiveness, or dependency
Self-destructiveness (alcohol/drug abuse, suicide attempts, reckless driving, illegal activities, etc.)
Difficulty with interpersonal relationships
Development of phobia regarding trauma
Avoidance of situations or activities that arouse recollection of the trauma
Social isolation/withdrawal, negative self-concept
Sleep disturbances, emotional disturbances

* This diagnosis was developed and submitted to NANDA by K. Tanaka.

Irritability, poor impulse control, or explosiveness
Loss of faith in people or the world/feeling of meaninglessness in life
Chronic anxiety and/or chronic depression
Somatic preoccupational/multiple physiological symptoms

Etiological, Contributing, Risk Factors

Situational (personal, environmental)

Natural-origin traumatic events, including floods, earthquakes, volcanic eruptions, storms, avalanches, epidemics (may be of human origin), or other natural disasters that are overwhelming to most people

Human-origin traumatic events, such as wars, airplane crashes, serious car accidents, large fires, bombing, concentration camps, torture, assault, rape, industrial disasters (nuclear, chemical, or other life-threatening accidents), or other human-origin traumatic events that involve death and destruction or threat of such

Focus Assessment Criteria

Subjective Data

1. History of the trauma*
   - Ask if person was exposed to very stressful, disturbing situations like major earthquakes or floods, very serious accidents or fires, physical assault or rape, seeing other people killed or dead, being in war or heavy combat, or some other type of disaster during his/her life
   - List all traumas, including dates and duration
2. The person's responses to the traumatic event(s)
   - Ask about person's thoughts, feelings, or actions that he/she feels have been different since the traumatic experience to assess signs and symptoms of re-experiencing or numbing responses
   - Ask if person's general life-style/pattern has changed since the traumatic event(s) to assess any readjustment difficulties

Objective Data

Make observations and collect information from family members or other appropriate persons as possible
- Excessive verbalization of the traumatic events
- Preoccupation with trauma-reminders, such as sorting through pictures or other trauma-related objects
- Use of denial, distortion, minimization, exaggeration, disavowal, fantasy, or avoidance
- Evidence of indifference or dissociation to stimuli (questions, noise, activities around him/her)
- Sudden or significant behavioral/personality changes since the traumatic event

Principles and Rationale for Nursing Care

1. Trauma victims are identified as having specific health-related problems that need nursing care.

---

* The purpose of securing a history is to substantiate evidence of trauma and not to explore details of trauma. This should be done in an appropriate therapy session.

2. Trauma is defined in terms of the subjective experience of (an) overwhelming event(s) that cannot be dealt with or assimilated in the usual way.
3. Traumatic situations differ from ordinary experience in that they involve realistic danger of physiological or psychological destruction that could mobilize fear of death.
4. A traumatic event may affect only a single person or many people at once, and it may be of human origin (*i.e.*, rape or wars) or natural origin (*i.e.*, avalanches or volcanic eruptions).
5. Because traumatic events of human origin are often characterized by indifference, negligence, or malice, they tend to result in more long-lasting, devastating effects when compared with natural-origin traumas.
6. Despite different types of traumatic events, there are commonly shared human responses: reexperiencing the trauma, reduced psychic and emotional functioning, and altered adaptation pattern and life-style.
7. Horowitz conceptualized these phenomena and postulated a phasic tendency in human responses to traumatic events.
   - The initial response to trauma is to survive and function in the immediate life-threatening situation by using all resources.
   - The powerful coping method of "numbing" is used to reduce psychological and emotional impact.
   - However, in an attempt to master the traumatic experience, intrusive recollection or reenactment of the trauma erupts into conscious awareness.
   - There is a pattern of oscillation between "numbing" and intrusive reactions peculiar to each individual.
   - Gradually, the individual works through the trauma by employing a broader perception and rationale for the event and the aftermath.
   - Finally, such an experience is assimilated into a meaningful whole that is congruent with basic beliefs and values.
8. Severity of trauma is associated with intensity, duration, and frequency of the traumatic experience.
9. It involves a complex interaction of environmental conditions and the person's subjective experiences such as degree of warning, threat to life, exposure to the grotesque, bereavement, displacement, and moral conflict about the role of the survivor.
10. Individual characteristics, such as early childhood experience, developmental phase, and character strength, may affect the outome of responses to trauma.
    - Unresolved childhood conflicts may be reactivated by the current trauma.
    - Age can be a crucial factor because trauma can interrupt a stage of human development.
    - Individual coping resources are important when one is confronted by a traumatic situation, and they will influence the effectiveness of adaptation.
11. The process of working through the trauma may be interrupted when there is a lack of support of additional stresses.
12. Cultural background also plays an important role in defining how a survivor deals with trauma.
13. Nurses need to explore their own feelings about traumas they encounter before attempting to intervene effectively with trauma victims.
14. The nurse may not see every symptom of trauma response, particularly when a victim is coping with "numbing."
15. Short-term trauma crisis intervention should begin as soon as victims are identified.
16. Follow-up counseling and long-term support therapy in the community should be arranged.

17. Victims need to work through trauma at their own pace; for some, it may take a lifetime.

Children

1. Children's responses to trauma depend on the nature and the extensiveness of the trauma, their developmental age, and the response of significant others.
2. Nursing assessment should include children's symbolic or nonverbal language communication.
3. Play therapy, such as writing, drawing, telling stories, or playing with dolls, should be offered so that the children can act out, express feelings, and/or communicate their experience safely (see Appendix IX).

Post-Trauma Response
Related to The Subjective Experience of (an) Overwhelming Traumatic Event(s)

Assessment
See Defining Characteristics

Outcome Criteria

Short-term goals

The person will
- Report a lessening of reexperiencing of numbing symptoms
- Acknowledge the traumatic event and begin to work with the trauma by talking over the experience and expressing feelings such as fear, anger, and guilt
- Identify and make connection with support persons/resources

Long-term goals

The person will
- Assimilate the experience into a meaningful whole and go on to pursue his/ her life as evidenced by goal setting

---

Interventions

A. Determine if the person has experienced (a) traumatic event(s)
- When interviewing the person, secure a quiet room where there will be no interruptions but easy access to other staff in case of management problems
- Be aware that talking about a traumatic experience may cause significant discomfort to the person

- If the person becomes too anxious, the assessment should be discontinued and the person helped to regain control of the distress or provided with other appropriate intervention

B. Assess for the responses

- Evaluate the severity of the responses and the effects on current functioning level

C. Assist person to decrease extremes of reexperiencing or numbing symptoms

- Provide a safe, therapeutic environment where the person can regain control
- Stay with the person and offer support during an episode of high anxiety (see *Anxiety* for additional information)
- Assist the person to control impulsive acting-out behavior by setting limits, promoting ventilation, and redirecting excess energy into physical exercise activity (gym, walking, jogging, etc.) (See *Potential for Self-harm* and *Potential for Violence* for additional information)
- Reassure the person that these feelings/symptoms are often experienced by the individuals who underwent such traumatic events
- Recognize that psychic/emotional numbness cushions the person's emotional impact

D. Assist person to acknowledge the traumatic event and begin to work through the trauma by talking over the experience and expressing feelings such as fear, anger, and guilt

- Provide a safe, structured setting for the person to describe the traumatic experience and to express feelings
- Explain to the person that talking about the traumatic event may intensify the symptoms (nightmares, flashbacks, painful emotions, feeling of numbness, etc.)
- Assist the person to proceed at an individual pace
- Listen attentively with empathy and unhurried manner
- Assist the person to talk about trauma, to understand what has occurred, and to validate the reality of personal involvement
- Help the person to ventilate feelings associated with the traumatic event and to become aware of the link between the experience and anger, depression, or anxiety
- Assist the person to differentiate reality from fantasy and to look back and talk about the areas of his/her life that have been changed
- Recognize and support cultural and religious values in dealing with the traumatic event

E. Assist person to identify and make connections with support persons and resources

- Help person to identify his/her strength and resources
- Explore available support system
- Assist person to make connections with support and resources according to his/her needs
- Assist person to resume old activities and begin some new ones

F. Assist children to understand and to integrate the experience in accordance with their developmental stage

- Assist child to describe the experience and to express his/her feelings (fear, guilt, rage, etc.) in safe, supportive places, such as play therapy sessions
- Provide accurate information and explanations to the child in terms he/she can understand

- Provide family counseling to promote family members' understanding of the child's needs

G. Assist family/significant others
- Assist them to understand what is happening to the victim
- Encourage ventilation of their feelings
- Provide counseling sessions and/or link them with appropriate community resources as necessary

H. Provide nursing care appropriate to each individual's traumatic experience and needs (see *Rape Trauma Syndrome* for additional information, if relevant)

I. Provide or arrange follow-up treatment where person can continue to work through the trauma and to integrate the experience into new ego synthesis

References/Bibliography

American Psychiatric Association: Quick Reference to the Diagnostic Criteria from DSM-III-R. Washington, DC, 1987

Benner P et al: Stress and coping under extreme conditions. In Dimsdale JE (ed): Survivors, Victims, and Perpetrators, Essays on the Nazi Holocaust. New York, Hemisphere Publishing Co, 1982

Burgess A, Holmstrom LL: Rape trauma syndrome. Am J Psychiatry, 131(9):981–986, 1974

Burgess AW et al: Child Molestation: Assessing impact in multiple victims. Arch Psychiatr Nurs 1(1):33–39, 1987

Card J: Epidemiology of PTSD in a national cohort of Vietnam veterans. J Clin Psychol 43(1):6–17, 1987

Catherall DR: The support system and amelioration of PTSD in Vietnam veterans. Psychotherapy, 23(3):472–482, 1986

Chodoff P: The German concentration camp as a psychological stress. Arch Gen Psychiatry, 22:78–87, 1970

Egendorf A et al: Legacies of Vietnam. Washington, DC, U.S. Government Printing Office, 1981

Gleser GC et al: Prolonged Psychosocial Effects of Disaster: A Study of Buffalo Creek. New York, Academic Press, 1981

Goodwin J: The etiology of combat-related post-traumatic disorders. In Williams T (ed): Post-Traumatic Stress Disorders: A Handbook for Clinicians. Cincinnati, OH: The Disabled American Veterans, 1987

Green B et al: A conceptual framework for post-traumatic stress syndromes among survivor groups. In Figley, CR (ed): Trauma and Its Wake. New York, Brunner/Mazel Publishers, 1985

Holmstrom LL, Burgess AW: Development of diagnostic categories: Sexual trauma. Am J Nurs 75(8):1288–1291, 1975

Horowitz, MJ: Stress Response Syndromes, 2nd ed. New York, Aronson, Inc, 1986

Horowitz MJ: Stress response syndromes: A review of post-traumatic and adjustment disorders. Hosp Community Psychiatry 37(3):241–248, 1986

Lenehan GP: Emotional impact of trauma. Nurs Clin North Am 21(4):729–740, 1986

Lifton RJ: Death in Life: Survivors of Hiroshima. New York, Vintage Books, 1969

Lifton RJ, Olson E: The human meaning of total disaster: The Buffalo Creek experience. Psychiatry, 39:1–18, 1976

Logue JN et al: A study of health and mental health status following a major natural disaster. Research in Community and Mental Health 2:217–274, 1981

Newman CF: Children of disaster: Clinical observations at Buffalo Creek. Am J Psychiatry, 133:306–312, 1976

Paul EA, O'Neill J: American nurses in Vietnam: Stressors and aftereffects. Am J Nurs 86(5):526, 1986

Perry RW, Lindell MK: The psychological consequences of natural disaster: A review of research on American communities. Mass Emergencies 3:105–115, 1978

Powell BJ, Penick EC: Psychological distress following a natural disaster: A one-year follow-up of 98 flood victims. J Community Psychol 11:269–276, 1983

Scurfield RM: Post-trauma stress assessment and treatment: Overview and formulations. In Figley CR (ed): Trauma and Its Wake. New York, Brunner/Mazel, 1985

Shore JH et al: The Mount St. Helens stress response syndrome. In Shore JH (ed): Disaster Stress Studies: New Methods and Findings. Washington, DC: American Psychiatric Press, Inc, 1986

Terr LC: Psychic trauma in children and adolescents. Psychiatr Clin North Am 8(4):815–835, 1985

Zimmerman ML et al: Art and group work: Interventions for multiple victims of child molestation. Arch Psychiatr Nurs 1(1):40–46, 1987

Rape Trauma Syndrome

Definition

Rape trauma syndrome: A state in which the individual experiences a forced, violent sexual assault (vaginal or anal penetration) against his or her will and without his or her consent. The trauma syndrome that develops from this attack or attempted attack includes an acute phase of disorganization of the victim and family's life-style and a long-term process of reorganization of life-style.*

> **Author's Note:** The use of causative or contributing factors with this category is needless because the etiology is always rape. Thus, the second part of the diagnostic statement is omitted; however, the individual's report of the rape can be added to the statement. For example, *Rape Trauma Syndrome* as evidenced by the report of a sexual assault and sodomy on June 22 and multiple facial bruises (refer to ER record for description).

Defining Characteristics

Major (must be present)
Reports or evidence of sexual assault

Minor (may be present)
If the victim is a child, parent(s) may experience similar responses

Acute Phase
Somatic responses
  Gastrointestinal irritability (nausea, vomiting, anorexia)
  Genitourinary discomfort (pain, pruritus)
  Skeletal muscle tension (spasms, pain)
Psychological responses
  Denial
  Emotional shock
  Anger
  Fear—of being alone or that the rapist will return (a child victim will fear punishment, repercussions, abandonment, rejection)
  Guilt
  Panic on seeing assailant or scene of the attack
Sexual responses
  Mistrust of men (if victim is a woman)
  Change in sexual behavior

Long-term Phase
Any response of the acute phase may continue if resolution does not occur.

* Holmstrom L, Burgess AW: Development of diagnostic categories: Sexual traumas. Am J Nurs 75:1288–1291, 1975

Psychological responses
Phobias   Anxiety
Nightmares or sleep disturbances   Depression

Focus Assessment Criteria

Subjective Data (must be recorded)
1. History of the assault
      Time and place of rape
      Identity or description of assailant
      Sexual contact (type, amount, coercion, weapon)
      Witnesses, if any
      Activities that may alter evidence (changing clothes, bathing, urinating, douching)
2. Sexual history
      Date of last menses   Contraceptive use
      Menstrual history   Date of last sexual contact
      History of venereal disease
3. Response to the assault during acute phase
      Assess person and family for
            Somatic symptoms
            Psychological symptoms
            Sexual reactions
      Assess child for
            Understanding of the event
            Knowledge of the identity of the molester
            Possibility of previous assaults
      Assess parent(s), spouse, others for
            Understanding of the event
            Ability to help the victim cope
            Ability to cope
4. Response to the assault during long-term phase
      Assess person and family for psychological symptoms and sexual reactions

Objective Data
1. Observe for injury (ecchymoses, lacerations, abrasions)
      Gastrointestinal system   Genitourinary system
         (mouth, anus, abdomen)   Skeletal muscle system
2. Assess the emotional responses
      Crying   Detachment
      Hysteria   Composure
      Withdrawal

Principles and Rationale for Nursing Care

General
1. Of the violent crimes, rape is the second most frequent (Uniform Crime Reports). It is estimated that 50–90% of rape cases are unreported. (Hilberman)
2. Rape is a crime using sexual expression to humiliate or degrade the victim. (Foley) The victim's right of privacy, sense of security, safety, and well-being are always violated. (McCombie)

3. Rape is a crime that must be reported by health care providers.
4. Our past culture (and some subcultures today) supported that: (Heinrich)
   - "A woman's rightful place in society is to fulfill man's destiny"
   - "Women are property of men and are responsible for retaining value" (therefore, women who allow themselves to get raped are bad)
   - "Women are important to men, as symbols of their power and status and prizes of prowess"
5. Some myths about rape are: (Heinrich)
   - The rapist is a sexually unsatisfied man unable to control his urges.
   - Committing rape is a one-time incident, representing a momentary lapse in judgment.
   - Rapists are strangers.
   - Rape is provoked by the victim.
   - Only promiscuous women get raped.
   - Rapes happen to women out alone at night. If a woman stays home, she will be safe.
   - Women cannot be raped against their will—the rape can be avoided by resistance.
   - Most rapes involve black men and white women.
   - Women respect men for overpowering them; they may even enjoy the rape.
   - Rapists are mentally ill or retarded, and therefore not responsible for their acts.
6. Victims, families, society, and caregivers who subscribe to these myths may not view themselves as victims or recognize the criminality of rape, may not seek help, or may be denied supportive interventions. (Heinrich)
7. Russell reported, in a random sample of 930 families, that 44% admitted experiencing rape or attempted rape. Only 8% reported it to the police.
8. The medicolegal examination serves to assess the condition of the victim and to gather documentary evidence. It consists of a general examination; oral, pelvic, and rectal exams; a culture for sperm and venereal diseases; serum pregnancy test; blood typing; and a drug and alcohol screen. Obvious debris is placed in separate envelopes. Dried sperm is collected. The victim's pubic hair and head hair is combed, and samples are placed in separate envelopes. Fingernail scrapings are placed in separate envelopes for each hand. (Heinrich)
9. Rape Crisis Centers provide rape victims and significant others with information regarding the medical examination, police interrogation, and court procedures; with escort service to hospital, police department, and courts; and with counseling.
10. Rape Crisis Centers work in the community to educate the public on rape and rape prevention, improve the response of hospitals and the police to rape victims, and improve rape-related legislation.
11. Nurses need to explore their own feelings about rape before attempting to intervene effectively with rape trauma victims. The nurse's responses to rape victims can be anxiety and overcompensation, denial of the event, condescending, anger, coercing, blaming, helplessness, and/or overinvolvement.
12. The nurse may not see every symptom of rape trauma syndrome with each rape victim.
13. Short-term rape crisis intervention should begin during the acute phase.
14. During the acute phase, hospital emergency rooms and crisis intervention centers are two places where the nurse may encounter the rape victim.
15. Nurses should consider pre-existing conditions of the rape trauma (*i.e.,* physical or psychiatric illnesses; substance abuse) that may lead to compound reactions.
16. Acute symptoms overlap with long-term symptoms of rape trauma syndrome.

17. Follow-up intervention is usually counselor-initiated.
18. Nurses in community settings can teach primary prevention concepts by reviewing with clients measures to take to reduce the possibility of rape.
19. The rape victim will resolve the rape trauma event at her/his own readiness.

Children

1. When working with young rape trauma victims, nurses should be cognizant of individual developmental levels, because the impact of the event will vary according to the child's developmental stage.
2. The child's reaction is dependent on age, degree of physical trauma, relationship to assailant, and parental (caretaker) reaction.
3. The assailant of a child is most likely someone the child knows, and the assaults have occurred for a period of time within the child's own home or neighborhood.
4. The pelvic exam can be more traumatic than the assault. Explaining the procedure and allowing the child to handle the equipment (speculum) may reduce the fear
5. Play therapy should be an integral part of the treatment regimen. Guidelines for play therapy are presented in Appendix IX. Use dolls that have genitalia for play therapy for rape victims; rag dolls can have genitalia attached. The child will then act out the assault with dolls of appropriate sex (a boy victim can use two male dolls). Puppets are also beneficial for play therapy.

Outcome Criteria

Short-term goals

The person will
• Share feelings
• Describe rationale and treatment procedures
• Identify members of support system and utilize them appropriately

Long-term goals

The person will
• Return to precrisis level of functioning
The child will:
• Discuss the assault
• Express feelings concerning the assault and the treatment
The parent(s), spouse, or significant other will
• Discuss their response to the assault
• Return to precrisis level of functioning

Interventions

The interventions for rape trauma syndrome are listed for usefulness under the three types of responses: psychological, sexual, and somatic. The nurse must assess and intervene with each response for each victim.

Psychological Responses

A. Assess for psychological responses
1. General
    Phobias, nightmares

Denial, emotional shock
Anger, fear, anxiety
Depression, guilt
2. Subjective
Expressions of numbness, shame, self-blame
3. Objective
Crying
Silence
Trembling hands
Excessive bathing (seen particularly with child or adolescent)
Avoiding interaction with others (staff, family)

B. Assist to identify major concerns (psychological, medical, legal) and her/his perception of the help she/he needs. (Heinrich)
1. Explain the care and examination she/he will experience (refer to principles for specifics)
   • Conduct the exams in an unhurried manner
   • Explain every detail prior to action
   • If this is the person's first pelvic exam, explain the position and the instruments
   • Discuss the possibility of pregnancy and a sexually transmitted disease and treatments available.
2. Explain the legal issues and police investigation (Heinrich)
   a. Explain the need to collect specimens for future possible court use
   b. Explain that the choice to report the rape is the victim's
   c. If the police interview is permitted
      • Negotiate with victim and police for an advantageous time
      • Explain to victim what kind of questions will be asked
      • Remain with the victim during the interview; do not ask questions or offer answers
      • "If the officer is insensitive, intimidating, offensive in manner or asks improper questions, discuss this with the officer in private. If the behavior continues, use proper channels and make a complaint."

C. Eliminate or reduce psychological responses where possible
1. Promote trusting relationship
   • Stay with person during acute stage or arrange for other support
   • Brief person on police and hospital procedures during acute stage
   • Assist person during medical examination and explain all procedures in advance
   • Help person to meet personal needs (bathing *after* examination and evidence has been acquired)
   • Listen attentively to person's requests
   • Maintain unhurried attitude toward person and family
   • Avoid rescue feelings toward person
   • Maintain nonjudgmental attitude
   • Support person's beliefs and value system and avoid labeling
   • Initiate play therapy with a child to explain treatments and allow child to express feelings
2. Whenever possible, provide crisis counseling within one hour of rape trauma event
   • Ask permission to contact the rape crisis counselor
   • Be flexible and individualize approach according to person's needs
   • Observe person's behavior carefully and record objective data

- Encourage victim to verbalize thoughts/feelings/perceptions of the event
- Discuss her/his treatment as victim; express empathy
- Assess person's verbal style (expressive, controlled)
- Discuss with person previous coping mechanism
- Explore available support system; involve significant others if appropriate
- Assess stress tolerance
- Reassure person about manner in which she/he reacted
- Explore with person her/his strengths and resources
- Convey to person confidence in her/his ability to return to prior level of functioning
- Assist person in decision-making and problem-solving; involve person in own treatment plan
- Help restore person's dignity by calmly exploring basis for feelings together
- Reassure person that these feelings/symptoms—fear of rapist, fear of death, guilt, loss of control, shame, short attention span, anger, anxiety, phobias, depression, flashbacks, embarrassment, and eating/sleeping pattern disturbances—are often experienced by rape trauma victims
- Respect victim's right; honor wishes to restrict unwanted visitors and offer privacy when appropriate
- Explain to person that this experience will disrupt his/her life and feelings that occurred during acute phase may recur; encourage person to proceed at his/her own pace
- Offer explanation of any papers that need to be signed
- Briefly counsel family and friends at their level
  a. Share with them the immediate needs of the victim for love and support
  b. Encourage them to express their feelings and ask questions
3. Support person's efforts to overcome feelings
- Change residence and/or telephone number
- Use objects that symbolize safety (nightlight)
- Take a trip
- Turn to support system
- Plan one day at a time
- Avoid highly stressful situations
- Engage in diversional activities
- Use previous coping mechanisms that proved effective

D. Fulfill medical–legal responsibilities by documenting: (Heinrich)
  a. History of rape (date, time, place)
  b. Nature of injuries, use of force, weapons used, threats of violence or retribution, restraints used
  c. Nature of assault (fondling, oral, anal, vaginal penetration, ejaculation, use of condom)
  d. Post-assault activities (douching, bathing/showering, gargling, urinating, defecating, changing clothes, eating or drinking)
  e. Present state (use of drugs, alcohol)
  f. Medical history, tetanus immunization status, gynecological history (last menstrual period), last voluntary intercourse
  g. Emotional state, mental status
  h. Examination findings, smears/cultures taken, blood tests, evidence collected, and photographs (if appropriate)
  i. Document to whom, when, and what evidence is delivered

E. Proceed with follow-up until victim is in control of reactions and feelings

1. Before person leaves hospital, provide card with information about follow-up appointments and names and telephone numbers of local crisis and counseling centers
2. Plan home visit or telephone call
3. Arrange for legal or pastoral counseling if appropriate
4. Recommend and make referrals to psychotherapist, mental health clinic, citizen action and community group advocacy-related services

Sexual Responses

A. Assess for sexual responses

1. General
   Fear of intercourse
   Parents' fear that assault will affect child's future sexual health
2. Subjective
   Mistrust of men
3. Objective
   Change in sexual behavior
   Lack of sexual desire (especially if victim never had intercourse before)

B. Promote helping relationship

- Encourage person to express feelings openly
- Provide accepting atmosphere
- Reassure person that her/his symptoms are frequently experienced by rape trauma victims
- Offer feedback to person on feelings verbalized
- Encourage person to recognize positive responses or support from sexual partner or members of opposite sex
- Discuss with person possible fear of rejection by significant others
- Discuss potential anxiety about resuming sexual relations with partner
- Explore sexual concerns with patient

C. Proceed with referrals

- Recommend couple therapy
- Recommend sexual counseling

Somatic Responses

A. Assess for somatic responses

Gastrointestinal irritability
Genitourinary discomfort
Rectal discomfort
Skeletal muscle tension
Vaginal discharge
Bruising and edema
Reports of

Headaches	Nausea
Fatigue	Pain
Itching	Burning on urination
Anorexia	

B. Eliminate or reduce somatic symptomatology

1. Gastrointestinal irritability
   a. Anorexia
      - Offer small, frequent feedings
      - Provide appealing foods
      - Record intake
      - Refer to *Altered Nutrition* if anorexia is prolonged
   b. Nausea
      - Avoid gas-forming foods
      - Restrict carbonated beverages
      - Observe for abdominal distention
      - Offer antiemetic as per physician's order
2. Genitourinary discomfort
   a. Pain
      - Assess pain for quality and duration
      - Monitor intake and output
      - Inspect urine and external genitalia for bleeding
      - Listen attentively to person's description of pain
      - Give pain medication as per physician's order (see *Altered Comfort*)
   b. Discharge
      - Assess amount, color, and odor of discharge
      - Allow person time to wash and change garments after initial examination has been completed
   c. Itching
      - Encourage bathing in cool water
      - Avoid use of detergent soaps
      - Avoid touching area causing discomfort
3. Skeletal muscle tension
   a. Headaches
      - Avoid any sudden change of person's position
      - Approach person in calm manner
      - Slightly elevate bed (unless contraindicated)
      - Discuss with person pain-reducing measures that have been effective in the past
   b. Fatigue
      - Assess present sleeping patterns if altered (see *Sleep Pattern Disturbance*)
      - Discuss with person precipitating factors for sleep disturbance and try to eliminate these factors if possible
      - Provide frequent rest periods throughout the day
      - Avoid interruptions during sleep
      - Avoid stress-producing situations
   c. Labile emotional responses
      - Provide person with emotionally secure environment
      - Discuss person's daily routines and adhere to them as much as possible
      - Avoid any sudden movements and approach in calm manner
      - Provide frequent quiet periods throughout the day
4. Generalized bruising and edema
   - Avoid constrictive garments
   - Handle affected body parts gently
   - Elevate affected body part if edema is present
   - Apply cool, moist compress to edematous area the first 24 hours, then warm compress after 24 hours

- Encourage person to verbalize discomfort
- Record presence and location of bruises, lacerations, edema, or abrasion

C. Proceed with health teaching with person and family

1. Gastrointestinal irritability
   - Explain to person side-effects of DES (diethylstilbestrol): nausea and vomiting; vaginal spotting when discontinued
2. Genitourinary discomfort
   - Advise person against scratching area causing discomfort
3. Skeletal muscle tension
   - Explain to person potential causes of discomfort
   - Explain to person measures that may help release tension
   - Teach person relaxation methods (see Appendix X)
   - Explain to person that these symptoms are often experienced by rape trauma victims

References/Bibliography

Burgess AW: Rape trauma syndrome: A nursing diagnosis. Occup Health Nurs 33(8):405–406, 419–422, 1985

Burgess AW, Holstrom LL: Rape trauma syndrome. Am J Psychiatry 131(9):981–986, 1974

Colao F et al: Therapists coping with sexual assault. Women and Therapy 2(2–3):205–214, 1983

Foley T, Darvies M: Rape: Nursing Care of Victims. St. Louis, CV Mosby, 1983

Heinrich L: Care of the female rape victim. Nurse Pract 12(11):9, 1987

Hicks C: Survivors advocate . . . Dealing with rape victims . . . The potential role of nurses. Nurs Time 81(19):26, 1985

Hilberman E: The Rape Victim. New York, Basic Books Inc, 1976

Kilpatrick D: Rape victims: Detection, assessment and treatment. The Clincial Psychologist 36(4):92–95, 1983

Ledray LE: Home Accommodation to Self-Determination; Nursing's Role in the Development of Health Care Policy; A Nursing Developed Model for the Treatment of Rape Victims . . . A Nursing Research-demonstration Project; ANA Publications, American Academy of Nursing, No. 6-153:68–76, 1982

Lenehan G et al: Rape victim protocol and chart for use in the emergency department. J Emerg Nurs 9(2):83–90, 1983

Longo RE: Sexual assault of handicapped individuals. J Rehabil 47:24–25, 1981

McCahill T et al: The Aftermath of Rape. Lexington, MA, DC Heath and Co, 1979

McCombie S: The Rape Crisis Intervention Handbook. New York, Plenum Press, 1980

Moore J: Rape: The double victim. Nurs Times 81(19)24–25, 1985

The problem of rape on campus. Project on the Status and Education of Women. Washington, DC, Association of American Colleges, 1978

Russell D: The prevalence and incidence of forcible rape and attempted rape of females. Victimology 7(1–4):81–93, 1982

Underwood MM: The crisis of rape: A community response. Community Ment Health J 19(3):227–230, 1983

Uniform Crime Reports for the United States, Federal Bureau of Investigation, US Department of Justice, Washington DC, 1984

Wertheimer A: Examination of the rape victim. Postgrad Med 71(3):173–180, 1982

Children

Benedict MI: Selected perinatal factors and child abuse. Am J Public Health 75(7):780–781, 1985

Burgess AW: Advancing the science of victimology. J Psychosoc Nurs Ment Health Serv 23(1): 35–38, 1985

Dodd KZ: Looking for empathy . . . Mother of a six year old boy. Nursing 12(12):112, 1982

Furniss T: Mutual influence and interlocking professional–family process in the treatment of child sexual abuse and incest. Child Abuse Negl 7(2):207–223, 1983

Hunka CD: Self-help therapy in Parents Anonymous. J Psychosoc Nurs Ment Health Serv 23(7):24–32, 1985

Kelley SJ: Drawings: Critical communications for sexually abused children. Pediatr Nurs 11(6):421–426, 1985

Lahiff ME: Family stress. Nursing (Oxford) 2(20):580–581, 1983

Pownall M: Health visting: A family affair? . . . Sexual abuse of children. Nurs Times 81(43):60–61, 1985

Powerlessness

Related to **Hospitalization**

Definition
Powerlessness: The state in which an individual or group perceives a lack of personal control over certain events or situations

> **Author's Note:** Most individuals are subject to feelings of powerlessness in varying degrees in various situations. This diagnostic category can be used to describe individuals who respond to loss of control with apathy, anger, or depression. Prolonged states of powerlessness may lead to hopelessness.

Defining Characteristics

Major (must be present)
Overt of covert expressions of dissatisfaction over inability to control situation (*e.g.*, illness, prognosis, care, recovery rate)

Minor (may be present)
Refuses or is reluctant to participate in decision-making

Apathy	Anxiety	Acting-out behavior
Aggressive behavior	Uneasiness	Depression
Violent behavior	Resignation	

Etiological, Contributing, Risk Factors

Pathophysiological
Any disease process, acute or chronic, can cause or contribute to powerlessness. Some common sources are

> Inability to communicate (CVA, Guillain-Barré, intubation)
> Inability to perform activities of daily living (CVA, cervical trauma, myocardial infarction, pain)
> Inability to perform role responsibilities (surgery, trauma, arthritis)
> Progressive debilitating disease (multiple sclerosis, terminal cancer)
> Mental illness
> Substance abuse
> Obesity
> Disfigurement

Situational (personal, environmental)
> Lack of knowledge
> Personal characteristics that highly value control (*e.g.*, internal locus of control)
> Hospital or institutional limitations

Some control relinquished to others	Not consulted regarding decisions

No privacy	Social displacement
Altered personal territory	Relocation
Social isolation	Insufficient finances
Lack of explanations from caregivers	Sexual harassment

Maturational

Adolescent: Dependence on peer group, independence from family
Young adult: Marriage, pregnancy, parenthood
Adult: Adolescent children, physical signs of aging, career pressures, divorce
Elderly: Sensory deficits, motor deficits, losses (money, significant others)

Focus Assessment Criteria

Because powerlessness is a subjective state, all inferences made regarding a person's feelings of powerlessness must be validated. The nurse will assess each individual to determine his usual level of control and decision-making and the effects that losing elements of control have had on him.

Subjective Data

1. Decision-making patterns
    "How would you describe your usual method of making decisions (career, financial, health care)?"

    Make them alone
    Consult with others for advice (who?)
    Allow others to make them for me (spouse? children? others?)
2. Individual and role responsibilities
    "What responsibilities did you have
        . . . as a school child and adolescent?"
        . . . at home?"
        . . . at work?"
        . . . in community and religious organizations?"
3. Perception of control
    a. "How would you describe your ability—high, moderate, fair, or poor—to control or cure your present health problem?" (e.g., diabetes mellitus, aphasia, activity intolerance, obesity)
    b. "To what do you attribute your (high, moderate, fair, poor) ability to control?"
        Preventive measures

Good nutrition	Stress management
Weight control	Exercise program

Others

Physician	Significant others
Nurses	Peer group

No control

Fate	Luck

Objective Data

1. Participation in grooming and hygiene care (when indicated)

Actively seeks involvement	Reluctant to participate
Requires encouragement	Refuses to participate

2. Information-seeking behaviors

Actively seeks information and literature from others concerning condition	Requires encouragement to ask questions
	Expresses lack of interest
Refuses to receive information	

3. Response to limits placed on decision-making and self-control behaviors

Acceptance	Depression
Apathy	Anger
	Withdrawal
Attempts to circumvent limits	
Ignores limits	
Increases attempts to exercise control	

Principles and Rationale for Nursing Care

1. One manifestation of alienation is powerlessness. Powerlessness is a subjective feeling.
2. An individual's response to loss of control depends on the meaning of the loss, individual patterns of coping, personal characteristics (psychological, sociological, cultural, spiritual), and the response of others.
3. Each individual, whether well or ill, has a desire for control.
4. Feelings of powerlessness are sometimes appropriate.
5. Powerlessness can have a negative effect on learning.
6. Powerlessness exists with a constant feeling of anxiety.
7. Children can gain control (mastery) over threatening situations by participating in play therapy (see Appendix IX).
8. Attempting to meet the developmental needs of the child can reduce the anxiety of powerlessness (see *Altered Growth and Development*)
9. Health care providers may frequently deny economically, socially, or educationally deprived individuals opportunities for decision-making.
10. Powerlessness is very closely related to but not synonymous with the concept of external vs. internal locus of control.
11. A person with internal locus of control believes he can affect his outcome by actively manipulating himself or the environment. Examples of internal behavior are participating in a regular exercise program, acquiring printed literature about a new diagnosis, or learning assertive skills.
12. A person with external locus of control believes that affecting his outcome is outside his control and attributes what happens to him to others or to fate. Examples of external behavior are losing weight because of fear of physician's response and blaming others for his present position (*e.g.*, depression, anger).
13. Internally controlled persons motivate themselves, while externally controlled persons usually need others to motivate them. Young children are usually externally controlled but can be taught to be internally controlled. For example, a child can be taught to keep a daily chart record of the nutrients needed daily and his intake of them to assist him to understand the concept of good nutrition and to encourage him to take responsibility for his eating patterns.
14. Individuals possessing internal locus of control may experience the loss of decision-making ability more profoundly than individuals possessing external locus of control.

15. Loss of or decrease in power in one area may be counterbalanced by the introduction of a new source of power or support by an increase in a present one.
16. Powerlessness is part of a continuum with hopelessness and helplessness.

Powerlessness
Related to Hospitalization

Author's Note: This specific diagnosis should be restricted to use for individuals exhibiting objective data or as a potential for individuals at high risk for developing powerlessness, *e.g.*, individuals with high internal locus of control.

Assessment

Subjective Data
The person reports
  Feelings of lack of control
  Statements such as
    "There is nothing I can do"   "I hate to bother you but . . . "
    "I'm no good now"   "Cannot think straight"
    "What do I know"

Objective Data

Anger	Depression	Lack of participation
Sadness	Hostility	in regimen
Apathy	Regressive behaviors	Distortions of reality

Outcome Criteria

The person will
- Identify factors that can be controlled by him
- Make decisions regarding his care, treatment, and future when possible

---

Interventions

A. Assess for causative and contributing factors
  Lack of knowledge
  Previous inadequate coping patterns (*e.g.*, depression; for discussion, see *Ineffective Individual Coping Related to Depression*)
  Unsatisfactory health care provider's routines
  Locus of control (internal or external)

B. Eliminate or reduce contributing factors if possible

1. Lack of knowledge
   - Increase effective communication between person and health care provider
   - Explain all procedures, rules, and options to person
   - Allow time to answer questions; ask him to write questions down so as not to forget them
   - Provide children with
     a. Opportunities to make decisions (*e.g.,* setting time for bath, holding still for injection)
     b. Specific play therapy (see Appendix IX) before and after a traumatic situation (refer to *Altered Growth and Development* for specific interventions for age-related developmental needs)
   - Provide a specific time (10–15 minutes) each shift that person knows can be used to ask questions or discuss subjects as desired
   - Keep person informed about condition, treatments, and results
   - Anticipate questions/interest and offer information
   - While being realistic, point out positive changes in person's condition, such as serum enzymes decreasing after myocardial infarction or surgical incision healing well
   - Be an active listener by allowing person to verbalize concerns and feelings; assess for areas of concern
   - Provide consistent staffing
   - Single out one nurse to be responsible for 24-hour plan of care, and provide opportunities for person and family to identify with this nurse
   - Contact self-help support groups if available (*e.g.,* mastectomy, ostomy clubs, paraplegics)

2. Unsatisfactory health care provider's routines
   Provide opportunities for individual to control decisions
   - Allow person to manipulate surroundings, such as deciding what is to be kept where (shoes under bed, picture on window)
   - Keep needed items within reach (call bell, urinal, tissues)
   - Do not offer options if none exist (*e.g.,* a deep IM Z-tract injection must be rotated)
   - Discuss daily plan of activities and allow person to make as many decisions as possible about it
   - Increase decision-making opportunities as person progresses
   - Respect and follow individual's decision if you have given him options
   - Record person's specific choices on care plan to ensure that others on staff acknowledge preferences ("Dislikes orange juice," "Take showers," "Plan dressing change at 7:30 prior to shower")
   - Keep promises
   - Provide opportunity for person and family to express feelings
   - Provide opportunities for person and family to participate in care
   - Be alert for signs of paternalism/maternalism in health care providers (*e.g.,* making decisions for clients)
   - Plan a care conference to allow staff to discuss methods of individualizing care; encourage each nurse to share at least one action that she discovered a particular individual liked
   - Shift emphasis from what one cannot do to what one can do
   - Set goals that are short-term, behavioral, practical, and realistic (walk 5 more feet every day; then in 1 week, client can walk to television room)

- Provide daily recognition of progress
- Praise gains/achievements

3. Locus of control
   a. Assess the person's usual response to problems (see Focus Assessment Criteria)

   Internal control (seeks to change own behaviors or environment to control problems)

   External control (expects others or other factors—fate, luck—to control problems)

   b. Provide person with internal locus of control the needed information to alter behavior or environment
      - Explain the problem as explicitly as the individual requests
      - Explain the relationship of prescribed behavior and outcome (*e.g.,* need for salt restriction, the physiological effects of exercise, the effects of bed rest on impaired cardiac function)

   c. Monitor a person with external locus of control to encourage participation
      - Have him keep a record for you (*e.g.,* his food intake for 1 week; weight loss chart; exercise program—type and frequency; medications taken)
      - Use telephone contact to monitor if feasible
      - Provide explicit written directions to follow (*e.g.,* meal plans; exercise regimen—type, frequency, duration; speech practice lessons—for aphasia)
      - Teach significant others methods to manipulate behaviors, if appropriate
      - Provide reward for each goal/step reached

4. Assist client in deriving power from other sources
   - Give permission to use other power sources to both client and significant others
   - Self-help groups
   - Support groups
   - Offer referral to religious leader
   - Provide privacy and support for other measures client may request (*e.g.,* meditation, imagery, special rituals)

C. Initiate health teaching and referrals as indicated (social worker, psychiatric nurse/physician, visiting nurse, religious leader, self-help groups)

References/Bibliography

Booth RL: Power: A negative or positive force in relationships. Nurs Adm Q 7(4):10–20, 1985

Bulechek G, McCloskey J: Nursing Interventions: Treatments for Nursing Diagnosis. Philadelphia, WB Saunders, 1985

Carlson C, Blackwell B: Behavioral Concepts and Nursing Interventions, 2nd ed. Philadelphia, JB Lippincott, 1978

Current Practice in Critical Care, vol 1. St. Louis, CV Mosby, 1979

Feather NT: Attribution of responsibility and valence of success and failure in relation to initial confidence and task performance. J Pers Soc Psychol 13:129–144, 1969

Hickey T: Powerlessness. In Carnevali DL, Patrick M (eds): Nursing Management for the Elderly. Philadelphia, JB Lippincott, 1979

Johnson DE: Powerlessness: A significant determinant in patient behavior. Journal of Nursing Education 6(2):39–44, 1967

Kleinke CL: Self-Perception, The Psychology of Personal Awareness. San Francisco, WH Freeman, 1978

Kritek PB: Patient power and powerlessness. Supervisor Nurse 12(6):26–34, 1981

Lamare EK: Communicating personal power through nonverbal behavior. J Nurs Adm 15(4):38–41, 1985

Lowerly B, DuCutte J: Disease-related learning and disease control in diabetes as a function of locus of control. Nurs Res 25(5):358–362, 1976

Roberto SL: Behavioral Concepts and Nursing Throughout the Life Span. Englewood Cliffs, NJ, Prentice-Hall, 1978

Rotter JB: Generalized expectancy for internal vs. external control of reinforcement. Psychology Monograph 80(609):1–28, 1966

Seeman M: On the meaning of alienation. Am Social Rev 24(6):783–791, 1959

Smith FB: Patient power. Am J Nurs 85(11):1260–1262, 1985

Stephenson CA: Powerlessness and chronic illness: Implications for nursing. Baylor Nursing Educator 1(1):17–23, 1979

Wilkinson MB: Power and the identified patient. Perspect Psychiatr Care 17(6):248–253, 1979

Respiratory Function, Potential Altered*

Related to **Immobility**

Related to **Environmental Allergens**

Ineffective Airway Clearance

Related to **(Specify)**

Ineffective Breathing Patterns

Related to **(Specify) as Manifested by Hyperventilation Episodes**

Impaired Gas Exchange

* This diagnostic category is not currently on the NANDA list but has been included for clarity or usefulness.

Respiratory Function, Potential Altered

Definition

Potential altered respiratory function (AIRF): The state in which the individual is at risk of experiencing a threat to the passage of air through the respiratory tract and to the exchange of gases (O_2–CO_2) between the lungs and the vascular system.

> **Author's Note:** This diagnostic category has been added by the author to describe a state in which there is a potential that the entire respiratory system may be affected, not just isolated areas such as airway clearance or gas exchange. Smoking, allergy, and immobility are examples of factors that affect the entire system and thus make it incorrect to say Impaired Gas Exchange Related to Immobility, since immobility also affects airway clearance and breathing patterns. The diagnoses *Ineffective Airway Clearance* and *Ineffective Breathing Patterns* can be used when the nurse can definitely alter the contributing factors that are influencing respiratory function, such as ineffective cough, immobility, or stress. The nurse is cautioned not to use this diagnostic category to describe acute respiratory disorders, which are the primary responsibility of medicine and nursing together (*i.e.*, collaborative problems). Such problems can be labeled *Potential Complication: Acute hypoxia* or *Potential Complication: Pulmonary edema*. When an individual's immobility threatens multiple systems, integumentary, musculoskeletal, vascular, as well as respiratory, the nurse should use *Potential for Disuse Syndrome* to describe the entire situation.

Defining Characteristics

Risk factors that can change respiratory function (see Etiological, Contributing, Risk Factors)

Etiological, Contributing, Risk Factors

The codes IAC (Ineffective Airway Clearance) and IBP (Ineffective Breathing Patterns) are used to indicate factors specific to those diagnoses. Factors without a code relate to all diagnostic categories.

Pathophysiological

Excessive or thick secretions (IAC)
    Infection (IAC)
Neuromuscular impairment
    Diseases of the nervous system   CNS depression
       (*e.g.,* Guillain-Barré syndrome,   CVA (stroke)
      MS, myasthenia gravis)
Allergic response
Hypertrophy or edema of upper airway structures—tonsils, adenoids, sinuses (IAC)

Treatment-related

Medications (narcotics, sedatives, analgesics)

Anesthesia, general or spinal (IAC, IBP)
Suppressed cough reflex (IAC)
Decreased oxygen in the inspired air
Bed rest or immobility

Situational (personal, environmental)

Surgery or trauma
Pain, fear, anxiety
Fatigue
Mechanical obstruction (IAC)
Improper positioning (IAC)
Altered anatomic structure (IAC)
    Tracheostomy
Aspiration
Extreme high or low humidity (IAC)
Smoking
Mouth breathing (IAC, IBP)
Perception/cognitive impairment (IAC)
Severe nonrelieved cough (IAC, IBP)
Exercise intolerance

Maturational

Neonate: Complicated delivery, prematurity, cesarean birth, low birth weight
Infant/child: Asthma or allergies, increased emesis (potential for aspiration), croup,
    cystic fibrosis, small airway
Elderly: Decreased surfactant in the lungs, decreased elasticity of the lungs, immo-
    bility, slowing of reflexes

Focus Assessment Criteria

Subjective Data

1. History of symptoms (*e.g.,* pain, dyspnea, cough)
        Onset? Precipitated by what?
        Description? Relieved by what?
        Effects on other body functions
            Gastrointestinal (nausea, vomiting, anorexia, constipation)?
            Genitourinary (impotence, kidney function)?
            Circulatory (angina, tachycardia/bradycardia, fluid retention)?
            Neurosensory (thought processes, headache)?
            Musculoskeletal (muscle fatigue, atrophy)?
        Effects on life-style
            Occupation   Social/sexual functions
            Role functions   Financial status
2. Presence of contributing or causative factors
        Smoking ("pack years": number of packs per day times number of smoking years)
        Allergy (medication, food, environmental factors—dust, pollen, other)
        Trauma, blunt or overt (chest, abdomen, upper airway, head)
        Surgery/pain
            Healing incision of chest/neck/head/abdomen
            Recent intubation
        Environmental factors

    Toxic fumes (cleaning agents, smoke)
    Extreme heat or cold
    Daily inspired air, work and home (humid, dry, level of pollution, level of
        pollens)
    Infection
3. Current drug therapy
    What? How often? When was last dose taken?
    Effect on symptoms?
4. Medical/surgical history
    Cardiac disease
    Pulmonary disease
5. For infants only, history of:
    Immaturity? Low birth weight?
    Cesarean birth? Complicated delivery?
    Family history of sudden infant death syndrome (SIDS)?

Objective Data
Respiratory
1. Description
    Rate (per minute)
        Slowed   Increased
    Rhythm
        Regular   Smooth
        Irregular   Uneven
    Depth
        Decreased   Symmetrical
        Increased   Variable
        Asymmetrical   Even
    Type
        Regular   Hyperpnea
        Tachypnea   Splinted/guarded
        Bradypnea   Kussmaul
        Apnea   Cheyne-Stokes
2. Cough
        Raspy   Productive
        Barking   Dry
        Painful
3. Sputum

Color	*Character*	*Amount*	*Odor*
Clear	Frothy	Small	None
Yellow	Watery	Moderate	Foul
White	Tenacious	Copious	Yeastlike
Greenish	Hemoptysic (bloody)		
Reddish (bloody)			
Brown specks			

4. Breath sounds (detected by auscultation: compare right upper and lower lobes to left
    upper and lower lobes; listen to all four quadrants of the chest)
        Diminished   Rales (crackles)
        Absent   Rhonchi (wheezes)
        Abnormal   Rubs (squeaks)

Circulatory
  Pulse

| Rate | Rhythm | Quality | Baseline |

  Blood pressure

| Usual | Present | Pulse pressure | Baseline |

  Skin color
    Within normal limits
    Pale
    Ashen

Ruddy
Cyanotic (central/peripheral)

Principles and Rationale for Nursing Care

General

1. Ventilation requires synchronous movement of the walls of the chest and abdomen. (Coordination and conscious control of breathing are key elements in teaching a person to breathe efficiently.) With *inspiration* the diaphragm moves downward, the intercostal muscles contract, the chest wall lifts up and out, the pressure inside the thorax lowers, and air is drawn in. *Expiration* occurs as air is forced out of the lungs by the elastic recoil of the lungs and the relaxation of the chest and diaphragm. Expiration is diminished in the elderly and with chronic pulmonary disease.
2. There are two phases of respiration. *External respiration* occurs in the lungs at the alveolar level (outside air to bloodstream). *Internal respiration* occurs between the systemic capillaries and the interstitial fluid (bloodstream to tissues; optimum perfusion needed).
3. A cough ("the guardian of the lungs") is accomplished by closure of the glottis and the explosive expulsion of air from the lungs by the work of the abdominal and chest muscles.
4. Lying flat causes the abdominal organs to shift toward the chest, thus crowding the lungs and making it more difficult to breathe.
5. Breath-holding can result in a "Valsalva" maneuver: a marked increase in intra-thoracic and intra-abdominal pressure, with profound circulatory changes (decreased heart rate, cardiac output, and blood pressure).
6. Hyperventilation (blowing off of CO_2) causes an acid–base imbalance and may result in temporary loss of consciousness (fainting).
7. The terms tachypnea, hyperpnea, hyperventilation, bradypnea, and hypoventilation are frequently confused. For our purposes, these terms will be defined as follows:
   Tachypnea: rapid, shallow respiratory rate
   Hyperpnea: rapid respiratory rate with increased depth
   Hyperventilation: increased rate or depth of respirations causing an alveolar ventilation that is above the body's normal metabolic requirements
   Bradypnea: slow respiratory rate
   Hypoventilation: decreased rate or depth of respiration, causing a minute alveolar ventilation that is less than the body's requirements

Oxygen Needs

1. An insufficient supply of oxygen reaching the tissues is called *hypoxia*. The effects of hypoxia upon vital signs are:

Vital Sign	*Early Hypoxia*	*Late Hypoxia*
Blood pressure	Rising systolic/falling diastolic	Falling
Pulse	Rising, bounding, arrhythmic	Falling, shallow, arrhythmic

Vital Sign	Early Hypoxia	Late Hypoxia
Pulse pressure	Widening	Widened/narrowed
Respirations	Rapid	Slowed/rapid

2. The clinical manifestations of hypoxia are:

Early Hypoxia	Late Hypoxia
Irritability	Seizures
Headache	Coma or brain tissue swelling
Confusion	Decreased cardiac output
Agitation	Oliguria or anuria
Pain	
Oliguria	

3. Infants consume three times more O_2 per kg of body weight than adults.
4. Hypoxia contributes to coma and shock. Oxygen demand is greater during febrile illness, exercise, pain, and physical and emotional stress.
5. Oxygen should be administered carefully (less than 3 per min) to people with a history of chronic CO_2 retention, for their drive to breathe is hypoxia.
6. Oxygenation is dependent upon the ability of the lungs to deliver oxygen to the blood and upon the ability of the heart to pump enough blood to deliver the oxygen to the microcirculation of the cells.

Potential Altered Respiratory Function
Related to Immobility

Assessment

Objective Data
Inability to turn self
Inability to ambulate
Presence of respiratory rales and diminished respiratory depth

---

Outcome Criteria

The person will
- Perform hourly deep breathing exercises (sigh) and cough sessions as needed
- Achieve maximum pulmonary function
- Relate importance of daily pulmonary exercises

Interventions

A. Assess causative factors
Pain, lethargy
Medical order of bedrest
Neuromuscular impairment

Lack of motivation (to ambulate; to cough and deep-breathe)
Decreased level of consciousness
Lack of knowledge

B. Eliminate or reduce causative factors if possible

1. Assess for optimal pain relief with minimal period of fatigue or respiratory depression
2. Encourage ambulation as soon as consistent with medical plan of care
   - If unable to walk, establish a regime for being out of bed in a chair several times a day (*i.e.,* one hour after meals and one hour before bedtime)
   - Increase activity gradually, explaining that respiratory function will improve and dyspnea will decrease with practice
3. For neuromuscular impairment
   - Vary the position of the bed, thus gradually changing the horizontal and vertical position of the thorax, unless contraindicated
   - Assist to reposition, turning frequently from side to side (hourly if possible)
   - Encourage deep breathing and controlled coughing exercises five times every hour
   - Teach individual to use blow bottle or incentive spirometer every hour while awake (with severe neuromuscular impairment, the person may have to be awakened during the night as well)
   - For child, use colored water in blow bottle; have him blow up balloons
   - Auscultate lung field every eight hours; increase frequency if altered breath sounds are present
4. For the person with a decreased level of consciousness
   - Position from *side to side* with set schedule (*e.g.,* left side even hours, right side odd hours); do not leave person lying flat on back
   - Position on right side after feedings (nasogastric tube feeding, gastrostomy) to prevent regurgitation and aspiration
   - Keep head of bed elevated 30° unless contraindicated

C. Prevent the complications of immobility

See specific diagnoses for interventions to prevent or treat the complications of immobility:
Potential for Disuse Syndrome
Sensory–Perceptual Alterations
Activity Intolerance
Diversional Activity Deficit

Potential Altered Respiratory Function
Related to Environmental Allergens

Assessment

Subjective Data
The person states
   "I'm allergic to . . ."
   " . . . gives me a rash"

"I have trouble breathing"
"I feel short of breath"
"I feel itchy"
"Something bit (stung) me"
"I have asthma"
History of ingestion of new food or drugs
Frequent ear infections

Objective Data

Hoarseness, wheezing/dyspnea
Coughing and sneezing, watery eyes and nose
Hives/rashes
Presence of stinger (bee)
Erythema
Edema

Outcome Criteria

The person will
• State causative allergens, if known
• State methods of avoiding allergens
• Relate the emotional aspects of the allergic response
• State the need to seek immediate medical attention for severe allergic response and demonstrate the use of hypodermic injection (for administration of epinephrine) if applicable

---

Interventions

A. Assess causative factors

Chronic allergy (known allergens such as molds, dust, pollen, food, others)
Stinging insect
Nonspecific (unknown) allergen

B. Provide the following health teaching

1. For chronic allergy to molds
   a. Avoid barns, cut grass, leaves, weeds, decaying or rotting vegetation, firewood, house plants, damp basements, attics, and crawl spaces
   b. Avoid eating marinated or aged foods (bread, flour, cheese, fruits, vegetables)
   c. Maintain household walls clean and dry
      • Be sure that there is adequate house drainage to keep walls dry
      • Check walls for black or grayish-blue mold spots
      • Wash walls with chlorine bleach solution to remove mold
   d. Maintain a dust-free environment, especially in the bedroom*
      • Empty room to the bare walls, including closets (store contents elsewhere if possible)

---

* It is difficult to keep one's home and work environment dust free, but special efforts can readily be made to keep the area where one sleeps free of dust.

- Scrub woodwork and floors
- Thereafter, dust and vacuum well daily and clean thoroughly once a week
- Keep bedroom furniture to a minimum (preferably wood, rather than stuffed furniture)
- Choose waxed, hardwood floors (no carpets)
- Use pull shades rather than venetian blinds at windows; do not use curtains or draperies
- Use closet to a minimum; keep it as dust free as the bedroom, and keep the door closed
- Use bedroom for sleeping only; if it is a child's bedroom, encourage play elsewhere
- Do not use stuffed toys
- Keep animals of fur or feathers out of the area
- Do not use fuzzy blankets or feather comforters; cotton bedspreads are preferred
- Launder bed linens frequently

e. Keep dust down throughout the entire house
- Use steam or hot-water heat if available
- Maintain a clean filter in furnace; use air conditioning if possible
- Cover hot-air furnace outlets with cheesecloth or have a filter installed; change filter frequently
- Avoid any room while it is being cleaned and do not handle any objects that may be dust collectors (such as books)
- Wear a mask while cleaning

2. For chronic allergy to pollen
- Reduce exposure as much as possible to trees (April–May), grass (May–July), weeds (mid–May to first frost)
- Use air conditioning with electrostatic filters
- Stay inside on windy days, avoiding drafts and cross-ventilation
- Use air conditioning in cars, and avoid extended rides
- Wear a dampened mask while cutting lawn
- Avoid strong odors (scents and perfumes)
- Do not drink ice-cold beverages or food (can cause spasms)
- Avoid granaries, barns, decaying materials, cut grass, weeds, dry leaves, firewood
- Try to arrange vacations during high pollen season in a low-pollen area such as the eastern seashore
- Be sure over-the-counter drugs such as antihistamines are approved by physician, for some may give the opposite intended effect

3. To avoid stinging insects (bees, wasps, yellow jackets, hornets)
- Do not wear brightly colored clothing (choose lighter colors such as white, light green, khaki)
- Keep hair short or tied back; avoid hair sprays, perfumes, and flappy clothing
- Wear shoes and socks
- Avoid riding horses or bicycles in areas where bees or wasps are plentiful (*e.g.,* fields of clover, flowers)
- Avoid mowing lawns, trimming hedges, or pruning trees during the insect season
- Carry an insect spray in the glove compartment of the car and keep one handy at home (attempts to swat or kill bees must be well planned, for a missed blow may infuriate the insect and make it more dangerous)
- If approached by a bee or wasp in the open, stay still or move back very slowly
- Each spring, have home and garden searched for new hornets', or bees' nests and

obtain professional assistance from an exterminator or fire department in eliminating them
4. For a severe allergic reaction where hives or any respiratory symptoms appear, or *if one has had a previous severe reaction to any kind of sting,* carry out the following procedure
   - Remove stinger if possible
   - Keep as quiet as possible (avoid panic)
   - Apply ice immediately
   - Use emergency bee-sting kit injection if available
   - Be driven to the nearest emergency room for *immediate* medical treatment and further observation (the person who merely suspects that a severe reaction may occur need not actually register, but should stay close by in case of an anaphylactic reaction)
5. General instructions for unknown or nonspecific allergies
   - Assess for introduction of new food or medication
   - Eliminate
      Fish and fish oils (cod-liver oil products)
      All kinds of nuts
      All fresh fruits and fresh vegetables (this elimination does not apply to cooked fruits and vegetables)
      Chocolate
      Eggs and food containing eggs
      Milk and foods containing milk
      Wheat and foods containing wheat
   - If you have an asthmatic response, practice conscious control of breathing (see *Ineffective Breathing Patterns* for technique)

Ineffective Airway Clearance

Definition
Ineffective airway clearance: The state in which the individual experiences a real or potential threat to respiratory status related to inability to cough effectively.

Defining Characteristics

Major (must be present)
Ineffective cough or
Inability to remove airway secretions

Minor (may be present)
Abnormal breath sounds
Abnormal respiratory rate, rhythm, depth

Etiological, Contributing, Risk Factors
See *Potential Altered Respiratory Function*

Principles and Rationale for Nursing Care
See *Potential Altered Respiratory Function*

Ineffective Airway Clearance
Related to (Specify)

Outcome Criteria

The person will
- Not experience aspiration
- Demonstrate effective coughing and increased air exchange in his lungs

---

Interventions

The nursing interventions for the diagnosis *Ineffective Airway Clearance* represent interventions for any individual with this nursing diagnosis, regardless of the etiological and contributing factors.

A. Assess for causative or contributing factors
   Inability to maintain proper position
   Ineffective cough
   Pain or fear of pain
   Viscous secretions (dehydration)
   Fatigue, weakness, drowsiness
   Lack of knowledge (of how to cough, and why it is important)
   Chronic, nonrelieved cough

B. Reduce or eliminate factors if possible
   1. Inability to maintain proper position
      - Refer to *Potential for Aspiration*
   2. Ineffective cough
      - Instruct person on the proper method of controlled coughing
         a. Breathe deeply and slowly while sitting up as high as possible
         b. Use diaphragmatic breathing
         c. Hold the breath for 3 to 5 seconds and then slowly exhale as much of this breath as possible through the mouth (lower rib cage and abdomen should sink down)
         d. Take a second breath, hold, and cough forcefully from the chest (not from the back of the mouth or throat), using two short forceful coughs

3. Pain or fear of pain
   a. Assess present analgesic regime
      - Administer pain medications as needed
      - Assess its effectiveness: Is the individual too lethargic? Is the individual still in pain?
      - Note time when person appears to have best pain relief with optimal level of alertness and physical performance: *This is the time for active breathing and coughing exercises.*
   b. Provide emotional support
      - Stay with person for the entire coughing session
      - Explain the importance of coughing after pain relief
      - Reassure person that suture lines are secure and that splinting by hand or pillow will minimize pain of movement
   c. Use appropriate comfort measures for site of pain
      - Splint abdominal or chest incisions with hand, pillow, or both
   d. For sore throat
      - Assess for adequate humidity in the inspired air
      - Consider warm saline gargle every 2 to 4 hours
      - Consider use of anesthetic lozenge or gargle, especially before coughing sessions*
      - Examine throat for exudate, redness, and swelling and note if it is associated with fever
      - Explain that a sore throat is common after anesthesia and should be a short-term problem
   e. Maintain good body alignment to prevent muscular pain and strain
      - Acquire and use extra pillows on both sides of person, especially the affected side, for support
      - Position person to prevent slouching and cramping positions of the thorax and abdomen; reassess positioning frequently
   f. Assess person's understanding of the use of analgesia to enhance breathing and coughing effort
      - Teach person during periods of optimal level of consciousness
      - Continually reinforce rationale for plan of nursing care ("I will be back to help you cough when the pain medicine is working and you can be most effective.")
4. Viscous (thick) secretions
   - Maintain adequate hydration (increase fluid intake to 2 to 3 quarts a day if not contraindicated by decreased cardiac output or renal disease)
   - Maintain adequate humidity of inspired air
5. Fatigue, weakness, drowsiness
   - Plan and bargain for rest periods ("Work to cough well now; then I can let you rest.")
   - Vigorously coach and encourage coughing, using positive reinforcement. ("You worked hard; I know it's not easy, but it is important.")
   - Be sure coughing session occurs at peak comfort period after analgesics, but not peak level of sleepiness
   - Allow for rest after coughing and before meals
   - For lethargy or decreased level of consciousness, stimulate person to breathe ("Take a deep breath.")

* May require a physician's order.

6. Lack of understanding or motivation (of how and why to cough)
   - Assess knowledge of reasons and method for coughing
   - Proceed with health teaching with constant reinforcement in principles of care
   - Acknowledge and encourage good individual effort and progress
7. For chronic, nonrelieved coughing
   - Minimize irritants in the inspired air (*e.g.,* dust, allergens)
   - Provide periods of uninterrupted rest
   - Administer Rx—cough suppressant, expectorant—as ordered by physician (withhold food and drink immediately after administration of meds for best results)
   - Relieve mucous membrane irritation through humidity (inhaling steam from shower, or sitting over pot of steaming water with a towel over the head, will loosen thick secretions and soothe the membranes)

C. Initiate health teaching and referrals as indicated

- Instruct parents on the need for child to cough, even if painful
- Allow adult and older child to listen to lungs; describe if clear or if rales are present
- Consult with respiratory therapist for assistance if needed

---

Ineffective Breathing Patterns

Related to **(Specify) as Manifested by Hyperventilation Episodes**

Definition

Ineffective breathing patterns: The state in which the individual experiences an actual or potential loss of adequate ventilation related to an altered breathing pattern.

Author's Note: This diagnostic category has little clinical utility except to describe situations that nurses definitively treat, such as hyperventilation. Individuals with periodic apnea and hypoventilation have a collaborative problem—*Potential Complication: Respiratory*—to indicate that the person is to be monitored for a variety of respiratory dysfunctions. If the person is more vulnerable to a specific respiratory complication, the collaborative problem then can be written as *PC: Pneumonia* or *PC: Pulmonary Embolism.* Hyperventilation is a manifestation of anxiety and/or fear. The nurse can use *Anxiety* or *Fear* related to (specify event) as manifested by hyperventilation as a more descriptive diagnosis.

Etiological, Contributing, Risk Factors

See *Potential Altered Respiratory Function*

Defining Characteristics (See also *Altered Respiratory Function*)

Major (must be present)
> Changes in respiratory rate or pattern (from baseline)
> Changes in pulse (rate, rhythm, quality)

Minor (must be present)
> Orthopnea
> Tachypnea, hyperpnea, hyperventilation
> Arrhythmic respirations
> Splinted/guarded respirations

Principles and Rationale for Nursing Care

See *Potential Altered Respiratory Function*

Ineffective Breathing Patterns:
Related to (Specify) as Manifested by Hyperventilation Episodes

Hyperpnea or hyperventilation is rapid breathing pattern that results in lowered arterial PCO_2.

Assessment

Subjective Data

The person states
> "I can't catch my breath"
> "My fingers tingle and my heart beats fast"
> "I feel dizzy (faint)"

History of existing emotional or physical stress
Fear of anxiety

Objective Data
> Tachypnea (forceful)   Rising blood pressure
> Tachycardia   Anxious facial expression
> Bounding pulse

Outcome Criteria

The person will
- Demonstrate an effective respiratory rate and experience improved gas exchange in the lungs
- Relate the causative factors, if known, and relate adaptive ways of coping with them

Interventions

A. Assess causative factors

Fear

Pain

Exercise/activity

B. Remove or reduce causative factors

1. Fear
   - Remove cause of fear, if possible
   - Reassure person that measures are being taken to ensure his safety
   - Distract person from thinking about his anxious state by having him maintain eye contact with you (or perhaps with someone else he trusts); say, "Now look at me and breathe slowly with me like this."
   - Consider use of paper bag as means of rebreathing expired air (expired CO_2 will be reinspired, thereby slowing respiratory rate)
   - See *Fear*

2. Pain
   - Determine location of discomfort
   - Use appropriate comfort measures (see *Altered Comfort*)
   - Encourage displacement of pain perception through concentration on more efficient breathing (*e.g.,* concentrating completely on air going in and out of lungs, giving plentiful oxygen to the body)
   - Stay with person and coach in taking slower, more effective breaths

3. Exercise/activity
   - Encourage slow deep breaths, pausing when ambulating for the first time after immobility or surgery
   - Encourage conscious control of breathing during exercise (slower, deeper, abdominal breathing)
   - See *Activity Intolerance* for additional interventions

C. Proceed with health teaching
   - Explain that one can learn to overcome hyperventilation through conscious control of breathing even when the cause is unknown
   - Discuss possible causes, physical and emotional, and methods of coping effectively (see *Anxiety*)

Impaired Gas Exchange

Definition

Impaired gas exchange: The state in which the individual experiences an actual or potential decreased passage of gases (oxygen and carbon dioxide) between the alveoli of the lungs and the vascular system.

Author's Note: This diagnostic category does not represent a situation for which nurses prescribe definitive treatment. Nurses do not treat impaired gas exchange, but nurses can treat the functional health patterns that decreased oxygenation can affect, such as activity, sleep, nutrition, or sexual function. Thus *Activity Intolerance* related to insufficient oxygenation for ADL better describes the nursing focus. If an individual is at risk or has experienced respiratory dysfunction, the nurse can describe the situation as *Potential Complication: Respiratory* or, even more specifically, as *PC: Emboli.*

Defining Characteristics (See also *Potential Altered Respiratory Function*)

Major (must be present)
Dyspnea on exertion

Minor (may be present)
Tendency to assume three-point position (sitting, one hand on each knee, bending forward)
Pursed-lip breathing with prolonged expiratory phase
Increased anteroposterior chest diameter, if chronic
Lethargy and fatigue
Increased pulmonary vascular resistance (increased pulmonary artery/right ventricular pressure)
Decreased gastric motility, prolonged gastric emptying
Decreased oxygen content, decreased oxygen saturation, increased pCO_2, as measured by blood gases
Cyanosis

References/Bibliography

Books and Articles

Aashika T: Evaluation of a community-based educational program for individuals with C.O.P.D. J Rehabil 46(2):23–27, 1980
Bates B: A Guide to Physical Examination. Philadelphia, JB Lippincott, 1979
Callahan M: A prudent pulmonary rehab program. Am J Nurs (85)12:1368–1369, 1985
Callahan M: COPD: A special post op challenge. RN 47(5):45–47, 1984
D'Agostino J: Teaching tips for living with COPD at home. Nursing 14(2):12:57, 1984
Ellmyer P: A guide to your patient's safe home use of oxygen. Nursing 12(1):54–57, 1982
Harimon A: Anaphylaxis can mean sudden death. Nursing 10(10):40–43, 1980
Harper RW: A Guide to Respiratory Care. Philadelphia, JB Lippincott, 1981
Hungel D, Madsen L: Acute and chronic asthma: A guide to intervention. Am J Nurs 80:1791–1795, 1980
Jacobs M: Protocol for C.O.P.D. Nurse Pract 4(6):11–28, 1979
Jecklin J: Positioning, percussion and vibrating patients for effective bronchial drainage. Nursing 9(3):64–70, 1979
Kaufman J, Woody J: C.O.P.D.—better living through teaching. Nursing 10(3):57–61, 1981
Kiriloff L, Tibals S: Drugs for asthma: A complete guide. Am J Nurs 83(1):55–61, 1981
Largerson J: The cough: Its effectiveness depends on you. Respiratory Care 27(4):418–434, 1982
Larter N: Cystic fibrosis. Am J Nurs 81(3):527–532, 1981
McCaully E: Breathing exercises as play for asthmatic children. Matern Child Nurs J 5(5):340–345, 1979
McCreary C, Watson J: Pickwickian syndrome. Am J Nurs 81(3):555, 1981

Mechanical ventilation: Patient assessment and nursing care–a programmed unit. Am J Nurs 80(12):2191–2217, 1980

Minis B: Helping your patient breathe easier after chest surgery. RN 47(12):25–29, 1984

Patrick M, Woods S et al: Medical–Surgical Nursing. Philadelphia. JB Lippincott, 1985

Pinney M: Foreign body aspiration. Am J Nurs 81(3):521–522, 1981

Pinney M: Pneumonia. Am J Nurs 81(3):517–518, 1981

Richard E, Shephard A: Giving up smoking: A lesson in loss theory. Am J Nurs 81(4):755–757, 1981

Rice V: Clinical hypoxia. Critical Care Nurse. 1(6):21–29, 1980

Rifas E: How you and your patient can manage dyspnea. Nursing 10(6):34–41, 1980

Simkins R: Asthma: Reactive airway disease. Am J Nurs 81(3):523–526, 1981

Simkins R: The crisis of bronchiolitis. Am J Nurs 81(3):515–516, 1981

Simkins R: Croup and epiglottitis. Am J Nurs 81(3):519–520, 1981

Sjoberg E: Nursing diagnosis and the COPD patient. Am J Nurs 83(2):244–248, 1983

Taylor D: Clinical applications. Assessing breath sounds. Nursing 3:60–63, 1985

Webber J: OTC (Over the Counter) Bronchodilators: What are the risks of relief in seconds? Nursing 10(1):34–39, 1980

Woolf CR: The Clinical Core of Respiratory Medicine. Philadelphia, JB Lippincott, 1981

Westra B: Assessment under pressure: When your patient says "I can't breathe." Nursing 14(5):34–39, 1984

Resources for the Consumer

Organizations

American Cancer Society, 777 3rd Avenue, New York, NY 10017

American Heart Association, 7320 Greenville Avenue, Dallas, TX 75231

American Lung Association, 1740 Broadway, New York, NY 10019

Cystic Fibrosis Foundation, 3091 Mayfield Road, Cleveland, OH 44118

SIDS Clearing House, Suite 600, 1555 Wilson Boulevard, Rosslyn, VA 22209

Literature

Tuhy J, Bither S: Breathing easy: Living with emphysema and chronic bronchitis. A manual for patients with chronic obstructive disease. Portland, Oregon Lung Association, 1977. Write for a copy: 830 Medical Arts Building, 1020 Southwest Taylor Street, Portland, OR 97205

Sources of Information on Allergy Control

Dickey Enterprises (environmentalists), 635 Gregory Road, Fort Collins, CO 80524; (303) 482-6001

Meridian, Bio-Medical (for pollen guide), 3278 Wadsworth Boulevard South, Denver, CO 80227; (303) 986-5555

Hollister-Stier Laboratories, Division of Cutter Laboratories, Inc., Box 3145, Terminal Annex, Spokane, WA 99220

Role Performance, Altered

Definition

Altered role performance: The state in which an individual experiences or is at risk for experiencing a disruption in the way one perceives one's role performance.

Author's Note: This diagnostic category had previously been a sub-category under *Self-Concept Disturbance*. The use of this category in its present state may prove problematic. If a woman were unable to continue her household responsibilities because of illness and these responsibilities were assumed by the other family members, the situations that may arise would better be described as *Potential Self-Concept Disturbance* related to Recent Loss of Role Responsibility secondary to Illness and Potential Impaired Home Maintenance Management related to Lack of Knowledge of Family Members. Until clinical research defines this category more definitively, use *Altered Role Performance* as an etiology for *Self-Concept Disturbance* or *Potential Impaired Home Maintenance Management*. Should the role disturbance relate to parenting *Parental Role Conflict* should be considered.

Defining Characteristics

Major (must be present)
Conflict related to role perception or performance

Minor (may be present)
Change in self-perception of role
Denial of role
Change in others' perception of role
Change in physical capacity to resume role
Lack of knowledge of role
Change in usual patterns of responsbility

Self-Care Deficit:

Feeding Self-Care Deficit

Related to **(Specify)**

Bathing Self-Care Deficit

Related to **(Specify)**

Dressing/Grooming Self-Care Deficit

Related to **(Specify)**

Toileting Self-Care Deficit

Related to **(Specify)**

Total Self-Care Deficit*

Related to **(Specify)**

Definition

Self-care deficit: The state in which the individual experiences an impaired motor function or cognitive function, causing a decreased ability to feed, bathe, dress, and/or toilet himself.

Defining Characteristics

Major (one of the following must be present)

1. Self-feeding deficits
   Unable to cut food
   Unable to bring food to mouth
2. Self-bathing deficits (includes washing entire body, combing hair, brushing teeth, attending to skin and nail care, and applying makeup)
   Unable or unwilling to wash body or body parts
   Unable to obtain a water source
   Unable to regulate temperature or water flow
3. Self-dressing deficits (including donning regular or special clothing, not night-clothes)
   Impaired ability to put on or take off clothing
   Unable to fasten clothing
   Unable to groom self satisfactorily
   Unable to obtain or replace articles of clothing
4. Self-toileting deficits
   Unable or unwilling to get to toilet or commode

* This diagnostic category is not currently on the NANDA list but has been included for clarity or usefulness.

Unable or unwilling to carry out proper hygiene
Unable to transfer to and from toilet or commode
Unable to handle clothing to accommodate toileting
Unable to flush toilet or empty commode
5. Total
Unable to perform any self-care activities

Etiological, Contributing, Risk Factors

Pathophysiological

Neuromuscular impairment
Autoimmune alterations (arthritis, multiple sclerosis)
Metabolic and endocrine alterations (diabetes mellitus, hypothyroidism)
Nervous system disorders (Parkinsonism, myasthenia gravis, muscular dystrophy, Guillain-Barré)
Lack of coordination
Spasticity or flaccidity
Muscular weakness
Partial or total paralysis (spinal cord injury, stroke)
CNS tumors
Increased intracranial pressure
Musculoskeletal disorders
Atrophy
Muscle contractures
Connective tissue diseases (systemic lupus erythematosus)
Edema (increased synovial fluid)
Visual disorders
Glaucoma
Cataracts
Diabetic/hypertensive retinopathy
Ocular histoplasmosis
Cranial nerve neuropathy
Visual field deficits

Treatment-related

External devices (casts, splints, braces, IV equipment)
Surgical procedures
Fractures
Tracheostomy
Gastrostomy
Jejunostomy
Ileostomy
Colostomy

Situational (personal, environmental)

Immobility
Trauma
Nonfunctioning or missing limbs
Coma

Maturational

Elderly: Decreased visual and motor ability, muscle weakness

Focus Assessment Criteria

Self-feeding abilities
    Swallowing
    Chewing
    Using utensils and cutting food
Self-bathing abilities
    Undressing to bathe
    Reaching water source
    Differentiating water
      temperatures
Self-dressing abilities
    Putting on or taking off
      necessary clothing
    Selecting appropriate clothing
Self-toileting abilities
    Getting to toilet and undressing
    Sitting on toilet
    Rising from toilet

Selecting foods
Seeing

Obtaining equipment (water,
  soap, towels)
Washing body parts

Retrieving appropriate clothing
Fastening clothing

Cleaning self/flushing toilet
Redressing
Performing proper hygiene
  (washing hands)

Principles and Rationale for Nursing Care

General

1. The concept of self-care emphasizes each person's right to maintain individual control over his own pattern of living. (This applies to both the ill individual and the well individual.)
2. Regardless of handicap, people should be given privacy and treated with dignity while performing self-care activities.
3. Self-care does not imply allowing the person to do things for himself as planned by the nurse but, rather, encouraging and teaching the person to make his own plans for optimal daily living.
4. Mobility is necessary to meet one's self-care needs and to maintain good health and self-esteem.
5. Cleanliness is important for comfort, for positive self-esteem, and for social interactions with others.
6. Inability to care for oneself produces feelings of dependency and poor self-concept. With increased ability for self-care, self-esteem increases.
7. Disability often causes denial, anger, and frustration. These are valid emotions that must be recognized and addressed.
8. It is acceptable for a limited period of time to be dependent on others to provide basic physiological and psychological needs.
9. Regression in ability to perform self-care activities may be a defense mechanism to threatening situations.
10. Neglect of an extremity refers to the memory loss of the presence of an extremity (*e.g.,* a person who has had a stroke or brain injury resulting in partial paralysis may ignore the arm or leg on the affected side of the body).

Endurance

1. The endurance or ability of the individual to maintain a given level of performance is influenced by the ability to use oxygen to produce energy (related to the optimal functioning of the heart, respiratory, and circulatory systems) and the functioning of

the neurological and musculoskeletal systems. Thus, individuals with alterations in these systems have increased energy demands or a decreased ability to produce energy.

2. Stress is energy consuming; the more stressors an individual has, the more fatigue he will experience. Stressors can be personal, environmental, disease-related, and treatment-related. Examples of possible stressors follow.

Personal	*Environmental*	*Disease-Related*	*Treatment-Related*
Age	Isolation	Pain	Walker
Support system	Noise	Anemia	Medications
Life-style	Unfamiliar setting		Diagnostic studies

3. The signs and symptoms of decreased oxygen in response to an activity—*e.g.,* self-care, mobility—are:

   Sustained increased heart rate 3 to 5 minutes after ceasing the activity or a change in the pulse rhythm

   Failure of systolic blood pressure reading to increase with activity, or a decrease in value

   Decrease or excessive increase in respiratory rate and dyspnea

   Weakness, pallor, cerebral hypoxia (confusion, incoordination)

4. Refer to Principles of Nursing Care under *Activity Intolerance* for additional information.

Teaching/Relearning

1. Optimal patient education promotes self-care. To teach effectively the nurse must determine what the learner perceives as his own needs and goals, determine what the nurse feels are his needs and goals, and then work to establish mutually acceptable goals.
2. Offering the individual choices and including him in planning his own care reduces feelings of powerlessness; promotes feelings of freedom, control, and self-worth; and increases the person's willingness to comply with therapeutic regimens.
3. The following key elements promote relearning of self-care tasks:

   Providing a structured, consistent environment and routine

   Repeating instructions and tasks

   Teaching and practicing tasks during periods of least fatigue

   Maintaining a familiar environment and teacher

   Using patience, determination, and a positive attitude (by both learner and teacher)

   Practicing, practicing, practicing

Feeding Self-Care Deficit
Related to (Specify)

Assessment

Subjective Data
The person reports

Problems with eating ("I can't feed myself."; "I'm too tired to eat."; "Could you help me with my food?")
Pain

Objective Data

Impaired visual acuity
Mental lethargy
Poor oral hygiene (lack of teeth or poorly fitting dentures; oral injury, ulcer, deformity)
Drooling or facial paralysis
Uncoordination
Inability to use hands to grip a device to move food to mouth
Absence of gag reflex

Outcome Criteria

The person will
- Demonstrate increased ability to feed self *or*
- Report that he is unable to feed self
- Demonstrate ability to make use of adaptive devices, if indicated
- Demonstrate increased interest and desire to eat
- Describe rationale and procedure for treatment
- Describe causative factors for feeding deficit

Interventions

A. Assess causative factors

Visual deficits (blindness, field cuts, poor depth perception)
Affected or missing limbs (casts, amputations, paresis, paralysis)
Cognitive deficits (aging, trauma, CVA)

B. Provide opportunities to relearn or adapt to activity

1. Common nursing interventions for feeding
   - Ascertain from person or family members what foods the person likes or dislikes
   - Have meals taken in the same setting: pleasant surroundings that are not too distracting
   - Maintain correct food temperatures (hot foods hot, cold foods cold)
   - Provide pain relief, since pain can affect appetite and ability to feed self
   - Provide good oral hygiene before and after meals
   - Encourage person to wear dentures and eyeglasses
   - Place person in the most normal eating position suited to his physical disability (best is sitting in a chair at a table)
   - Provide social contact during eating
   - See *Altered Nutrition: Less Than Body Requirements*
2. Specific interventions for people with sensory/perceptual deficits
   - Encourage the person to wear prescribed corrective lenses
   - Describe location of utensils and food on tray or table
   - Describe food items to stimulate appetite

- For perceptual deficits, choose different-colored dishes to help distinguish items (*e.g.,* red tray, white plates)
- Ascertain person's usual eating patterns and provide food items according to preference (or arrange food items in clocklike pattern); record on care plan the arrangement used (*e.g.,* meat, 6 o'clock; potatoes, 9 o'clock; vegetables, 12 o'clock)
- Encourage eating of "finger foods" (*e.g.,* bread, bacon, fruit, hot dogs) to promote independence
- Avoid placing food to blind side of person with field cut, until visually accommodated to surroundings; then encourage him to scan entire visual field

3. Specific interventions for people with missing limbs
   - Provide for eating environment that is not embarrassing to individual and allow sufficient time for the task of eating
   - Provide only the amount of supervision and assistance necessary for relearning or adaptation
   - To enhance maximum amount of independence, provide necessary adaptive devices

      Plate guard to avoid pushing food off plate
      Suction device under plate or bowl for stabilization
      Padded handles on utensils for a more secure grip
      Wrist or hand splints with clamp to hold eating utensils
      Special drinking cup
      Rocker knife for cutting

   - Assist with set-up if needed, opening containers, napkins, condiment packages; cutting meat; buttering bread
   - Arrange food so person has adequate amount of space to perform the task of eating

4. Specific interventions for people with cognitive deficits
   - Provide isolated, quiet atmosphere until person is able to attend to eating and is not easily distracted from the task
   - Supervise feeding program until there is no danger of choking or aspiration
   - Orient person to location and purpose of feeding equipment
   - Avoid external distractions and unnecessary conversation
   - Place person in the most normal eating position he is physically able to assume
   - Encourage person to attend to the task, but be alert for fatigue, frustration, or agitation
   - Provide one food at a time in usual sequence of eating until person is able to eat the entire meal in normal sequence
   - Encourage person to be tidy, to eat in small amounts, and to put food in unaffected side of mouth if paresis or paralysis is present
   - Check for food in cheeks
   - Refer to *Impaired Swallowing* for additional interventions

C. Initiate health teaching and referrals as indicated

1. Assess to assure that both person and family understand the reason and purpose of all interventions
2. Proceed with teaching as needed
   - Maintain safe eating methods
   - Prevent aspiration
   - Use appropriate eating utensils (avoid sharp instruments)
   - Test temperature of hot liquids and wear protective clothing (*e.g.,* paper bib)
   - Teach use of adaptive devices

Bathing Self-Care Deficit
Related to (Specify)

Assessment

Objective Data
Impaired visual acuity
Impaired hearing acuity
Impaired upper limb movement
Inability to use hands
Uncoordinated movements or spasticity
Presence of restrictive devices (splints, casts, braces, traction equipment)
Decreased mental alertness

Subjective Data
The person states
"I can't wash myself"
"I don't want (need) a bath"
"I'm too tired (weak) to wash myself"
"It hurts"

Outcome Criteria

The person will
- Perform bathing activity at expected optimal level *or*
- Report satisfaction with accomplishments despite limitations
- Relate feeling of comfort and satisfaction with body cleanliness
- Demonstrate ability to use adaptive devices
- Describe causative factors of bathing deficit
- Relate rationale and procedures for treatment

Interventions

A. Assess causative factors
Visual deficits (blindness, field cuts, poor depth perception)
Affected or missing limbs (casts, amputations, paresis, paralysis, arthritis)
Cognitive deficits (aging, trauma, CVA)

B. Provide opportunities to relearn or adapt to activity
1. General nursing interventions for inability to bathe
   - Bathing time and routine should be consistent to encourage greatest amount of independence
   - Encourage person to wear prescribed corrective lenses or hearing aid
   - Keep bathroom temperature warm; ascertain individual's preferred water temperature
   - Provide for privacy during bathing routine

- Observe skin condition during bathing
- Provide all bathing equipment within easy reach
- Provide for safety in the bathroom (nonslip mats, grab bars)
- When person is physically able, encourage use of either tub or shower stall, depending upon which facility is at home (the person should practice in the hospital in preparation for going home)
- Provide for adaptive equipment as needed
  a. Chair or stool in bathtub or shower
  b. Long-handled sponge to reach back or lower extremities
  c. Grab bars on bathroom walls where needed to assist in mobility
  d. Bath board for transferring to tub chair or stool
  e. Safety treads or nonslip mat on floor of bathroom, tub, and shower
  f. Washing mitts with pocket for soap
  g. Adapted toothbrushes
  h. Shaver holders
  i. Hand-held shower spray
- Provide for relief of pain that may affect ability to bathe self*

2. Specific interventions for bathing for people with visual deficits
   - Place bathing equipment in location most suitable to individual
   - Avoid placing bathing equipment to blind side if person has a field cut and is not visually accommodated to surroundings
   - Keep call bell within reach if person is to bathe alone
   - Give the visually impaired individual the same degree of privacy and dignity as any other person
   - Verbally announce yourself before entering or leaving the bathing area
   - Observe the person's ability to locate all bathing utensils
   - Observe the person's ability to perform mouth care, hair combing, and shaving tasks
   - Provide place for clean clothing within easy reach

3. Specific interventions for bathing for people with affected or missing limbs
   - Bathe early in morning or before bed at night to avoid unnecessary dressing and undressing
   - Encourage person to use a mirror during bathing to inspect the skin of paralyzed areas
   - Encourage the person with amputation to inspect remaining foot or stump for good skin integrity
   - For limb amputations, bathe stump twice a day and be sure it is dry before wrapping it or applying prosthesis
   - Provide only the amount of supervision or assistance necessary for relearning the use of extremity or adaptation to the handicap
   - For lack of sensation, encourage use of the affected area in the bathing process (an individual tends to forget the existence of body parts in which there is no sensation)

4. Specific interventions for bathing people with cognitive deficits
   - Provide a consistent time for the bathing routine as part of a structured program to help decrease confusion
   - Keep instructions simple and avoid distractions; orient to purpose of bathing equipment

* May require a physician's order.

- If person is unable to bathe the entire body, have him bathe one part until he does it correctly; give positive reinforcement for success
- Supervise activity until person can safely perform the task unassisted
- Encourage attention to the task, but be alert for fatigue that may increase confusion
- Apply firm pressure to the skin when bathing; it is less likely to be misinterpreted than a gentle touch
- Use a warm shower or bath to help a confused or agitated person to relax

C. Initiate health teaching and referrals as indicated

- Communicate to staff and family the person's ability and willingness to learn
- Teach use of adaptive devices
- Ascertain bathing facilities at home and assist in determining if there is any need to make adaptations; refer to occupational therapy or social service for help in obtaining needed home equipment
- Teach to use tub or shower stall, depending on type of facility at home
- If person is paralyzed, instruct him or his family to demonstrate complete skin check on key areas for redness (buttocks, bony prominences)
- Teach to maintain a safe bathing environment

Dressing/Grooming Self-Care Deficit
Related to (Specify)

Assessment

Subjective Data

The person reports
"I can't dress myself"
"I don't want to get dressed"
"It hurts to dress myself"
"I'm too tired to get dressed"

Objective Data

Impaired visual acuity
Inability to use hands
Spasticity, weakness, lack of coordination
Presence of restrictive devices (traction, casts, splints, braces)
Disheveled appearance or inappropriate dress
Decreased mental alertness
Inability to dress self

Outcome Criteria

The person will
- Demonstrate increased ability to dress self *or*
- Report the need of having someone else assist him in performing the task
- Demonstrate ability to learn how to use adaptive devices to facilitate optimal independence in the task of dressing
- Demonstrate increased interest in wearing street clothes
- Describe causative factors for dressing deficit
- Relate rationale and procedures for treatments

Interventions

A. Assess causative factors

Visual deficits (blindness, field cuts, poor depth perception)
Affected or missing limbs (casts, amputations, arthritis, paresis, paralysis)
Cognitive deficits (aging, trauma, CVA)

B. Provide opportunities to relearn or adapt to activity

1. Common nursing interventions for self-dressing
   - Encourage person to wear prescribed corrective lenses or hearing aid
   - Promote independence in dressing through continual and unaided practice
   - Choose clothing that is loose fitting, with wide sleeves and pant legs and front fasteners
   - Allow sufficient time for dressing and undressing, since the task may be tiring, painful, or difficult
   - Plan for person to learn and demonstrate one part of an activity before progressing further
   - Lay clothes out in the order in which they will be needed to dress
   - Provide dressing aids as necessary (some commonly used aids include dressing stick, Swedish reacher, zipper pull, buttonhook, long-handled shoehorn, and shoe fasteners adapted with elastic laces, Velcro closures, or flip-back tongues; all garments with fasteners may be adapted with Velcro closures)
   - Encourage person to wear ordinary or special clothing rather than nightclothes
   - Increase participation in dressing by medicating for pain 30 minutes before it is time to dress or undress, if indicated*
   - Provide for privacy during dressing routine
   - Provide for safety by ensuring easy access to all clothing and by ascertaining individual's performance level
2. Specific interventions for dressing people with visual deficits
   - Allow person to ascertain the most convenient location for clothing, and adapt the environment to best accomplish the task (*e.g.,* remove unnecessary barriers)
   - Verbally announce yourself before entering or leaving the dressing area
   - Avoid placing clothing to the blind side if person has a field cut, until he is visually accommodated to surroundings; then encourage him to turn head to scan entire visual field

* May require a physician's order.

- Apply adaptive devices (*e.g.,* hand splints) before dresing activity
- Consult or refer to Physical or Occupational Therapy for teaching application of prosthetics to missing limbs
3. Specific interventions for dressing for people with cognitive deficits
    - Make a consistent dressing routine to provide a structured program to decrease confusion
    - Keep instructions simple and repeat them frequently, avoid distractions
    - Introduce one article of clothing at a time
    - Encourage attention to the task; be alert for fatigue, which may increase confusion

C. Initiate health teaching and referrals as indicated

1. Assess understanding and knowledge of individual and family for above instructions and rationale
2. Proceed with teaching as needed
    - Communicate the individual's ability and willingness to learn to staff and family members
    - Teach use of adaptive devices and techniques that are specific to each disability
    - Teach to maintain a safe dressing environment
    - Attempt to be noncritical in correcting errors

Toileting Self-Care Deficit
Related to (Specify)

Assessment

Subjective Data

The person states
    "I can't go to the toilet"
    "It hurts"
    "I can't get out of bed (walk, move)"
    "I can't get to the bathroom in time"
    "I wet myself"
    "I can't control my bowels"

Objective Data

    Impaired visual acuity
    Decreased mental alertness
    Weakness, lack of coordination
    Spasticity
    Presence of restrictive devices (traction, casts, splints, braces)
    Immobility

Outcome Criteria

The person will
- Demonstrate increased ability to toilet self *or*
- Report that he is unable to toilet self
- Demonstrate ability to make use of adaptive devices to facilitate toileting
- Describe causative factors for toileting deficit
- Relate rationale and procedures for treatment

Interventions

A. Assess causative factors

Visual deficits (blindness, field cuts, poor depth perception)
Affected or missing limbs (casts, amputations, paresis, paralysis)
Cognitive deficits (aging, trauma, CVA)

B. Provide opportunities to relearn or adapt to activity

1. Common nursing interventions for toileting difficulties
   - Encourage person to wear prescribed corrective lenses or hearing aid
   - Obtain bladder and bowel history from individual or significant other (see *Altered Bowel Elimination* or *Altered Patterns of Urinary Elimination*)
   - Ascertain communication system person uses to express the need to toilet
   - Maintain bladder and bowel record to determine toileting patterns
   - Provide for adequate fluid intake and balanced diet to promote adequate urinary output and normal bowel evacuation
   - Promote normal elimination by encouraging activity and exercise within the person's capabilities
   - Avoid development of "bowel fixation" by less frequent discussion and inquiries about bowel movements
   - Be alert to possibility of falls when toileting person (be prepared to ease him to floor without causing injury to either of you)
   - Achieve independence in toileting by continual and unaided practice
   - Allow sufficient time for the task of toileting to avoid fatigue (lack of sufficient time to toilet may cause incontinence or constipation)
   - Avoid use of indwelling catheters and condom catheters to expedite bladder continence (if possible)
2. Specific interventions for toileting for people with visual deficits
   - Keep call bell easily accessible so person can quickly obtain help to toilet; answer call bell promptly to decrease anxiety
   - If bedpan or urinal is necessary for toileting, be sure it is within person's reach
   - Avoid placing toileting equipment to the blind side of an individual with field cut (when he is visually accommodated to surroundings, you may suggest he search entire visual field for equipment)
   - Verbally announce yourself before entering or leaving toileting area
   - Observe person's ability to obtain equipment or get to the toilet unassisted
   - Provide for a safe and clear pathway to toilet area
3. Specific interventions for toileting for people with affected or missing limbs
   - Provide only the amount of supervision and assistance necessary for relearning or adapting to the prosthesis

- Encourage person to look at affected area or limb and use it during toileting tasks
- Encourage useful transfer techniques taught by Occupational or Physical Therapy (the nurse should familiarize herself with planned mode of transfer)
- Provide the necessary adaptive devices to enhance the maximum amount of independence and safety (commode chairs, spill-proof urinals, fracture bedpans, raised toilet seats, support side rails for toilets)
- Provide for a safe and clear pathway to toilet area

4. Specific interventions for toileting for people with cognitive deficits
- Offer toileting reminders every 2 hours, after meals, and before bedtime
- When person is able to indicate the need to toilet, begin toileting at 2 hour intervals, after meals, and before bedtime
- Answer call bell immediately to avoid frustration and failure to be continent
- Encourage wearing ordinary clothes (many confused individuals are continent while wearing regular clothing)
- Avoid the use of bedpans and urinals; if physically possible, provide a normal atmosphere of elimination in bathroom (the toilet used should remain constant to promote familiarity)
- Give verbal cues as to what is expected of the individual, and give positive reinforcement for success
- Work to achieve daytime continency before expecting nighttime continency (nighttime incontinence may continue after daytime continency has returned)
- See *Altered Patterns of Urinary Elimination* for additional information on incontinence

C. Initiate health teaching and referrals as indicated

1. Assess the understanding and knowledge of the individual and significant others of foregoing interventions and rationale
- Communicate person's ability and willingness to learn to staff and family
- Maintain a safe toileting environment
- Reinforce knowledge of transferring techniques
- Teach use of adaptive devices
- Ascertain home toileting needs and refer to Occupational Therapy or Social Services for help in obtaining necessary equipment

Total Self-Care Deficit
Related to (Specify)

Definition

Self-care deficit, total: The state in which the individual experiences an inability to perform any self-care activities.

Assessment

Objective Data

Presence of severe nervous system disorder (MS, Alzheimer's disease)
Coma
Total paralysis

Outcome Criteria

The person will
- Demonstrate optimal hygiene after care is provided

Interventions

Refer to interventions under the following diagnoses, as indicated:
Feeding Self-Care Deficit
Bathing Self-Care Deficit
Dressing Self-Care Deficit
Toileting Self-Care Deficit
Diversional Activity Deficit
Powerlessness
Potential for Injury
Potential Altered Oral Mucous Membrane
Potential for Disuse Syndrome

References/Bibliography

Books

American Nurses Association Division on Medical-Surgical Nursing Practice and the Association of Rehabilitation Practice: Standards of Rehabilitation Nursing Practice. Kansas City, American Nurses Association, 1977

Guidelines for Stroke Care. Public Health Service Publ. No. 76-14017. Washington, DC. U.S. Department of Health Education and Welfare, 1976

Hirschberg GG, Lewis L, Vaughan P: Rehabilitation. 2nd ed. Philadelphia, JB Lippincott, 1976

Martin N, Holt NB, Hicks D: Comprehensive Rehabilitation Nursing. New York, McGraw-Hill, 1981

Palmer M, Tonis J: Manual for Functional Training. Philadelphia, FA Davis, 1980

Sine RD et al: Basic Rehabilitation Techniques. Rockville, MD, Aspen Systems Corp, 1981

Articles

Aged

Barton EM: Etiology of dependence in older nursing home residents during morning care: The role of staff behavior. J Pers Soc Psychol 10(3):423–431, 1980

Garvan P, Lee M, Lloyd K et al: Self-care applied to the aged. New Jersey Nurse 10(1):3–6, 1980

Hirschfield MJ: Self-care potential: Is it present? The elderly. J Gerontol Nurs 11(8):28–34, 1985

Karl CA: The effect of an exercise program on self-care activities for the institutionalized elderly. J Gerontol Nurs 8(5):282–285, 1982

Leering C: A structural model of functional capacity in the aged. J Am Geriatr Soc 27(7):314–316, 1979

Lundsren-Lindquist B et al: Functioning studies in 79 year olds. I. Performance in hygiene activities. Scand J Rehabil Med 15(3):109–115, 1983

Rameizl P: Cadet; A self care assessment tool. Geriatr Nurs 4(6):377–378, 1983

Rodgers JC, Snow T: An assessment of the feeding behaviors of the institutionalized elderly. Am J Occup Ther 36(6):373–380, 1982

Warshaw GA et al: Functional disability in the hospitalized elderly. JAMA 248(7):847–850, 1982

Amputee

Weiss-Lambrou R et al: Brief or new: Toilet independence for the severe bilateral upper limb amputee. Am J Occup Ther 39(6):397–399, 1985

Brain Injury

Panikoff LB: Recovery trends of functional skills in the head-injured adult. Am J Occup Ther 37(11):735–743, 1983

Talmage EW, Collins GA: Physical abilities after head injury: A retrospective study. Phys Ther 63(12):2007–2010, 1983

General

Allen C, Bennett A: One step at a time to relearn self-help skills. Nurs Mirror 158(15): Clinical Forum II–IV, 1984

Alteri CA: The patient with myocardial infarction: Rest prescriptions for activities of daily living. Heart Lung 14(4):355–360, 1984

Ciuca R, Bradish J, Trombly SM: Active range of motion exercises: A handbook. Nursing 8(8):45–49, 1978

Gardiner R: Getting the right piece in the right place: Home aids. Community Outlook 10(2):39–42, 1979

Gould MT: Nursing diagnoses concurrent with multiple sclerosis. J Neurosurg Nurs 15(16):339–345, 1983

Lerner JF, Alexander J: Activities of daily living: Reliability and validity of gross vs specific ratings. Arch Phys Med Rehabil 62(4):161–166, 1981

Levin LS: Patient education and self-care: How do they differ? Nurs Outlook 26(3):170–175, 1978

Meissner SF: Evaluate your patient's level of independence. Nursing 10(9):72–73, 1980

Newton A: Clothing: A positive part of the rehabilitation process. J Rehabil 42(4):18–22, 1976

Orem DE: A concept for self-care for the rehabilitation process. Rehabil Nurs 10(3):33–36, 1985

Reeder JM: Help your disabled patient be more independent. Nursing 14(11):43, 1984

Ross T: Nursing process: Activities of living. Nurs Mirror 156(6):28–29, 1983

Staff PH: ADL assessment. Scand J Rehab Med (Suppl) 31, 153–157, 1980

Sullivan IJ: Self-care model for nursing. ANA Pub. No. G-147, 57–68, 1980

Walter KM: Techniques and concepts: Independent living. Perceptions by professionals in rehabilitation. J Rehabil 46(3):57–63, 1980

Yep JO: Tools for aiding physically disabled individuals increase independence in dressing. J Rehabil 43(5):39–41, 1977

Spinal Cord Injury

Panchal PD: Rehabilitation of the patient with spinal cord injury. Curr Probl Surg 17(4):254–262, 1980

Rogers JC, Figone JJ: Traumatic quadriplegia: Follow-up study of self-care skills. Arch Phys Med Rehabil 61(7):316–321, 1980

Stauffer S: A master plan for teaching the patient with spinal cord injury. RN 42(7):55–60, 1979

Stroke and Brain Injury

Adler MK: Stroke rehabilitation: Is age a determinant? J Am Geriatr Soc 28(11):499–503, 1980

Dzau RE, Bochme AR: Stroke rehabilitation: A family-team education approach. Arch Phys Med Rehab 59(5):236–239, 1978

Rogers EJ: Goals in hemiplegia care. J Am Geriatr Soc 28(11):497–498, 1980

Stonington HH: Rehabilitation in cerebrovascular diseases. Primary Care 7(3):87–106, 1980

Self-Concept Disturbance*

Body Image Disturbance

Related to **(Specify)**

Personal Identity Disturbance

Self-Esteem Disturbance

* This diagnostic category is not currently on the NANDA list but has been included for clarity or usefulness.

Chronic Low Self-Esteem

Related to **(Specify)**

Situational Low Self-Esteem

Related to **(Specify)**

Definition

Self-concept Disturbance: The state in which the individual experiences or is at risk of experiencing a negative state of change about the way he feels, thinks, or views himself. It may include a change in body image, self-esteem, role performance, or personal identity.

> **Author's Note:** *Self-Concept Disturbance* represents a broad category under which more specific categories fall. Initially the nurse may not have sufficient clinical data to validate a more specific category as *Chronic Low Self-Esteem* or *Body Image Disturbance,* thus *Self-Concept Disturbance* can be used until more specific categories can be supported with data.

Defining Characteristics

Since a self-concept disturbance may include a change in any one or combination of its four component parts (body image, self-esteem, role performance, personal identity), and since the nature of the change causing the alteration can be so varied, there is no "typical" response to this diagnosis. Reactions may include:

Refusal to touch or look at a body part
Refusal to look into a mirror
Unwillingness to discuss a limitation, deformity, or disfigurement
Refusal to accept rehabilitation efforts
Inappropriate attempts to direct own treatment
Denial of the existence of a deformity or disfigurement
Increasing dependence on others
Signs of grieving: weeping, despair, anger
Refusal to participate in own care or take responsibility for self-care (self-neglect)

Self-destructive behavior (alcohol, drug abuse)
Displaying hostility toward the healthy
Withdrawal from social contacts
Changing usual patterns of responsibility
Showing change in ability to estimate relationship of body to environment

Etiological, Contributing, Risk Factors

A self-concept disturbance can occur as a response to a variety of health problems, situations, and conflicts. Some common sources follow.

Pathophysiological

Chronic disease
Loss of body part(s)
Loss of body function(s)
Severe trauma

Treatment-related

Hospitalization: chronic or terminal illness
Surgery

Situational (personal, environmental)

Divorce, separation from, or death of a significant other
Loss of job or ability to work
Pain
Obesity
Pregnancy
Immobility or loss of function
Need for nursing home placement

Maturational

Infant and preschool: Deprivation
Young adult: Peer pressure, puberty
Middle aged: Signs of aging (graying or loss of hair), reduced hormonal levels (menopause)
Elderly: Losses (people, function, financial, retirement)

Other

Women's movement
Sexual revolution

Focus Assessment Criteria

Self-concept disturbance is manifested in a variety of ways. An individual may respond with an alteration in another life process (see *Spiritual Distress, Fear, Ineffective Individual Coping*). The nurse should be aware of this and utilize the assessment data to ascertain the dimensions affected.

It may be difficult for the nurse to identify the cues and make the inferences necessary to diagnose a self-concept disturbance. Each individual reacts differently to loss, pain, disability, and disfigurement. Therefore, the nurse should determine an individual's usual reactions to problems and feelings about himself before attempting to diagnose a change.

Subjective Data
Self Views
 "Describe yourself"
 "What do you like most/least about yourself?"
 "What do others like?"
 "What do you/others want to change about you?"
 "What do you enjoy?"
 "Has being ill affected how you see yourself?"
Identity
 "What personal achievements have given you satisfaction?"
 "What are your future plans?"
Role Responsibilities
 "What do you do for a living? Job responsibilities? Home responsibilities?"
 "Are these satisfying?"
 If the person has had a role change, how has it affected life-style and relationships?
Stress Management
 "How do you manage stress?"
 "To whom do you go for help with a problem?"
 Substance abuse?
 Exercise
 Religious convictions
 Problem-solving approach
Support System
 "Any problems in current relationships?"
 "How does your family feel about your illness?" "Do they understand?"
 "Does your family regularly discuss problems?"
Somatic Problems
 "Do you feel fearful, anxious or nervous?"
 "Ever have panic spells?"
 "Ever feel like you are falling apart? Dizziness? Aches and pains? Shortness of breath? Palpitations? Urinary frequency? Nausea/Vomiting? Sleep problems? Fatigue? Loss of sexual interest?"
Affect and Mood
 "How do you feel now?"
 "How would you describe your usual mood?"
 "What things make you happy/upset?"
 "Have you ever thought of harming yourself?
Body Image
 "What do you like most/least about your body?"
 "What parts are most important to you?"
 "Before you were sick, how did you feel about people who were sick or disabled?"
 "What do you understand to be your health problem?"
 "What limitations do you think will result?"
 "How do you feel about this illness/disability?"
 "Has it changed the way you feel about yourself or the way others respond to you?"
 Children may be able to draw self-portraits.

Objective Data
General Apperance
 Facial expression

Affect
Hygiene (cleanliness)
Grooming (clothes, hair, make-up)
Dress (condition, appropriateness)
Thought Processes/Content
    Orientation
    Feelings of depersonalization
    Appropriate
    Rambling
    Suspicious
    Homicidal/Suicidal Ideation
    Sexual preoccupation
    Delusions (grandeur, persecution, reference, influence, or bodily sensations)
    Difficulty concentrating
    Slowed thought processes
Behavior
    Aggressiveness
    Hyperactivity
    Delinquency
    School problems
    Social withdrawal
    Ability for self-care
    Communication Patterns
        With significant others
            Relates well
            Hostile
            Dependent
            Demanding
        Physical impairment to communication (*e.g.*, deafness, aphasia, trach)
        Cultural variations in communication (*e.g.*, use of gestures, touch, etc)
        Decision-making ability
            Indecisive
            Procrastination
    Nutritional Status
        Appetite
        Eating patterns
        Weight (gain/loss)
    Rest/Sleep Pattern
        Recent change
        Early wakefulness
        Insomnia

Principles and Rationale for Nursing Care

General

1. Both the client and the nurse have their own personal self-concept. To deal effectively with others, the nurse must be aware of her own behavior, feelings, attitudes, and responses.
2. Self-concept involves a person's feelings, attitudes, and values and affects his reactions to all experiences.

3. Self-concept is learned. A child's concept of self, for example, emerges as a result of changes occurring during earlier developmental stages.
4. The concept of self includes components of body image, self-esteem, role performance, and personal identity.
5. Body image is the mental idea a person has of his body. It is based on past as well as present experience. It is composed of the interrelated phenomena of body surface and depth and the attitudes, emotions, and personality reactions of the individual to his body. It is flexible and subject to change.
6. Alterations in the components of self-concept are described as follows:
   Body image: Viewing oneself differently as a result of actual or perceived changes in body structure or function
   Self-esteem: Lack of confidence in ability to accomplish that which is desired
   Role performance: Inability to perform those functions and activities expected of a particular role in a given society
   Personal identity: Disturbance in perception of self ("Who am I?")
7. A nurse's attitude can hinder or facilitate the individual's adaptation to an alteration in self-concept.
8. Intrusive procedures can threaten an individual's sense of wholeness. The nurse should provide a great deal of emotional support during procedures that increase a person's sense of vulnerability.
9. Body image changes constantly. There is often a time lag between the actual body change and the change in body image. The nurse must be aware that during this lag the individual may reject both the diagnosis and the education and treatment prescribed.
10. Body image is influenced during pregnancy in relation to biologic, psychological, and role changes.

Children

1. The child's development of body image is based on his own body, which is influenced by present and past perceptions of his body, his physiological functioning, his developmental maturation, and the response of others to him.
2. The child strives to master conflicts, and his success or lack of success will influence his pattern for coping throughout his life.
3. The child has periods of decreased self-esteem during the primary grades and again during adolescence.
4. The process of acquiring autonomy, independence, and individuality requires that the child have periods of separation from family even though they may cause anxiety.
5. In order to develop and maintain self-esteem, children need to feel worthwhile, different in some way, and superior and more lovable than any other child.
6. Disturbances in body image are encountered in prepubescent and pubescent children who are either early or late maturing, since children at this age are most comfortable when they are just like their peers.
7. The development of a positive body image by age is charted below.

Age	*Developmental Task*
Birth to 1 year	Learns to tolerate small frustrations Learns to trust
1 to 3 years	Learns to like body Learns mastery of 　Motor skills 　Language skills 　Bowel training

Age	Developmental Task
3 to 6 years	Learns initiative
	Learns sex typing
	Identifies with parent models
	Increases skills (motor language)
6 to 12 years	Develops a sense of industry
	Has a clear sex role identification
	Learns peer interaction
	Develops academic skills

8. A child learns to see himself the way he is seen by his parents or significant others.
9. The child's personality evolves as the child responds to his changing body and to the environment.

Loss of Body Part

1. The loss of a body part of function is followed by a period of grief and mourning. The grief is similar to that following the loss of any valued object.
2. The process of mourning for the loss of a body part of function may include feelings of helplessness, loneliness, sadness, guilt, and anger. The stages of adaptation to loss include shock and disbelief, anger, depression, and eventual adaption (see *Grieving*).
3. Reorganization of an altered body image is a process of recognition, acceptance, and resolution.

Self-Esteem

1. Self-esteem evolves from a comparison between the self-concept and self-ideal. The greater the congruency, the higher the self-esteem. (Stuart and Sundeen)
2. Self-esteem is derived from one's own perceptions of competency and efficacy and from appraisals of others.
3. High self-esteem is rooted in unconditional acceptance as an innately worthy person. (Stuart and Sundeen)
4. Persons with high self-esteem tend to attribute failures or any threatening event to external causes (beyond their control—diet, stress, medication, trauma), unlike persons with low self-esteem, who tend to attribute failure or any threatening event to internal causes. (Tenner and Herzberger)
5. Low self-esteem may be an indicator of susceptibility to depression.
6. Low self-esteem can be a trait in some individuals that is stable over time. For others it can be initiated by a broad range of stressful situations. (Tenner and Herzberger)
7. As self-esteem declines, so does a person's belief that he can exert control over his environment. Likewise, as personal control is perceived to decrease, so does self-esteem. (Taft)
8. In response to a threat to a person's self-concept, self-esteem is protected through three cognitive processes:
   a. Searching for meaning in the experience
   b. Regaining mastery over the event
   c. Self-enhancement ("How am I managing as compared to others?") (Taylor)
9. A variety of variables interact to produce a decline in self-esteem in the elderly, including negative societal attitudes, decreased social interactions and decreased power and control over the environment. (Taft)
10. Increased social interaction through involvement in groups will enable one to receive social and intellectual stimulation (Taft), which will enhance self-esteem.

11. Attributing failure to a lack of ability (internal cause) leads to decreased expectations and motivation. (Antaki and Brewin)
12. The adolescent's self-esteem is closely linked to his body image. The changes the adolescent's body is undergoing increase the vulnerability of his self-esteem. (Miller)

Outcome Criteria

The person will
- Describe changes in feelings regarding self

Interventions

Nursing interventions for the variety of problems that might be associated with a diagnosis of *Self-Concept Disturbance* are very similar.

A. Establish a trusting nurse/client relationship

- Encourage person to express his feelings, especially about the way he feels, thinks, or views himself
- Encourage person to ask questions about his health problem, his treatment, his progress, his prognosis
- Provide reliable information and reinforce information already given
- Clarify any misconceptions the person has about himself, his care, or his caregivers
- Avoid negative criticism
- Provide privacy and a safe environment

B. Assess for signs and symptoms

(Utilize the focus assessment criteria to isolate signs and symptoms. Refer to the defining characteristics of *Self-Esteem Disturbance, Body Image Disturbance* and *Altered Role Performance*. After confirmation, utilize the interventions under the category.)

C. Initiate health teaching as indicated

- Teach person what community resources are available, if needed (*e.g.,* mental health centers, such self-help groups as Reach for Recovery, Make Today Count)

Body Image Disturbance

Related to **(Specify)**

Definition

Body image disturbance: The state in which an individual experiences or is at risk to experience a disruption in the way one perceives one's body image.

Defining Characteristics

Major (must be present)

> Verbal or nonverbal negative response to actual or perceived change in structure and/or function

Minor (may be present)

> Not looking at body part
> Not touching body part
> Hiding or overexposing body part
> Change in social involvement
> Negative feelings about body feelings of helplessness, hopelessness, powerlessness
> Preoccupation with change or loss
> Refusal to verify actual change
> Depersonalization of part or loss

Etiological, Contributing, Risk Factors

Pathophysiological

> Chronic disease
> Loss of body part
> Loss of body function
> Severe trauma

Treatment-Related

> Hospitalization
> Surgery
> Chemotherapy
> Radiation

Situational

> Pain
> Obesity
> Pregnancy
> Infertility
> Immobility
> Cultural influences

Maturational

    Adolescent: puberty
    Middle age: signs of aging (graying, menopause)
    Elderly: loss of function

Focus Assessment Criteria

See *Self-Concept Disturbance*

Principles and Rationale for Nursing Care

See *Self-Concept Disturbance*

Body Image Disturbance
Related to (Specify)

Assessment

See Defining Characteristics

Outcome Criteria

The person will
- Share feelings about how he views himself
- Achieve or maintain control of his body
- Begin to assume role-related responsibilities
- Develop confidence in his ability to accomplish what is desired

---

Interventions

A. Establish a trusting nurse/client relationship

- Encourage person to express his feelings, especially about the way he feels, thinks, or views himself
- Encourage person to ask questions about his health problem, his treatment, his progress, his prognosis
- Provide reliable information and reinforce information already given
- Clarify any misconceptions the person has about himself, his care, or his caregivers
- Avoid negative criticism
- Provide privacy and a safe environment

B. Promote social interaction

- Assist person to accept help from others
- Avoid overprotection, but limit the demands made on the individual
- Encourage movement
- Support family as they adapt

- Encourage visits from peers and significant others
- Encourage contact (letters, telephone) with peers and family
- Encourage involvement in unit activities
- Provide opportunity to share with persons going through similar experiences

C. Provide specific interventions in selected situations

1. Pregnancy
   - Encourage the woman to share her concerns
   - Attend to each concern if possible or refer her to others for assistance
   - Discuss the challenges and changes that pregnancy and motherhood bring
   - Encourage her to share expectations: her own and those of her significant others
   - Assist her to identify sources for love and affection
   - Provide anticipatory guidance to both parents-to-be regarding
     a. Fatigue and irritability
     b. Appetite swings
     c. Gastric disturbances (nausea, constipation)
     d. Back and leg aches
     e. Changes in sexual desire
     f. Mood swings
     g. Fear (for self, for unborn baby, of loss of attractiveness, of inadequacy as a mother)
   - Encourage the mutual sharing of concerns between spouses

2. Hospitalized child
   a. Prepare child for hospitalization, if possible, with an explanation and a visit to the hospital to meet personnel and examine the environment
   b. Provide child with opportunities to share fears, concerns, anger (see Appendix IX for play therapy guidelines)
      - Acknowledge the normalcy of these fears, concerns, anger
      - Correct child's misconceptions (*e.g.,* that he's being punished; that his parents are angry)
      - Encourage family to stay with or visit child, despite the child's crying when they leave; teach them to provide accurate information as to when they will return to reduce fears of abandonment
      - Allow parents to help with care
   c. Assist child to understand his experiences
      - Provide child with an explanation ahead of time, if possible
      - Explain sensations and discomforts of condition, treatments, and medications
      - Encourage crying
   d. Maintain sense of intactness during periods of immobility
      - Encourage movement, no matter how slight
      - During bath, ask child to identify body parts: "Where is your leg?"
      - Allow child access to mirror to provide visualization of body

3. Loss of body part of function
   - Assess the meaning of the loss for the individual and significant others, as related to visibility of loss, function of loss, and emotional investment
   - Expect the individual to respond to the loss with denial, shock, anger, and depression
   - Be aware of the effect of the responses of others to the loss; encourage sharing of feelings between significant others
   - Allow individual to ventilate his feelings and to grieve
   - Utilize role-playing to assist with sharing; if person says, "I know my husband

will not want to touch me with this colostomy," take the husband's role and discuss her colostomy, then switch roles so she can act out her feelings about her husband's response

- Explore realistic alternatives and provide encouragement
- Explore strengths and resources with person
- Assist with the resolution of a surgically created alteration of body image
  a. Replace the lost body part with prosthesis as soon as possible
  b. Encourage viewing of site
  c. Encourage touching of site
- Teach about the health problem and how to manage
- Begin to incorporate person in care of operative site
- Gradually allow person to assume full self-care responsibility, if feasible
- Teach person to monitor own progress (Miller)
- Refer to *Sexual Dysfunction* for additional information if indicated

4. Changes associated with chemotherapy. (Cooley)
- Discuss the possibility of hair loss, absence of menses, temporary or permanent sterility, decreased estrogen levels, vaginal dryness, mucosititis
- Encourage to share concerns, fears and their perception of the impact of these changes on their life
- Explain where hair loss may occur (head, eyelashes, eyebrows, auxiliary hair, pubic and leg hair)
- Explain that hair will grow back after treatment but may change in color and texture
- Select a wig prior to hair loss, wear it before hair loss. Consult a beautician for tips on how to vary the look, (*e.g.,* combs, clips, etc.)
- Encourage the wearing of scarves, turbans when wig is not on.
- Teach to minimize the amount of hair loss by
  a. Avoiding excessive shampooing, using a conditioner twice weekly
  b. Patting hair dry gently
  c. Avoiding electric curlers, dryers and curling irons
  d. Avoiding pulling hair with bands, clips or bobby pins
  e. Avoiding hair spray and hair dye
  f. Using wide-tooth comb, avoiding vigorous brushing
- Refer to American Cancer Society for information regarding new or used wigs. Inform them that the wig is a tax-deductible item
- Discuss the difficulty that others (spouse, friends, coworkers) may have with visible changes
- Encourage the person to initiate calls and contacts with others who may be having difficulty
- Encourage the person to ask for assistance of friends, relatives. Ask person if the situation were reversed, what he or she would want to do to help a friend.
- Allow significant others opportunities to share their feelings and fears
- Assist significant others to identify positive aspects of the client and ways this can be shared
- Provide information regarding support groups for couples

D. Initiate health teaching as indicated

- Teach person what community resources are available, if needed (*e.g.,* mental health centers, such self-help groups as Reach for Recovery, Make Today Count)
- Teach wellness strategies (see *Health-Seeking Behaviors*)

Personal Identity Disturbance

Definition

Personal identity disturbance: The state in which an individual experiences or is at risk of experiencing an inability to distinguish between self and nonself.

> **Author's Note:** This diagnostic category is a subcategory under *Self-Concept Disturbance*. Until clinical research defines and differentiates this category from others, refer to *Self-Concept Disturbance* or *Altered Growth and Development* for assessment criteria and interventions.

Defining Characteristics

See Defining Characteristics for *Self-Concept Disturbance* or *Altered Growth and Development*.

Self-Esteem Disturbance

Definition

Self-esteem disturbance: The state in which an individual experiences or is at risk of experiencing negative self-evaluation about self or capabilities.

> **Author's Note:** Self-Esteem is one of the four components of Self-Concept. *Self-Esteem Disturbance* is the general diagnostic category. *Chronic Low Self-Esteem* and *Situational Low Self-Esteem* represent specific types of *Self-Esteem Disturbances*, thus involving more specific interventions. Initially the nurse may not have sufficient clinical data to validate a more specific diagnosis as *Chronic Low Self-Esteem* or *Situational Low Self-Esteem*. Refer to the major defining characteristics under these categories for validation.

Defining Characteristics*

Overt or covert
- Self-negating verbalization
- Expressions of shame of guilt
- Evaluates self as unable to deal with events
- Rationalizes away/rejects positive feedback and exaggerates negative feedback about self
- Hesitant to try new things/situations
- Denial of problems obvious to others
- Projection of blame/responsibility for problems
- Rationalizes personal failures
- Hypersensitivity to slight criticism
- Grandiosity

Etiological, Contributing, Risk Factors

Self-Esteem Disturbance can be either an episodic event or a chronic problem. Failure to resolve a problem or multiple sequential stresses can result in chronic low self-esteem. Those factors, which occur over time and are associated with chronic low self-esteem, are indicated by chronic low self-esteem (CLSE).

Pathophysiological

Loss of body parts
Loss of body function(s)
Disfigurement (trauma, surgery, birth defects)

Situational (personal, environmental)

Hospitalization
Loss of job or ability to work
Death of significant other
Separation from significant other
Increase/decrease in weight
Pregnancy
Unemployment
Financial problems
Relationship problems
    Marital discord   Step-parents
    Separation   In-laws
Failure in school
History of ineffective relationship with own parents (CLSE)
History of abusive relationships (CLSE)
Unrealistic expectations of child by parent (CLSE)
Unrealistic expectations of self (CLSE)
Unrealistic expectations of parent by child (CLSE)
Parental rejection (CLSE)
Overpassiveness (CLSE)
Inconsistent punishment (CLSE)

* Source: Norris J, Kunes-Connell M: Self-esteem disturbance: A clinical validation study. In McLane A, (ed): Classification of Nursing Diagnoses: Proceedings of the Seventh Conference. St. Louis, CV Mosby, 1987

Legal difficulties
Institutionalization
> Mental health facility
> Jail

Orphanage
Halfway house

Cultural influences
> Ethnic group

Minority

Drug/alcohol abuse by self or family member

Maturational

Infant/toddler/preschool
> Lack of stimulation (CLSE)
> Separation from parents/significant others (CLSE)
> Restriction of activity (CLSE)
> Inadequate parental support (CLSE)
> Inability to trust significant other (CLSE)

School-age
> Loss of significant others
> Failure to achieve grade level objectives
> Loss of peer group

Adolescent
> Loss of independence and autonomy
> Disruption of peer relationships
> Disruption in body image
> Interruption of intellectual achievement
> Loss of significant others
> Career choices

Middle age
> Signs of graying
> Menopause
> Career pressures

Elderly
> Losses (people, function, financial, retirement)

Focus Assessment Criteria

See *Self-Concept Disturbance*

Principles and Rationale for Nursing Care

See *Self-Concept Disturbance*

Chronic Low Self-Esteem

Related to **(Specify)**

Definition

Chronic low self-esteem: The state in which an individual experiences long-standing negative self-evaluation about the self's capabilities.

Defining Characteristics*

Major (80–100%)

Long-standing or chronic
 Self-negating verbalization
 Expressions of shame/guilt
 Evaluates self as unable to deal with events
 Rationalizes away/rejects positive feedback and exaggerates negative feedback about
  self
 Hesitant to try new things/situations

Minor (50–79%)

 Frequent lack of success in work or other life events
 Overly conforming, dependent on others' opinions
 Lack of eye contact
 Nonassertive/passive
 Indecisive
 Excessively seeks reassurance

Etiological, Contributing, Risk Factors

See *Self-Esteem Disturbance*

Principles and Rationale for Nursing Care

See *Self-Esteem Disturbance*

Chronic Low Self Esteem
Related to (Specify)

Assessment
See Defining Characteristics

Outcome Criteria

The individual will
 • Verbalize realistic perceptions of self
 • Identify positive aspects about self
 • Interact appropriately with others
 • Participate in activities

---

 * Source: Norris J, Kunes-Connell M: Self-esteem disturbance: A clinical validation study. In McLane A, (ed): Classification of Nursing Diagnoses: Proceedings of the Seventh Conference, St. Louis, CV Mosby, 1987

Interventions

1. Assist the person to reduce his present anxiety level
   - Be supportive, nonjudgmental
   - Accept silence, but let him know you are there
   - Orient as necessary
   - Clarify distortions; do not use confrontation
   - Be aware of your own anxiety and avoid communicating it to the individual
   - Refer to *Anxiety* for further interventions
2. Enhance the person's sense of self
   - Be attentive
   - Respect his personal space
   - Validate your interpretation of what he is saying or experiencing ("Is this what you mean?")
   - Help him to verbalize what he is expressing nonverbally
   - Use communication that helps to maintain his own individuality ("I" instead of "we")
   - Pay attention to person, especially new behavior
   - Provide encouragement as a task or skill is attempted
   - Provide realistic positive feedback on accomplishments
   - Teach person to consensually validate with others
   - Respect need for privacy
   - Provide consistency among staff (Miller)
3. Assist person in expressing his thoughts and feelings
   - Use open-ended statements and questions
   - Encourage expression of both positive and negative statements
   - Use movement, art, and music as means of expression
   - If person has impaired reality-testing ability, refer to *Altered Thought Processes* for further interventions
4. Provide opportunities for positive socialization
   - Encourage visits/contact with peers and significant others (letters, telephone)
   - Be a role model in one-to-one interactions
   - Involve in activities, especially when strengths can be utilized
   - Do not allow person to isolate self (refer to *Social Isolation* for further interventions)
   - Involve in supportive group therapy
   - Teach social skills as required (Refer to *Impaired Social Interaction* for further interventions)
   - Encourage participation with others sharing similar experiences
5. Set limits on problematic behavior such as aggression, poor hygiene, ruminations and suicidal preoccupation. Refer to *Potential for Self Harm* and/or *Potential for Violence* if these are assessed as problems
6. Provide for development of social and vocational skills
   - Reinforce confidence as person demonstrates new skills
   - Refer for vocational counseling
   - Involve in volunteer organizations
   - Encourage participation in senior citizens groups
   - Arrange for continuation of education (*e.g.,* literacy class, GEDs, vocational training, art/music classes)
7. Assist in self-exploration as anxiety and trust permit
   - Identifying positive self-evaluation
   - Assessing self-appraisal
   - Refer to *Situational Low Self-Esteem* for specific interventions

Situational Low Self-Esteem

Related to **(Specify)**

Definition

Situational low self-esteem: The state in which an individual who previously had positive self-esteem experiences negative feelings about self in response to an event (loss, change).

> **Author's Note:** Although situational low self-esteem is an episodic event, repeated occurrences and/or the continuation of these negative self-appraisals over time can lead to chronic low self-esteem. (Willard)

Defining Characteristics*

Major (80–100%)
- Episodic occurrence of negative self-appraisal in response to life events in a person with a previous positive self-evaluation
- Verbalization of negative feelings about self (helplessness, uselessness)

Minor (50–79%)
- Self-negating verbalizations
- Expressions of shame/guilt
- Evaluates self as unable to handle situations/events
- Difficulty making decisions

Etiological, Contributing, Risk Factors

See *Self-Esteem Disturbance*

Principles and Rationale for Nursing Care

See *Self-Esteem Disturbance*

Situational Low Self-Esteem
Related to (Specify)

Assessment

See Defining Characteristics

* Source: Norris J, Kunes-Connell M: Self-esteem disturbance: A clinical validation study. In McLane A, (ed): Classification of Nursing Diagnoses: Proceedings of the Seventh Conference. St. Louis, CV Mosby, 1987

Outcome Criteria

The person will
- Identify positive aspects of self
- Express a positive outlook for the future
- Analyze his own behavior and its consequences
- Identify ways of exerting control and influencing outcomes

Interventions

1. Assist the individual in identifying and expressing feelings
   - Be empathetic, nonjudgmental
   - Listen. Do not discourage expressions of anger, crying, and so forth
   - What was happening when he began feeling this way?
   - Clarify relationships between life events
2. Assist in identifying positive self-evaluations
   - How has he handled other crises?
   - How does he manage anxiety, exercise, withdrawal, drinking/drugs, talking
   - Reinforce adaptive coping mechanisms
   - Examine and reinforce positive abilities and traits (*e.g.,* hobbies, skills, school, IPRs, appearance, loyalty, industriousness, etc.)
   - Help individual accept both positive and negative feelings
   - Do not confront defenses
   - Communicate confidence in person's ability
   - Involve person in mutual goal-setting
3. Explore relationship between behavior and self-appraisals
   - Encourage examination of current behavior and its consequences. (*e.g.,* dependency, procrastination, isolation)
   - Assist in mutually identifying faulty perceptions
   - Assist in identifying unrealistic expectations
   - Help to identify negative automatic thoughts ("I will never be able to do this.")
   - Examine if person is overgeneralizing ("If I can't do this, then I'm a failure at everything.")
   - Assist in identifying own responsibility and control in a situation (*e.g.,* when continually blaming others for problems)
4. Assess and mobilize current support system
   - Does he live alone? Employed?
   - Does he have available friends and relatives?
   - Is the church a support?
   - Has he previously used community resources?
   - Refer to Vocational Rehabilitation for retraining
   - Support returning to school for further training
   - Assist in involving in local volunteer organizations (senior citizens employment, Foster Grandparents, local support groups)
   - Arrange continuation of school studies for students
5. Assist individual in learning new coping skills
   - Teach about how persons respond to a life change
   - Let him know he is not alone
   - Assist in identifying options (*e.g.,* saying no, time off)
   - Refer to Appendix VII, Guidelines for Problem-Solving and Crisis intervention

- Refer to Appendix X for Stress Management techniques
- Encourage trail of new behavior
- Reinforce the belief that the individual does have control over the situation

6. Assist person in managing specific problems

Rape—refer to *Rape Trauma Response*

Loss—refer to *Grieving*

Hospitalization—refer to *Powerlessness* and *Parental Role Conflict*

Ill family member—refer to *Altered Family Processes*

Change or loss of body part—refer to *Body Image Disturbance*

Depression—refer to *Ineffective Individual Coping* and *Hopelessness*

Domestic violence—refer to *Ineffective Family Coping*

References/Bibliography

Antaki C, Bruoin C (eds): Attributions and Psychological Change. Academic Press, London, 1982

Bille D: The role of body image in patient compliance and education. Heart Lung 6(1):143–147, 1977

Brundage DJ: Altered body image. In Phipps WJ, Long B, Woods N (eds): Medical-Surgical Nursing: Concepts and Clinical Practice. St. Louis, CV Mosby, 1979

Burnside I: I, me and the self: Self-esteem in later life. In Burnside I et al (eds): Psychosocial Caring Throughout the Life Span. New York, McGraw-Hill, 1979

Combs AW, Avilla DL, Purkey WW: Self-concept: Product and producer of experience. In Arkoff A, (ed): Psychology and Personal Growth, pp 8–21. Boston, Allyn and Bacon, 1980

Crouch MA, Straub V: Enhancement of self-esteem in adults. Family Community Health 6(2):76–78, 1983

Donovan M, Pierce S: Cancer Care Nursing. New York, Appleton-Century-Crofts, 1976

Gilberts R: The evaluation of self-esteem. Family Community Health (8):29–49, 1983

Gruendemann BJ: The impact of surgery on body image. Nurs Clin North Am 10(4):635–643, 1975

Harris M: Helping the person with an altered self-image. Geriatr Nurs 7(2):90–92, 1986

Jackson DW: The adolescent and the hospital. Pediatr Clin North Am 20(4):903, 1973

Meisenhelder JB: Self-esteem: A closer look at clinical interventions. Int Journal Nurs Stud 22(2):127–135, 1985

McCloskey JC: How to make the most of body image theory in nursing practice. Nursing 6(6):68–72, 1976

McGrory A: A Well Model Approach to Care of the Dying Client. New York, McGraw-Hill, 1978

Miller S: Promoting self-esteem in the hospitalized adolescents: Clinical interventions. Issues of Comprehensive Pediatric Nursing 10(3):187–194, 1987

Murray R: The concept of body image. Nurs Clin North Am 7(4):593–707, 1972

Norris J, Kunes–Connell M: Self-esteem disturbance. Nurs Clin North Am 20(12): 745–761, 1985

Reasoner RW: Enhancement of Self-esteem in children and adolescents. Family Community Health 6(2):51–63, 1983

Roberts S: Behavioral Concepts and Nursing Throughout the Life Span. Englewood Cliffs, NJ, Prentice-Hall, 1978

Rubin R: Body image and self-esteem. Nursing Outlook 16(6):20–23, 1968

Showalter JE, Lord RD: The hospitalized adolescent. Children 18(4):127–132, 1971

Stuart G, Sundean S: Principles and Practice of Psychiatric Nursing, 3th ed. St. Louis, CV Mosby, 1987

Taft LB: Self-esteem in later life: A nursing perspective. Adv Nurs Sci 8(1):77–84, 1985

Taylor S: Adjustment to threatening events: A theory of cognitive adaptation. Am Psychol 38(8):1161–1173, 1983

Tennen H, Herzberger S: Depression, self-esteem and the absence of self-protective attributional biases. J Pers Soc Psychol 52(2):72–80, 1987

Self-Harm, Potential for*

Related to **(Specify)**

Definition
Potential for self-harm: A state in which an individual is at risk for inflicting direct harm on himself or herself.

> **Author's Note:** If the individual is experiencing hopelessness, refer also to *Hopelessness*. If this is a chronic response, refer also to *Ineffective Coping*.

Defining Characteristics
Suicidal ideation

Minor (may be present)
Severe stress
Depression
Hallucinations/delusions
Hostility
Substance abuse
Low self-esteem

Hopelessness
Acute agitation
Poor impulse control
Lack of a support system
Helplessness

Etiological, Contributing, Risk Factors
Potential for self-harm can occur as a response to a variety of health problems, situations, and conflicts. Some sources are:

Pathophysiological
Terminal illness
Chronic illness (*e.g.,* diabetes,
  hypertension)

Alcoholism
Organic mental disorder
Chronic pain

Treatment-related
Dialysis
Insulin injections or any ongoing
  treatments

Chemotherapy/radiation
Ingestion of prescribed or
  nonprescribed drugs

Situational
Parental/marital conflict
Job loss
Divorce/separation
Threatened or actual financial loss

Depression
Death of significant other
Loss of status, prestige
Someone leaving home

* This diagnostic category is not currently on the NANDA list but has been included for clarity or usefulness.

Alcoholism/drug abuse in family
Wish to reunite with loved one who
   has died
Inadequate coping skills

Child abuse
Threat of abandonment by
   significant other

Maturational

Adolescent: Separation from family, peer pressure, role changes, identity crisis, loss
   of significant support person
Adult: Marital conflict, parenting, loss of family member, role changes
Elderly: Retirement, social isolation, loss of spouse

Focus Assessment Criteria

Information must be gathered from the individual and at least one significant other.

Subjective Data

1. Psychological status
   a. Assess for feelings of:
      Hopelessness
      Isolation/abandonment
      Anger, hostility

      Helplessness
      Guilt, shame
      Suicide as a viable alternative
   b. Assess for presence of:
      Persecutory delusions
      Confusion/disorganization

      Hallucinations
      Poor impulse control
   c. Recent changes in behavior
   d. History of psychiatric problems:
      Outpatient treatment
      Previous attempts
      • Number
      • Recency
      • Lethality

      Hospitalization
2. Medical status
   Acute or chronic illness—how is it affecting life?
   Has person consulted MD in past 6 months?
   History of alcoholism/drug abuse?
3. Sources of stress in current environment
   Job change/loss
   Failure in work/school
   Threat of financial loss
   Divorce/separation

   Death of significant other
   Illness/accident
   Threat of criminal prosecution
   Alcohol/drug use in family
4. Coping strategies (past and present)
   Assess ability of individual and family to cope with repeated stresses
   Available resources
   Level of impulse control
   Taking unnecessary risks (drugs, alcohol)
5. Support system
   a. Who is relied on during periods of stress?
      Are they available?
      Their reaction to current situation:
      • Denial of problem
      • Not receptive to helping now
      • Anger, guilt

- Helplessness, frustration
- Concern and willingness to help
b. Personal and financial resources
    Employment   Financial problems
    Housing
6. Suicide Ideation
    a. Have you ever thought of ending your life?
    b. Assess for a suicide plan:
        Method: Is there a specific plan (pills, wrist-slashing, shooting, etc.); plans for rescue?
        Availability: Is the method accessible? Is access easy or difficult?
        Specificity: How specific is plan?
        Lethality: How lethal is the method?

Objective Data

1. General appearance
    Facial expression   Dress
    Posture
2. Behavior during interview
    Withdrawn   Quiet
    Hostile   Cooperative
    Hopeless
3. Communication pattern (subjective/objective)
    Content
        Appropriate   Tangential/allusive
        Denial of problem   Suspicions
        Delusions (grandeur,   Hopelessness ("It's hopeless; it's
          persecution)   the end of the road")
        Suicidal thoughts ("I may as   Negative cognitive set
          well be dead"; "I wish I
          were dead")
    Flow of thought
        Appropriate   Jumps from one topic to another
        Blocking of ideas   Unable to come to a decision
        Ideas loosely connected   Unable to see alternatives (tunnel
                                          vision)
    Rate of speech
        Appropriate   Reduced
        Excessive   Pressured
    Reaction of significant others
        Ignoring suicidal expressions   Anger at expressions
        Leaving or turning away
          following expression
4. Activities of daily living
    Capable of caring for self   Impaired ability to care for self
5. Nutritional status
    Weight (increased, decreased)   Appetite
6. Sleep/rest pattern
    Recent change   Early wakefulness
    Insomnia   Sleeps too much

7. Personal hygiene
    Cleanliness
    Grooming

Clothes (condition, appropriateness)

8. Motor activity
    Within normal limits
    Decreased
    Repetitive

Increased
Agitated

9. Evidence of self-harm
    Wrist slashes
    Burns on body
    Broken bones

Eye enucleation
Gunshot wound
Overdose

Principles and Rationale for Nursing Care

See also *Hopelessness*

General

1. Self-destructive behavior ranges from indirect acts (obesity, noncompliance with medical treatment) to direct acts of self-destruction.
2. Indirect self-destructive behavior has the potential to be harmful and result in death; however, the person is unaware of this potential.
3. With direct self-destructive behavior, usually referred to as suicidal, the intent is death, and the individual is aware.
4. Suicidal behavior is an attempt to escape from intolerable life stressors that have accumulated over time. It is a response to intense feelings of hopelessness.
5. Both the individual and the family have exhausted their resources.
6. A suicidal crisis happens both to the individual and to the person's support system.
7. Suicide may be seen as a viable alternative both by the individual and by significant others.
8. Situations that contribute to suicidal behavior include depression, loss (significant other, job, finances), debilitating disease, and alcohol/drug abuse.
9. Persons exhibiting poor reality testing, delusions, and poor impulse control are at high risk. Alcohol and drugs tend to lower impulse control.
10. When assessing suicidal behavior in children, one must consider age-appropriateness of the behavior (*e.g.,* self-biting, head-banging in toddlers vs. in an older child).
11. Depression may be masked by a wide range of physical complaints in children: school phobias, daydreaming, and social withdrawal.
12. Suicidal individuals are usually ambivalent about the decision. Staff can work with the positive goals to effect a change in attitude.
13. Changes in behavior (*e.g.,* giving away possessions) may signal an increase in risk. Individuals may appear to be better just prior to an attempt. This may be due to feelings of relief after making a decision.
14. Older men will seldom seek help from mental health agencies. Families, senior citizen centers, clergy, and physicians are the network that can most readily identify the potential problem.
15. Demographic factors can serve the caregiver in identifying people who are at risk for suicidal behavior:
   - Suicide increases with age to a peak at about 50 years for white males.
   - Adolescents also represent a high-risk group.
   - More women attempt suicide, but men complete suicide more often.
   - Unemployment and frequent job changes are associated with an increased risk.

- Alcohol is associated with a high risk.
- The greater the satisfaction with social relationships, the lower the risk will be; thus, divorce, separation, and widowhood increase the risk.
- Previous attempts place the person in a high-risk group, since they are likely to repeat the attempt.
16. The more resources are available, the more likely the crisis can be effectively managed. This includes personal support systems, employment, physical and mental abilities, finances, and housing.
17. Some individuals use suicide attempts as a way to cope with stress. The more frequent the attempts and the more lethal, the higher is the current risk.
18. In order to assess more accurately the risk for suicide, the caregiver must question the person directly. Ask simple, straightforward questions. The more specific, more lethal, more available the means, the higher is the present risk. The most lethal methods in our culture are shooting and hanging. The least lethal is wrist-slashing.
19. Long-term suicide risk exists for some people. This can be assessed best by evaluating:
    - Their coping strategies when confronted with stress
    - Their life-style—is it stable or unstable?
    - The specificity and lethality of the plan
20. Interventions are based on the type of risk the person presents. Long-term treatment is often more difficult to institute than emergency care.
21. Caregivers can become immobilized or drained by the acutely suicidal person. Feelings of hopelessness are often communicated to the caregiver. Self-awareness and use of consultation can help prevent negative consequences.
22. Use verbal and nonverbal clues to assess risk, since seriously suicidal persons may deny suicidal thoughts.
23. Levels of risk can be assessed as low or high. Not all of the following parameters are necessarily present in any one individual.

High

Adolescent or over 45	Male
Divorced, separated, widowed	Isolated socially
Professional worker	Unemployed or lack of stable job history
Chronic or terminal illness	
Delusions/hallucinations	Severe depression
Hopelessness/helplessness	Severe anxiety
Intoxicated or addicted	Multiple attempts
Frequent or constant suicidal thoughts	With a specific plan, method is highly lethal
Means—readily available	

Low

25–45 years of age or under 12	Female
Married	Socially active
Blue-collar worker	Employed
No serious medical problems	Infrequent substance abuse
No specific plan, or has a plan with low lethality	Thoughts are fleeting (if person has a vague plan)

High-risk elderly

1. Caucasian males over 65 years old have a suicide rate twice the rate for all age groups. (US Bureau of the Census)

2. The self-esteem of older men is negatively affected by retirement, loss of vigor, and loss of a meaningful role. (Boxwell)
3. The elderly tend to complete suicide when attempted. The rate of attempts to completion is 4 to 1 while for younger persons, the ratio is approximately 15 to 1. (McIntosh)

Potential for Self-Harm
Related to (Specify)

Assessment
See Defining Characteristics

Outcome Criteria

The person will
- not harm self
- accept help from significant others and community
- use effective coping mechanisms in handling stress

Interventions

A. Assist the person in reducing his present risk for self-destruction

1. Assess level of present risk (see Principles and Rationale for Nursing Care for specific differentiation)

| High | Moderate | Low |

2. Assess level of long-term risk

| Life-style | Lethality of plan | Usual coping mechanisms |

3. Provide a safe environment based on level of risk

Immediate management for high-risk person
- Acutely suicidal persons should be admitted to a closely supervised environment.
- Although it is impossible to create a completely safe environment, removal of dangerous objects and close observation convey a nonverbal message of concern to the individual. Restrict glass, nail files, scissors, nail polish remover, mirrors, needles, razors, soda cans, plastic bags, lighters, electric equipment, belts, hangers, knives, tweezers, alcohol, guns.
- Meals should be provided in a closely supervised area, usually on the unit or in individual's own room
    Ensure adequate food and fluid intake
    Use paper/plastic plates and utensils
    Check to be sure all items are returned on the tray
- When administering oral medications, check to ensure that all medications are swallowed.

- Designate a staff member to provide checks on the person as designated by institution's policy. Provide relief for the staff member.
- Restrict the individual to the unit unless specifically ordered by physician. When off unit, provide a staff member to accompany the person.
- Instruct visitors on restricted items. Ensure that they do not give the person food in a plastic bag for example.
- Restricted items may be used by individual in presence of staff, depending on level of risk. Acutely suicidal persons should not be allowed access to such items.
- The acutely suicidal person may be required to wear a hospital gown to prevent elopement. As risk decreases, client may be allowed own clothing.
- Room searches should be done periodically according to institution policy.
- Utilize seclusion and restraint if necessary (refer to *Potential for Violence* for discussion).
- Notify police if the person elopes and is at risk for suicide.
- When the individual is being constantly observed, he is not to be allowed out of sight even though privacy is lost.

4. Notify all staff that this person is at risk for self-harm.
   - Use both written and oral communication
5. Make a no-suicide contract with the individual (include family if person is at home).
   - Use a written contract
   - Mutual agreement
     "I will not kill myself" or "I will not accidentally or intentionally take medicine except according to instructions." "I will talk to a staff member about my thoughts when suicidal ideas increase."

B. Help build self-esteem

- Be nonjudgmental and empathetic
- Be aware of own reactions to the situation
- Provide genuine praise
- Encourage interactions with others
- Divert attention to external world (*e.g.,* odd jobs)
- Convey sense that he is not alone (use group or peer therapy)
- Seek out person for interactions
- Set limits by informing of rules
- Use firm, consistent approach
- Provide planned daily schedules to persons with low impulse control

C. Assist in identifying and contacting support system

- Inform family and significant others
- Enlist support
- Do not provide false reassurance that behavior will not recur
- Point out vague or unclear messages from individual or support system
- Encourage an increase in social activity

D. Assist individual in developing positive coping mechanism

- Refer to *Anxiety, Ineffective Individual Coping,* and *Hopelessness* for further interventions
- Encourage appropriate expression of anger and hostility
- Set limits on ruminations about suicide or previous attempts
- Assist in recognizing predisposing factors: "What was happening before you started having these thoughts?"

- Facilitate examination of life stresses and past coping mechanisms
- Explore alternative behaviors
- Anticipate future stresses and assist in planning alternatives
- Use appropriate behavior modification techniques for noncompliant, resistive persons
- Help identify negative thinking patterns and direct person to practice altering these patterns
- Involve person in planning the treatment goals and evaluating progress

E. Initiate health teaching and referrals when indicated

- Provide teaching that will prepare person to deal with life stresses (relaxation, problem-solving skills, how to express feelings constructively)
- Refer for peer or group therapy
- Refer for family therapy, especially when child or adolescent is involved
- Teach family limit-setting techniques
- Teach family constructive expression of feelings
- Instruct significant others in how to recognize an increase in risk: change in behavior, verbal, nonverbal communication, withdrawal, signs of depression
- Supply phone number of 24-hour emergency hotlines
- Refer to vocational training if appropriate
- Refer to halfway houses or other agencies as appropriate
- Refer to ongoing psychiatric follow-up
- Refer to senior citizen centers or other agencies to increase leisure time activities.

References/Bibliography

Blythe M, Pearlmutter D: The suicidal watch: A re-examination of maximum observation. Perspect Psychiatr Care 21(3):90–93, 1983

Boxwell A: Geriatric Suicide, The Preventable Death. Nurse Pract 13(6):10–14, 1988

Gilead M, Muliak J: Adolescent suicide: A response to developmental crisis. Perspect Psychiatr Care 21(3):94–101, 1983

Hatton C, Valente S: Assessment of suicidal risk. In Suicide: Assessment and Intervention.

McIntosh JL: Suicide among the elderly: Levels and trends. Am J Orthopsychiatry 55(4):2, 288–293, 1985

Richman J: Family Therapy for Suicidal People. New York, Springer-Verlag, 1986

U.S. Bureau of the Census: Statistical Abstracts of the United States: 1985, 105th ed., pp 75–79. Washington, DC, 1984

Valente S: The suicidal teenager. Nursing 15(12):47–50, 1985

Whall A: Suicide in older adults. J Gerontol Nurs 11(8):40, 1985

Sensory—Perceptual Alterations

Related to **Sensory Overload**

Definition

Sensory—perceptual alterations: A state in which the individual/group experiences or is at risk of experiencing a change in the amount, pattern, or interpretation of incoming stimuli.

> **Author's Note:** The category *Sensory—Perceptual Alterations* has six subcategories–visual, auditory, kinesthetic, gustatory, tactile, and olfactory.
>
> When an individual has a visual or hearing deficit, how does the nurse intervene with the diagnosis *Sensory Perceptual Alterations: visual related to effects of glaucoma?* What would the outcome criteria be? The nurse should assess for the individual's response to the visual loss and specifically label the response, not the deficit.
>
> *Sensory—Perceptual Alterations* is more clinically useful without the addition of the sensory deficit. Examples of responses to sensory deficits may be:
>
> | | |
> |---|---|
> | Visual: | Potential for Injury |
> | | Self-care Deficit |
> | Auditory: | Impaired Communication |
> | | Social Isolation |
> | Kinesthetic: | Potential for Injury |
> | Olfactory: | Altered Nutrition |
> | Tactile: | Potential for Injury |
> | Gustatory: | Altered Nutrition |
>
> *Altered Thought Processes* describes an individual with altered cognition and perception influenced by coping problems different from *Sensory—Perceptual Alterations,* which describes an individual with altered perception and cognition influenced by physiological functions and stimuli from the environment.

Defining Characteristics

Major (must be present)

Inaccurate interpretation of environmental stimuli and/or
Negative change in amount or pattern of incoming stimuli

Minor (may be present)

Disoriented in time or place
Disoriented about people
Altered ability to problem-solve
Altered behavior or communication
    pattern
Sleep pattern disturbances

Restlessness
Reports auditory or visual
    hallucinations
Fear
Anxiety
Apathy

Etiological, Contributing, Risk Factors

Many factors in an individual's life can contribute to sensory–perceptual alterations. Some common factors are listed below.

Pathophysiological

Sensory organ alterations (visual, gustatory, hearing, olfactory, and tactile deficits)
Neurological alterations
  Cerebrovascular accident (CVA)   Neuropathies
  Encephalitis meningitis
Metabolic alterations
  Fluid and electrolyte imbalance   Acidosis
  Elevated blood urea nitrogen   Alkalosis
    (BUN)
Impaired oxygen transport
  Cerebral   Respiratory
  Cardiac   Anemia
Musculoskeletal changes
  Paraplegia   Quadriplegia

Treatment-related

Amputation
Medications (sedatives, tranquilizers)
Surgery (glaucoma, cataract, detached retina)
Physical isolation (reverse isolation, communicable disease, prison)
Radiation therapy
Immobility
Mobility restrictions (bedrest, traction, casts, Stryker frame, Circoelectric bed)

Situational (personal, environmental)

Social isolation (terminal or infectious patient)
Pain
Stress
Environment (noise pollution, ICU)

Focus Assessment Criteria

Subjective Data

1. History of symptoms
     The person reports
       Difficulty concentrating   Fatigue or irritability
       Anxiety   Unusual sensations
     Onset and description
       Precipitated by?   Frequency?
       Relieved by?
2. Assess for presence or history of
     Recent surgery   Change in biorhythm pattern
     Recent hospitalization   Mobility restrictions
     Neurological impairment   Social isolation
     Sensorry organ deficit   Substance abuse (drugs, alcohol)

Objective Data

1. Assess sensory acuity
   Visual
   > Snellen chart
   > Newspaper clippings and large lettered index cards
   > Aids (contact lenses, glasses)

   Auditory
   > Observation of client during normal conversation
   > Use of hearing aids

   Tactile
   > Thermal sensation
   > Sensitivity

   Olfactory/gustatory
2. Assess for the presence of factors that contribute to sensory-perceptual alterations
   > Sensory deprivation (isolation, lack of visitors)
   > Sensory overload (noise, personnel)
   > Physiological alterations
   > Medication (side-effects, toxic levels)
   > Sleep deprivation
   > Fluid, electrolyte, nutritional imbalances
   > Crisis, fears, losses

Principles and Rationale for Nursing Care

1. Receiving (reception) and accurately interpreting (perception) incoming stimuli from the environment are essential for survival.
2. People receive information via their five senses. Deficits in one or more senses can alter perception.
3. The five senses can be organized into close (olfactory, gustatory, and tactile) and distant (auditory and visual). When an individual is deprived of a distant sense, he becomes more dependent on the close senses. A blind person will develop a keener sense of touch than a sighted person.
4. Individuals adapt to the stimuli from their internal and external environments. The capacity for this adaptation varies with individuals and also varies at times in the same individual.
5. A disruption in the quality or quantity of incoming stimuli can affect an individual's physiological, emotional, cognitive, and affective domains.
6. Manifestations of sensory deprivation vary with an individual's adaptation ability. Some common manifestations are generalized anxiety, perceptual distortions, inability to think and reason, distortion of time sense, vivid imagery, and illusions and hallucinations.
7. The quality and quantity of sensory input are reduced by immobility or confinement.
8. The elderly are more prone to develop sensory deprivation due to loneliness, physical isolation, and the increased incidence of chronic disabilities experienced during this life stage.
9. An illness state may decrease the efficiency of the sensory organs and thus alter an organism's capacity for adequate reception and perception of information.
10. Sensory overload produces the problem of sensory bombardment and also blocks out meaningful stimuli, thus concurrently producing sensory deprivation.
11. Refer to Principles and Rationale for Nursing Care for *Altered Thought Processes* for additional information.

Sensory–Perceptual Alterations
Related to Sensory Overload

Assessment

Subjective Data

The person reports
Visual imagery
Nightmares
Difficulty concentrating
Color perception changes
Alteration in the size and contour of objects
Hallucinations

Objective Data

(Occurs in an environment with excessive stimuli)
Mood alterations
Sleep pattern disturbances
Poor appetite
Evidence of lack of self-care
Delusions

Outcome Criteria

The person will
- Demonstrate decreased symptoms of sensory overload as evident by (specify)
- Identify and eliminate the potential risk factors if possible
- Describe the rationale for the treatment modality

Interventions

A. Assess causative and contributing factors

Altered sleep and rest pattern (refer to *Sleep Pattern Disturbance*)
Pain (refer to *Altered Comfort*)
Excessive noise or light
Critical care unit activity
Health care facility routines
Unfamiliar environment (different culture of language)

B. Reduce or eliminate causative and contributing factors where possible

1. Excessive noise or light
   - Cover nonessential blinking lights at bedside with tape
   - Dim lights at night
   - Encourage use of blindfolds
   - Decrease noise output

   a. Shut off nonessential alarms
   b. Encourage use of earplugs
   c. If possible, limit the use of flasher, etc., during sleep hours
   d. Turn off unnecessary equipment
   e. Position person away from direct source of noise if possible
   f. Curtail nonessential personnel conversation
   g. Avoid loud noises
   h. Discourage television after 10 P.M.
  • Share with person the source of the noise
  • Discuss the use of a radio with earplugs to provide soft, relaxing music
  • Share with personnel the need to reduce noise and provide individuals with uninterrupted sleep for at least 2 to 4 hours' duration
 2. Unfamiliar environment
  • Attempt to reduce fears and concerns by explaining equipment, its purpose and noises
  • Encourage person to share his perceptions of noises
  • Enlist the aid of an interpreter to explain the environment to person who does not speak English

C. Promote reorientation
 1. Orient to all three spheres (person, place, time)
  • Address person by name
  • Introduce yourself frequently
  • Identify the place
  • Identify the time
     "Good morning Mr. Jones. I am Mary Smith. I will be your nurse today."
     "Where are you Mr. Jones? You are in the hospital."
     "Today is May sixth and it is eight thirty in the morning."
 2. Explain all activities
  • Offer simple explanations of each task
  • Allow person to handle equipment related to the task
  • Allow him to participate in task, such as washing his face
  • Acknowledge when you leave and when you will return

D. Promote movement
 • Encourage person to remain out of bed as much as possible (eat meals in chair)
 • Teach person to perform isometric and isotonic exercises when in bed
 • Encourage person to change his position frequently, even if it is just lifting one side off a surface by rolling slightly
 • To encourage walking, choose a destination to reach or give the walk a purpose (walking to the lounge for breakfast)

E. Utilize measures to prevent injury
 • Keep side rails in place and bed in lowest position
 • Place call bell in convenient location
 • Refer to *Potential for Injury* for additional interventions

F. Assist person to differentiate reality from fantasy
 • Refer to *Altered Thought Processes Related to Inability to Evaluate Reality* for additional interventions

References/Bibliography

Bolin RH: Sensory deprivation: An overview. Nurs Forum 13(3):240–258, 1974

Burnside I: Nursing and the Aged. New York, McGraw-Hill, 1981

Chodil J, Williams B: The concept of sensory deprivation. Nurs Clin North Am 5(3):453–465, 1970

Dodd MJ: Assessing mental states. Am J Nurs 78:1501–1503, 1978

Downs F: Bed rest and sensory deprivation. Am J Nurs 74:434–438, 1974

Drummond LK, Scarbrough D: A practical guide to reality orientation: A treatment approach for confusion and disorientation. Gerontologist 18(12):568–573, 1978

Gimbel P: The pathology of boredom and sensory deprivation. Psychiatric Nursing 16(5):12–13, 1975

Kintzel KC: Advanced Concepts in Clinical Nursing, 2nd ed. Philadelphia, JB Lippincott, 1977

Murray R, Huelskoetter M, O'Driscoll D: The Nursing Process in Later Maturity. Englewood Cliffs, NJ, Prentice-Hall, 1980

Nowakowski L: Disorientation—signal or diagnosis? Journal of Gerontological Nursing 6(4):197–202, 1980

Schultz P: Sensory Restriction: Effects on Behavior. New York, Academic Press, 1965

Severtsen B: Sensory impairment: Its effects on the family. In Hymovich D, Barnard M (eds): Family Health Care, pp 293–304. New york, McGraw-Hill, 1979

Shelby S: Sensory deprivation. Image 10(2):49–55, 1978

Solomon L: Sensory Deprivation. Cambridge, MA, Harvard University Press, 1961

Trockman G: Caring for the confused or delirious patient. Am J Nurs 78:1495–1499, 1978

Wyness MA: Perceptual dysfunction: Nursing assessment and management. J Neurosci Nurs 17(2):105–110, 1985

Zubek S: Sensory Deprivation: Fifteen Years of Research. New York, Appleton-Century-Crofts, 1969

Sexuality Patterns, Altered

Sexual Dysfunction

> **Author's Note:** *Altered Sexuality Patterns* is a broad diagnostic category that encompasses sexual identity, sexuality, and sexual function. *Sexual Dysfunction* describes dissatisfaction with sexual function.
>
> Sexual health is the integration of somatic, emotional, intellectual and social aspects of sexual being in ways that are enriching and that enhance personality, communication, and love (World Health Organization).

Sexuality Patterns, Altered

Related to **Ineffective Coping**

Related to **Change or Loss of Body Part**

Related to **Prenatal and Postpartum Changes**

Definition

Altered sexuality patterns: The state in which an individual experiences or is at risk of experiencing a change in sexual health.

Defining Characteristics

Major (must be present)
Identification of sexual difficulties, limitations, or changes

Etiological, Contributing, Risk Factors
An alteration in sexual patterns can occur as a response to a variety of health problems, situations, and conflicts. Some common sources are indicated below.

Pathophysiological
Endocrine
    Diabetes mellitus
    Decreased hormone production
    Myxedema
    Hyperthyroidism
    Addison's disease
    Acromegaly
Genitourinary
    Chronic renal failure
    Premature or retarded ejaculation
    Priapism
    Chronic vaginal infection
    Decreased vaginal lubrication
    Vaginismus
    Altered structures
    Venereal disease
Neuromuscular and skeletal
    Arthritis
    Multiple sclerosis
    Amyotrophic lateral sclerosis
    Disturbances of nerve supply to brain, spinal cord, sensory nerves, and autonomic nerves
Cardiorespiratory
    Myocardial infarction
    Congestive heart failure
    Peripheral vascular disorders
    Chronic respiratory disorders
Cancer
Liver disease

Treatment-related
Medications
Radiation treatment
Altered self-concept from change in appearance (trauma, radical surgery)

Situational (personal, environmental)
Partner
    Unwilling
    Uninformed
    Abusive
    Not available
    Separated
    Divorced
Environment
    Unfamiliar
    No privacy
    Hospital
Stressors
    Job problems
    Financial worries
    Conflicting values
    Religious conflict
Lack of knowledge
Fatigue
Obesity
Pain
Alcohol ingestion

Drug abuse
Fear of failure (sexual)
Fear of pregnancy
Depression
Anxiety
Guilt
Fear of sexuality transmitted diseases

Maturational

Ineffective role models
Negative sexual teaching
Absence of sexual teaching
Aging (separation, isolation)

Focus Assessment Criteria

Guidelines in Taking a Sexual History

Take sexual history in a private, relaxed setting to ensure confidentiality
Do not judge the individual by your own norms
Permit the individual to refuse to answer
Clarify vocabulary
Strive to be open, warm, objective, unembarrassed, and reassuring
Assume the individual has had some form of sexual experience
Several interviews may be necessary to complete the history

Subjective Data

1. General
   Age, sex, marital status
   Quality of relationship with significant other
   Number of children and siblings
   Religious and cultural background
   Job and financial status
   Medical and surgical history
   Drug therapy (present and past—type, dosage, frequency)
2. Sexual knowledge and attitudes
   Source of sexual information
   Knowledge of anatomy and physiology
   Childhood sexual experiences (parental influence, religious influence, masturbation)
   Attitudes concerning sexual variations
   Myths and taboos
   Menstruation
   Birth control methods
3. Sexual function
   Usual pattern
   Present pattern
   Satisfaction (individual, partner)
   Erection problems for male (attaining, sustaining)
   Ejaculation problems for male (premature)
4. Sexual problem
   Description

Onset (when, gradual, sudden)

Pattern over time (increased, decreased, unchanged)

Person's concept of cause

Knowledge of problem by others (physician, support system)

Past diagnostic studies and treatments

Expectations

5. School-aged child*

Knowledge

"What is the difference between boys and girls?"

"What do you know about having babies?"

"Who taught you? At what age?"

Body changes

"Is your body changing in any way? How? Why?"

"How do you feel about these changes?"

Masturbation

"Almost everyone touches their body; how do you feel about this?"

6. Adolescent

Knowledge and attitudes

"What were your parent's attitudes toward sex, nudity, and touching?"

"Were these subjects discussed in your home?"

"How are babies made?"

"What are some methods of birth control?"

Body changes

"Is your body changing in any way? How? Why?"

"How do you feel about these changes?"

Sexual activity

"Some young people are sexually active; how do you feel about that?"

Principles and Rationale for Nursing Care

General

1. All humans are sexual beings. Sexuality is an integral part of one's identity.
2. Sexuality encompasses how one feels about oneself and how one interacts with others. Sexual function is the choice an individual makes in the manner or form of how he or she will express sexuality. Sexuality and sexual function are influenced by age, marital status, value system, knowledge, sexual patterns, resources (social, economic, geographic), culture, physical health, and emotional health.
3. Sexual health care is often given low priority by nurses. In promoting sexual health the nurse generalist can:

Utilize the PLISSIT model for treatment of sexual problems. The nurse is encouraged to intervene at the level at which she or he is comfortable and knowledgeable (Annon)

Permission—convey to client and significant others that you are willing to discuss sexual thoughts and feelings

(e.g., "Have you experienced or do you expect to experience a problem with sexual function because of your condition?")

Limited Information—provide client/significant others with information regarding the effects certain situations (pregnancy), conditions (cancer), and treatments (medications), have or can have on sexuality and sexual function

---

* Data that relate to children or adolescents may be more appropriately labeled *Disturbance in Self-Concept or Altered Health Maintenance related to Lack of Knowledge of Sexuality*

Specific Suggestions—provide specific instructions that can facilitate positive sexual functioning (*e.g.,* coital positions for women with arthritis)

Intensive Therapy—these interventions are referrals to nurses with advanced knowledge of sex therapy or to therapists; if surgical interventions are indicated, selected referrals are initiated (*e.g.,* penile implants)

4. If nurses utilized the first three levels of interventions of the PLISSIT model, 70% of clients would receive the counseling they need. The remaining 30% would need referral to a therapist specializing in sexual counseling (Shipes and Lehr).

5. The characteristics of a sexually healthy person are (Lion):
   • A positive body image despite the body's packaging (as opposed to the Madison-Avenue attitude)
   • Acceptance of sexual and body functions as normal and natural
   • Valid knowledge about human sexuality and sexual functioning
   • Recognition and acceptance of own sexual feelings
   • Effective interpersonal relationships (respect for self and others)
   • Acceptance of mistakes in self and others

6. The nurse must educate herself regarding sexuality and sexual health through the life span. She must examine her own beliefs and feelings regarding sexuality and sexual function and what is considered to be sexually normal and abnormal.

7. Sexuality and sexual function are not restricted solely to the young and healthy.

8. Sexual gratification is an individual matter. It encompasses self-pleasure and giving pleasure to others.

9. Sexual expression is not limited to intercourse. It includes closeness, touching, and one's approach to others.

10. Satisfaction and gratification can be experienced from responses to interactions other than sexual organ interaction.

11. Sexual preferences are an individual matter. Homosexuality is not a diagnosis unless the person sees it as a problem. In such a situation another nursing diagnosis might be more appropriate; for example, *Self-Concept Disturbance.*

12. Sexual expression is essential for complete well-being and should be nutured in all age groups.

13. Masturbation can be a necessary outlet for sexual release.

14. Individuals must have the opportunity to make their own decisions regarding sexual function.

15. Individuals decide what is normal for them. Mutually satisfying acts between consenting adults are considered normal.

16. Male sexual function can be negatively influenced by physiological factors that interfere with:
   Circulation (leukemia, diabetes mellitus)
   Oxygen transport (cardiac, respiratory)
   Neurotransmission (prostatectomy)
   CNS function (CVA)

17. Female sexual function can be negatively influenced by physiological factors that interfere with:
   Lubrication (aging, radiation)
   Assuming position for coitus (arthritis, MS)

18. As stress increases, there is a negative influence on sexual performances that conversely increases stress.

19. Sexual options available to the cord-injured person are influenced (Woods) by sexual value system, previous sexual function, upper-extremity muscle strength, presence

of hip flexors and extensors, presence of appliances (casts, catheters) and availability of a caring partner.

20. Cord injuries do not usually affect fertility. Paraplegic females can become pregnant and deliver vaginally.

Cancer and Sexuality

Factors that contribute to alterations in sexuality and sexual function in cancer clients are:

1. The contrast between perceptions of cancer (fear of death, disfigurement) and sexuality (vitality, beauty)
2. Uncertainty about the future leads to insecurity and regression; free expression and spontaneity may be hindered
3. The role changes or reversals that may occur (*e.g.,* when the female cannot continue housekeeping functions or the primary supporter cannot work); sexually defined gender roles can be disrupted
4. Social isolation may result from fears of family and friends
5. The disease process and/or the treatments (chemotherapy, radiotherapy, immunotherapy, surgical interventions) can impose pain, fatigue, separation, and economic difficulties
6. Surgical intervention and drug therapy can interfere physiologically with sexual function (*i.e.,* abdominal–perineal resection, narcotics)

Pregnancy and Sexuality

1. Barring complications, a pregnant woman is free to engage in sexual activity with her partner to the extent that it is comfortable and desired
2. Pregnant women have varying degrees of sexual desire during pregnancy
   a. Some women are very sexually excitable
   b. Some women are not very desirous of sex
   c. Libido changes by large degrees during different stages of pregnancy
   d. A woman's body image affects her sexuality (If thinness is an attribute, then many pregnant women are confused about changing size)
   e. A woman's attitude toward her body can influence her partner's sexual attraction toward her
3. Pregnancy is a time of stress for both man and woman; to deny physical closeness at a time when both partners are struggling can add to tension and alienation
4. The postpartum period is a time of self-doubt. For the first 6 weeks, a new mother feels lost, overwhelmed, tired, depressed, ignorant, and isolated. Her self-esteem as well as her sexuality may suffer
5. A high number of divorced persons relate marital difficulties beginning during pregnancy or shortly after the arrival of their first child

Aging and Sexuality

1. Aging influences sexual anatomy and physiology, but the elderly person is physically able to engage in sexual activity.
2. Decreased levels of hormones influence tissue elasticity. Females have decreased tone in breasts, thinning and loss of elasticity of the vaginal wall, and shortening of its length. Males experience decreased production of spermatozoa, decreased ejaculation force, and smaller, less firm testicles.
3. The need for intimacy and love may be more critical for the elderly who are experiencing diminishing meaningful relationships.

4. Past sexual function (enjoyment, interest, frequency) are predicators of sexual activity for the aging.

Drugs and Sexuality

1. Drugs can influence sexual function positively and negatively. Table II-16 illustrates their effects.

Altered Sexuality Patterns
Related to Ineffective Coping

Ineffective coping (associated with sexual dysfunction) is the difficulty or inability to adapt to stressors or changes in the life-style that negatively influence sexual function.

Assessment

Subjective Data

The person reports
Multiple stressors that are accompanied by altered sexual function

Job-related stress	Death of partner or significant
Financial worries	other
Relocation	Job change
Divorce	Disability of spouse
Separation from partner	

Feelings

Depression	Frustration
Anxiety	Impaired or absent libido
Severe fatigue	

Outcome Criteria

The person will
- Identify stressors in life
- Identify constructive coping patterns
- Resume previous sexual activity

Interventions

A. Assess for causative factors

Job change or problems
Financial worries
Relocation
Divorce or separation from partner
Death of significant other

Table II-16. **Drugs That Alter Sexual Behavior**

Drug	Probable Effects
Antihypertensives Guanethidine (Ismelin) Reserpine (Serpasil) Mecamylamine (Inversine) Trimetaphan (Arfonad) Spironolactone (Aldactone) Methyldopa (Aldomet) Phenoxybenzamine (Dibenzyline) Clonidine (Catapres) Propranolol (Inderal) Pargyline (Eutonyl) Captopril (Capoten)	Produce vasodilation and decreased cardiac output; depress CNS Cause impotence in men and decreased vaginal lubrication in women
Antidepressants Imipramine (Tofranil) Desipramine (Norpramin, Pertofrane) Amitryptyline (Elavil) Maprotilene (Ludiomil) Doxepin (Sinequan) Trazodone (Desyrel) Nortriptyline (Aventyl) Protriptyline (Vivactil) Phenelzine sulfate (Nardil) Tranylcypromine sulfate (Parnate)	Peripheral blockage of nervous innervation of sex glands May have positive effect, since they decrease depression
Antihistamines Diphenhydramine (Benadryl) Promethazine (Phenergan) Chlorpheniramine (Chlor-Trimeton)	Block parasympathetic nervous innervation of sex glands
Antispasmodics/Anticholinergics Methantheline (Banthine) Glycopyrrolate (Robinul) Hexocyclium (Tral) Poldine (Nacton) Diphenoxylate hydrochloride with atropine (Lomotil)	Inhibit parasympathetic innervation of sex glands
Sedatives and Tranquilizers Chlorpromazine (Thorazine) Prochlorperazine (Compazine) Thioridazine (Mellaril) Mesoridazine (Serentil) Chlordiazepoxide (Librium) Diazepam (Valium) Phenoxybenzamine (Dibenzyline) Chlorprothixene (Taractan) Haloperidol (Haldol) Oxazepam (Serax) Fluphenazine (Prolixin)	Block autonomic innervation of sex glands May have positive effect because they produce tranquilization and relaxation May have negative effect influencing libido

(continued)

Table II-16.   **Drugs That Alter Sexual Behavior** *(continued)*

Drug	*Probable Effects*
Oral Contraceptives	Remove fear of pregnancy
Alcohol	In small amounts, may increase libido
	In large amounts, impairs neural reflexes involved in erection and ejaculation
	Chronic use may cause impotence
Narcotics	Central sedation causes impotence in chronic users
Cancer chemotherapy agents	Possible temporary sterility or neurotoxicity in males, causing impotence
Estrogen	Suppresses sexual function in males
Diuretics	Chronic use may cause impotence
Ethacrynic acid (Edecrin)	
Furosemide (Lasix)	

Severe fatigue
Depression
Disability of spouse

B. Assist person in modifying life-style to reduce stress
   • Encourage identification of present stressors in life; group as those he can control and those he cannot

Can Control	*Cannot Control*
Personal lateness	Report due
Involvement in community activities	Daughter's illness

   • Assist in analyzing the problem
        What is it?
        Who or what is responsible?
        What are the options?
        What are the advantages and disadvantages of each option?

C. Identify alternative methods for dispersing sexual energy when partner is unavailable or unwilling
   • Utilize masturbation, if acceptable to individual
   • Teach the physical and psychological benefits of regular physical activity (at least 3 times a week for 30 minutes)—yoga, walking or running, exercise (aerobics, dance) (see *Altered Health Maintenance,* for an exercise program)
   • If partner is deceased, explore opportunities to meet and socialize with others (night school, singles club, community work)
   • See Appendix VII for problem-solving techniques

D. Initiate health teaching and referrals as indicated
     Marriage counselor
     Psychiatrist or psychologist

Sex therapist
Social service (for assistance with job, financial, housing, or family problems)

Altered Sexuality Patterns
Related to Change or Loss of Body Part

Assessment

Subjective Data
The person reports
    An altered sexual function
    Feelings of undesirability
    Partner unwilling to look at affected part
    Partner's change in usual responses (social, sexual)

Objective Data
    Withdrawn behavior
    Depression
    Unwillingness to acknowledge loss
    Unwillingness to look at affected area

Outcome Criteria

The person will
- Discuss the loss or change in body part
- Report on desire to resume sexual activity

Interventions

A. Assess causative or contributing factors
Anatomic disruptions from surgery (mastectomy, hysterectomy, uterostomal surgery, prostatectomy, amputation)
Pregnancy
Obesity
Trauma (burns, scarring)
Chronic disease

B. Assess individual's self-esteem (Howard-Ruben)
See also *Self-Esteem Disturbance* and *Body Image Disturbance*
    Functional ability
        What can he (she) do?
    Appearance
        How does one perceive his/her looks?

Interpersonal
Who are the social and intimate relations?
Achievement
What achievements have been accomplished at work, school, etc.?
Identification
What spiritual, ethical, social, cultural, or moral influences are in one's life?

C. Assess the stage of adaptation of the individual and his partner to the loss (denial, depression, anger, resolution; see *Grieving*)

D. Encourage individuals to share concerns
- Explain the normalcy of the foregoing responses to loss
- Explain the need to share concerns with partner
    The imagined response of partner
    The fear of rejection
    Fear of future losses
    Fear of physically hurting partner
- Maintain modesty and privacy
- Help individual realize that his body changes are acceptable by spending time with him
- Encourage the couple to discuss the strengths of their relationship and to assess the influence of the loss on their strengths

E. Encourage person to resume sexual activity as close to previous pattern as possible
- Suggest that intercourse be resumed as soon as possible
- Advise modifying positions because of alteration
- Teach the use of pillows to provide comfort (mastectomy, amputation)
- Caution the person against covering the affected body part (delays confronting the actual or perceived fear)
- Teach techniques to control drainage or odor prior to sexual activity (change colostomy bag or dressing; utilize a light scent such as aftershave or perfume)
- Encourage the individual or couple to read about various sexual techniques and responses (see Bibliography)
- Encourage individuals to experiment and enjoy each other

F. Initiate health teaching and referrals as indicated; discuss with individuals or couples the availability of self-help groups
Reach for Recovery (post-mastectomy)
Encore program (post-mastectomy)
United Ostomy Association

Altered Sexuality Patterns
Related to Prenatal and Postpartum Changes

Assessment

Subjective Data
The person reports
> Altered sexual function
> Feelings of undesirability
> Partner's change in usual sexual and social responses

Outcome Criteria

The person will
- Share concerns
- Express increased satisfaction with sexual patterns

Interventions

A. Assess the sexual patterns during and after pregnancy (Reeder)

> How does the pregnancy make you feel? (asked of both partners)
> How do you feel about changes in appearance?
> How do you feel about changes in emotions?
> How do you feel about one another's experience of the pregnancy?
> What are your feelings about sex during pregnancy?
> Has the pregnancy made many changes in your life and sexual relationship?
> What have you heard about what you should or should not do sexually during pregnancy?
> Have you experienced any physical difficulties with intercourse during pregnancy?
> Are there any concerns or worries about your sexual relationship during pregnancy or afterwards?
> How do you think having a baby will change your life? How do you plan to manage these changes?
> How do you feel physically?
> What medications do you take?
> Have you had any recent changes in your health?

Postpartum

> Have you resumed sexual activity?
> Are you concerned about conceiving again?
> Has breast-feeding altered your sexual relationship?
> How has the baby affected your sexuality?
> Is your episiotomy healed and comfortable during intercourse?
> Have you experienced a lack of lubrication since delivery?

B. Assess contributing factors

1. Body changes

2. Change in sex drive
3. Fatigue
4. Emotional lability
   a. Anxieties about taking on parental responsibilities
   b. Grief from separating from childhood
   c. Anxiety about outcome of pregnancy
   d. Ambivalence about having a baby
   e. Guilt about desiring sex when pregnancy has been achieved (religious, social pressure)
   f. Fear of dependency
   g. Fear of loss of current status (career, freedom)
   h. Self-doubt
5. Fear of damaging fetus
6. Dyspareunia in pregnancy
7. Dyspareunia in postpartum
8. Guilt due to baby
   Afraid to let go and enjoy sex lest something happen to baby
9. Influence of others
   Relatives (mother, in-laws)
      Attitudes related to pregnancy and child care
   Partner
      Intrusion on time together
   Baby
      Intrusion on time (nursing, care)
10. Fear of pregnancy
11. Breast-feeding (see *Ineffective Breast-feeding*)

C. Reduce or eliminate contributing factors

1. Body changes
   • Provide literature or suggested reading list for person to read to establish knowledge of normalcy of pregnancy and changes
   • Refer to community resources
   • Early pregnancy classes
   • Childbirth preparation classes
   • Suggest alternative sexual positions for later pregnancy
      Side-lying
      Positions for vaginal entry
         Woman kneeling
         Woman standing
         Woman on hands and knees
         Woman on top
   • Postpartum changes
      Provide literature
      Give reassurance about these changes
         Episiotomy
         Lubrication
         Uterine resolution
         Flabby abdominal musculature
         Breast engorgement
      Reassure that this is a temporary state and will resolve in 2 to 3 months
      Refer to postpartum exercise class

2. Change in sex drive
   - Reassure that sexual attitudes change throughout pregnancy from feeling very desirous of sex to wanting only to be cuddled. Support acceptance of whatever pleasuring may be desired. Encourage flexibility and alternative sexual patterns (*e.g.,* oral sex, mutual masturbation, fondling, stroking, massage, vibrators)
3. Fatigue
   - Acknowledge this as factor especially during first trimester and again during last month
   - Can be a major contributor to postpartum sexual problem
   - Encourage patient to make time for her relationship, in sexual as well as other contexts
   - Ask for help
   - Hire sitter, etc.
4. Emotional lability
   Encourage woman and/or partner to discuss emotions
   Listen—allow time for person to elaborate on feelings
   Reassure that these feelings are normal
   Refer to reading material
   Refer to other pregnant couples for verification
   Relate your own experiences, if appropriate
5. Fear of damaging fetus
   Reassure that unless problems exist (preterm labor, previous early loss, bleeding or rupture of membrane) intercourse is allowed until labor begins
   Refer to physician for reassurance
   Explore misinformation. Use anatomical charts to show protection of baby in uterus
   Inform that orgasm causes contractions that are not harmful and will subside
6. Dyspareunia in pregnancy
   Explore what pain is experienced and when
   Suggest alternative positions
      Woman on top
      Side-lying
      Posterior–vaginal entry
   Suggest use of water-soluble lubricant
   Refer to physician if pain continues
7. Postpartum issues
   Dyspareunia in postpartum
   - Explore what pain is experienced and under what circumstances
   - Assess healing of episiotomy
   - Suggest varied positions
   - Suggest use of water-soluble lubricant (nursing women report reduced vaginal lubrication during entire nursing experience)
   - Teach person to identify her pelvic floor muscles and strengthen them with exercise
      a. "For posterior pelvic floor muscles, imagine you are trying to stop the passage of stool and tighten your anus muscles without tightening your legs or your abdominal muscles"
      b. "For anterior pelvic floor muscles, imagine you are trying to stop the passage of urine, tighten the muscles (back and front) for four seconds, and then release them; repeat ten times, four times a day" (can be increased to four times an hour if indicated)

- Instruct person to stop and start the urinary stream several times during voiding
- Refer to physician if pain continues

8. Guilt due to baby

Encourage discussion; reassure that these feelings are normal; allow time to elaborate

Expression of these feelings will often create a release and relaxation

Include partner in discussion (both may have similar feelings they have not felt free to express to one another)

Refer to postpartum support groups

Refer to psychological or social assistance if pathology is observed

9. Influence of others

Encourage discussion of mother/woman relationship

Does woman see her mother as a sexual being?

Does she now feel confused about her roles as mother vs. sex partner?

Reassure that identity confusion is common

Refer to postpartum discussion groups

Allow to express feelings concerning changes in life

Refer to postpartum support group

Include partner in discussion (perhaps at a later time)—let both parties talk about adjustment and pressures that interfere with relating sexually and otherwise

10. Fear of pregnancy

Encourage discussion

Explore contraceptive choices

Refer to nurse practitioner or gynecologist for contraception

Inform patient that breast-feeding does not provide effective contraception

Pre-pregnancy contraceptive devices may no longer fit

Oral contraceptives are contraindicated while nursing

D. Initiate health teaching and referrals

1. Teach couples to abstain from intercourse and seek the advise of their health care provider if any of the following situations are present (Zlatnik):
   - Vaginal bleeding
   - Premature dilation
   - Multiple pregnancy
   - Engaged fetal head or lightening
   - Placenta previa
   - Rupture of membranes
   - History of premature delivery
   - History of miscarriage
2. Refer to suggested references for printed material
3. Refer to counselor if resolution is not achieved

Sexual Dysfunction

Related to **Unknown Etiology as Manifested by Erectile Problems**
Related to **Physiological Limitations**

Definition

Sexual dysfunction: The state in which an individual experiences or is at risk of experiencing a change in sexual function that is viewed as unrewarding or inadequate.

Defining Characteristics

Major

Verbalization of problem with sexual function
Reports limitations on sexual performance imposed by disease or therapy

Minor

Fears future limitations on sexual performance
Misinformed about sexuality
Lacks knowledge about sexuality and sexual function
Value conflicts involving sexual expression (cultural, religious)
Altered relationship with significant other
Dissatisfaction with sex role (perceived or actual)

Etiological, Contributing, Risk Factors

See *Altered Sexuality Patterns*

Focus Assessment Criteria

See *Altered Sexuality Patterns*

Sexual Dysfunction
Related to Unknown Etiology
as Manifested by Erectile Problems

Erectile dysfunction is the inability to achieve or sustain an erection for satisfying intercourse.

Assessment

Subjective Data
The person states he is unable to have or sustain an erection

Objective Data
Monitoring of nocturnal penile tumescence to determine if erection occurs during REM sleep

---

Outcome Criteria

The person will
- Relate a return to satisfying sexual relationships

Interventions

A. Assess causative or contributing factors

Degenerative physiological factors
　　Neurological (diabetes mellitus, multiple sclerosis)
　　Circulatory (severe anemia, arteriosclerosis)
Trauma (surgical injury)
　　Spinal cord injury or lesion
　　Prostatectomy
　　Arteriofemoral bypass
　　Sympathectomy
　　Abdominal-perineal resection
Chemical influences
　　Alcohol
　　Drugs (see Table II-16)
Psychogenic influences
　　Almost any stressor

B. Discuss with individual and significant other the varied etiologies of temporary impotence

- Convey the normalcy of the situation
- Relate the interrelationship of stress and the ability to perform sexually
- Review with individual any changes that may have occurred in his life (*e.g.*, financial, career, significant other, health)
- Assist with constructive problem-solving (see Appendix VII)
- Identify stress reduction techniques that can be incorporated into his life (see Appendix X)
- Assist individual or couple to examine their relationships
　　What are the benefits of the relationship?
　　How can each person improve the relationship?
　　How does the couple handle conflicts?
- Refer individuals or couples to professional counseling when indicated
- See *Sexual Dysfunction Related to Ineffective Coping* for additional interventions

C. Facilitate or enhance sexual expression in individuals with irreversible impotence
- Explain the cause of the impotence, if known
- Discuss alternate means for sexual satisfaction for self and partner (vibrator, touching, oral–genital techniques, body massage); consider past sexual experiences prior to giving specific techniques
- Refer to pertinent literature in bibliography for specific information
- Explain penile implants, function, limitations, surgical procedure, and cost
- Refer to a urologist for further details

D. Initiate health teaching and referrals when appropriate (sex therapy, psychotherapy)

Sexual Dysfunction
Related to Physiological Limitations

Assessment

Subjective Data
The person reports the following as interfering with sexual function

Chest pain	Fatigue
Shortness of breath	Decreased vaginal secretions
Joint pain	Paralysis

Objective Data
Dyspnea
Joint deformities
Paralysis

Outcome Criteria

The person will
- Identify practices that conserve energy and oxygen requirements during sexual activity
- Describe the rationale for interventions
- Report sexual activity that is satisfying

Interventions

A. Assess causative or contributing factors
Limited oxygen reserve

Decreased cardiac output
Pain
Inability to assume positions
Inability to experience sensations at genitourinary level

B. Teach techniques to

1. Reduce oxygen consumption
   - Do not lie flat
   - Use oxygen during sexual activity if indicated
   - Engage in sexual activity after IPPB treatment or postural drainage
   - Plan sexual activities for time of day person is most rested
   - Utilize positions for intercourse that are comfortable and permit unrestricted breathing (side to side; compromised individual on top)
2. Reduce cardiac workload
   - Cardiac patients should avoid sexual activity
       In extremes of temperature
       Directly after eating or drinking
       When intoxicated
       When tired
       With unfamiliar partner (when other stressors are present, *e.g.*, alcohol, fatigue)
   - Rest before engaging in sexual activity (mornings are best)
   - Cardiac patients should terminate sexual activity if chest discomfort or dyspnea occurs
3. Reduce or eliminate pain
   - If vaginal lubrication is decreased, use a water-soluble lubricant
   - Refer person with vaginismus to gynecologist
   - Take medication for pain before beginning sexual activity
   - Use whatever relaxes individual before beginning sexual activity (hot packs, hot showers)
4. Teach techniques for intercourse for individuals with specific alterations
   a. Inability to abduct hip joints (woman)
      - Posterior vaginal entry
      - Woman supine with hips abducted and pillow under thigh and knee
      - Woman supine with knees flexed
      - Woman kneeling with posterior vaginal entry by partner
      - Woman standing with posterior vaginal entry by partner
   b. Spinal cord injury
      - Consider that the sexual options available are dependent on the values and extent of injury
      - Modify positions if necessary (quadriplegic, partner on top; paraplegic can assume most positions)
      - If partner must initiate all pelvic thrusting then partner must assume the top position
      - Water beds amplify pelvic movements
      - Individuals with chronic urinary tract infections should be taught to wash well and empty the bladder completely before sexual activity to prevent infecting partner
      - Individuals with Foley catheters can lubricate with a water-soluble jelly and tape catheter to their penis or leg. It is, however, better to remove the catheter if possible

   c. Pregnant woman
      • Discuss the effects of stress, fatigue, and the other changes that pregnancy and motherhood bring on libido and sexual function
      • Allow her to verbalize her concerns and beliefs about pregnancy and coitus
      • Advise that coital positions may need to be varied according to the woman's contour (side-lying during 8th and 9th months)
      • Orgasms from intercourse or masturbation should be discouraged if spotting or bleeding occurs, fetal membranes rupture prematurely, or there is a repeated history of miscarriage
      • Vaginal discomfort during coitus can be reduced with the use of a water-soluble lubricant
      • Intercourse can usually be resumed after delivery when the woman is comfortable participating
5. Promote the stimulation of alternate senses and perceptions
   • The use of erotic material may help prepare the individual for sexual response
   • Encourage techniques to pleasure partner that provide satisfaction for individual (vibrators, touching, oral–genital intercourse, body massaging, anal stimulation)

C. Provide health teaching and referrals when indicated

   • Partner must be included in counseling and teaching to be aware of limitations
   • Encourage individual to consult others with similar alterations for an exchange of information
   • Refer individual and partner to pertinent literature and organizations (see Bibliography)

References/Bibliography

Adams G: The sexual history as an integral part of the patient history. Matern Child Nurs J 1(3):170–175, 1976
Annon JS: The PLISS + Model: A proposed conceptual scheme for the behavioral treatment of sexual problems. J Sex Educ Ther 2(1):211–215, 1976
Baxter R: Sex counseling and the spinal cord injured patient. Nursing 8(9):46–52, 1978
Calderone M, Johnson E: Family Book About Sexuality. New York, JB Lippincott, 1981
Carey P: Temporary sexual dysfunction in reversible health limitations. Nurs Clin North Am 10(3):575–585, 1975
Comfort A: Sexual Consequences of Disability. Philadelphia, GF Stickley, 1978
Comfort J, Comfort A: The Facts of Love, Living, Loving and Growing Up. New York, Crown Publishers, 1979
Cooley M, Yeomans A, Cobb S: Sexual reproductive issues for women with Hodgkin's disease, part II, Application of PLISSIT model, Cancer Nurs 9(5):248–255, 1986
Davies H: Sexual dysfunction in diabetes: Psychogenic and physiologic factors. Medical Aspects of Human Sexuality 12(3):48–53, 1978
Evans R, Halar EM, DiFreece AB et al: Multidisciplinary approach to sex education of spinal cord injured patients. Phys Ther 56(6):541–545, 1976
Falk G, Falk UA: Sexuality and the aged. Nursing Outlook 10(1):51–55, 1980
Hickman B: All about sex—despite dialysis. Am J Nurs 77:606–609, 1977
Hill L, Smith N: Self-Care Nursing, chap 15. Englewood Cliffs, NJ, Prentice-Hall, 1985
Hogan R: Human Sexuality: A Nursing Perspective. New York, Appleton-Century-Crofts, 1980
Howard-Ruben J: Sexual dysfunction related to disease process and treatment. In McNally J, Stair J, Somerville E (eds): Guidelines for Cancer Nursing Practice, p 268. Orlando, FL, Grune & Stratton, 1985
Kennerly S: What I learned about mastectomy. Am J Nurs 77:1430–1432, 1977

Kolodney RC, Masters WH, Johnson VE et al: Textbook of Human Sexuality for Nurses. Boston, Little, Brown, 1979

Krozy R: Becoming comfortable with sexual assessment. Am J Nurs 78(6):1036–1038, 1978

Lamb M, Woods N: Sexuality and the cancer patient, Cancer Nurs (4):137–144, 1981

Lion E: Human Sexuality in the Nursing Process. New York, John Wiley & Sons, 1982

Macrae I, Henderson M: Sexuality and irreversible health limitations. Nurs Clin North Am 10(3):587–597, 1975

Masters WH, Johnson VE: Human Sexual Inadequacy. Boston, Little, Brown, 1970

Masters WH, Johnson VE: The Pleasure Bond. Boston, Little, Brown, 1970

Mims FH, Sevenson M: A model to promote sexual health care. Nurs Outlook 26(2):121–125, 1978

Mooney T: Sexual Options for Paraplegics and Quadriplegics. Boston, Little, Brown, 1975

Muscari M: Obtaining the adolescent sexual history, Pediatr Nurs, 13(5):307–310, 1987

Peach E: Counseling sexually active very young adolescent girls. Matern Child Nurs J 5(3):191–195, 1980

Pettyjohn RD: Health care of the gay individual. Nurs Forum 17(4):367–371, 1979

Pogoncheff E: The gay patient—what not to do. RN 42(4):46–48, 1979

Schwarz-Appelbaum J, Dedrick J, Jusinius K et al: Nursing care plans: Sexuality and treatment of breast cancer. Oncol Nurs Forum 11(6):16–24, 1984

Shipes E, Lehr S, Sexuality and the male cancer patient. Cancer Nurs 5:375–381, 1982

Siemens S, Brandzel R: Sexuality: Nursing Assessment and Intervention. Philadelphia, JB Lippincott, 1982

Schiller P: The nurse's role as sex counselor. Nurs Care 10(7):10–13, 1977

Steinke E, Bergen B: Sexuality and aging. J Gerontol Nurs 12(6):6–10, 1986

Watts RJ: Sexuality and the middle-aged cardiac patient. Nurs Clin North Am 11(2):349–359, 1976

Wood R, Rose R: Penile implants for potency. Am J Nurs 78(2):229–231, 1978

Woods NF: Human Sexuality in Health and Illness, 2nd ed. St. Louis, CV Mosby, 1979

Zlatnik FJ, Burmeistey LF: Reported Sexual Behavior in Late Pregnancy. Selected Medicine, 27(3):627–632, 1982

Sex in Pregnancy and Postpartum

Bing E, Colman L: Making Love During Pregnancy. New York, Bantam Books, 1977

Brenner P, Greenberg M: The impact of pregnancy on marriage. Med Aspects Human Sexuality 2:15–22, 1977

Falicov CJ: Sexual adjustment during first pregnancy and postpartum. Am J Obstet Gynecol 117(7):991–1000, 1973

Friday N: My Mother Myself. New York, Dell, 1980

Masters W, Johnson V: Human Sexual Response. Boston, Little, Brown & Co, 1966

Perkins RP: Sexuality in pregnancy: What determines behavior? Obstet Gynecol 59(2):189–198, 1982

Reeder S, Mastroianni L, Martin L: Maternity Nursing, p 197. Philadelphia, JB Lippincott, 1983

SIECUS (Sex Information and Education Council of the U.S.): Sexual relations during pregnancy and the post-delivery period. Study Guide No. 6, 1974

Solberg DA, Butler J, Wagner NN: Sexual behavior in pregnancy. N Engl J Med 288(5):1098–1103, 1973

Tolor A, DiGrazia PV: Sexual attitudes and behavior patterns during and following pregnancy. Arch Sex Behav 5(6):539–551, 1976

Zalk SR: Psychosexual conflicts in expectant fathers. In Blum BL (ed): Psychological Aspects of Pregnancy, Birthing and Bonding, chap 11. Human Sciences Press, NY, 1980

Resources Literature for the Consumer

"Sex Can Help Arthritis" (pamphlet), available from the Arthritis Foundation (local chapters)

Sex and Spinal Cord Injured, Superintendent of Documents, U.S. Government Printing Office, Washington, DC 20402

Sex Information and Education Council of the United States, 80 Fifth Avenue, New York, NY 10011

Bibliographies for professionals and the general public (*e.g.*, aging, disabilities, children)

Planned Parenthood, Publications Section, 810 Seventh Avenue, New York, NY 10019

American Cancer Society, 77 Third Avenue, New York, 10017

American Fertility Society, 1608 14th Avenue South, Birmingham, AL 35205

National Clearinghouse for Family Planning Information, P.O. Box 2225, Rockville, MD 20852

United Ostomy Association, 1111 Wilshire Boulevard, Los Angeles, CA 90017

"Sex Education for Adolescents," American Library Association, Order Department, 50 East Huron Street, Chicago, IL 60611

Public Affairs Pamphlets, 381 Park Avenue South, New York, NY 10016 (many inexpensive pamphlets for parents; send for free catalog)

Sleep Pattern Disturbance

Related to **(Specify)**

Definition

Sleep pattern disturbance: The state in which the individual experiences or is at risk of experiencing a change in the quantity or quality of his rest pattern as related to his biological and emotional needs.

Defining Characteristics

Adults

Major (must be present)

Difficulty falling or remaining asleep

Minor (may be present)

Fatigue on awakening or during the day
Dozing during the day
Agitation
Mood alterations

Children

Sleep disturbances in children are frequently related to fear, enuresis, or inconsistent responses of parents to child's requests for changes in sleep rules, such as requests to stay up late.

Reluctance to retire
Frequent awakening during the night
Desire to sleep with parents

Etiological, Contributing, Risk Factors

Many factors in an individual's life can contribute to sleep pattern disturbances. Some common factors are listed below.

Pathophysiological

Impaired oxygen transport
Angina
Peripheral arteriosclerosis
Respiratory disorders
Circulatory disorders
Impaired elimination (bowel or bladder)
Diarrhea
Constipation
Incontinence
Retention
Dysuria
Frequency
Impaired metabolism
Hyperthyroidism
Gastric ulcers
Hepatic disorders

Treatment-related

Immobility (imposed by casts, traction)
Medications

Tranquilizers	Steroids
Sedatives	Soporifics
Hypnotics	MAO inhibitors
Antidepressants	Anesthetics
Antihypertensives	Barbiturates
Amphetamines	

Situational (personal, environmental)

Lack of exercise
Pain
Anxiety response
Pregnancy
Life-style disruptions

Occupational	Sexual
Emotional	Financial
Social	

Environmental changes

Hospitalization (noise, disturbing roommate, fear)	Travel

Focus Assessment Criteria

Subjective Data

1. History of symptoms
   Complaints of

Sleeplessness	Depression
Anxiety	Fear (nightmares, dark,
Irritability	maturational situations)

   Onset and duration
   Location
   Description

Precipitated by what?	Aggravated by what?
Relieved by what?	

2. Sleep requirements
   In order to establish the amount of sleep an individual needs, have him go to bed and sleep until he wakes in the morning (without an alarm clock). This should be done for a few days and the average of the total sleeping hours calculated— with the subtraction of 20 to 30 minutes, which is the time most people need to fall asleep.
3. Sleep patterns (present, past)
   Usual bedtime and arising time
   Difficulty in getting to sleep, staying asleep, awakening
   Reasons for difficulty
   Use of sleep aids or rituals

Warm bath	Pillows
Drink or food (milk, wine)	Position
Medications	Toy, book

   Naps (frequency, length)

Objective Data

Physical characteristics
   Drawn appearance (pale, dark circles under eyes, puffy eyes)
   Yawning
   Dozing during the day
   Decreased attention span

Principles and Rationale for Nursing Care

General

1. The average adult requires approximately 20 minutes to fall asleep.
2. The amount of sleep a person needs varies with life-style, health, and age.
3. The average amount of sleep needed according to age follows (William):

Age	Hours of Sleep
Newborn	10.5 to 23
6 months	12 to 16
Over 6 months to 4 years	12 to 13
5 to 13 years	7 to 8.5
13 to 21 years	7 to 8.75
Adults under 60	6 to 9
Adults over 60	7 to 8

4. The quality of sleep and the ability to fall asleep and remain asleep for a sufficient period are a direct measurement of the physiological, psychological, and spiritual health of the individual.
5. Age affects the amount of time spent in each stage of sleep as well as the amount of time one needs to engage in sleep in order to replenish body energies. The neonate spends the greatest amount of time sleeping, and spends the most time in REM sleep (see numbers 5 and 6 under *Physiological*).
6. Older adults require the same or slightly less sleep than younger adults but can experience a decreased intensity of sleep related to nighttime wakenings.
7. Moderate sleep deprivation can produce behaviors of withdrawal, depression, memory lapses, apathy, irritability, confusion, and even hallucinations.
8. Fear (of recurrent nightmares, the dark) may interfere with sleep or create a reluctance to go to sleep.
9. Depression usually influences sleep in the form of initial insomnia (difficulty getting to sleep). Depressed individuals may then increase their sleeping hours (daytime and nighttime).
10. The use of sedatives to induce sleep also inhibits other mental and physical activities (respiration, cognition, circulation, digestion, elimination).
11. Chronic insomnia and chronic use of hypnotics reflect ineffective individual coping and require intensive therapeutic interventions.
12. Use of hypnotics by the elderly is usually contraindicated because of decreased renal function, which increases the toxicity of the drug. If sedatives are required, antihistamines will provide the needed sedation with fewer adverse side-effects.
13. There is no evidence that naps decrease nighttime sleep. Some older persons may need naps to restore their energy (Hayter).

Children

1. Children need to understand nighttime and be assisted to prepare for it. Preparation for bedtime involves switching the child from activity to bedtime gradually. It is a time for calmness, reassurance, and closeness.

2. Sleep problems in older infants and preschool children are identified as difficulty getting to sleep, inadequate daytime sleep, and inadequate night sleep (Edgil).
3. Children should be helped to learn that their beds are safe places to be in.

Physiological

1. Sleep is a restorative and recuperative process that facilitates cellular growth and the repair of damaged and aging body tissues.
2. The sleep process is hypothesized to be dependent on the action of the reticular activating system. Impulses are transported to the reticular activating system where epinephrine is secreted. Brain stem activity is therefore increased. It is speculated that after a period of time the impulses become fatigued, decreasing their output, and sleep spreads throughout the body.
3. There are different levels of sleep at which the various body tissues relax and rejuvenate. Each level has its own structure and function.
   Stage I: The individual becomes very drowsy and his musculature relaxes
   Stage II: Progressive muscular relaxation occurs, with decreasing cerebral activity
   Stage III: Physiological alterations become evident—vital signs become depressed, gastrointestinal function accelerates to facilitate cellular metabolism, and venous dilation occurs to accelerate the exchange of cellular metabolites
   Stage IV: The individual is in a deep sleep pattern; body functions decrease to an extremely depressed level of functioning
4. The entire sleep cycle is completed in an interval of 70 to 100 minutes and repeats itself frequently during the course of the sleep pattern. During stages I and II the sleeper can be awakened by relevant stimuli, but in stages III and IV the stimuli must be louder and stronger to awaken the sleeper.
5. Sleep can be divided into two major kinds: rapid eye movement (REM) and nonrapid eye movement sleep.
6. REM is the active phase of the sleep cycle that appears at the end of stage I. This phase is characterized by increased irregular vital signs, penile erections, flaccid musculature, and the release of adrenal hormones. REM sleep occurs approximately four to five times a night and is essential to one's sense of well-being.
7. During sleep the basal metabolic rate and the volume of urine production is decreased, but the secretion of sweat and gastric juice is increased.

Pregnancy

1. Pregnant women require increased periods of sleep because of physical and emotional stressors.
2. Insomnia during pregnancy is influenced by conflicts and anxieties of pregnancy and impending motherhood, fetal activity, musculoskeletal discomforts, and abdominal pressure.

Sleep Pattern Disturbance
Related to (Specify)

Assessment

See Defining Characteristics

Outcome Criteria

The person will
- Describe factors that prevent or inhibit sleep
- Identify techniques to induce sleep
- Report an optimal balance of rest and activity

Interventions

Since a variety of factors can disrupt sleep patterns, the nurse should consult the index for specific interventions to reduce certain factors (*e.g.,* pain, anxiety, fear). The following suggests general interventions for promoting sleep and specific interventions for selected clinical situations.

A. Identify causative contributing factors

Pain (see *Altered Comfort*)
Fear (see *Fear*)
Stress or anxiety (see *Anxiety*)
Immobility or decreased activity
Pregnancy
Urinary frequency or incontinence (see *Altered Patterns of Urinary Elimination*)
Unfamiliar or noisy environment

B. Reduce or eliminate environmental distractions and sleep interruptions

1. Noise
   - Close door to room
   - Pull curtains
   - Unplug telephone
   - Provide soft music (*e.g.,* a radio with earplugs)
   - Eliminate 24-hour lighting
   - Provide night lights
   - Decrease the amount and kind of incoming stimuli (*e.g.,* staff conversations)
   - Cover blinking lights with tape
   - Reduce the volume of alarms and televisions
   - Place with compatible roommate if possible
2. Interruptions
   - Organize procedures to provide the fewest number of disturbances during sleep period (*e.g.,* when individual awakens for medication also administer treatments and obtain vital signs)
   - Avoid unnecessary procedures during sleep period
   - Limit visitors during optimal rest periods (*e.g.,* after meals)
   - If voiding during the night is disruptive, have person limit his nighttime fluids and void before retiring

C. Increase daytime activities as indicated
   - Establish with person a schedule for a daytime program of activity (walking, physical therapy)

- Limit amount and length of daytime sleeping if excessive (*i.e.,* more than 1 hour)
- Provide others to communicate with person and stimulate wakefulness

D. Provide comfort measures to induce sleep

- Assess with person, family, or parents the usual bedtime routine—time, hygiene practices, rituals (reading, toy)—and adhere to it as closely as possible
- Encourage or provide p.m. care
  - Bathroom or bedpan
  - Personal hygiene (mouth care, bath, shower, partial bath)
  - Clean linen and bedclothes (freshly made bed, sufficient blankets)
- Utilize sleep aids
  - Desired bedtime snack (avoid highly seasoned and high-roughage foods)
  - Reading material
  - Back rub or massage
  - Soft music or tape-recorded story
- Utilize pillows for support (painful limb, pregnant or obese abdomen, back)

Children

- Explain night to the child (stars and moon)
- Discuss how some people (nurses, factory workers) work at night
- Compare the contrast that when night comes for them, day is coming for other people somewhere else
- If a nightmare occurs, encourage the child to talk about it if possible. Reassure child that it is a dream, even if it seems so real. Share with child that you have dreams too
- Provide child with a nightlight and/or a flashlight to use to give him control over the dark
- Reassure child that you will be nearby all night
- Avoid allowing child to sleep with parents or parents to sleep in child's bed. Stay with child for a while (*e.g.,* sit on bed or chair, rub child's back)

E. Reduce the potential for injury during sleep

- Utilize side rails if needed
- Place bed in low position
- Provide adequate supervision
- Provide night lights
- Place call bell within reach
- Ensure that an adequate length of tubing is available for turning (IV tubing, Levin tube)

F. Provide health teaching and referrals as indicated

- Teach the importance of regular exercise for at least one-half hour three times a week (if not contraindicated) to reduce stress and promote sleep (walking, running, aerobic dance and exercise)
- Teach the pregnant woman
  - Not to stand when she can sit
  - To elevate feet when sitting
  - Not to sit when she can lie down
  - To adjust her schedule to provide for an afternoon rest (*e.g.,* upon returning home from work)
- Explain to person and significant others the causes of sleep/rest disturbance and possible ways to avoid them
- Explain interventions that relieve symptoms

References/Bibliography

Edgil A, Wood K, Smith D: Sleep problems of older infants and preschool children. Pediatr Nurs 11:88–89, 1985

Erman MK: Insomnia management. J Enterostom Ther 12(6):210–213, 1985

Fass G: Sleep, drugs, and dreams. Am J Nurs 71(12):2316–2320, 1971

Grant DA, Klell C: For goodness' sake—let your patient sleep! Nursing 4(11):54–57, 1974

Hayter J: The rhythm of sleep. Am J Nurs 80(3):457–461, 1980

Hayter J: To nap or not to nap. Geriatr Nurs 2:104–106, 1985

Hilton BA: Quality and quantity of patient's sleep and sleep disturbing factors in a respiratory intensive care unit. J Adv Nurs 1(3):453–468, 1976

Kleitman N: Sleep and Wakefulness. Chicago, University of Chicago Press, 1963

William D: Sleep and disease. Am J Nurs 71(12):2321–2324, 1971

Woods N: Patterns of sleep in post-cardiotomy patients. Nurs Res 2(4):437–452, 1972

Zareau SC et al: Sleep disorders: Insomnia. Nurse Pract 10(8):16–17, 1985

Zelechowski G: Helping your patient sleep. Planning instead of pills. Nursing 7(5):63–65, 1977

Zelechowski G: Sleep and the critically ill. Crit Care Update 6(2):5–13, 1979

Zwillich CW: Uncovering the mysteries of sleep. Arch Intern Med 138(2):195, 1978

Social Isolation

Related to **(Specify)**

Definition

Social isolation: The state in which the individual or group experiences a need or desire for contact with others but is unable to make that contact.

> **Author's Note:** Social isolation is a negative state of aloneness. It is a subjective state that exists whenever a person says it does and is perceived as imposed by others. Social isolation is *not* the voluntary solitude that is necessary for personal renewal, nor is it the creative aloneness of the artist or the loneliness—and possible suffering—one may experience as a result of seeking individualism and independence (*e.g.*, moving to a new city, going away to college).

Defining Characteristics

Since social isolation is a subjective state, all inferences made regarding a person's feelings of aloneness must be validated. Because the causes vary and people show their aloneness in different ways, there are no absolute cues to this diagnosis.

Major (must be present)

Expressed feelings of aloneness and/or
Desire for more contact with people

Minor (may be present)

Time passing slowly ("Mondays are so long for me")
Inability to concentrate and make decisions
Feelings of uselessness
Doubts about ability to survive
Feeling of rejection
Behavior changes
  Increased irritability or restlessness
  Underactivity (physical or verbal)
  Inability to make decisions
  Increased signs and symptoms of illness (a change from previous state of good
    health)
  Appearing depressed, anxious, or angry
  Postponing important decision-making
  Failure to interact with others nearby
  Sleep disturbance (too much sleep or insomnia)
  Change in eating habits (overeating or anorexia)

Etiological, Contributing, Risk Factors

A state of social isolation can result from a variety of situations and health problems that are related to a loss of established relationships or to a failure to generate these relationships. Some common sources follow.

Pathophysiological

Obesity

Cancer (disfiguring surgery of head or neck, superstitions of others)

Physical handicaps (paraplegia, amputation, arthritis, hemiplegia)

Emotional handicaps (extreme anxiety, depression, paranoia, phobias)

Incontinence (embarrassment, odor)

Communicable diseases (Acquired Immunodeficiency Syndrome [AIDS], hepatitis)

Situational (personal, environmental)

Death of a significant other

Divorce

Extreme poverty

Hospitalization or terminal illness (dieing process)

Moving to another culture (*e.g.,* unfamiliar language)

Drug or alcohol addiction

Homosexuality

Loss of usual means of transportation

Maturational

Child: Child in protective isolation or with a communicable disease

Elderly: Sensory losses, motor losses, loss of significant others

Principles and Rationale for Nursing Care

1. A person does not have to be alone to feel socially isolated. The physically handicapped are frequently ignored, for example.
2. Social isolation can result in intense feelings of loneliness and suffering.
3. The suffering associated with social isolation is not always visible. To diagnose this state, nurses must first be able to identify those persons at risk.
4. The lonely or isolated person often aggravates his condition by suffering alone. The lonely tend to shun each other.
5. The isolated person may resign himself to his situation and never seek companionship. He may deny his own feelings.
6. For the socially isolated, certain times (*e.g.,* nighttime or sundown) are harder to bear than others.
7. Persons who feel isolated may communicate and be communicated with in only the most concrete terms. "Hello, how are you?" "Do you want to eat?"
8. Illness may be the only legitimate way a socially isolated individual can get attention.
9. Hospitalization, which involves separation and isolation from the familiar and the secure, can cause feelings of loneliness.
10. A hospitalized child may have feelings of abandonment.
11. Aging can be an isolating experience.
12. The socially isolated are usually not able to initiate or coordinate various isolation reduction activities on their own behalf.
13. Sensory deficits rate highest on the list of problems in the elderly that have the potential for causing social isolation (Bernardini).
14. The functional ability of a person's senses has a strong influence on his/her perception of the world, his behavior, and the behavior of others toward him/her (Yurick).

High-risk Elderly

1. Elderly persons are at high risk for social isolation because there often are fewer natural opportunities for being among people. Retirement from work, difficulty securing transportation, health problems that restrict visiting, sensory deficits making communication laborious or frustrating, or isolation from the mainstream in institutions (hospitals or nursing homes) each can significantly limit the natural encounters an elderly client would have with people.

2. Family roles become altered and stressed when parents become dependent on their children, and children begin to assume traditional parental tasks or decision-making. To help elderly individuals meet their affiliative needs and increase satisfaction with social encounters, it is suggested that small groups be formed to promote interaction (rather than large noisy crowds) and that one or two meaningful relationships (confidante) be encouraged.

Focus Assessment Criteria

The nurse must listen attentively to hear what the patient is telling her or him. She or he must also make astute observations of behavior if an accurate nursing diagnosis is to be made and appropriate interventions identified.

Subjective Data

1. Social resources (support)

   "Who lives with you?"

   "About how many times did you talk to someone—friends, relatives or others—on the telephone in the past week (either you called them or they called you)?" If subject has no phone, question as follows:

   "How many times during the past week did you spend some time with someone who does not live with you; that is, you went to see them, or they came to visit you, or you went out to do things together?"

   "How many times in the past week did you visit with someone, either with people who live here or people who visited you here?"

   To whom does the person turn in time of need?

   Are there friends or neighbors on whom he relies for such things as meals and transportation?

   "Do you see your relatives and friends as often as you want to, or are you somewhat unhappy about how little you see them?"

   If institutionalized: "In the past year, about how often did you leave here to visit your family and/or friends for weekends or holidays, or to go on shopping trips or outings?"

2. Feelings of loneliness

   Does the person feel lonesome (isolated)?

   Why does he think he feels this way?

   Can he describe this feeling of loneliness?

   Are there times (holidays or other occasions) when this feeling is more painful?

   When during a 24-hour period does he feel most alone (morning, afternoon, evening, or during the night)?

   What does he do to relieve this feeling?

3. Desire for more human contact

   Who does the person think could help relieve this feeling of isolation?

   What kind of relationships would he like? (Same sex or opposite sex? Same age? Someone with same situational or maturational problem?)

Is he willing to make the effort to meet new people and go to new places?

What kind of group activities does he most enjoy? (Travel? A religious service or activity?)

Has divorce or death (of spouse, child, sibling, friend, pet) occurred recently?

Has the person moved away from vicinity of significant other? (Living alone increases the likelihood of loneliness)

4. Barriers to social contacts

Does the person lack knowledge of resources available, where to meet others, how to initiate conversation with strangers?

Is he housebound? (Illness or incapacity—lack of mobility on steps or curbs—and weather hazards can physically isolate the elderly, as does loss of usual transportation, living in dangerous area, and lack of access to public transportation)

Are there changes in the person's sensory ability (tactile sense, hearing, visual acuity, ability to write letters)?

5. Change in living arrangement

Has the person moved recently (to nursing home or child's home, to an apartment, to a strange location)?

Objective Data

Esthetic problems

Mutilating surgery

Odor (*e.g.,* ulcerating tumor)

Extreme obesity

Incontinence

Social Isolation
Related to (Specify)

Assessment

See Defining Characteristics

Outcome Criteria

The person will
- Identify the reasons for his feelings of isolation
- Discuss ways of increasing meaningful relationships
- Identify appropriate diversional activities

Interventions

The nursing interventions for a variety of contributing factors that might be associated with a diagnosis of social isolation are very similar.

A. Identify causative and contributing factors

(See Focus Assessment Criteria)

B. Reduce or eliminate causative and contributing factors

1. Promote social interaction
   - Support the individual who has experienced a loss as he works through his grief (see *Grieving*)
   - Validate the normalcy of grieving
   - Encourage person to talk about his feelings of loneliness and the reasons they exist
   - Mobilize person's support system of neighbors and friends
2. Decrease barriers to social contact
   - Assist with identification of transportation options
   - Determine available transportation in the community (public, church-related, volunteer)
   - Determine if person must be taught how to use alternate transportation (*e.g.*, drive a car)
   - Identify activities that help keep people busy, especially during times of high risk of loneliness (see *Diversional Activity Deficit*)
   - Assist with the development of alternate means of communication for persons with compromised sensory ability (*e.g.*, amplifier on phone; see *Impaired Communication Related to Hearing Loss*)
   - Assist with the management of esthetic problems, (*e.g.*, consult enterostomal therapist if ostomy odor is a problem; teach those with cancer to control odor of tumors by packing area with yogurt or pouring in buttermilk, then rinsing well with saline solution)
   - Assist person in locating stores that sell clothing especially made for those who have had disfiguring surgery (*e.g.*, mastectomy)
   - Refer to *Altered Patterns of Urinary Elimination* for specific interventions to control incontinence
3. Identify strategies to expand the world of the isolated
   Senior centers and church groups
   Foster grandparent program
   Day care centers for the elderly
   Retirement communities
   House sharing
   College classes opened to older persons
   Pets
   Telephone contact

C. Initiate referrals as indicated

   Community-based groups that contact the socially isolated
   Self-help groups for clients isolated due to specific medical problems (Reach to Recovery, United Ostomy Association)
   Wheelchair groups

References/Bibliography

Bernardini L: Effective communication as an intervention for sensory deprivation in the elderly client. Top Clin Nurs 1(4):72–81, 1985

Burnside IM: Nursing and the Aged. New York, McGraw-Hill, 1976

Carnevali D, Patrick M: Nursing Management for the Elderly. Philadelphia, JB Lippincott, 1979

Decker S, Kinzel S: Learned helplessness and decreased social interactions in elderly disabled persons. Rehabil Nurs 10(2):31–33, 1985

Eliopoulos C (ed): Health Assessment of the Older Adult. Menlo Park, CA, Addison-Wesley, 1984

Glassman-Feibusch B: The socially isolated elderly. Geriatr Nurs 2(1):28–31, 1981

Lynch JJ: The Broken Heart: The Medical Consequences of Loneliness. New York, Basic Books, 1979

Ravish T: Prevent social isolation before it starts. J Gerontol Nurs 11(10):10–13, 1985

Roberts SL: Behavioral Concepts and the Critically Ill Patient. Englewood Cliffs, NJ, Prentice-Hall, 1976

Roberts SL: Behavioral Concepts and Nursing Throughout the Life Span. Englewood Cliffs, NJ, Prentice-Hall, 1978

Yurick A et al: The Aged Person and the Nursing Process, 2nd ed, p 341. Norwalk, CT, Appleton-Century-Crofts, 1984

Social Interactions, Impaired

Related to **(Specify) Secondary to Chronic Illness**

Definition

Impaired social interaction: The state in which individual experiences or is at risk of experiencing negative, insufficient, or unsatisfactory responses from interactions.

Defining Characteristics

Major (must be present)

Reports inability to establish and/or maintain stable, supportive relationships

Minor (may be present)

Lack of motivation
Severe anxiety
Dependent behavior
Hopelessness
Delusions/hallucinations
Disorganized thinking
Lack of self-care skills

Distractibility/inability to
  concentrate
Social isolation
Superficial relationships
Poor impulse control
Difficulty holding a job
Lack of self-esteem

Etiological, Contributing, Risk Factors

Impaired social interactions can result from a variety of situations and health problems that are related to the inability to establish and maintain rewarding relationships. Some common sources are:

Pathophysiological

Loss of body function
Hearing deficits
Mental retardation
Terminal illness
Loss of body part

Visual deficits
Speech impediments
Chronic illness (Crohn's disease,
  renal failure, epilepsy)
Psychiatric disorders

Treatment-related

Surgical disfigurement
Dialysis
Reaction to medication

Situational (personal, environmental)

Depression
Language/cultural barriers
Social isolation
Lack of vocational skills
Substance abuse

Anxiety
Divorce/death of spouse
Institutionalization
Thought disturbances

Maturational

>Child/adolescent: Altered appearance, speech impediments, separation from family
>Adult: Loss of ability to practice vocation
>Elderly: Death of spouse, retirement

Focus Assessment Criteria

Subjective Data

1. Interaction patterns and skills
    a. Job-related
        Job-seeking and interviewing skills
        - Able to identify own job-related assets
        - Dresses appropriately
        - Asks appropriate questions
        - Identifies employment sources
        - Ability to complete an application
        Employment status
        - Employed
        - Unemployed
        Employment history
        - Length of employment
        - Reasons for leaving (problems with co-workers or supervisors)
        - Frequency of job changes
        Interactions with co-workers
        - Contacts outside work
    b. Living arrangements
        Ability to live cooperatively with others
        - Ability to participate with others in group tasks; such as food preparation, cleaning
        - Performs assigned tasks
        - Adequacy of personal hygiene
        - How does he handle conflict?
        - Dependability
        Residential patterns
        - Where?—family, group home, boarding house, institution
        - How long?
        - Frequency of relocation
        - Reasons for relocation
        Assess social isolation (see *Social Isolation*)
    c. Leisure/recreation
        "What do you do with your free time?"
        "Who do you share your time with?"
        Attendance at any structured activity?
        What interferes with participating in recreational activities?
        Preference for individual or group activity?
2. Recent life stress (Krauss and Slavinsky)
    Explore each of the following:
    - Emergencies (*e.g.,* police, fire)
    - Health (*e.g.,* others in household)
    - Financial (*e.g.,* increase or decrease in income, increased debt)
    - Job (*e.g.,* change in responsibility)

- Relationships (*e.g.,* new, broken)
- Treatment (*e.g.,* change in medications, therapist)
3. Support system
    Assess availability and responses of others
        Family and significant others
        - Fearful
        - Frustrated
        - Guilty
        - Angry
        - Embarrassed
        - Hopeless
        Relationships
        - Does he have friends?
        - Does he initiate friendship?
        Health care system
        - Frequency of contact
        - Frequency of admissions
        - Variety of services used
        - Compliance with prescribed treatment—kept appointments, medications
4. Coping skills
    How does he respond to stress, conflict?
    Substance abuse
    Aggression (verbal or physical)
    Suicide
    Withdrawal
5. Legal history
    Arrests and convictions

Objective Data

1. General appearance
    Facial expression (*e.g.,* sad, hostile, expressionless)
    Dress (*e.g.,* meticulous, disheveled, seductive, eccentric)
    Personal hygiene
        Cleanliness
        Grooming
        Clothes (appropriateness, condition)
2. Communication pattern
    During interview

Quiet	Withdrawn
Hostile	Cooperative
Apathetic	Hyperactive
Elated	

    Content

Appropriate	Sexually preoccupied
Rambling	Delusions
Suspicious	Obsessions
Denial of problem	Homicidal or suicidal plans

    Flow of thought

Appropriate	Blocking (unable to finish an idea)
Circumstantial (unable to get to the point)	Jumps from one topic to another
	Indecisive

Rate of speech
    Appropriate   Reduced
    Excessive   Pressured
3. Relationship skills
    Able to listen and respond appropriately
    Has conversational skills
    Does not seek interactions
    Withdrawn/preoccupied with self
    Shows dependency
    Demanding/pleading
    Hostile
        Barriers to satisfactory relationships
- Social isolation
- Severe depression
- Panic attacks
- Thought disturbances
- Chronic mental illness
- Preoccupation with illness

Principles and Rationale for Nursing Care

General

1. Social competence is the ability of the individual to interact effectively with his environment.
2. Effective reality testing, ability to problem-solve, and a variety of coping mechanisms are necessary for the individual to be socially competent.
3. Both the individual and the environment contribute to impaired functioning. A person may be able to function in one environment or situation and not in others.
4. Adequate social functioning is most often associated with conjugal living and a stable occupation.

Chronic Mental Illness

1. Chronic mental illness is characterized by recurring episodes over a long period of time.
2. The extent to which the individual is impaired in role performance varies. The extent of impairment is related to social inadequacy.
3. Alterations in thought processes may interfere with the individual's ability to engage in appropriate social or occupational role behavior.
4. Dependency is one of the most consistent features presented. It may be seen through multiple readmissions requiring a large amount of clinician's time, resistance to discharge, resistance to any change including medication, and refusal to leave home.
5. The origins of impaired social interactions in the chronically mentally ill vary. For some, it is the result of poor reality testing. If a person is unable to perceive reality accurately, it is difficult to manage everyday problems. For others, it may be the result of social isolation or the loss of interpersonal skills due to long-term institutionalization.
6. The chronically mentally ill person usually has no friends, is socially isolated and engages in little community activity.
7. Deinstitutionalization has decreased the number of institutionalized individuals and decreased the median length of hospital stay, thus changing the character of today's chronically ill population. There is now an emerging group of individuals 18 to 35

years old who are distinctly different from the older institutionalized adults, in that their lives reflect a transient existence and multiple hospital admissions versus stable, long-term residence in a state hospital.

8. The young chronically ill patients exhibit problems with impulse control (*e.g.,* suicidal gestures, legal problems, alcohol/drug intoxication), disturbances in affect (*e.g.,* anger, argumentativeness, belligerence), and poor reality testing especially when under stress.

9. The population of young chronically ill people varies from system-dependent, poorly motivated persons to system-resistant persons with low frustration tolerance and refusal to acknowledge problems.

10. Despite the variations, most have several factors in common (Pepper, Ryglewicz, and Kirshner):
    - Difficulty in maintaining stable supportive relationships—most have transient, unstable relationships with marginally functional people
    - Repeated errors in judgment—seen in their inability to learn from their experiences and the inability to transfer knowledge from one situation to another
    - Vulnerability to stress—those experiencing stress are at greater risk for relapse
    - Patterns of social interaction are demanding, hostile, and manipulative, which produces negative reactions among caregivers

11. Many chronically ill individuals return to their families after a period of hospitalization.

12. Both the individuals and families are under stress. The individual's behaviors that strain the family include their excessively demanding behavior, social withdrawal, lack of conversation, and minimal leisure interests. The family also affects the individual's ability to survive in the community by either supportive or nonsupportive behaviors.

13. Skills learned in one situation are not transferred to another, so that skills are best taught in the environment in which the person will be functioning.

14. Passivity or lack of motivation is a part of the illness and thus should not be simply accepted by the caregivers. Caregivers must use an assertive approach in which the treatment is "taken to the person" rather than waiting for him to participate (Test and Stein).

15. Treatment approaches which do not rely on verbal skills are more successful. Examples are coaching, modeling, and reinforcements for positive behaviors.

16. Chronically mentally ill persons often lose their jobs, not because of inability to do job tasks, but because of deficits in emotional and interpersonal functions (Anthony).

Impaired Social Interactions
Related to (Specify) Secondary to Chronic Illness

Assessment

Subjective Data
Psychiatric history
    Hospitalized several times
    Relapse in last year

Use of several facilities and a variety of treatments ("revolving door")
Use of other social agencies
Medication
    Recent changes
    Patient response
    Problem with compliance
Suicidal ideation or attempts
History of assaults or property destruction
Examination of symptoms associated with recent life stress
    Residence change or problem
    Employment problem
    Medication change
    Problem among family members
    Medical problem
    Financial change
    Relationship change
Obstacles to community functioning
    Poor personal hygiene
    Expects self-reliance
    Lacks leisure-time activities
    Inappropriate behavior in public
    Legal problems
    Unemployed
    Unstable, transient residences
    Social isolation

Objective Data

Thought disturbances
Inappropriate dress
Lack of conversational skills
Preoccupation with self
Noncompliant with previous treatment
Demanding, hostile, manipulative
Low motivation
Dependent

Outcome Criteria

The person will
- Identify problematic behavior that deters socialization
- Substitute constructive behavior for disruptive social behavior (specify)

The family will
- Describe strategies to promote effective socialization

Interventions

A. Provide support for the maintenance of basic social skills and reduce social isolation

(Refer to *Social Isolation* for further interventions)
1. Provide an individual, supportive relationship

- Assist person in managing life stresses
- Focus on present and reality
- Help to identify how stress precipitates problems
- Support healthy defenses
- Help to identify alternative courses of action
- Assist in analyzing approaches that work best

2. Provide supportive group therapy
   - Focus on here and now
   - Establish group norms which discourage inappropriate behavior
   - Encourage testing of new social behavior
   - Use snacks or coffee to decrease anxiety during sessions
   - Role-model certain accepted social behaviors (*e.g.,* responding to a friendly greeting versus ignoring it)
   - Foster development of relationships among members through self-disclosure and genuineness
   - Use questions and observations to encourage persons with limited interaction skills
   - Encourage members to validate their perception with others
   - Identify strengths among members and ignore selected weaknesses
   - Activity groups, drop-in socialization centers can be used for some individuals

3. Monitor medication compliance
   - Use small groups or scheduled individual sessions
   - Question individual regarding side-effects and symptom exacerbation (do not expect person to self-monitor)

4. Be assertive with persons who are unmotivated or passive
   - Contact the person when he fails to attend a scheduled appointment, job interview, etc.
   - Do not wait for person to want to participate

5. Hold persons accountable for their own actions
   - Treat as responsible citizens
   - Allow decision-making, but may have to outline limits
   - Do not allow them to use their illness as an excuse for their behavior
   - Set consequences and enforce when necessary, including encounters with law

6. Allow individual to be dependent as necessary

7. Utilize a wide variety of agencies and services (medical, psychiatric, vocational, social, residential)
   - Services must be coordinated by one agency (individual will not be able to coordinate for self)
   - Case managers have been successful in providing linkage
   - Programs must be flexible and culturally relevant

B. Decrease problematic behavior

1. Impaired reality testing (refer to *Altered Thought Processes*)
2. Lack of leisure-time activities (refer to *Diversional Activity Deficit*)
   - Companionship program
   - Day treatment centers
3. Social isolation (refer to *Social Isolation*)
4. Hostility and violent outbursts (refer to *Anxiety* and *Potential for Violence*)
5. Suicidal threats or attempts (refer to *Potential for Self-Harm*)
6. Manipulation
   - Use limit-setting (refer to section on anger in *Anxiety*)
   - Be aware of own reactions

C. Provide for development of social skills

- Identify the environment in which social interactions are impaired
    Living
    Learning
    Working
- Provide instruction in the environment where person is expected to function when possible (*e.g.*, accompany to job site, work with person in own residence)
- Combine verbal instructions with demonstration and practice
- Be firm in setting parameters of appropriate social behaviors such as punctuality, attendance, managing illnesses with employers, dress, etc.
- Use group as a method of discussing work-related problems
- Use sheltered workshops and part-time employment depending on person's level where success can best be achieved
- Give positive feedback; use verbal and behavioral reinforcers
- Convey a "can-do" attitude

D. Assist family and community members in understanding and providing support

1. Provide factual information concerning illness, treatment, and progress to family members
2. Validate family members' feelings of frustration in dealing with daily problems
3. Provide guidance on overstimulating or understimulating environments
4. Allow families to discuss their feelings of guilt and how their behavior affects the person
5. Develop an alliance with family
6. Arrange for periodic respite care
7. Provide support to landlords, shopkeepers, and anyone else with whom person has contact
    - Provide information on mental illness
    - Teach them relationship skills needed to manage person (*e.g.*, direct, firm, simple directions; use of modeling)
    - Give person name and number he can call when problems arise
    - Provide this education as the need arises with specific individuals

E. Initiate health teaching and referrals as indicated

1. Teach individual (McFarland):
    - Responsibilities of his/her role as a client (making requests clearly known, participating in therapies)
    - To outline activities of the day and to focus on accomplishing them
    - How to approach others in order to communicate
    - To identify which interactions encourage others to give him/her consideration and respect
    - To identify how he/she can participate in formulating family roles and responsibility to comply
    - To recognize signs of anxiety and methods to relieve them
    - To identify his/her positive behavior and to experience satisfaction with himself in selecting constructive choices
2. Teach basic coping skills necessary to live independently (home management, personal hygiene, financial management, transportation skills)
3. Teach or refer for assertive skill training
4. Teach basic conversational skills

5. Teach job-seeking skills
6. Teach parenting skills
7. Refer to a variety of social agencies; however, coordination and continuity to be maintained by one agency
8. Refer for supportive family therapy as indicated
9. Refer families to local self-help groups
10. Provide numbers for crisis intervention services

References/Bibliography

Anthony WA: The Principles of Psychiatric Rehabilitation, Baltimore, University Park Press, 1980

Bachrach L: Young adult chronic patients: An analytical review of the literature. Hosp Community Psychiatry 33(6):189–197, 1982

Krauss J: The chronic psychiatric patient in the community—A model of care. Nurs Outlook 308–314, 1980

Krauss J, Slavinsky A: The Chronically Ill Psychiatric Patient and the Community. Oxford, Blackwell Scientific, 1982

McFarland G, Wasli E: Manipulation in nursing diagnoses and process. In Psychiatric Mental Health Nursing, p 92. Philadelphia, JB Lippincott, 1986

Pepper B, Ryglewicz H, Kirshner M: The uninstitutionalized generation: A new breed of psychiatric patient. Pepper B, Ryglewicz H (eds): In New Directions for Mental Health Services: The Young Adult Chronic Patient No. 14. San Francisco, Jossey-Bass, June 1982

Test MA, Stein L: Practical guidelines for the community treatment of markedly impaired patients. Community Ment Health J 12(31):72–82, 1976

Spiritual Distress

Related to **Inability to Practice Spiritual Rituals**

Related to **Conflict Between Religious or Spiritual Beliefs and Prescribed Health Regimen**

Related to **Crisis of Illness/Suffering/Death**

Definition

Spiritual distress: The state in which the individual or group experiences or is at risk of experiencing a disturbance in the belief or value system which provides strength, hope and meaning to life.

Defining Characteristics

Major (must be present)
Experiences a disturbance in belief system

Minor (may be present)
Questions credibility of belief system
Demonstrates discouragement or despair
Is unable to practice usual religious rituals
Has ambivalent feelings (doubts) about beliefs
Expresses that he has no reason for living
Feels a sense of spiritual emptiness
Shows emotional detachment from self and others
Expresses concern—anger, resentment, fear—over meaning of life, suffering, death
Requests spiritual assistance for a disturbance in belief system

Etiological, Contributing, Risk Factors

Pathophysiological
Loss of body part or function
Terminal illness
Debilitating disease
Pain
Trauma
Miscarriage, stillbirth

Treatment-related
Abortion   Isolation
Surgery   Amputation
Blood transfusion   Medications
Dietary restrictions   Medical procedures

Situational (personal, environmental)

Death or illness of significant other

Embarrassment at practicing spiritual rituals

Hospital barriers to practicing spiritual rituals

Restrictions of intensive care

Confinement to bed or room

Lack of privacy

Lack of availability of special foods/diet

Beliefs opposed by family, peers, health care providers

Childbirth

Divorce, separation from loved one

Focus Assessment Criteria

Subjective Data

The following questions may be included as part of the psychosocial nursing assessment for individuals and families.

1. "Is religion or God important to you?"

If answer is *yes,* "To what religion do you belong?" or "In what do you believe?"

If *no,* "Do you find a source of strength or meaning in another area?"

2. "What effect do you expect your illness (hospitalization) to have on your spiritual practices or beliefs?"

3. "Are there any religious books (statues, medals, services, places) that are especially important to you?"

4. Do you have a special religious leader (priest, pastor, rabbi)?"

5. "How can I help you maintain your spiritual strength during this illness (hospitalization)?" (*e.g.,* contact spiritual leader, provide privacy at special times, request reading materials)

Objective Data

1. Present practices

Assess for

The presence of religious or spiritual articles (clothing, medals, texts)

Visits from religious leader

Visits to religious place of worhsip (chapel)

Requests for spiritual counseling or assistance

2. Response to interview on spiritual needs

Assess for the presence of anxiety, doubt, anger, depression

Principles and Rationale for Nursing Care

1. All people have a spiritual dimension, whether or not they participate in formal religious practices.

2. The practice of nurses should not violate their own moral, ethical, spiritual, or religious values.

3. The nature of the spiritual care an individual receives may directly affect the speed and quality of his recovery from illness.

4. An individual is a spiritual person even when disoriented, confused, emotionally ill, delirious, or cognitively impaired.

5. Religion influences attitudes and behavior related to right and wrong, family, child-rearing, work, money, politics, and many other functional areas.

6. The nurse's spiritual and religious background will influence her feelings about the spirituality and religion of her patients.
7. To deal effectively with a person's spiritual needs, the nurse must recognize her own beliefs and values, acknowledge that these values may not be effective for others, and set her own values aside when helping the individual meet his perceived spiritual needs.
8. The value of prayers or spiritual rituals to the believer is not affected by whether or not they can be scientifically "proved" to be beneficial.
9. Do not deny a request to see a spiritual leader except in case of extreme emergency (leader may even be sent to O.R. or treatment room if necessary).
10. The nurse should function as an advocate in recognizing and respecting the individual's spiritual needs, which may sometimes be overlooked or ignored by other health professionals.
11. In order to assist people in spiritual distress, the nurse must know certain beliefs and practices of the various spiritual groups found in this country. Table II-17 provides information on the beliefs and practices that are most directly related to health and illness. It is intended as a quick reference only. Major religions, denominations, and spiritual groups are arranged alphabetically. Denominations with similar practices and restrictions are grouped together. No attempt is made to discuss the broad beliefs and philosophies of the selected groups; see the bibliography for such in-depth information.

Spiritual Distress
Related to Inability to Practice Spiritual Rituals

Assessment

Subjective Data
The person expresses one or more of the following feelings related to spiritual belief system

Anxiety	Embarrassment
Guilt	Sense of loss
Depression	Grief

Requests spiritual articles, reading materials, sacraments, services, etc.
Questions others about their spiritual rituals.
Person requests changes in medical regimen or hospital protocols to allow practice of spiritual rituals.

Objective Data
Cannot go to religious services or place of worship
Cannot maintain religious diet or fast
Is separated from religious or spiritual articles, clothing, texts, etc.
Is unable to say prayers or meditate
Is unable to maintain usual contact with spiritual leader or members of spiritual group

(*text continues on page 720*)

Table II-17.   **Overview of Religious Beliefs**

Agnostic
Beliefs
  It is impossible to know if God exists (specific moral values may guide behavior)

Armenian
See Eastern Orthodox

Atheist
Beliefs
  God does not exist (specific moral values may guide behavior)

Baptist, Churches of God, Churches of Christ, and Pentecostal (Assemblies of God, Foursquare Church)
Illness
  Some practice laying on of hands, divine healing through prayer
  May request Communion
  Some prohibit medical therapy
  May consider illness divine punishment or intrusion of Satan
Diet
  No alchohol (mandatory for most)
  No coffee, tea, tobacco, pork, or strangled animals (mandatory for some)
  Some fasting
Birth
  Opposes infant baptism
Text
  Bible
Beliefs
  Some practice glossolalia (speaking in tongues)

Buddhist
Illness
  Considered trial that develops the soul
  May wish counseling by priest
  May refuse treatment on holy days (1/1, 1/16, 2/15, 3/21, 4/8, 5/21, 6/15, 8/1, 8/23, 12/8, 12/31)
Diet
  Strict vegetarianism (mandatory for some)
  Discourages use of alcohol, tobacco, and drugs
Death
  Last-rite chanting by priest
  Death leads to rebirth, may wish to remain alert and lucid
Texts
  Buddha's sermon on the "eightfold path"
  The Tripitaka, or "three baskets" of wisdom
Beliefs
  Cleanliness is of great importance

Church of Christ
See Baptist

Church of Christ, Scientist
Illness
  Caused by errors in thought and mind
    May oppose drugs; IV fluid; blood transfusions; psychotherapy; hypnotism; physical examinations; biopsies; eye, ear, and blood-pressure screening; and other medical and nursing interventions
  Accepts only legally required immunizations
    May desire support from a Christian Science reader or treatment by a Christian Science nurse or practitioner (a list of these nonmedical practitioners and nurses may be found in the *Christian Science Journal*)

(continued)

Table II-17. **Overview of Religious Beliefs** (continued)

Church of Christ, Scientist (continued)
Death
  Autopsy permitted only in cases of sudden death
Text
  Science and Health With Key to the Scriptures by Mary Baker Eddy

Church of God
See Baptist

Confucian
Illness
  The body was given by one's parents and should therefore be well cared for
  May be strongly motivated to maintain or regain wellness
Beliefs
  Respect for family and older persons very important

Cults (variety of groups, usually with living leader)
Illness
  Most practice faith healing
  May reject modern medicine and condemn health personnel as enemies
  Therapeutic compliance and follow-up are generally poor
  Illness may represent wrong thinking or inhabitation by Satan
Beliefs
  Expansion of cult through conversions important
  May depend on cult environment for definition of reality

Eastern Orthodox (Greek Orthodox, Russian Orthodox, Armenian)
Illness
  May desire Holy Communion, laying on of hands, anointing, or sacrament of Holy Unction
  Most oppose euthanasia and favor every effort to preserve life
  Russian Orthodox males should be shaved only if necessary for surgery
Diet
  May fast Wednesdays, Fridays, during Lent, before Christmas, or for 6 hours before Communion
    (seriously ill are exempted)
  May avoid meat, dairy products, and olive oil during fast (seriously ill are exempted)
Birth
  Baptism 8 to 40 days after birth, usually by immersion (mandatory for some)
  May be followed immediately by confirmation
    Greek Orthodox only: If death of infant is imminent, nurse should baptize infant by touching
    the forehead with a small amount of water three times
Death
  Last rites and administration of Holy Communion (mandatory for some)
  May oppose autopsy, embalming, and cremation
Texts
  Bible
  Prayer book
Religious articles
  Icons (pictures of Jesus, Mary, saints) are very important
  Holy water and lighted candles
  Russian Orthodox wears cross necklace which should be removed only if necessary
Other
  Greek Orthodox opposes abortion
  Confession at least yearly (mandatory for some)
  Holy Communion 4 times yearly; Christmas, Easter, 6/30, and 8/15 (mandatory for some)
  Dates of holy days may differ from Western Christian calendar

(continued)

Table II-17. **Overview of Religious Beliefs** *(continued)*

Episcopal
Illness
  May believe in spiritual healing
  May desire confession and Communion
Diet
  May abstain from meat on Fridays
  May fast during Lent or before Communion
Birth
  Infant baptism is mandatory (nurse may baptize infant when death is imminent by pouring water
    on forehead and saying, "I baptize thee in the name of the Father, the Son, and the Holy
    Ghost")
Death
  Last rites optional
Texts
  Bible
  Prayer book

Friend (Quaker)
No ministers or priests; direct, individual, inner experience of God is vital
Diet
  Most avoid alcohol and drugs and favor practice of moderation
Death
  Many do not believe in afterlife
Beliefs
  Pacifism important; many are conscientious objectors to war

Greek Orthodox
See Eastern Orthodox

Hindu
Illness
  May minimize illness and emphasize its temporary nature
  Considered important only as it affects spiritual quest
  Illness or injury may represent sins committed in previous life
Diet
  Various doctrines, many vegetarian; many abstain from alcohol (mandatory for some)
Death
  Seen as rebirth; may wish to be alert
  Priest ties thread around neck or wrist of body—do not remove
  Water is poured into mouth, and family washes body
  Cremation preferred
Beliefs
  Self-control, self-discipline, and cleanliness emphasized
  Opposes artificial insemination
Texts
  Vedas
  Upanishads
  Bhagavad-Gita
Worship
  Usually in home
  May involve various images, statues, and symbols of gods
  May include use of water, fire, lights, sounds, natural objects, special postures, and gestures

Jehovah's Witness
Illness
  Opposes blood transfusions and organ transplantation (mandatory)
  May oppose other medical treatment and all modern science

(continued)

Table II-17. **Overview of Religious Beliefs** (continued)

Jehovah's Witness (continued)
Opposes faith healing
Opposes abortion
Diet
Refuses foods to which blood has been added; may eat meats that have been drained

Jew (Judaism)
Illness
Medical care emphasized
Rabbinical consultation necessary for donation and transplantation of organs
May oppose surgical procedures on the Sabbath (sundown Friday to sundown Saturday);
seriously ill are exempted
May prefer burial of removed organs or body tissues
May oppose shaving
May wear skull cap and socks continuously, believing head and feet should be covered
Diet
Fasting for 24 hours on holy days of Yom Kippur (in September or October) in Tisha Bab (in
August)
Matzo replaces leavened bread during Passover week (in March or April)
May observe strict Kosher dietary laws (mandatory for some) that prohibit pork, shellfish, and
the eating of meat and dairy products at same meal or with same dishes (milk products,
served first, can be followed by meat in a few minutes; reverse is not Kosher); seriously ill are
exempted
Birth
Ritual circumcision 8 days after birth (mandatory for some)
Fetuses are buried
Death
Ritual burial society members wash body
Burial as soon as possible
Opposes cremation
Many oppose autopsy and donation of body to science
Most do not believe in afterlife
Generally oppose prolongation of life after irreversible brain damage
Texts
Torah (first five books of Old Testament)
Talmud
Prayer book
Religious articles
Menorah (seven-branched candlestick)
Yarmulke (skull cap, may be worn continuously)
Tallith (prayer shawl worn for morning prayers)
Tefillin, or phylacteries (leather boxes on straps containing scripture passages)
Star of David (may be worn around neck)

Lutheran, Methodist, Presbyterian
Illness
May request Communion, anointing and blessing, or visitation by minister or elder
Generally encourages utilization of medical science
Birth
Baptism by sprinkling or immersion of infants, children, or adults
Death
Optional last rites or scripture reading

Mennonite
Illness
Opposes laying on of hands
May oppose shock treatment and drugs

(continued)

Table II-17. **Overview of Religious Beliefs** (continued)

Methodist
See Lutheran

Mormon (Church of Jesus Christ of Latter-day Saints)
Illness
  Comes from breaking laws of health or failing to keep God's commandments
  May desire Sacrament of the Lord's Supper to be administered by a Church Priesthood holder
  Divine healing through laying on of hands
  May prohibit medical therapy
  Church may provide financial support during illness
Diet
  Prohibits alcohol, tobacco, and hot drinks (tea and coffee)
  Sparing use of meats
Birth
  No infant baptism
Death
  Baptism of dead (mandatory), sometimes with living person as proxy
  May preach Gospel to the dead
  Opposes cremation
Texts
  Bible
  Book of Mormon
Religious articles
  Special undergarment worn by some men should not be removed if possible (seriously ill are
    exempted)

Muslim (Islamic, Moslem) and Black Muslim
Illness
  Opposes faith healing
  May be noncompliant due to fatalistic view (illness is God's will)
  Group prayer may be helpful—no priests
  Favors every effort to prolong life
Diet
  Pork prohibited
  May oppose alcohol and traditional Black American foods (corn bread, collard greens)
  Fasts sunrise to sunset during Ramadan (9th month of Muslim year—falls different time each
    year on Western calendar); seriously ill are exempted
Birth
  Circumcision practiced with accompanying ceremony
  Aborted fetus after 130 days is treated as human being
Death
  Confession of sins before death, with family present if possible
  Family follows specific procedure for washing and preparing body, which is then turned to face
    Mecca
  May oppose autopsy
Texts
  Koran (scriptures)
  Hadith (traditions)
Prayer
  Five times daily—upon rising, midday, afternoon, early evening, and before bed—facing Mecca
    and kneeling on prayer rug
  Ritual washing after prayer
Beliefs
  All activities (including sleep) restricted to what is necessary for health
  Personal cleanliness very important
  All Muslims: gambling and idol worship prohibited

(continued)

Table II-17. **Overview of Religious Beliefs** (continued)

Pentecostal
See Baptist

Presbyterian
See Lutheran

Roman Catholic
Illness
  Allowed by God because of man's sins but not considered personal punishment
  May desire confession (penance) and Communion
  Anointing of sick for all seriously ill patients (some patients may equate this with "Last Rites"
    and assume they are dying)
  Donation and transplantation of organs permitted
  Burial of amputated limbs (mandatory for some)
Diet
  Fasting or abstaining from meat mandatory on Ash Wednesday and Good Friday (seriously ill
    are exempted); optional during Lent and on Fridays
  Fasts from solid food for 1 hour and abstains from alcohol for 3 hours before receiving Communion
(mandatory) (seriously ill are exempted)
Birth
  Baptism of infants and aborted fetuses mandatory (nurse may baptize in case of imminent death
    by sprinkling water on the forehead and saying, "I baptize thee in the name of the Father, of
    the Son, and of the Holy Spirit")
Death
  Anointing of sick (mandatory)
  Extraordinary artificial means of sustaining life are unnecessary
Texts
  Bible
  Prayer book
Religious articles
  Rosary, crucifix, saints' medals, statues, holy water, lighted candles
Other
  Attendance at mass required (seriously ill are exempted) on Sundays or late Saturday and on
    holy days (1/1, 8/15, 11/1, 12/8, 12/25, and 40 days after Easter)
  Sacrament of Penance at least yearly (mandatory)
  Opposes abortion

Russian Orthodox
See Eastern Orthodox

Scientologist
Illness
  Believes that "becoming clear" can affect physical and mental health, control weight, etc.
  May refuse psychiatric treatment
  May request visit by minister, pastoral counselor, or confessor
Text
  Scientology: The Fundamentals of Thought by L. Ron Hubbard

Seventh-Day Adventist (Advent Christian Church)
Illness
  May desire baptism or Communion
  Some believe in divine healing
  May oppose hypnosis
  May refuse treatment on the Sabbath (sundown Friday to sundown Saturday)
  Healthful diet and life-style are stressed
Diet
  No alcohol, coffee, tea, narcotics, or stimulants (mandatory)
  Some abstain from pork, other meat, and shellfish

(continued)

Table II-17. **Overview of Religious Beliefs** *(continued)*

Seventh-Day Adventist (Advent Christian Church) *(continued)*
Birth
　Opposes infant baptism
Text
　Bible, especially Ten Commandments and Old Testament

Shinto
Illness
　May believe in prayer healing
　Great concern for personal cleanliness
　Physical health may be valued due to emphasis on joy and beauty of life
　Family extremely important in giving care and providing emotional support
Beliefs
　Worships ancestors, ancient heroes, and nature
　Traditions emphasized
　Esthetically pleasing area for worship important

Silva Mind Control
Type of meditation utilizing various relaxation techniques
Illness
　Believes "sensory projection" can diagnose and cure illness
　All problems are solved through programming the mind for positive action, utilizing dreams and
　　visual exercises

Taoist
Illness
　Illness is seen as part of the health/illness dualism
　May be resigned to and accepting of illness
　May consider medical treatment as interference
Death
　Seen as natural part of life
　Body is kept in house for 49 days
　Mourning follows specific ritual patterns
Text
　Tao-te-ching by Lao-tzu
Beliefs
　Esthetically pleasing area for meditation important

Transcendental Meditation (TM)
Form of nonreligious meditation useful in relieving stress
Meditate for 20 minutes once or twice a day using a mantra (special word)
Illness
　Some evidence that TM is useful in treating insomnia, hypertension, obesity

Unitarian Universalist
Illness
　Reason, knowledge, and individual responsibility are emphasized, so may prefer not to see clergy
Birth
　Most do not practice infant baptism
Death
　Prefers cremation

Zen
Meditation utilizing lotus position (many hours and years are spent in meditation and
　contemplation); goal is to discover simplicity
Illness
　May wish consultation with Zen master

Cannot read religious materials
Cannot assume normal position for prayer or meditation

Outcome Criteria

The person will
- Continue spiritual practices not detrimental to health
- Express decreasing feelings of guilt and anxiety
- Express satisfaction with spiritual condition

Interventions

A. Assess causative and contributing factors

Lack of knowledge of religious restrictions or demands

Fear of imposing upon or antagonizing medical and nursing staff with requests for spiritual rituals

Embarrassment regarding spiritual beliefs or customs (especially common in adolescents)

Separation from articles, texts, or environment of spiritual significance

Limitations related to disease process or treatment regimen (*e.g.*, cannot kneel to pray due to traction; cannot vocalize prayers due to laryngectomy)

Lack of transportation to spiritual place or service

B. Eliminate or reduce causative and contributing factors, if possible

1. Fear of imposing upon others
   - Communicate acceptance of various spiritual beliefs and practices
   - Convey nonjudgmental attitude
   - Acknowledge importance of spiritual needs
   - Express willingness of health care team to help in meeting spiritual needs
2. Embarrassment
   a. Provide privacy and quiet as needed for daily prayer, for visit of spiritual leader, and for spiritual reading and contemplation
      - Pull curtains or close door
      - Turn off television and radio
      - If possible, ask desk to hold telephone calls
   b. Contact spiritual leader to clarify practices and perform religious rites or services if desired
      - Communicate with spiritual leader regarding person's condition
      - Prevent interruption during visit, if possible
      - Provide table or stand covered with clean white cloth (for most religious statues, etc.; see Table II-17)
      - Chart result of visit
      - Address Roman Catholic, Orthodox, and Episcopal ministers as "Father"; other Christian ministers as "Pastor"; Jewish rabbis as "Rabbi"
   c. Maintain diet with spiritual restrictions when not detrimental to health (see Table II-17)
      - Consult with dietitian

- Allow fasting for short periods if possible*
- Change therapeutic diet*
- Have family or friends bring special food, if possible
- Have members of spiritual group supply meals to individual at home
- Be as flexible as possible in serving methods, times of meals, etc.
3. Separation from articles, texts, or environment of spiritual significance
    a. Question individual about missing religious or spiritual articles or reading material (see Table II-17)
       - Obtain missing items from clergy in hospital, spiritual leader, family, or members of spiritual group
       - Treat these articles and books with respect
       - Allow person to keep spiritual articles and books within reach as much as possible, or where they can be easily seen
       - Protect from loss or damage (*e.g.,* medal pinned to patient's gown can be lost in laundry)
       - Recognize that articles without overt religious meaning may have spiritual significance for individual (*e.g.,* wedding band)
       - Utilize spiritual texts in large print, in Braille, or on tape when appropriate
    b. Provide opportunity for individual to pray with others or be read to by members of own religious group or member of the health care team who feels comfortable with these activities
       - Jews and Seventh-Day Adventists would find Psalms 23, 34, 42, 63, 71, 103, 121, and 127 appropriate
       - Christians would also appreciate I Corinthians 13, Matthew 5:3–11, Romans 12, and the Lord's Prayer
4. Lack of transportation
    - Take person to chapel or quiet environment on hospital grounds
    - Arrange transportation to church or synagogue for individual in home
    - Provide access to spiritual programming on radio and television when appropriate
5. Encourage spiritual rituals not detrimental to health (see Table II-17)
    - Encourage children to maintain bedtime or before-meal prayer rituals
    - Assist individuals with physical limitations in prayer and spiritual observances (*e.g.,* help to hold rosary; help to kneeling position, if appropriate)
    - Assist in habits of personal cleanliness
    - Avoid shaving if beards are of spiritual significance
    - Make special arrangements for burial of limbs or body organs
    - Perform baptism for critically ill infant
    - Allow family or spiritual leader to perform ritual care of body
    - Make arrangements as needed for other important spiritual rituals (*e.g.,* circumcisions, séance)

* May require a physician's order.

Spiritual Distress
Related to Conflict Between Religious or Spiritual Beliefs and Prescribed Health Regimen

Assessment

Subjective Data

The person expresses one or more feelings related to spiritual beliefs

Anxiety	Depression
Guilt	Fear of God
Grief	Fear of physician
Sense of loss	Dream about angry God or
Doubt	minister
Sense of powerlessness	Ambivalence in decisions
Trapped feeling	

Objective Data

Questions or refuses therapeutic regimen
Agrees to morally or ethically unacceptable therapy
Frantically seeks advice or support for decision-making
Questions others about their beliefs and values
Experiences insomnia or nightmares
Objects to prescribed or legally required medical procedures (autopsy, blood transfusion, immunization) that conflict with personal spiritual beliefs
Objects to prescribed diet or medication that conflicts with spiritual dietary restrictions

---

Outcome Criteria

The person will
- Express religious or spiritual satisfaction
- Express decreased feelings of guilt and fear
- Relate he is supported in his decision regarding his health regimen
- State that conflict has been eliminated or reduced

Interventions

A. Assess causative and contributing factors (see Table II-17)

Lack of information about or understanding of spiritual restrictions
Lack of information about or understanding of health regimen
Informed, true conflict
Parent conflict regarding treatment of child
Lack of time before emergency treatment or surgery for deliberation

B. Eliminate or reduce causative and contributing factors, if possible

1. Lack of information about spiritual restrictions
   - Have spiritual leader discuss restrictions and exemptions as they apply to those who are seriously ill or hospitalized
   - Provide reading materials on religious and spiritual restrictions and exemptions
   - Encourage person to seek information from and discuss restrictions with others in spiritual group
   - Chart results of these discussions
2. Lack of information about health regimen
   - Provide accurate information about health regimen, treatments, medications
   - Explain the nature and purpose of therapy
   - Discuss possible outcomes without therapy; be factual and honest but do not attempt to frighten or force person to accept treatment
3. Informed, true conflict
   a. Encourage individual and physician to consider alternate methods of therapy* (*e.g.,* utilization of Christian Science nurses and practitioners; special surgeons and techniques for surgery without blood transfusions)
   b. Support individual making informed decision—even if decision conflicts with own values
      - Consult own spiritual leader
      - Change patient assignment so person can be cared for by nurse with compatible beliefs
      - Arrange for discussions among health care team to share feelings
4. Parent conflict regarding treatment of child
   - If parents refuse treatment of child, follow interventions under *a* and *b* above
   - If treatment is still refused, physician or hospital administrator may obtain court order appointing temporary guardian to consent to treatment*
   - Call spiritual leader to support parents (and possibly child)
   - Encourage expression of negative feelings
5. Emergency treatment
   - Provide as little treatment as possible for Christian Scientists, cult members, etc. (see Table II-17)
   - Delay treatment if possible until spiritual needs have been met (*e.g.,* receiving last rites before surgery)*; send spiritual leader to treatment room or O.R. if necessary
   - Anticipate reaction and provide support when individual chooses to accept or is forced to accept spiritually unacceptable therapy
      a. Depression, withdrawal, anger, fear
      b. Loss of will to live
      c. Reduced speed and quality of recovery

* May require a physician's order.

Spiritual Distress
Related to Crisis of Illness/Suffering/Death

Assessment

Subjective Data

The person asks one or more questions similar to the following:
"What did I do to deserve this?"
"Why is this happening to me?"
"Is this God's will?"
"How can God love me and still allow me to suffer?"
"Is my faith too weak?"
"Does God exist?"

The person expresses one or more of the following feelings related to spiritual beliefs:

Doubt	Anger	Depression
Ambivalence	Alienation	Emptiness
Regret	Worthlessness	Shame
Guilt	Apathy	Fear

Objective Data

Shows symptoms of depression and withdrawal
Experiences disturbances in sleep/rest patterns
Cries frequently
Questions others about their belief systems
Refuses to see or speak to spiritual leader
Reduces participation in religious/spiritual activities

Outcome Criteria

The person will
- Express his feelings related to change in beliefs
- Describe spiritual belief system positively
- Express desire to perform religious/spiritual practices
- Describe satisfaction with meaning and purpose of illness/suffering/death

---

Interventions

A. Assess causative and contributing factors

Failure of spiritual beliefs to provide explanation/comfort during crisis of illness/suffering/impending death
Doubting quality or strength of own faith to deal with current crisis
Anger toward God/spiritual beliefs for allowing/causing illness/suffering/death

B. Eliminate or reduce causative and contributing factors, if possible

1. Failure of spiritual beliefs to provide explanation/comfort during crisis of illness/suffering/impending death

- Communicate that you take spiritual concerns seriously by being available to listen to feelings, questions, etc.
- Give "permission" to discuss spiritual matters with nurse by bringing up subject of spiritual welfare if necessary
- Use questions about past beliefs and spiritual experiences to assist person in putting this life event into wider perspective
- Assist person to begin problem-solving process and move toward new spiritual understandings if necessary
- Offer to contact usual or new spiritual leader
- Offer to pray/meditate/read with client if you are comfortable with this, or arrange for another member of health care team if more appropriate
- Provide uninterrupted quiet time for prayer/reading/meditation on spiritual concerns

2. Doubting quality of own faith to deal with current illness/suffering/death
   - Be available and willing to listen when client expresses self-doubt, guilt, or other negative feelings
   - Silence and/or touch may be useful in communicating the nurse's presence and support during times of doubt or despair
   - Suggest process of "life review" to identify past sources of strength or spiritual support
   - Guided imagery or meditation to reinforce faith/beliefs
   - Offer to contact usual or new spiritual leader

3. Anger toward God/spiritual beliefs for allowing or causing illness/suffering/death
   - Express to person that anger toward God is a common reaction to illness/suffering/death
   - Help client recognize and discuss feelings of anger
   - Allow client to problem-solve to find ways to express and relieve anger
   - Offer to contact usual spiritual leader
   - Offer to contact other spiritual support person (such as pastoral care, hospital chaplain, etc.) if person cannot share feelings with usual spiritual leader

References/Bibliography

Ballou RO (ed): The Portable World Bible. New York, Viking Press, 1944

Conrad NL: Spiritual support for the dying. Nurs Clin North Am 20(2):415–425, 1985

Ellis D: Whatever happened to the spiritual dimension? Canadian Nurse 9(9):42–43, 1980

Fehring RJ, McLane AM: Value belief–Spiritual distress. In Clinical Nursing, pp 1843–1857. St. Louis, CV Mosby, 1986

Fish S, Shelly J: Spiritual Care: The Nurse's Role. Downer's Grove, Intervarsity Press, 1978

Henderson V, Nite G: Worship. In Principles and Practice of Nursing, 6th ed. New York, Macmillan, 1978

Highfield MF, Cason C: Spiritual needs of patients: Are they recognized? Cancer Nurs 6(3):187–192, 1983

Kennedy R: The International Dictionary of Religion, New York, Crossroad, 1984

Miller JF: Inspiring hope. Am J Nurs 85(1):22–25, 1985

Murray R, Zentner J: Religious influences on the person. In Nursing Concepts for Health Promotion, 2nd ed. Englewood Cliffs, NJ, Prentice-Hall, 1979

Pumphrey JB: Recognizing your patients' spiritual needs. Nursing 7(12):64–70, 1977

Rosten L (ed): Religions of America. New York, Simon & Schuster, 1975

Ryan J: The neglected crisis. Am J Nursing 84(10):1257–1258, 1984

Shannon M: Spiritual needs and nursing responsibility. Imprint 10(12):23, 1980

Smith H: The Religions of Man. New York, Harper & Row, 1958

Stoll RI: Guidelines for spiritual assessment. Am J Nurs 79:1574–1577, 1979

Thought Processes, Altered

Related to **(Specify) as Manifested by Inability to Evaluate Reality**

Related to **Factors Related to Aging**

Definition

Altered thought processes: A state in which an individual experiences a disruption in such mental activities as conscious thought, reality orientation, problem solving, judgment, and comprehension.

Author's Note: *Altered Thought Processes* is a state in which an individual experiences a disruption in such mental activities as conscious thought, reality orientation, problem-solving, judgments and comprehension related to coping (personality, mental) disorders. Cognitive function is influenced by physiological functions, stimuli from environment, and the person's emotional status. *Altered Thought Processes* describes an individual with altered cognition and perception influenced by coping problems; it differs from *Sensory–Perceptual Alterations,* which describes an individual with altered perception and cognition influenced by physiological functions and stimuli from the environment.

Defining Characteristics

Major (must be present)
Inaccurate interpretation of stimuli, internal and/or external

Minor (may be present)

Cognitive defects, including abstraction, memory
Suspiciousness
Delusions
Hallucinations
Distractibility
Lack of consensual validation

Language disturbances, *e.g.,* echolalia, neologism
Confusion/disorientation
Ritualistic behavior
Social isolation
Dependency
Impulsivity

Etiological, Contributing, Risk Factors

Pathophysiological
Personality and mental disorders related to
Alteration in biochemical compounds
Genetic disorder
Progressive dementia

Situational (personal, environmental)*

Depression or anxiety
Substance abuse (alcohol, drugs)
Fear of the unknown
Actual loss (of control, routine, income, significant others, familiar object or sur-
roundings)
Unclear communication
Emotional trauma
Rejection or negative appraisal by others
Negative response from others
Isolation

Maturational*

Adolescent: Peer pressure, conflict, separation
Adult: Marital conflict, family additions or deaths
Elderly: Isolation

Focus Assessment Criteria

Acquire data from client and significant others

Subjective Data

1. History of the individual
    Life-style
        Interests
        Work history
        Coping patterns (past and
            present)
        Support system (availability)

        Strengths and limitations
        Previous level of functioning and
            handling stress

    History of medical problems and treatments (medications)
    Activities of daily living (ability and desire to perform)
2. History of symptoms (onset and duration)
    Acute or chronic
    Sudden or gradual

    Continuous or intermittent?
    Time of day
3. History of unusual sensations and thought productions
    Precipitating factors
    Frequency and duration
    Routine time of occurrence

    Description in individual's own
        words
4. Assess for presence of
    Feelings of
        Extreme sadness and
            worthlessness
        Guilt for past actions
        Apprehension in various
            situations
        Being rejected or isolated

        Living in an unreal world
        Mistrust or suspiciousness of
            others
        Others' making him do and say
            things
        Excessive self-importance

* These situational and maturational factors should not be considered causative or contributive
unless they are present in an individual with a history of coping disorders.

Fears

That others will harm him	Of falling apart
That mind is being controlled by external agents	Of thoughts racing
	Of being held prisoner
Of being unable to cope	Body is rotting or not there

Difficulty concentrating

Senses difficulty grasping particular circumstances or events

States he is unable to follow what is being said

Hallucinations (visual, auditory, gustatory, olfactory, tactile—includes an objective component)

5. Orientation

Person

"What is your name?"	"What is your occupation?"

Time

"What season is it?"	"What month is it?"

Place

"Where are you?"	"Where do you live?"

6. Problem-solving ability

"What would you do if the phone rang?"

"What is the difference between the doctor and the president?"

Objective Data (includes a subjective component)

1. General appearance

Facial expression (alert, sad, hostile, expressionless)

Dress (meticulous, disheveled, seductive, eccentric)

2. Behavior during interview

Withdrawn	Cooperative
Hostile	Quiet
Apathetic	

3. Communication pattern

Content

Appropriate	Lacking content
Rambling	Sexual preoccupations
Suspicious	Delusionary (grandeur,
Denying problem	persecution, reference,
Homicidal plans	influence, control,
Suicidal ideas	or bodily sensations)

Flow of thought

Appropriate	Loose connection of ideas
Blocking (unable to finish idea)	Jumps from one topic to another
Circumstantial (unable to get to point)	Unable to come to conclusion, be decisive

Rate of speech

Appropriate	Reduced
Excessive	Pressured

Nonverbal behavior

Affect appropriate to verbal content	Gestures, mannerisms, facial grimaces
Affect inappropriate to verbal content	Posture

4. Interaction skills
    With nurse
        Inappropriate
        Relates well
        Withdrawn/preoccupied
    With significant others
        Relates with all (some) family
            members
        Hostile toward one (all) members

Shows dependency
Demanding/pleading
Hostile

Does not seek interaction
Does not have visitors

5. Activities of daily living
    Emotionally capable of self-care

Physically capable of self-care

6. Nutritional status
    Appetite
    Eating patterns

Weight (within normal limits,
    decreased, increased)

7. Sleep/rest pattern
    Recent change
    Sleeps too much or too little

Early wakefulness
Insomnia

8. Personal hygiene
    Cleanliness (body, hair, teeth)
    Grooming (clothes, hair, makeup)

Clothes (condition,
    appropriateness)

9. Motor activity
    Within normal limits
    Increased
    Decreased

Agitated
Repetitive

Principles and Rationale for Nursing Care

General

1. Thought is a functioning process of the brain that integrates every individual's daily living experiences.
2. Cognitive processes are the mental processes related to reasoning, comprehension, judgment, and memory.
3. Cognitive function is influenced by physiological functions, stimuli from the environment, and the person's emotional state.
4. The cognitive processes of remembering and perception are influenced by the individual's current needs and interests as well as his fund of knowledge.
5. Development of cognitive abilities follows a systematic pattern of maturational experiences and requires varied perceptual stimulation.
6. A disruption in the quality and quantity of incoming stimuli can affect an individual's thought processes.
7. Psychological equilibrium is enhanced when the individual is able to think clearly and rationally; emotional tension may interfere with rational thinking and behavior.
8. An individual's psychological equilibrium is influenced by his cognitive function, including his perceptions, opinions, attitudes, and beliefs.
9. Actual events frequently become reorganized and reinterpreted individually so that they are substantially changed and distorted during the process of remembering.
10. The ability to conceptualize develops relatively slowly and requires contact with others; the development of concrete concepts precedes the development of abstract concepts.

Reality

1. Reality testing is the objective evaluation and judgment of the world outside the self, differentiated from one's thoughts and feelings.
2. Reality testing is determined by early life experiences and by significant people in one's life.
3. Delusions—fixed false beliefs—and hallucinations originate during extreme emotional stress when one is unable to cope and reflect underlying feelings.
4. Delusions include those of

    Grandeur: An exaggerated sense of importance of identity or of ability

    Persecution: A sense that one is being harassed

    Reference: Belief that the behavior of others refers to oneself

    Influence: Exaggerated sense of power over others

    Control: Sense that one is being manipulated by others

    Bodily sensations: Belief that one's organs are diseased despite contrary evidence

    Infidelity: Belief, due to pathological jealousy, that one's lover is unfaithful
5. Delusions arise when the person attempts to alter reality. First, he denies his own feelings, then projects those feelings onto the environment and finally he must explain this to others.
6. The fundamental feelings being projected by suspicious and grandiose clients are inadequacy and worthlessness.
7. Hallucinations are perceptions that arise from within the person's own thoughts. He actually hears, sees, feels or tastes the phenomenon.
8. Hallucinations are meeting underlying needs (*e.g.,* loneliness, anxiety, self-worth), and until a person can substitute other activities, he may be unwilling to "give these up."
9. Not only are the connections between words disturbed, but the words often have a different meaning to the person than is generally accepted.
10. The person may spend much time in his fantasy world, which leads to a lack of consensual validation of language.
11. Verbal assaults are expressions of fear and anxiety and should not be taken personally.
12. Disorganized thinking often leads to regression in behavior, disturbed communication, and difficulty in interactions with others.

High-risk Elderly

1. Thinking ability, arithmetic ability, memory, judgment, and problem-solving are measured in the elderly to give a general index of overall cognitive ability. Short-term memory may decline somewhat, but long-term memory often remains intact.
2. Intelligence does not alter, perhaps until the very later years, but the person needs more time to process information. Reaction time increases as well. There may be some difficulty in learning new information because of increased distractibility, decrease in concrete thinking, and difficulty solving new problems. However, older persons usually compensate for these deficiencies by taking more time to process the information, screening out distractions, and using extreme care in making decisions. Marked cognitive decline is usually attributed to disease processes such as atherosclerosis, loss of neurons, and other pathological changes.
3. Elderly persons are vulnerable to acute confusion when their ability to compensate for stressors, physiologically or psychologically, is compromised. Failure to adapt to changes in the external and internal environment results in confusion. Adaptation can be assessed in the following categories:
    a. Compromised brain function (CHF, anemia, pneumonia, hypoglycemia, fluid and electrolyte imbalance, hypotension, toxic drug reactions)

b. Sensory–perceptual problems (decreased vision, hearing, information processing)
c. Disruption in pattern and meaning (unable to cope with chronic stress-producing situations)
d. Altered normal physiologic states (problems in eating, sleeping, or elimination, pain, etc.)
e. True dementias (senile dementia of the Alzheimer type, multi-infarct dementia, etc.) (Wolanin and Phillips, 1981)

Altered Thought Processes
Related to (Specify)

The inability to evaluate reality is an inability to differentiate one's thoughts and feelings from the actualities of the outside world.

Assessment

Subjective Data

Expresses mistrust
Feels he is being controlled
Fears falling apart
Fears objects are communicating
States he sees, hears, feels, tastes something that is not there

Expresses hostility: "Everyone is against me"
Has difficulty concentrating
Accuses others of making him do things
States body parts are rotting or missing

Objective Data

Mood alterations
Poor judgment
Regression (childlike behavior)
Disturbed communication
Inappropriate laughter, grinning
Delayed verbal responses
Eye movements
Increased verbal/motor activity
Sleep disturbances

Overreaction to stimuli
Arrogant
Seclusive
Reduced fluid/food intake
Social isolation
Altered interpersonal interactions
Poor impluse control
Poor hygiene/grooming

Outcome Criteria

The person will
• Identify situations that evoke anxiety
• Express delusional material less frequently
• Communicate clearly with others
• Describe problems in relating with others
• Differentiate between reality and fantasy
• Describe the rationale for treatment

Interventions

A. Promote communication that enhances the person's sense of integrity

1. Encourage open, honest dialogue
   - Approach in a calm, nurturing manner
   - Persevere, be consistent
   - Be open and share with the person
   - Discuss expectations and demands
   - Recognize when person is testing the trustworthiness of others
   - Avoid making promises that cannot be fulfilled
   - Initial staff contact minimal and brief with suspicious person; increase time as suspiciousness decreases
   - Explain if appointments cannot be kept
   - Verify your interpretation of what person is experiencing ("I understand you are fearful of others")
   - Be an attentive listener; note both verbal and nonverbal messages
   - Help individual verbalize what person indicates nonverbally
   - Utilize terminology that is familiar and evokes little anxiety
   - Recognize the importance of body posture, facial expression, and tone of voice
   - Present information in a matter-of-fact way that is least likely to be misinterpreted; do not use humor or bantering with suspicious persons
   - Utilize communication that helps person maintain his own individuality (*e.g.,* "I" instead of "we")
   - Eliminate whispered comments or incomplete explanations that encourage fantasy interpretation
2. Maintain client's personal space
   - Do not touch person until you have developed an ongoing trusting relationship
   - Talk to the person in open space; avoid small rooms or offices

B. Assist person to differentiate between own thoughts and reality

1. Validate the presence of hallucinations
   - Observe for verbal and nonverbal cues—inappropriate laughter, delayed verbal response, eye movements, moving lips without sound, increased motor movements, grinning.
     "Are you hearing/seeing something now?"
     "What's happening now?"
   - Assist person in observing thoughts and feelings as they relate to the underlying need(s) being met
     "Has this happened before?"
     "What were you doing/thinking?"
     "You were lonely?"
2. Focus on here-and-now
   - Direct the focus from delusional expression to discussion of reality-centered situations
   - Encourage person to validate his thoughts by sharing them with significant others
   - Avoid derogation or belittling when person misinterprets stimuli or is delusional; do not laugh or make fun of him
   - Encourage person to identify and focus on his strengths, not his weaknesses
   - Encourage differentiation of stimuli arising from inner sources from those from outside (*e.g.,* in response to "I hear voices," say: "Those are the voices of people on TV" or "I hear no one speaking now; they are your own thoughts")

- Avoid the impression that you confirm or approve reality distortions; tactfully express doubt
- Focus on reality-oriented aspects of the communication (*e.g.*, if person states, "The TV is controlling my mind," the nurse can say, "How does it make you feel when others try to control you?")
- Set limits for discussing repetitive delusional material ("You've already told me about that; let's talk about something realistic")
- Teach person to relearn to focus attention on real things and people
- Identify the underlying needs being met by the delusions/hallucinations
- Help person become aware that his needs are being expressed in fantasy and teach more appropriate ways to meet these needs (*e.g.*, aggression expressed through delusion of persecution can be put into constructive activity such as hammering metal objects)
- Do not automatically dismiss physical complaints; however, do not express undue concern

C. Assist the person with disordered thinking in communicating more effectively
- Ask for the meaning of what is said; do not assume that you understand
- Validate your interpretation of what is being said ("Is this what you mean?")
- Clarify all global pronouns—we, they ("Who is *they*?")
- Refocus when person changes the subject in the middle of an explanation or thought
- Tell the person when you are not following his train of thought
- Do not mimic or restate words, phrases that you do not understand
- Teach the person to consensually validate with others

D. Encourage a more mature level of functioning
1. Assist person to set limits on his own behavior
   - Discuss alternative methods of coping (*e.g.*, taking a walk instead of crying)
   - Confront person with the attitude that regression is not acceptable behavior
   - Help delay gratification (*e.g.*, "I want you to wait 5 minutes before you repeat your request for help in making your bed")
   - Encourage person to achieve realistic expectations
   - Pace expectations to avoid frustration
2. Encourage and support person in the decision-making process
   - Help person review options and the advantages and disadvantages of each option
   - Assist in structuring daily living activities (*e.g.*, help schedule bath time before activity hour)
   - Compliment the person who assumes more responsibility
   - Show patience and understanding when a mistake is made
   - Provide opportunity for person to contribute to his own treatment plan
   - Help establish future goals that are realistic; examine problems in achieving a goal and suggest various alternatives
3. Assist person to differentiate between needs and demands
   - Explain the difference between needs and demands (*e.g.*, food and clothing are needs; expectations that others dress and feed him, if he can do it, are demands)
   - Assist person to examine the effects of his behavior on others; encourage a change in behavior if it evokes negative responses
   - Teach negotiation to achieve needs and goals
   - Help person ask for what he wants and tell others how he feels

- Help person realize that failure of others to meet his needs and demands is not always related to their regard for him

E. Provide person with opportunities for positive socialization

1. Help him share on a one-to-one basis
   - Be warm, honest, and sincere in interactions
   - Demonstrate that you accept him
   - Recognize that some people deny the need for close relationships
   - Be sensitive to behaviors that indicate resistance to interpersonal involvement
   - Help person know you recognize his uneasiness in social situations ("It must be difficult for you")
   - Use touch judiciously if person fears closeness
2. Help person recognize behaviors that stimulate rejection
   - Identify activities that reduce interpersonal anxiety (*e.g.*, exercise, controlled breathing exercises; see Appendix X)
   - Set limits firmly and kindly on destructive behavior
   - Allow expression of negative emotions, verbally or in constructive activity
   - Avoid argument or debate about delusional ideas or destructive behavior
   - Help person accept responsibility for responses he elicits from others
   - Encourage discussion of problems in relating after visits with family members
   - Help person test new skills in relating to others in role-playing situations
3. Refer to impaired socialization for further interventions

F. Promote physical well-being and prevent injury

1. Explain and monitor medication regimen
   - Assess person's ability to remember to take medications
   - Assist person to remember to take medications by color coding each bottle with a sticker and writing out the times of the day that medications are prescribed for, with the appropriate color sticker next to the time
   - Teach about the purpose of medications and their side-effects
   - Encourage person to report all physical symptoms
   - Encourage person to take prescribed medication, especially antipsychotic (*e.g.*, lithium)
   - Check to ensure that medication was swallowed. If you have doubts about patient taking oral medications (*e.g.*, failure to improve), change to concentrate
   - Extremely suspicious and hostile persons should begin on concentrate, so that you will not have to check mouth and increase distrust
   - Do not mix medications with food
2. Monitor nutritional intake
   - Observe eating habits (amount, selection, frequency, food preferences and dislikes, appetite)
   - Note weight gain or loss
   - Discuss adequate nutrition in relation to activity level
   - Allow person to choose food he especially likes; contract with individual who eats predominantly snack foods (*e.g.*, "If you eat one egg you can order a doughnut")
   - Note delusions regarding food or body that might interfere with nutritional intake
   - Encourage increased calorie intake for hyperactive person
   - Provide finger foods that can be eaten on-the-run (*e.g.*, sandwiches)
   - Allow choices in foods (may prefer to eat food brought in by family, in unopened packages, fruit, etc.)
   - Refer to *Altered Nutrition* for additional interventions

3. Assess ability for self-care activities
   - Identify areas of physical care for which person needs assistance (sleep and rest, nutrition, bathing, dressing, elimination, exercise)
   - Note person's motivation and interest in appearance
   - Teach skills required to assume responsibility for self-care
   - Assist person in planning his daily routines in order to foster independence and responsibility
   - Monitor for sleep disturbances
   - Provide a single room for extremely suspicious person
   - Suggest leaving the light on
   - Give nonstimulating drinks with a snack at bedtime
   - Assess the need for a sleeping medication
   - If appropriate, arrange to give last dose of antipsychotic medication at bedtime (*e.g.*, BID medication—give AM and HS)
   - Refer to *Self-Care Deficit* for additional interventions

G. Reduce the potential for violence to self and others

1. Provide a minimally stimulating environment
   - Reduce incidence of bright colors and loud noises
   - Be short, concise, and matter-of-fact
   - Be consistent
   - May need to assign staff responsible for developing trusting relationship
   - Avoid large groups
2. Provide activities in which he will be successful
   - Avoid competitive sports
   - Suspicious persons are often good managers
   - Involve in activities for a short time period
3. Allow ventilation of hostility (as long as it is not combative/destructive)
   - Be nonjudgmental
   - Do not personalize
4. Assess for signs indicative of aggression ("Those Russian spies are going to attack me tonight")
   - Refer to *Potential for Violence* for further interventions
5. Identify cues to suicide
   - Sudden changes in mood or behavior
   - Report of plan to harm himself
   - Report of voices directing person to harm himself or others
   - Observe closely for changes in behavior; increase vigilance
   - Share with personnel the individual's potential for self-harm
   - Refer to *Potential for Self-harm* for further interventions.
6. Interview family and note approaches that have been beneficial in the past in controlling aggression
7. Reduce anxiety and develop a sense of safety through a climate of care and concern

H. Initiate health teaching and referrals as indicated

- Anticipate difficulties in adjusting to community living; discuss concerns about returning to community and elicit family reaction to individual's discharge
- Provide health teaching that will prepare person to deal with life stresses (methods of relaxation, problem-solving skills, how to negotiate with others, how to express feelings constructively)
- Review signs and symptoms of recurrent illness that indicate impending maladjustment

- Refer to other professions for assistance
  - To occupational therapist to learn leisure-time activities
  - To industrial therapist to improve or learn new job skills
  - To social worker to discuss living arrangements, financial problems, or family negotiations
- Supply telephone number and address of local mental health clinic
- Inform individual of social agencies that offer help in adjusting to community living
  1. General social agencies
     Mental health and mental retardation centers
     Mental Health Association
     HELP (alternative to mental health center)
     Family Service (family counseling)
     Drug rehabilitation centers
  2. Specific social agencies
     Alcoholics Anonymous
     Gray Panthers
     Suicide Crisis Intervention Center
     Synanon
     Contact

Altered Thought Processes
Related to Factors Related with Aging

Factors associated with aging are social isolation, losses (motor, sensory, object, person), attitudes and responses of others, and physiological disorders that can be reduced or eliminated.

Assessment

Subjective Data

The person expresses
  Fear
  Persecution
  Seeing objects or persons that others cannot see
  Hearing voices that others cannot hear

Objective Data

Change in the person's usual response to stimuli
  Talks to persons not present
  Restless
  Combative
  Withdrawn
  Lack of animation
  Unsmiling
  Rambling
  Shouting

Outcome Criteria

The person will
- Demonstrate contact with reality as evident by (specify)
- Demonstrate an increase in self-care activities

Interventions

A. Assess for etiological and contributing factors

1. Physiological factors

Decreased function (respiratory, renal, endocrine, cerebral, circulatory, sensory—vision, hearing)

Sleep and rest imbalance

Fluid and electrolyte imbalance (potassium, sodium; dehydration)

Nutritional imbalance

Medication (overdose, side-effects)

2. Situational factors

Sensory overload (hospitalization)

Sensory deprivation (hospitalization, isolation)

Fear of unknown, fear of loss

Actual loss of control, income, significant others, familiar objects and surroundings

Significant others/caregiver factors

Attitude toward aging

Beliefs about confusion

Communication patterns (tone, speed, volume, content)

B. Assess history of the confusion (onset and duration)

Acute or chronic

Sudden or gradual

Continuous or intermittent

Time of day

C. Determine the amount and type of stimuli needed by the individual in the context of his usual life-style

Usual day routine

Work history

Available support systems

Coping patterns

Strengths and limitations

D. Reduce and eliminate reversible physiological factors

1. Monitor physiological functions (electrolytes, circulation, urine output)
2. Maintain optimal physiological functioning
   - Encourage person to remain out of bed as much as possible
   - Teach person to perform isometric and isotonic exercises when in bed
   - Encourage person to change position frequently even if it is just lifting one side off a surface by rolling slightly (see *Activity Intolerance* for specific interventions)

- To encourage walking, choose a destination or give the walk a purpose (*e.g.,* walk to the lounge for breakfast)
- Encourage dietary and fluid intake necessary for metabolic requirements (refer to *Altered Nutrition* and *Fluid Volume Deficit*)
- Promote optimal acuity of hearing and vision (*e.g.,* assess adequacy and function of aids [glasses, hearing aids])
- Provide interventions to ensure adequate periods of sleep
- Discourage the use of sedatives in older individuals (refer to *Sleep Pattern Disturbance*)
- Assess person's response to medications
  - a. Identify signs and symptoms of overdose
  - b. Identify compromised physiological functions that may contribute to such side-effects as toxic levels of medications (*e.g.,* decreased renal function, which may cause certain drugs to accumulate to toxic levels)
  - c. Consult pharmacist for possible adverse interactions of two or more drugs
  - d. Consult with physician to review present medication regimen and person's response

E. Promote communication that contributes to the person's sense of integrity
  1. Examine attitudes about aging (in self, caregivers, significant others)
  2. Maintain standards of empathetic, respectful care
     - Be an advocate when other caregivers are insensitive to the individual's needs
     - Function as a role model with co-workers
     - Provide other caregivers with up-to-date information on aging and reality orientation
     - Expect empathetic, respectful care and monitor its administration
  3. Reduce unessential stimuli, if possible
     - Attempt to assign same caregivers to person
     - Avoid changing rooms
     - Explain procedures and activities prior to event; show equipment
     - Do not move person's belongings; keep them where he can see and use them
  4. Attempt to obtain information that will provide useful and meaningful topics for conversations (likes, dislikes; interests, hobbies; work history)
  5. Encourage significant others and caregivers to speak slowly and at an average volume (unless hearing deficits are present), as one adult to another, with eye contact, and as if expecting person to understand
  6. Provide respect and promote sharing
     - Pay attention to what person is saying
     - Pick out meaningful comments and continue talking
     - Call person by name and introduce yourself each time a contact is made; utilize touch if welcomed
     - Use name the person prefers; avoid "Pops" or "Mom," which can increase confusion and are unacceptable
     - Convey to person that you are concerned and friendly (through smiles, an unhurried pace, humor, and praise; do not argue)

F. Provide sensory input that is sufficient and meaningful
  1. Keep person oriented to time and place
     - Refer to time of day and place each morning
     - Provide person with a clock and calendar large enough to see

- Provide person with opportunity to see daylight and dark through a window or take person outdoors
- Single out holidays with cards or pins (*e.g.*, wear a red heart for Valentine's Day)
2. Encourage family to bring in familiar objects from home (photographs, afghan)
   - Ask person to tell you about the picture
   - Focus on familiar topics
3. Discuss current events, seasonal events (snow, water activities); share your interests (travel, crafts)
4. Assess if person can perform an activity with his hands (*e.g.*, latch rugs, wood crafts)
   - Provide reading materials, audio tapes, puzzles (manual, computer, crossword)
   - Encourage person to keep his own records if possible (*e.g.*, intake and output)
   - Provide tasks to perform (addressing envelopes, occupational therapy)
5. If hallucinations and delusions persist, refer to *Altered Thought Processes for specific interventions*
6. In teaching a task or activity—for example, eating—break it into small, brief steps by giving only one instruction at a time
   - Remove covers from food plate and cups
   - Locate napkin and utensils
   - Add sugar and milk to coffee
   - Add condiments to food (sugar, salt, pepper)
   - Cut foods
   - Proceed with eating
7. Explain all activities
   - Offer simple explanations of tasks
   - Allow individuals to handle equipment related to each task
   - Allow individual to participate in task, such as washing his face
   - Acknowledge that you are leaving and say when you will return

G. Increase person's self-esteem

- Allow former habits (*e.g.*, reading in the bathroom)
- Encourage the wearing of dentures
- Assist with removal of facial hair
- Ask family to provide spending money
- Ask person his usual grooming routine and encourage him to follow it
- Provide privacy at all times; when it is necessary to expose a body surface, take precautions to cover all other areas (*e.g.*, if washing a back, use towels or blankets to cover legs and front torso)
- Provide for personal hygiene according to person's preferences (hair grooming, showers or bath, nail care, cosmetics, deodorants and fragrances)

H. Promote a well role

- Discourage the use of nightclothes during the day; have person wear shoes, not slippers
- Encourage self-care and grooming activities
- Have person eat meals out of bed, unless contraindicated
- Promote socialization during meals (*e.g.*, set up lunch for four individuals in lounge)
- Plan an activity each day to look forward to (*e.g.*, bingo, ice-cream-sundae gathering)

I. Do not endorse confusion
  - Never agree with confused statements
  - Direct person back to reality; do not allow him to ramble
  - Adhere to the schedule; if changes are necessary, advise person of them
  - Avoid talking to co-workers about other topics in person's presence
  - Provide simple explanations that cannot be misinterpreted
  - Remember to acknowledge your entrance with a greeting and your exit with a closure ("I will be back in ten minutes")

J. Utilize various modalities to promote stimulation for the individual
  1. Music therapy
     - Provide soft, familiar music during meals
     - Arrange group song fests
     - Play music during other therapies (physical, occupational)
     - Have person exercise to music
     - Encourage construction of simple instruments and have individuals play them in a rhythm band
     - Organize guest entertainment
     - Use client-developed songbooks (large print and decorative covers)
  2. Recreation therapy
     - Encourage arts and crafts (knitting and crocheting)
     - Suggest creative writing
     - Provide puzzles
     - Organize group games
  3. Remotivation therapy
     a. Organize group sessions into five steps (Dennis):
        Step 1: Climate of Acceptance (approx. 5 min)
            Relaxed atmosphere with introductions of leaders and participants
            Provide large-letter name tags and names on chairs
            Maintain assigned places for every session
        Step 2: Creating a Bridge to Reality (approx. 15 min)
            Use a prop (visual, audio, song, picture, object, poem) to introduce theme of session
        Step 3: Sharing the World We Live In (approx. 15 min)
            Group members discuss the topic
            Stimulation of senses should be promoted
        Step 4: Appreciation of the Work of the World (approx. 20 min)
            Discussion of how the topic relates to their past experiences (work, leisure)
        Step 5: Climate of Appreciation (approx. 5 min)
            Each member is thanked individually
            Announcement of the next session's topic and meeting date
     b. Use associations and analogies
        "If ice is cold, then fire is . . . ?"
        "If day is light, then night is . . . ?"
     c. Topics for remotivation sessions are chosen based on suggestions from group leaders and the interest of the group. Examples are pets, bodies of water, canning fruits and vegetables, transportation, holidays (Janssen).
  4. Sensory training
     - Stimulate vision (with mirrors, brightly colored items of different shape, pictures, colored decorations, kaleidoscopes)
     - Stimulate smell (with flowers, coffee, cologne)

- Stimulate hearing (ring a bell, play records)
- Stimulate touch (sandpaper, velvet, steel wool pads, silk, stuffed animals)
- Stimulate taste (spices, salt, sugar, sour substances)

K. Prevent injury to the individual

1. Discourage the use of restraints; explore other alternatives
   - Put person in a room with others who can help watch him
   - Enlist aid of family or friends to watch person during confused periods
   - If person is pulling out tubes, use mitts instead of wrist restraints
2. Refer to *Potential for Injury* for strategies for assessing and manipulating the environment for hazards.

References/Bibliography

Arnold HM: Working with schizophrenic patients. Four A's: A guide to one-to-one relationships. Am J Nurs 76:941–943, 1976

Bayer M: The multipurpose room: A way-out outlet for staff and clients. J Psychiatr Nurs 18(10):35–37, 1980

Dennis H: Remotivation therapy groups. In Burnside IM (ed): Working With the Elderly Group Process and Techniques, 2nd ed. Monterey, CA, Jones & Bartlett, 1984

Dixon B: Intervening when the patient is delusional. J Psychiatr Nurs 7(1):25–34, 1969

Janssen J, Giberson D: Remotivation therapy. J Gerontol Nurs 14(6):31–34, 1988

Knowles RD: Disputing irrational thought. Am J Nurs 81:735, 1981

Kreigh H, Perko J: Psychiatric and Mental Health Nursing: A Commitment to Cure and Concern, pp 195–203. Reston, VA, Reston Publishing, 1979

Libow L: A rapidly administered, easily remembered mental status evaluation: FROMAJE. In Libow L and Sherman (eds): The Core of Geriatric Medicine, pp 84–85. St. Louis, CV Mosby, 1981

O'Brien J: Teaching psychiatric inpatients about their medications. J Psychiatr Nurs 17(10):30–32, 1979

Ozuna J: Alterations in mentation: Nursing assessment and intervention. J Neurosurg Nurs 17(1):65–70, 1985

Pullinger WF Jr: Remotivation. Am J Nurs 60(5):682–685, 1960

Schroeder PJ: Nursing interventions with patients with thought disorders. Perspect Psychiatr Care 17(1):32–39, 1979

Schwartzman ST: The hallucinating patient and nursing intervention. J Psychiatr Nurs 13(6):23–28, 33–36, 1976

Slater MC: Altered levels of consciousness: Impaired thought processes. In Snyder M (ed): A Guide to Neurological and Neurosurgical Nursing, pp 157–188. New York, John Wiley & Sons, 1983

Smith JE: Improving drug knowledge. J Psychiatr Nurs 19(4):1916–1918, 1981

Stuart G, Sundeen S: Principles and Practice of Psychiatric Nursing, 2nd ed. St. Louis, CV Mosby, 1983

Torrey EF: Surviving Schizophrenia: A Family Manual. New York, Harper & Row, 1983

Wolanin M, Phillips L: Confusion: Prevention and Care. St. Louis, CV Mosby, 1981

Resources for the Consumer

Literature

Powell LS, Courtice K: Alzheimer's Disease: A Guide for Families, Menlo Park, CA, Addison-Wesley, 1983

Tissue Integrity, Impaired*

Related to **Mechanical Destruction**
Related to **Chemical Destruction**

Skin Integrity, Impaired

Related to **Immobility: Potential**
Related to **Pressure, Shear, Friction, Maceration**

Oral Mucous Membrane, Altered

Related to **Inadequate Oral Hygiene or Inability to Perform Oral Hygiene**
Related to **(Specify) as Manifested by Stomatitis**

*This diagnostic category was developed and submitted to NANDA by the Clinical Nurse Specialist Group, Harper Hospital, in the Detroit Medical Center.

Impaired Tissue Integrity

Related to **Mechanical Destruction**
Related to **Chemical Destruction**

> **Author's Note:** *Impaired Tissue Integrity* is the broad category under which the more specific diagnostic categories of *Impaired Skin Integrity* and *Impaired Oral Mucous Membranes* fall. Since tissue is composed of epithelium, connective tissue, muscle, and nervous tissue, *Impaired Tissue Integrity* correctly describes some pressure ulcers that are deeper than the dermis. *Impaired Skin Integrity* should be used to describe potential or actual disruptions of epidermal and dermal tissue only. If an individual is at risk for damage to corneal tissue, the nurse can use the diagnosis *Potential Impaired Corneal Tissue Integrity related to* (for example: to corneal drying and lower lacrimal production secondary to unconscious state).
>
> If an individual is immobile and multiple systems are threatened, respiratory, circulatory, musculoskeletal as well as integumentary, the nurse can use *Potential for Disuse Syndrome* to describe the entire situation.

Definitions

Impaired tissue integrity: A state in which an individual experiences or is at risk for damage to the integumentary, corneal, or mucous membranous tissues of the body.

Defining Characteristics

Major (must be present)

Disruptions of corneal, integumentary, or mucous membranous tissue, invasion of body structure (incision, dermal ulcer, corneal ulcer, oral lesion)

Minor (may be present)

Lesions (primary, secondary)	Dry mucous membrane
Edema	Leukoplakia
Erythema	Coated tongue

Etiological, Contributing, Risk Factors

Pathophysiological

Autoimmune alterations
    Lupus erythematosus
    Scleroderma

Metabolic and endocrine alterations
  Diabetes mellitus
  Hepatitis
  Cirrhosis
  Renal failure
  Jaundice
  Cancer
  Thyroid dysfunction
Nutritional alterations
  Obesity   Emaciation
  Dehydration   Malnutrition
  Edema
Impaired oxygen transport
  Peripheral vascular alterations
  Venous stasis
  Arteriosclerosis
  Anemia
  Cardiopulmonary disorders
Medications (steroid therapy)
Psoriasis
Eczema
Infections
  • Bacterial (impetigo, folliculitis, cellulitis)
  • Viral (herpes zoster [shingles], herpes simplex, gingivitis, acquired immune deficiency syndrome [AIDS])
  • Fungal (ringworm [dermatophytosis], athlete's foot, vaginitis)
Dental caries/periodontal disease

Treatment-related

NPO status
Therapeutic extremes in body temperature
Therapeutic radiation
Surgery
Drug therapy (local and systemic)
  Steroids
Imposed immobility related to sedation
Mechanical trauma
  Therapeutic fixation devices
    Wired jaw
    Traction
    Casts
    Orthopedic devices/braces
  Inflatable or foam donuts
  Torniquets
  Footboards
  Restraints
  Dressings, tape, solutions
  External urinary catheters
  Nasogastric tubes
  Endotracheal tubes

Oral prostheses/braces
Contact lenses

Situational (personal, environmental)

Chemical trauma
    Excretions
    Secretions
    Noxious agents/substances
Environmental
    Radiation—sunburn   Bites (insect, animal)
    Temperature   Inhalants
    Humidity   Poisonous plants
    Parasites
Immobility
    Related to pain, fatigue, motivation, cognitive, sensory, or motor deficits
Depression
Allergies
Inadequate personal habits (hygiene, dental, dietary, sleep)
Body build, weight distribution, bony prominences, muscle mass, range of motion, joint mobility
Stress
Occupation
Pregnancy

Maturational

Infants/children: Diaper rash, childhood diseases (chickenpox)
Elderly: Dry skin, thin skin, loss of skin elasticity, loss of subcutaneous tissue

Focus Assessment Criteria

Subjective Data

1. History of Symptoms
    a. Onset
    b. Precipitated by what?
    c. Relieved by what?
    d. Frequency?
    e. Effects on life-style
           Occupation
           Financial
           Role functions
           Sexual/social
2. History of exposure (if allergy is suspected)
        Carrier of contagious disease
        Chemicals, paints, cleaning agents, plants, animals
        Heat or cold
3. Medical, surgical, and dental history, use of tobacco, alcohol
4. Current drug therapy
        What drugs? How often? When was last dose taken?
        Effects on symptoms

5. Factors contributing to the development or extension of tissue destruction (assess for)

Skin deficits
    Dryness
    Edema
    Obesity
    Thinness
    Excessive perspiration
    Aging skin (dry, thin, loss of elasticity, subcutaneous tissue)

Mucous membrane deficits
    Mouth pain
    Bleeding gums
    Coated tongue
    Oral lesions or ulcers
    Oral plaque
    Dryness

Corneal deficits
    Absence of blink reflex
    Corneal ulcers
    Ptosis
    Excessive tearing
    Diminished tearing
    Contact lens wear
    Sensory deficits

Impaired oxygen transport
    Edema
    Anemia
    Peripheral vascular disorders
    Arteriosclerosis
    Venous stasis
    Cardiopulmonary disorders

Chemical/mechanical irritants
    Radiation
    Incontinence (feces, urine)
    Oral prostheses
    Casts, splints, braces
    Contact lenses

Nutritional deficits
    Protein deficiencies
    Vitamin deficiencies
    Mineral deficiencies
    Dehydration

Systemic disorders
    Infection
    Diabetes mellitus
    Cancer
    Hepatic or renal disorders

Sensory deficits
    Brain or cord injury
    Decreased level of consciousness
    Confusion
    Neuropathy
    Visual or taste alterations

Immobility

Objective Data*

Tissue Characteristics

1. Skin

Color	Texture	Turgor	Vascularity
Pigment	Coarse	Good	Bruising
Pallor	Thick	Poor	Bleeding
Cyanosis	Thin		Angioma
Jaundice			Petechiae
Flushed			Purpura
			Telangiectasis

Moisture	Temperature
Dry	Cool, <98.6°
Moist	Warm, >98.6°
Normal	Normal

2. Lesions (primary, secondary; see Table II-18)
   - Type   Shape
   - Location   Size
   - Distribution   Drainage
   - Color
3. Circulation
   - Is erythema present?
   - Does the skin blanch when pressure is applied?
   - Does erythema subside within 30 minutes after pressure is removed?
4. Edema
   - Note degree and location
   - Palpate over bony prominences for sponginess (indicates edema)
5. Oral mucous membrane
   - Refer to Focus Assessment for *Altered Oral Mucous Membrane* category

Principles and Rationale for Nursing Care

Tissue Physiology

1. Tissues are groupings of specialized cells that unite to perform specific functions. The human body is composed of four basic types of tissue: epithelial, connective tissue (including skeletal tissue and blood), muscle, and nervous tissue.
2. The epithelial tissue is a continuous layer of cells that either covers an outside body surface or lines an inside lumen or cavity. Epithelial tissue is classified by numbers of layers (simple—single layer; stratified—more than one layer) and by shapes of the surface cells (squamous, or flat; cuboidal, or cubes; columnar, or tall columns). All communication between the body and the outside world is through the epithelium. Under favorable conditions, the regeneration of epithelial tissue occurs rapidly by a process called epithelialization.
3. Connective tissue is the supporting, binding, and wrapping tissue of the body. It has few living cells and contains a great deal of nonliving intercellular material.

* Dark or black skin should be assessed in good light (daytime preferred). Palpation is usually more beneficial than observation. Borders of rashes can be felt and the skin surface can indicate increased warmth (inflammation) and tautness (edema) when palpated.

Table II-18.   **Primary and Secondary Lesions**

Primary	Secondary
Macules Circumscribed, flat discolorations of the skin Examples: freckles, flat nevi	**Scales** Dead epidermal cells that thicken and flake off Examples: dandruff, psoriasis
Papules Circumscribed, elevated, superficial, solid lesions that are smaller than 1 cm Examples: elevated nevi, warts	**Crusts** Dried exudate on the surface of the skin produced when skin is damaged Examples: impetigo, infected dermatitis
Nodules Solid elevation, usually greater than 1 cm in diameter, extend deeper into dermis than papules Examples: epitheliomas	**Fissures** Linear breaks in the tissue, sharply defined with abrupt walls Example: congenital syphilis, athlete's foot
Tumors Larger-than-1-cm, solid lesions with depth; they may be above, level with, or beneath the skin Example: tumor stage of mycosis fungoides	**Erosion** Loss of epidermis that does not extend into the dermis Example: abrasion
Plaques Circumscribed, elevated, superficial, solid lesions that are larger than 1 cm Examples: localized mycosis fungoides, neurodermatitis	**Ulcers** Localized areas of tissue destruction that may extend into the mucous membrane or through the epidermis, dermis, and underlying tissue Examples: venous ulcers of the legs, tertiary syphilis
Wheals Types of plaques; result is transient edema in dermis	**Scars** Formations of connective tissue replacing tissue lost through injury or disease Example: keloids
Vesicles Up-to-1-cm, circumscribed elevations of the skin or mucous membrane containing serous fluid Examples: early chickenpox, contact dermatitis	
Bullae Larger-than-1-cm, circumscribed elevations containing serous fluid Examples: pemphigus, second-degree burns	

Connective tissue is classified according to intercellular material (a gelatin-type ground substance and collagen, elastin, and reticular fibers) and by types of cells (fibroblasts, macrophages, reticular cells, mast cells, plasma cells, leukocytes, fat cells, and pigment cells). Connective tissue is found throughout the body as adipose tissue, ligaments, and loose or dense connective tissue. The fibroblasts of loose connective tissue reproduce rapidly, which aids in the healing of defects in other tissue that has less power to regenerate.

4. Muscle tissue is classified into three categories: involuntary, voluntary, and cardiac. Involuntary or smooth muscle tissue is found in muscles of internal organs, the gastrointestinal tract, the respiratory tract, the genitourinary tract, the lymphatics and blood vessels, and the pupils of the eye. Voluntary or striated muscle tissue is found in the body wall and extremities. Cardiac muscle tissue is found in the heart

wall and in portions of the pulmonary vein. Regeneration of muscle tissue takes place mainly by scar tissue formation.

5. Nervous tissue is found in the brain, spinal cord, and nerves throughout the body. Nervous tissue has the ability to transmit important information by way of chemical and electrical messages. Nerve cells do not regenerate by mitosis, but they do grow axons.

6. The external covering of the body is composed of epithelial tissue called the integument. Wherever the body exposes large openings to the outside, its outer covering changes from integument to an inner lining called mucous membrane, *e.g.*, mouth. Each layer of the integument has its counterpart in a complete mucous membrane. The integument includes both the skin and the subcutaneous tissue.

7. The skin is a complex organ consisting of two layers: the outer epidermis and the deeper dermis. The epidermis is approximately 0.04 mm thick, and the dermis is about 0.5 cm thick.

8. The epidermis functions as a barrier to protect inner tissues (from injury, chemicals, organisms); as a receptor for a range of sensations (touch, pain, heat, cold); as a regulator of body temperature through radiation (giving off heat), conduction (transfer of heat), and convection (movement of warm air molecules away from the body); as a regulator of water balance by preventing water and electrolyte loss; and as a receptor for vitamin D from the sun.

9. Essentially avascular, the multiple layers of epidermal cells progressively die as they reach the surface. Homeostasis of the skin surface is dependent on equilibrium between cell production and renewal, and cell destruction or loss.

10. Epidermal regeneration is depressed by a water-soluble mitotic inhibitor called chalone. Chalone levels are high during daytime stress and activity and lower during sleep. Healing is therefore promoted during rest and sleep.

11. Beneath the avascular epidermis lies the highly vascularized dermis. The dermis contains epithelial tissue, connective tissue, muscle, and nervous tissue. The dermis is rich in collagen, which imparts toughness to the skin. Hair follicles extend into the dermis and serve as islands of cells for rapid reepithelization of minor wounds. Sweat glands in the dermis contribute to control of body water and temperature. Small muscles within the dermis serve to produce goose pimples. Specialized dermal nerve endings for pain, touch, heat, and cold are irreplaceable once destroyed.

12. The subcutaneous tissue, which lies beneath the dermis, stores fat for temperature regulation and contains the remainder of the sweat glands and hair follicles.

13. Complex interactions between the dermis and epidermis carry messages to one another in case of injury requiring repair.

14. The skin's responses to antigens are capillary dilation (erythema), arteriole dilation (flare), and increased capillary permeability (wheal), which all contribute to localized edema, spasms, and pruritus.

15. Application of heat causes local vasodilation, which promotes healing but increases pruritus and edema.

16. Application of cold causes local vasoconstriction, which decreases edema and pruritus but retards healing.

17. Skin lesions can be described as primary or secondary. Primary lesions are the initial responses of the skin to an irritant. Secondary lesions result from changes that take place in primary lesions (see Table II-18).

18. Causes of tissue destruction can be mechanical, immunological, bacterial, chemical, and thermal. Mechanical destruction includes physical trauma or surgical incision. Immunological destruction occurs as an allergic response to an antigen. Bacterial

destruction results from an overgrowth of organisms. Chemical destruction results when a caustic substance maintains contact with unprotected tissue. Thermal destruction occurs when tissue is exposed to temperature extremes that are incompatible with cell life.

Wound Healing of Damaged Tissue

1. Wound healing is a complex sequence of events initiated by injury to the tissues. The components of wound healing are coagulation of bleeding, inflammation, epithelialization, fibroplasia and collagen metabolism, collagen maturation and scar remodeling, and wound contraction.
2. A wound must be considered in relation to the entire person. Major factors that affect wound healing are nutrition, vitamins, minerals, anemia, blood volume and tissue oxygenation, steroids and anti-inflammatory drugs, diabetes mellitus, chemotherapy, and radiation.
3. Wound healing requires the following intrinsic factors (Constantian):

    Increased protein–carbohydrate intake sufficient to prevent negative nitrogen balance, hypoalbuminemia, and weight loss

    Increased daily intake of vitamins and minerals

    Vitamin A, 10,000 IU to 50,000 IU

    Vitamin B_1, 0.5 mg to 1.0 mg per 1,000 diet calories

    Vitamin B_2, 0.25 mg per 1,000 diet calories

    Vitamin B_6, 2 mg

    Niacin, 15 mg to 20 mg

    Vitamin B_{12}, 400 mg

    Vitamin C, 75 mg to 300 mg

    Vitamin D, 400 mg

    Vitamin E, 10 IU to 15 IU

    Traces of zinc, magnesium, calcium, copper, manganese

    Adequate oxygen supply and the blood volume and ability to transport it
4. Wound healing occurs most efficiently with the following extrinsic factors:
    a. Humidity has been shown to affect the rate of epithelization and the amount of scar formation. A moist environment provides the optimum conditions for rapid healing.
    b. When wounds are left uncovered, epidermal cells must migrate under the scab and over the fibrous tissue below. When wounds are semi-occluded and the surface of the wound remains moist, epidermal cells migrate more rapidly over the surface.
    c. Moist wound healing may be promoted with the appropriate use of dressings. Wounds that are epidermal or dermal in depth may be mechanically protected and properly humidified by the use of semi-occlusive film dressings or hydrophilic barrier wafers. These dressings bathe the wound in serous exudate and do not adhere to the wound surface when they are removed. A physician's order may be required.

Impaired Tissue Integrity
Related to Mechanical Destruction

Assessment

Subjective
The person reports discomfort from physical trauma

Objective
Tissue deficits
- Drain site
- Ulcer
- Abrasion
- Erosion
- Laceration
- Avulsion

- Erythema
- Edema
- Inflammation
- Induration
- Drainage
- Necrosis

Mechanical factors
- Pressure
- Friction
- Shear
- Excessive moisture

Outcome Criteria

The person will
- Identify cause of mechanical tissue destruction
- Identify rationale for treatment
- Participate in plan to promote wound healing
- Demonstrate progressive healing of tissue

Interventions

A. Identify causative/contributing factors

Removal of adhesives
Pressure dressings
Nasogastric tubes
Endotracheal tubes
Skeletal prominences with little overlying soft tissue
Hard supporting sleep or sitting surfaces
Prolonged sitting or lying in same position
Dragging across bed linens
Sitting in Fowler's position
Bladder and bowel incontinence
Profuse diaphoresis
Cognitive, sensory, motor deficits

Fixation devices
 Skeletal traction
 Oral prostheses
Contact lens wear

B. Eliminate or reduce causative factors if possible

1. Assess for risk of mechanical tissue destruction
2. Encourage highest degree of mobility to avoid prolonged periods of pressure
3. For neuromuscular impairment
   - Teach patient/significant other appropriate measures to prevent pressure, shear, friction, maceration
   - Teach to recognize early signs of tissue damage
   - Change position at least every 2 hours around the clock
   - Frequently supplement full body turns with minor shifts in body weight
4. Keep patient clean and dry
5. Reduce environmental sources of pressure (drains, tubes, dressings)
6. Avoid stripping of epidermis when removing adhesives
7. Use pressure-dispersing devices as appropriate
8. Limit Fowler's position in high-risk patients
9. Avoid use of knee gatch on bed
10. Use lift sheet to reposition patient
11. Install overhead trapeze to allow patient increased mobility
12. Use sheepskin pad to reduce friction
See *Impaired Skin Integrity* for further interventions

Impaired Tissue Integrity
Related to Chemical Destruction

Assessment

Subjective Data
The person reports itching, burning pain from chemical trauma

Objective Data
Tissue deficits

Burn	Ulcer
Blister	Erythema
Excoriation	Inflammation
Erosion	Edema
Stoma	Drainage
Fistula	Exudate
Abscess	Necrosis

Chemical factors

Excretions	Body soap
Secretions	Mouth wash

Chemical irritant
Topical medication
Chemotherapy

Dental adhesive
Contact lens solution
Eye drops

Outcome Criteria

The person will
- Identify cause of chemical tissue destruction
- Identify rationale for treatment
- Participate in plan to promote wound healing
- Demonstrate progressive healing of tissue

Interventions

A. Identify causative/contributing factors

Uncontrolled fecal or urinary incontinence
Poorly fitting ostomy appliances resulting in peristomal excoriation
Uncontained draining fistulas or ulcers
Use of caustic topical solutions
Use of harsh soaps or mouth wash
Ingestion of acidic foods or fluids
Use of ophthalmic drops or solution
Chemotherapy—see *Altered Oral Mucous Membrane* for specific interventions

B. Eliminate or reduce causative factors if possible

1. Assess for risk of chemical tissue destruction
2. Devise method to contain bowel or bladder incontinence. See *Altered Patterns of Urinary Elimination* and *Altered Bowel Elimination* for specific interventions
3. Teach correct application of stoma pouch. See *Altered Health Maintenance Related to Lack of Knowledge of Ostomy Care* for specific interventions
4. Use stoma pouching techniques to contain drainage from fistulas/ulcers
5. Teach safe use of topical solutions; teach to test small amount of new product on inner aspect of arm
6. Recommend mild soaps that do not alter skin pH
7. Recommend saline mouth washes
8. Follow intake of acidic food or fluid with several glasses of water
9. Refer drug reactions to physician; stop use immediately if untoward effects occur
10. Teach use of protective gloves/clothing when using chemical products in occupational setting

Skin Integrity, Impaired

Related to **Immobility: Potential**

Related to **Pressure, Shear, Friction, Maceration**

Definition

Impaired skin integrity: A state in which the individual experiences or is at risk for damage to the epidermal and dermal tissue.

Defining Characteristics

Major (must be present)

Disruptions of epidermal and dermal tissue

Minor (may be present)

Denuded skin
Erythema
Lesions (primary, secondary)
Pruritus

Etiological, Contributing, Risk Factors

See *Impaired Tissue Integrity*

Focus Assessment Criteria

See *Impaired Tissue Integrity*

Principles and Rationale for Nursing Care

(See also *Impaired Tissue Integrity*)

1. Pressure is a compressing force on a given area. If pressure against soft tissue is greater than intracapillary blood pressure (approximately 32 mm Hg), the capillaries will be occluded, and the tissue will be damaged as a result of hypoxia.
2. Shear is a mechanism by which one layer of tissue moves in one direction and another layer moves in the opposite direction. If the skin sticks to the bed linen and the weight of the sitting body makes the skeleton slide down inside the skin, the subepidermal capillaries may become angulated and pinched resulting in decreased perfusion of the tissue.
3. Friction is the physiologic wearing away of tissue. If the skin is rubbed against the bed linens, the epidermis can be denuded by abrasion.
4. Maceration is a mechanism by which the tissue is softened by prolonged wetting or soaking. If the skin becomes waterlogged, the epidermis is easily eroded.
5. Pressure relief is the one consistent intervention that must be included in all pressure ulcer treatment plans.
6. The choice of products to relieve pressure is best made by actually measuring the

tissue interface pressure between a bony prominence and an external supporting surface. A product should reduce the external pressure below the amount of pressure required to keep the capillaries open. A pressure-relieving surface must not be able to be fully compressed by the body. In order to be effective, a support surface must be capable of first being deformed and then redistributing the weight of the body across the surface. Comfort is not a valid criterion for determining adequate pressure relief.

Potential Impaired Skin Integrity
Related to Immobility

Assessment

Subjective Data
The person reports fatigue, discomfort over bony prominence, inability to move or turn

Objective Data
Imposed bed rest or immobility
Contributing factors
    Skin deficits
    Impaired oxygen transport
    Nutritional deficit
    Cognitive deficits
    Motor deficits
    Sensory deficits
    Irritants
    Bowel or bladder incontinence

Outcome Criteria

The person will
- Express willingness to participate in prevention of pressure ulcers
- Describe etiology and prevention measures
- Explain rationale for interventions
- Demonstrate skin integrity free of pressure ulcers

Interventions

A. Identify persons who are at risk for developing pressure ulcers
    Assess for
        Skin deficits
            Dryness
            Edema
            Obesity
            Thinness
            Excessive perspiration

   Impaired oxygen transport
      Edema
      Anemia
      Peripheral vascular disorders
      Arteriosclerosis
      Cardiopulmonary disorders
   Chemical/mechanical/thermal irritants
      Radiation
      Incontinence (feces, urine)
      Casts, splints, braces
      Spasms
   Nutritional deficits
      Protein deficiencies
      Vitamin deficiencies
      Mineral deficiencies
      Dehydration
   Systemic disorders
      Infection
      Diabetes mellitus
      Cancer
      Hepatic or renal disorders
   Sensory deficits
      Neuropathy
      Confusion
      Head injury
      Cord injury
   Immobility

B. Attempt to reduce contributing factors in order to lessen the possibility of development of a pressure ulcer
1. Incontinence of urine or feces
   • Maintain sufficient fluid intake for adequate hydration (approximately 2500 ml daily, unless contraindicated); check mucous membranes in mouth for moisture and check urine specific gravity
   • Establish a schedule for emptying bladder (begin with q 2 hr)
   • If person is confused, determine what his incontinence pattern is and intervene before incontinence occurs
   • Explain problem to individual and secure cooperation for plan
   • When incontinent, wash perineum with a liquid soap that will not alter skin pH
   • Apply a protective barrier to the perineal region (incontinence film barrier spray or wipes)
   • Check person frequently for incontinence when indicated
   • For additional interventions, refer to *Altered Patterns of Urinary Elimination*
2. Immobility
   a. Encourage range-of-motion exercise and weight-bearing mobility, when possible, to increase blood flow to all areas
   b. Promote optimal circulation when in bed
      • Utilize repositioning schedule that relieves vulnerable area most often (*e.g.,* if vulnerable area is the back, turning schedule would be left side to back, back to right side, right side to left side, and left side to back); post "turn clock" at bedside

- Turn person or instruct him to turn or shift weight every 30 minutes to 2 hours, depending on other causative factors present and the ability of the skin to recover from pressure
- Frequency of turning schedule should be increased if any reddened areas that appear do not disappear within 1 hour after turning
- Position person in normal or neutral position with body weight evenly distributed (see Fig. II-4)
- Keep bed as flat as possible to reduce shearing forces; limit Fowler's position to only 30 minutes at a time
- Use foam blocks or pillows to provide a bridging effect to support the body above and below the high-risk or ulcerated area so that affected area does not touch bed surface. Do not use foam donuts or inflatable rings, since this will increase the area of pressure
- Alternate or reduce the pressure on the skin surface with:
  Foam mattresses
  Air mattresses
  Air fluidized beds
  Vascular boots to suspend heels
  c. Utilize enough personnel to lift person up in bed or chair rather than pull or slide skin surfaces. Have patient wear long-sleeved top and socks to reduce friction on elbows and heels.
  d. To reduce shearing forces, support feet with footboard to prevent sliding
  e. Promote optimum circulation when person is sitting
- Limit sitting time for person at high risk for ulcer development
- Instruct person to lift self using chair arms every 10 minutes if possible or assit person in rising up off the chair every 10 to 20 minutes, depending on risk factors present
- Do not elevate legs unless calves are supported, to reduce the pressure over the ischial tuberosities
- Pad chair with pressure-relieving device
  f. Inspect areas at risk of developing ulcers with each position change
  Ears
  Occiput
  Heels*
  Sacrum
  Scrotum
  Elbows
  Trochanter*
  Ischia
  Scapula
  g. Observe for erythema and blanching and palpate for warmth and tissue sponginess with each position change
  h. Use gentle massage over vulnerable areas with each position change. To avoid damaging the capillaries avoid deep massage.
3. Malnourished state
- Increase protein and carbohydrate intake to maintain a positive nitrogen balance; weigh the person daily and determine serum albumin level weekly to monitor status

---

*Areas with little soft tissue over a bony prominence are at greatest risk.

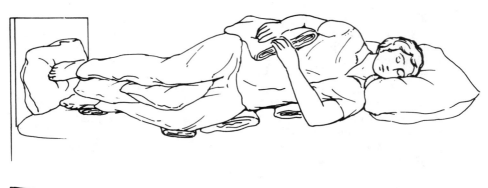

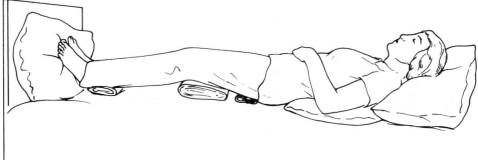

Fig. II-4   Positioning. (*Top*) Side-lying position. Pads are used above and below the trochanter and lateral malleolus to relieve pressure. (*Bottom*) Supine position. Pads are used above and below the sacrum and above the heels to relieve pressure. A pad above the knees prevents hyperextension of the knees and relieves pressure on the popliteal space.

- Ascertain that daily intake of vitamins and minerals is maintained through diet or supplements (see Principles for recommended amounts)
- See *Altered Nutrition: Less Than Body Requirements* for additional interventions
4. Sensory deficit
  - Inspect person's skin every 2 hours, since he will not experience discomfort
  - Teach person or family to inspect skin with mirror

C. Initiate health teaching as indicated
  - Instruct person and family in specific techniques to utilize at home to prevent pressure ulcers
  - Investigate use of long-term pressure-relieving devices for permanent disabilities

---

Impaired Skin Integrity
Related to Pressure, Friction, Shear, Maceration

This nursing diagnosis describes a dermal ulcer as an area of cellular necrosis (due to tissue hypoxia) resulting from pressure, friction, shear, or maceration.

Assessment

Subjective Data
The person may report no discomfort or may report pain or numbness

Objective Data
The following signs may be noted over a bony prominence (sacrum, heel) or under a cast or brace
Erythema
Elevated skin temperature
Reactive hyperemia
Blanching on pressure
Ulcer
Blister
Drainage
Tissue erosion
Tissue sponginess

Outcome Criteria

The person will
- Identify causative factors for pressure ulcers
- Identify rationale for prevention and treatment
- Participate in the prescribed treatment plan to promote wound healing
- Demonstrate progressive healing of dermal ulcer

Interventions
1. Identify the stage of pressure ulcer development
   Stage I: Nonblanchable erythema or ulceration limited to epidermis
   Stage II: Ulceration of dermis not involving underlying subcutaneous fat
   Stage III: Ulceration involving subcutaneous fat
   Stage IV: Extensive ulceration penetrating muscle and bone
2. Reduce or eliminate factors that contribute to the development or extension of pressure ulcers
   - Refer to *Potential Impaired Skin Integrity Related to Immobility*
3. Prevent extension of the ulcer in stages I, II, and III
   a. Wash reddened area gently with a mild soap, rinse area thoroughly to remove soap, and pat dry
   b. Gently massage healthy skin around the affected area to stimulate circulation; do not massage reddened area
   c. Protect the healthy skin surface with one or a combination of the following
      - Apply a thin coat of liquid copolymer skin sealant
      - Cover area with moisture-permeable film dressing
      - Cover area with a hydroactive wafer barrier and secure with strips of 1-inch microscope tape; leave in place for 4 to 5 days
   d. Increase dietary intake to promote wound healing
      - Initiate calorie count
      - Increase protein and carbohydrate intake to maintain a positive nitrogen

balance: weigh the person daily and determine serum albumin level weekly to monitor status

- Ascertain that daily intake of vitamins and minerals is maintained through diet or supplements (see Principles for recommended amounts)
- See *Altered Nutrition: Less Than Body Requirements* for additional interventions

4. Devise plan for pressure ulcer management using principles of moist wound healing
   - Assess status of pressure ulcer. Measure size of wound bed for baseline data. Assess color, odor and amount of drainage from wound. Also assess color of skin surrounding wound bed.
   - Debride necrotic tissue (collaborate with physician)
   - Flush ulcer base with sterile saline solution. Avoid use of harsh antiseptic solutions.
   - Protect granulating wound bed
   - Cover pressure ulcer with a sterile dressing that maintains a moist environment over the ulcer base (*e.g.,* film dressing, hydroactive wafer dressing, moist gauze dressing)
   - Avoid the use of drying agents (heat lamps, Maalox, Milk of Magnesia)
   - Monitor for clinical signs of wound infection
   - Measure pressure ulcer weekly to determine progress of wound healing
5. Consult with nurse specialist or physician for treatment of stage IV pressure ulcers
6. Initiate health teaching and referrals as indicated
   - Instruct person and family on care of ulcers
   - Teach the importance of good skin hygiene and optimum nutrition
   - Refer to community nursing agency if additional assistance at home is needed

Oral Mucous Membrane, Altered

Related to **Inadequate or Inability to Perform Oral Hygiene**
Related to **(Specify) as Manifested by Stomatitis**

Definition
Altered oral mucous membrane: The state in which an individual experiences or is at risk of experiencing disruptions in the oral cavity.

Defining Characteristics

Major (must be present)
Disrupted oral mucous membranes

Minor (may be present)

Coated tongue
Xerostomia (dry mouth)
Stomatitis
Oral tumors
Oral lesions

Leukoplakia
Edema
Hemorrhagic gingivitis
Purulent drainage

Etiological, Contributing, Risk Factors

Pathophysiological

Diabetes mellitus
Oral cancer
Periodontal disease
Infection
Herpes simplex

Gingivitis

Treatment-related

NPO >24 hours
Radiation to head or neck
Prolonged use of steroids or other immunosuppressives
Antineoplastic drugs
Endotracheal tube
Nasogastric tube

Situational (personal, environmental)

Chemical trauma
Acidic foods
Drugs
Noxious agents
Mechanical trauma
Broken or jagged teeth
Ill-fitting dentures
Braces
Malnutrition
Dehydration
Mouth breathing
Inadequate oral hygiene
Lack of knowledge
Fractured mandible

Alcohol
Tobacco

Focus Assessment Criteria

Subjective Data

1. The person complains of
    Mouth pain, irritation, or burning
    Xerostomia (dry mouth)
    Bad taste or odor in mouth
    Chewing difficulties
    Change in tolerance to temperatures of food (cold, hot)
    Change in tolerance to acidic or highly seasoned food
    Change in taste
    Poorly fitting dentures

2. History
>   Medical/surgical
>   Medication use (prescribed, over the counter)
>   Use of tobacco
>>   Type (cigarettes, pipe, cigars, snuff)
>>   Frequency (packs per day, how many years)
>   Use of alcohol
>>   Type
>>   Amount (daily, weekly)

3. Oral hygiene
>   Frequency of dental checkups
>   Personal hygiene
>>   "Describe your oral care procedure"
>>   Type of equipment (brush, floss)
>>   Frequency
>   Possible barriers to performing oral care
>>   Unable to hold standard brush
>>   Unable to close hand
>>   Limited arm movement
>>   Semicomatose
>>   Lack of knowledge

4. Nutritional status (refer to *Altered Nutrition* for specific assessment crtieria)
>   Daily intake of basic four food groups
>   Daily fluid intake
>   Difficulty in chewing or swallowing
>   Are certain foods avoided? Why?

Objective Data

1. Lips
>   Color
>   Presence of

Cracks	Blisters
Fissures	Ulcers/lesions

2. Tongue
>   Color
>   Presence of

Masses	Cracks, dryness
Lesions	Exudates
Hairy extensions	

3. Oral mucosa (gums, floor of mouth, inner cheeks, palate)
>   Color
>   Presence of

Bleeding	Plaques
Swelling	Lesions

4. Teeth
>   Presence of

Sharp edges	Looseness
Chips	Missing teeth
Cracks	

5. Dentures/prosthetics
>   Condition
>   Fit

Presence of
Sharp edges   Cracks
Loose parts   Chips

Principles and Rationale for Nursing Care

1. Oral health directly influences many activities of daily living (eating, fluid intake, breathing) and interpersonal relations (appearance, self-concept, communication).
2. The frequency of oral health maintenance will vary according to an individual's health status and self-care ability. All persons should have their teeth and mouths cleaned at least once after meals and at bedtime. High-risk persons (*e.g.,* persons with cancer and poorly nourished persons) should have oral assessments daily. Persons in chronic care settings should have oral assessment *at least* once a month.
3. Factors that contribute to oral disease are alcohol and tobacco (excessive use), microorganisms, inadequate nutrition (quantity, quality), inadequate hygiene, and trauma (ill-fitting dentures, sharp-edged teeth, sharp-edged prostheses, improper use of cleaning devices).
4. Many oral diseases begin quietly and are painless until significant involvement has taken place.
5. Plaque is microbial flora found in the mouth and is the primary factor contributing to dental cavities and periodontal disease. Daily removal of plaque through brushing and flossing can help prevent dental decay and disease.
6. Decreased salivary flow and increased viscosity of saliva reduce the removal of debris (food, bacteria) from the mouth.
7. Common causes of decreased salivation are dehydration, anemia, radiation treatment to head and neck, vitamin deficiencies, removal of salivary glands, allergies, and side-effects of drugs (*e.g.,* antihistamines, anticholinergics, phenothiazines, narcotics, chemotherapy).
8. Excessive use of hydrogen peroxide for mouth care may predispose to an oral yeast infection. Rinse afterward with normal saline.
9. Lemon and glycerine swabs should be used only on clean, healthy mouths as a source of refreshment for an NPO client.
10. Alcohol and tobacco are chronic irritants to oral mucosa and may lead to oral carcinoma.

Altered Oral Mucous Membrane
Related to Inadequate or Inability
to Perform Oral Hygiene

Assessment

Subjective Data
The person reports
Does not practice oral hygiene
Cannot perform oral hygiene

Objective Data
Pain
Burning
Coated tongue

Outcome Criteria

The person will
- Demonstrate integrity of the oral cavity
- Be free of harmful plaque to prevent secondary infection
- Be free of oral discomfort during food and fluid intake

Interventions

A. Assess for the presence of causative or contributing factors
Lack of knowledge
Lack of motivation
Impairment of use of hands
Fatigue
Altered consciousness

B. Discuss the importance of daily oral hygiene and periodic dental examinations
- Explain the relationship of plaque to dental and gum disease
- Evaluate the person's ability to perform oral hygiene
- Allow person to perform as much of his oral care as possible

C. Teach correct oral care
1. Have person sit or stand upright over sink (if unable to get to sink, place an emesis pan under the chin)
2. Remove and clean dentures and bridges daily
   - Fill wash bowl half full of water (place washcloth on bottom to keep denture from breaking if dropped)
   - Brush dentures with a denture brush or stiff hard toothbrush inside and outside; rinse in cool water before replacing
   - Stains and odors can be removed from dentures by soaking them overnight in 8 oz of water and 1 teaspoon of laundry bleach (avoid bleach on any appliance with metal)
   - Hard deposits can be removed by soaking dentures in white (not brown) vinegar overnight
   - If commercial liquid denture cleaners are used, brushing is still required
3. Floss teeth (q 24 hr)
   - With a piece of dental floss approximately 25 inches long, floss each tooth by wrapping the floss around the second and third fingers of each hand
   - Beginning with the back teeth, insert the floss between each tooth gently to prevent injuring the gum
   - Wrap floss around tooth, making a C, and gently pull floss up and down over the back of each tooth
   - Repeat this in reverse to floss the front of the tooth

- Remove the floss by either pulling straight up or by releasing one end and pulling the floss through (minor bleeding may occur)
- Allow the person to rinse
- Floss holders can be used by the person or the nurse to make flossing easier (back teeth cannot be reached with a floss holder)

4. Brush teeth (after meals and before sleep)
   - Use a soft toothbrush (avoid hard brushes) with a nonabrasive toothpaste or sodium bicarbonate (1 tsp in 8 oz of water; may be contraindicated in persons with sodium restrictions)
   - Brush back and forth or in a small circle, starting at the back of the mouth and brushing one or two teeth at a time
   - Gently brush tongue and inner sides of cheeks
   - Rinse with water

5. Inspect mouth for lesions, sores, or excessive bleeding

D. Perform oral hygiene on person who is unconscious or at risk for aspiration as often as needed

1. Preparation
   - Tell person what you are going to do
   - Turn person on his side, supporting back with pillow (protect bed with an absorbent pad)
   - Place a tongue blade or bite block to keep mouth open
   - Wear gloves to protect hands

2. Brushing procedure
   - For persons with their own teeth, brush following the procedure outlined in Nos. 3 and 4 above
   - Use a solution instead of toothpaste: hydrogen peroxide and water (1 to 4), sodium bicarbonate (1 tsp to 8 oz water), or normal saline solution (may be contraindicated in persons with sodium restrictions)
   - For persons with dentures, remove dentures and clean according to procedure in No. 2
   - Leave dentures out for persons who are semicomatose and store in water (in denture cup)
   - If gums are inflamed, use moist cotton-tipped applicators or soft foam Toothettes
   - Use a bulb syringe to rinse mouth; aspirate rinse with suction or use an aspirating toothbrush
   - Move tongue blade or bite block for access to other areas; do not put fingers on tops or edges of teeth
   - Brush tongue and inner cheek tissue gently
   - Pat mouth dry and apply lip lubricant
   - Gums and teeth should be lightly wiped four to six times a day to prevent drying (*e.g.,* swab with mineral oil or saline but use sparingly to prevent aspiration)

E. Initiate health teaching and referrals as indicated

1. Identify individuals who need toothbrush adaptations to perform own mouth care
   a. Difficulty closing hand tightly
      - Tape a wide elastic band to toothbrush tight enough to hold brush snugly in hand
   b. Limited hand mobility
      - Enlarge toothbrush handle with a sponge hair roller, wrinkled aluminum foil, or a bicycle handbar grip attached with a small amount of plaster of paris

    c. Limited arm movement
- Extend handle of standard toothbrush by attaching handle of an old toothbrush (after cutting off bristle end) to a new toothbrush with strong cord or plastic cement, or by attaching toothbrush to a plastic rod (the toothbrush can be curved by gently heating and then bending it)

2. Refer individuals with tooth and gum disorders to a dentist
3. Teach parents to
- Provide their child with fluoride supplements if not present in concentrations over 0.7 parts per million (ppm) in drinking water
- Avoid taking tetracycline drugs during pregnancy or giving to child during infancy
- Refrain from putting an infant to bed with a bottle of juice or milk
- Provide child with safe objects for chewing during teething
- Replace toothbrushes frequently (q 3 mo)
- Schedule dental checkups every 6 months after the age of 2 years

4. Teach child to
- Avoid highly sugared liquids and foods
- Drink water and extra fluid
- Brush teeth using fluoride toothpaste

Altered Oral Mucous Membrane
Related to (Specify) as Manifested by Stomatitis

Stomatitis is inflammation of the mucous membrane of the mouth, ranging from redness to ulcerations to hemorrhage.

Assessment

Subjective Data

The person reports
    Oral burning or pain
    Change in tolerance to food temperatures (cold, hot)
    Change in tolerance to acidic or highly seasoned food

Objective Data

    Erythema of oral mucosa (mild)
    Small areas of ulcerations or white patches (moderate)
    White patches over 25% of oral mucosa (moderate to severe)
    Hemorrhagic ulcerations (severe)

Outcome Criteria

The person will
- Be free of oral mucosa irritation or exhibit signs of healing with decreaed inflammation
- Demonstrate knowledge of optional oral hygiene

Interventions

A. Assess for the presence of causative or contributing factors

Lack of oral hygiene
Malnourishment
History of high alcohol intake and tobacco use
Chemotherapeutic drugs with mucous membrane toxicity
Radiation to head or neck
Immunosuppression
Dehydration
Steroid therapy

B. Teach individuals at risk to develop stomatitis preventive oral hygiene

1. Refer to *Altered Oral Mucous Membrane Related to Inadequate Oral Hygiene* for specific instructions on brushing and flossing
2. Instruct person to
   - Perform the regimen after meals and before sleep (if there is excessive exudate, perform regimen before breakfast also)
   - Avoid mouthwashes with high alcohol content, lemon/glycerine swabs, or prolonged use of hydrogen peroxide
   - Use an oxidizing agent to loosen thick, tenacious mucous (gargle and expectorate); for example, hydrogen peroxide and water ¼ strength (avoid prolonged use) or sodium bicarbonate 1 tsp in 8 oz warm water (can flavor these with mouthwash or one drop of oil of wintergreen)
   - Rinse mouth with saline solution after gargling
   - Apply lubricant to lips q 2 hr and PRN (*e.g.*, lanolin, A&D ointment, petroleum jelly)
   - Inspect mouth daily for lesions and inflammation and report alterations
3. For person who is unable to tolerate brushing or swabbing, teach to irrigate mouth (q 2 hr and PRN)
   - With baking soda solution (4 tsp in 1 l warm water) using an enema bag (labeled for oral use only) with a soft irrigation catheter tip
   - By placing catheter tip in mouth and slowly increasing flow while standing over a basin or having a basin held under chin
   - Remove dentures prior to irrigation and do not replace in person with severe stomatitis
4. Consult with physician for possible need of prophylactic antifungal or antibacterial agent

C. Promote healing and reduce progression of stomatitis

1. Inspect oral cavity three times daily with tongue blade and light; if stomatitis is severe, inspect mouth q 4 hr
2. Ensure that oral hygiene regimen is done q 2 hr while awake and q 6 hr (q 4 if severe) during the night
3. Use normal saline solution as a mouthwash unless crusts and debris are present; then use
   - Hydrogen peroxide and water ¼ strength; then rinse with saline solution
   - Sodium bicarbonate solute, 1 tsp in 8 oz water; then rinse with water
   - Alternate one of the above q 2 hr with saline rinses
4. Floss teeth only once in 24 hours
5. Omit flossing if excessive bleeding occurs and use extreme caution with persons with platelet counts of less than 50,000

D. Reduce oral pain and maintain adequate food and fluid intake

1. Assess person's ability to chew and swallow
2. Administer mild analgesic q 3–4 hr as ordered by physician
3. Instruct individual to
   - Avoid commercial mouth washes, citrus fruit juices, spicy foods, extremes in food temperature (hot, cold), crusty or rough foods, alcohol, mouth washes with alcohol
   - Eat bland, cool foods (sherbets)
   - Drink cool liquids q 2 hr and PRN
4. Consult with dietitian for specific interventions
5. Refer to *Altered Nutrition: Less Than Body Requirements Related to Anorexia* for additional interventions
6. Consult with physician for an oral pain relief solution
   - Xylocaine Viscous 2% oral swish and expectorant q 2 hr and before meals (if throat is sore, the solution can be swallowed; if swallowed, Xylocaine produces local anesthesia and may affect the gag reflex)
   - Mix equal parts of Xylocaine Viscous, 0.5 aqueous Benadryl solution, and Maalox, swish and swallow 1 oz of mixture q 2–4 hr PRN
   - Mix equal parts of 0.5 aqueous Benadryl solution and Kaopectate; swish and swallow q 2–4 hr PRN

E. Initiate health teaching and referrals as indicated

1. Teach person and family the factors that contribute to the development of stomatitis and its progression
2. Teach diet modifications to reduce oral pain and to maintain optimal nutrition
3. Have individual describe or demonstrate home care regimen

References/Bibliography

Agris J, Spira M: Pressure ulcers: Prevention and treatment. Clinical Symposia (CIBA) 31, 1979

Allman R, Laprade C, Noel L, Walker J, Moorer C, Dear M, Smith C: Pressure sores among hospitalized patients. Ann Intern Med 105(3):337–342, 1986

Bergstron N, Demuth PJ, Braden BJ: A clinical trial of the Braden Scale for predicting pressure sore risk. Nurs Clin North Am 22(2):417–428, 1987

Bergstron N, Braden BJ, Laguzza A, Holman V: The Braden Scale for predicting pressure sore risk. Nurs Res 36(4):205–210, 1987

Bruno P, Craven R: Age challenges to wound healing. J Gerontol Nurs 8(12):686–715, 1982

Constantian MB: Pressure Ulcers: Principles and Techniques of Management. Boston, Little, Brown & Co, 1980

Cooper DM, Watt RC, Alterescu V: Guide to Wound Care. Hollister Incorporated, 1983

David J: Tissue breakdown. Nurs Mirror 158(10)(suppl)i–xvi, 1984

Dossey L: The skin: What is it? In the integument. Top Clin Nurs 5(2)1–4, 1983

Elias H, Pauly JE, Burnes ER: Histology and Human Microanatomy, 4th ed. New York, John Wiley & Sons, 1980

Elliott TM: Pressure ulcerations. Am Fam Physician 25(2):171–180, 1982

Fowler E: Pressure sores: A deadly nuisance. J Gerontol Nurs 8(12):680–685, 1982

Goldstone LA, Goldstone JG: The Norton score: An early warning of pressure sores? J Adv Nurs 7(5):419–426, 1982

Gosnell DJ: Development of an instrument to assess client risk for pressure sores. In Waltz CF, Strickland O, (eds): Measurement of Clinical and Educational Nursing Outcomes: A Compendium of Tools for Research, Education and Practice. New York, Springer, 1987

Hilderly L: Skin care in radiation therapy: A review of the literature. Oncol Nurs Forum 10(1):51–56, 1983

Horsley J: Preventing Decubitus Ulcers. CURN Project. New York, Grune & Stratton, 1981

Humphry JP: Skin. In Broadwell D, Jackson B (eds): Principles of Ostomy Care. St Louis, CV Mosby, 1982

Krouskop TA: A synthesis of the factors that contribute to pressure sore formation. Med Hypotheses 11:255, 1983

Lasanti P: Altered integumentary functioning. In Mahoney EA, Flynn JP (eds): Handbook of Medical–Surgical Nursing, pp 203–228, New York, John Wiley & Sons, 1983

Maklebust JA, Mondoux LC, Sieggreen MY: Pressure relief characteristics of various support surfaces used in prevention and treatment of pressure ulcers. J Enterostom Ther 13(3):85–89, 1986

Maklebust J: Pressure ulcers: Etiology and prevention. Nurs Clin North Am 22(2):359–377, 1987

Maklebust J, Mondoux L, Sieggreen MY: Pressure relief characteristics of various support surfaces used in prevention and treatment of pressure ulcers. J Enterostom Ther 14(3):85–89, 1986

Maklebust J, Sieggreen MY, Mondoux L: Pressure relieving capabilities: A comparison of the SoF-Care cushion and the Clinitron bed. Unpublished.

Maklebust J, Sieggreen MY, Mondoux L, LaPlante J, Lenk D, Singer D, Cameron O: Pressure Ulcer Guidelines: Nursing Diagnoses and Management, 2nd ed. Detroit, Harper Grace Hospitals, 1987

Maklebust J, Brunckhorst L, Craccheolo-Caraway A, Ducharme M, Dundon R, Panfilla R, Parzuchowski J, Sieggreen M, Walthall S: Pressure ulcer incidence in high risk patients managed on a special three layered air cushion. Decubitus: A Compendium of Prevention and Treatment of Pressure Ulcers (in press)

Peacock EE: Wound Repair, 3rd ed. Philadelphia, WB Saunders, 1984

Parish LC, Witkowski JA, Crissey JT: The Decubitus Ulcer. New York, Masson, 1983

Pinchofsky-Devin GD, Kaminski MV: Correlation of pressure sores and nutritional status. J Am Geriatr Soc 34(3):435–440, 1986

Ringsdorf W, Cheraskin E: Vitamin C and human wound healing. Oral Surg 53(3):231–236, 1982

Ross LS: Oral Management of Patients Radiated to the Head and Neck. Detroit, The Oral Cancer Detection Center, Michigan Cancer Foundation, 1982

Rovee DT: Effect of local wound environment on epidermal healing. In Maibach HL, Rovee DT (eds): Epidermal wound healing, Chicago, Year Book Medical Publishers, 1972

Rudolph R, Noe JM: Chronic Problem Wounds. Boston, Little, Brown, & Co, 1983

Sauer G: Manual of Skin Diseases, 4th ed. Philadelphia, JB Lippincott, 1980

Schumann D: The Nature of wound healing. AORN J 35(6):1068–1077, 1982

Sieggreen MY, The healing of physical wounds. Nurs Clin North Am 22(2):439–447, 1987

Smith MD: Cellular growth. In Mahoney EA, Flynn JP (eds): Handbook of Medical–Surgical Nursing, pp 142–143, New York, John Wiley & Sons, 1983

Stotts NA: Predicting pressure ulcers in a surgical population. Heart Lung 17(6):641–647, 1988

Stotts NA, Paul SM: Pressure ulcer development in surgical patients. Decubitus: A Compendium of Prevention and Treatment of Pressure Ulcers 1(3):24–30, 1988

Sutton RL, Waisman M: The Practitioners' Dermatology. Tampa, FL, Medical Books, 1975

Willis J: Extended wear contact lenses and corneal ulcers. In FDA Drug Bulletin, DHHS, FDA, Rockville, MD, 16(1), 1986

Oral Mucous Membrane

Ariaudo A: How frequently must patients carry out effective oral hygiene procedures in order to maintain gingival health? J Periodontol 42(2):309–313, 1971

Beck S: Impact of a systematic oral care protocol on stomatitis after chemotherapy. Cancer Nursing 2:185–199, 1979

Bennett J: Oral health maintenance. In Carnevali D, Patrick M (eds): Nursing Management for the Elderly, pp 111–135. Philadelphia, JB Lippincott, 1981

Bruya M, Maderia N: Stomatitis after chemotherapy. Am J Nurs 75(8):1349–1352, 1975

Daeffler R: Oral hygiene measures for patients with cancer. Cancer Nursing 3(10):347–355, 1980; 3(12):427–432, 1980, 4(2):29–36, 1981

DeWalt E: Effect of timed hygienic measures on oral mucosa in a group of elderly subjects. Nurs Res 24(2):104–108, 1975

DeWalt E, Haines S: Effects of specified stressors on healthy oral mucosa. Nurs Res 18:22–27, 1969

Kloch J, Seidduth A: Oral hygiene instruction and plaque formation during hospitalization. Nurs Res 18:124–130, 1969

Lovelock DJ: Oral hygiene for patients in hospitals. Nursing Mirror 61(6):39–42, 1973

O'Leary TJ: Oral hygiene agents and procedures. J Periodontol 41:625–629, 1970

Passos J, Brand L: Effects of agents for oral hygiene. Nurs Res 15:196–202, 1966

Reitz M, Pope W: Mouth care. Am J Nurs 73:1728–1730, 1973

Schweiger J, Lang JW, Schweiger JW et al: Oral assessment: How to do it. Am J Nurs 80:654–657, 1980

Wiley S: Why lemon and glycerol? Am J Nurs 69:342–348, 1969

Ross LS: Oral Management of Patients Radiated to the Head and Neck. Detroit, The Oral Cancer Detection Center, Michigan Cancer Foundation, 1982

Tissue Perfusion, Altered (Specify)
(Renal, cerebral, cardiopulmonary, gastrointestinal, peripheral)

Tissue Perfusion, Altered Peripheral*

Related to **(Specify)**

Tissue Perfusion, Altered (Specify)
(Renal, cerebral, cardiopulmonary, gastrointestinal, peripheral)

Definitions

Altered tissue perfusion: The state in which the individual experiences or is at risk of experiencing a decrease in nutrition and respiration at the cellular level due to a decrease in capillary blood supply.

Author's Note: This diagnostic category is restricted in use to represent only diminished peripheral tissue perfusion situations in which nursing prescribes definitive treatment to reduce, eliminate, or prevent the problem. In the other situations of diminished cardiopulmonary, cerebral, renal, or gastrointestinal tissue perfusion, the nurse should focus on the functional abilities of the individual that are or may be compromised because of decreased tissue perfusion. The nurse should also monitor to detect for physiological complications of the decreased tissue perfusion and label these situations as collaborative problems. The following are

(Continued)

---

* Tissue perfusion is dependent upon many physical and physiological factors within the systems of the body and in the structures and functions of the cells. When an alteration in peripheral tissue perfusion exists, the nurse must take into account the nature of the alteration in perfusion. The two major components of the peripheral vascular system are the arterial and the venous systems. Signs, symptoms, etiology, and nursing interventions are different for problems occurring in each of these two systems and are therefore addressed separately when appropriate.

examples of a compromised functional health problem (nursing diagnosis) and a potential complication (collaborative problem) for an individual with compromised cerebral tissue perfusion:

Potential for Injury Related to Vertigo Secondary to Recent Head Injury (nursing diagnosis)

Potential Complication: increased intracranial pressure (collaborative problem) Refer to Chapter 2 for additional information on collaborative problems. For additional examples of nursing diagnoses and collaborative problems grouped under medical conditions refer to Carpenito LJ: Handbook of Nursing Diagnosis, 3rd ed. Philadelphia, JB Lippincott, 1989.

Tissue Perfusion, Altered Peripheral

Related to **(Specify)**

Definition

Altered peripheral tissue perfusion: The state in which an individual experiences or is at risk of experiencing a decrease in nutrition and respiration at the peripheral cellular level due to a decrease in capillary blood supply.

Defining Characteristics

Major (must be present)

Presence of one of the following types (see Principles for definitions):
  Claudication
  Rest pain
  Aching pain
Diminished or absent arterial pulses
Skin color changes
  Pallor (arterial)
  Cyanosis (venous)
  Reactive hyperemia (arterial)
Skin temperature changes
  Cooler (arterial)
  Warmer (venous)
Decreased blood pressure changes (arterial)
Capillary refill less than 3 seconds (arterial)

Minor (may be present)

Edema (venous)
Loss of sensory function (arterial)
Loss of motor function (arterial)

Tropic tissue changes (arterial)
Hard, thick nails
Loss of hair
Lack of lanugo (newborn)

Etiological, Contributing, Risk Factors

Pathophysiological

Vascular disorders

Arteriosclerosis	Leriche's syndrome
Hypertension	Raynaud's disease/syndrome
Aneurysm	Varicosities
Arterial thrombosis	Buerger's disease
Deep vein thrombosis	Sickle cell crisis
Collagen vascular disease	Cirrhosis
Rheumatoid arthritis	Alcoholism

Diabetes mellitus
Hypotension
Sympathetic stress response (vasospasm/vasoconstriction)
Blood dyscrasias (platelet disorders)
Renal failure
Cancer/tumor

Treatment-related

Immobilization
Presence of invasive lines
Pressure sites/constriction (Ace bandages, stockings)
Medications (diuretics, tranquilizers, anticoagulants)
Anesthesia
Blood vessel trauma or compression

Situational (personal, environmental)

Pregnancy
Heredity
Obesity
Diet (hyperlipidemia)
Anorexia/malnutrition
Dehydration
Dependent venous pooling
Hypothermia
Frequent exposure to vibrating tools/equipment
Tobacco use
Exercise

Maturational

Neonate
Immature peripheral circulation
Rh incompatibility (erythroblastosis fetalis)
Hypothermia
Elderly
Sensory–perceptual changes

Atherosclerotic plaques
Capillary fragility

Principles and Rationale for Nursing Care

Blood Pressure

1. Blood pressure (necessary for tissue perfusion) is dependent upon two factors: the force of the flow of blood (cardiac output), and the diameter of the blood vessel.
2. Blood pressure is affected by the sympathetic and parasympathetic nervous systems. The *sympathetic nervous system increases blood pressure* by increasing heart rate and ventricular contraction (thereby increasing cardiac output and increasing the force of blood flow) and by controlling the diameter of the arterioles and resistance of blood vessels (*i.e.,* blood vessel constriction). The *parasympathetic nervous system decreases blood pressure* by relaxation of the vessel walls and by vagal stimulation, causing a decreased heart rate (thereby decreasing cardiac output and decreasing the force of blood flow).
3. Blood pressure is dependent upon adequate circulating blood volume (*i.e.,* dehydration predisposes one to hypotension).
4. Constricted vessels cause a rise in blood pressure, while dilated vessels cause a drop in blood pressure.
5. *Systolic blood pressure* is dependent upon cardiac stroke volume (pressure within the vessels while the heart is contracting).
6. *Diastolic blood pressure* is dependent upon the condition of the vessels while the heart is at rest (vessel resistance).

Cellular Perfusion

1. Cellular nutrition and respiration are dependent on adequate blood flow through the microcirculation.
2. Adequate cellular oxygenation is dependent upon the following processes:
   The ability of the lungs to exchange air adequately (O_2–CO_2)
   The ability of the pulmonary alveoli to diffuse oxygen and carbon dioxide across the cell membrane to the blood
   The ability of the red blood cells (hemoglobin) to carry oxygen
   The ability of the heart to pump with enough force to deliver the blood to the microcirculation
   The ability of intact blood vessels to deliver blood to the microcirculation
3. Hypoxemia (decreased oxygen content of the blood) results in cellular hypoxia, which causes cellular swelling and contributes to tissue injury.
4. Obstruction of blood flow can be a result of
   Clot formation (thrombus)
   Embolus (air, fat, thrombi, other)
   Blood vessel injury (*e.g.,* trauma)
   Pressure upon the vessels (*e.g.,* tourniquet, edema)
   Structural changes in the vessels (*e.g.,* arteriovascular disease)
   Vasospasm
5. *Arterial* blood flow is enhanced by a *dependent* position and inhibited by an *elevated* position (gravity pulls blood downward, away from the heart).
6. *Venous* blood flow is enhanced by an *elevated* position and inhibited by a *dependent* position (gravity pulls blood downward toward the heart).
7. Immobility and venous stasis predispose one to thrombus and embolus production.

Focus Assessment Criteria
(See Tables II-18 and II-19)

Subjective Data
1. Symptoms
   Pain
   Temperature change
   Paresthesias
2. Medical history
   See Etiological, Contributing, Risk Factors
3. Risk factors
   Smoking
   Immobility
   Sedentary life-style
   Family history for heart disease, peripheral vascular disease, stroke, kidney disease
       or diabetes mellitus
   Stress (type A personality)
4. Medications
   Type
   Dosage
   Presence of side-effects
5. Psychosocial
   Occupation
   Family support

Table II-18. **Arterial Insufficiency vs. Venous Insufficiency: A Comparison of Subjective Data**

Symptom	Arterial Insufficiency	Venous Insufficiency
Pain		
Location	Feet, muscles of legs, toes	Ankles, lower legs
Quality	Burning, shocking, prickling, throbbing, cramping	Aching, tightness
Quantity	Increase in severity with increased muscle activity	Varies with fluid intake, use of support hose, and decreased muscle activity
Chronology	Brought on predictably by exercise	Greater in evening than in morning
Setting	Use of affected muscle groups	Increases during course of day with prolonged standing or sitting
Aggravating factors	Exercise	Immobility
	Extremity elevation	Extremity dependence
Alleviating factors	Cessation of exercise	Extremity elevation
	Extremity dependence	Compression stockings or Ace wraps
Paresthesia	Numbness, tingling, burning, decreased sensation	No change unless arterial system or nerves are affected

Table II-19. **Arterial Insufficiency vs. Venous Insufficiency: A Comparison of Objective Data**

Sign	Arterial Insufficiency	Venous Insufficiency
Temperature	Cool skin	Warm skin
Color	Pale on elevation, dependent rubor (reactive hyperemia)	Flushed, cyanotic
		Typical brown discoloration around ankles
Capillary filling	>3 seconds	Nonapplicable
Pulses	Absent	Present unless there is concomitant arterial disease
Movement	Decreased motor ability with nerve and muscle ischemia	Motor ability unchanged unless edema is severe enough to restrict joint mobility
Ulceration	Occurs on foot at site of trauma or at tips of toes (most distal to be perfused)	Occurs around ankle (area of greatest pressure from chronic venous stasis due to valvular incompetence)
	Ulcers are deep with well-defined margins	Ulcers shallow with irregular edges
	Surrounding tissue is shiny and taut with thin skin	Surrounding tissue edematous with engorged veins

Objective Data

1. Signs
   Color
   Temperature
   Pulses
   Pressures
   Motor activity
   Ulcerations
2. Diagnostic studies
   Noninvasive vascular studies
      Doppler ultrasound
      Exercise stress test
   Laboratory studies
      Serum lipid profile
      Platelet profile

A useful method of recording peripheral pulse volume is based on a scale from 0 to 4 as follows:

   0 = Absent, nonpalpable
 +1 = Thready, weak, fades in and out
 +2 = Present but diminished
 +3 = Normal, easily palpable
 +4 = Aneurysmal

Altered Peripheral Tissue Perfusion
Related to (Specify)

Statement Example: **Altered Peripheral Tissue Perfusion related to insufficient circulation for ADL secondary to Diabetes Mellitus**

Assessment

Rest pain (see preceding Defining Characteristics)
Diminished or absent arterial pulses

Outcome Criteria

The individual will
- Define own peripheral vascular problem in own words
- Identify factors that improve peripheral circulation
- Identify necessary life-style changes
- Identify medical regimen, diet, medications, activities that promote vasodilation
- Identify factors that inhibit peripheral circulation
- Report decrease in pain
- Describe when to contact physician/health care professional

---

Interventions

A. Assess causative and contributing factors

Underlying disease
Inhibited arterial blood flow
Inhibited venous blood flow
Fluid volume excess or deficit
Hypothermia or vasoconstriction
Activities related to symptom/sign onset

B. Promote factors that improve arterial blood flow

Keep extremity in a dependent position
Keep extremity warm (do not use heating pad or hot water bottle, since the individual with a peripheral vascular disease may have a disturbance in sensation and will not be able to determine if the temperature is hot enough to damage tissue; the use of external heat may also increase the metabolic demands of the tissue beyond its capacity
Reduce risk for trauma
    Change positions at least every hour
    Avoid leg crossing
    Reduce external pressure points (inspect shoes daily for rough lining)
    Avoid sheepskin heel protectors (they increase heel pressure and pressure across dorsum of foot)
    Encourage range-of-motion exercises

Plan a daily walking program
  Instruct individual in reasons for program
  Teach individual to avoid fatigue
  Instruct to avoid increase in exercise until assessed by physician for cardiac
    problems
  Reassure individual that walking does not harm the blood vessels or the muscles;
    "walking into the pain," resting and resuming walking, assists in developing
    collateral circulation
Discuss cessation of smoking (see *Altered Health Maintenance Related to Tobacco
  Use*)

C. Promote factors that improve venous blood flow

1. Elevate extremity above the level of the heart (may be contraindicated if severe
   cardiac or respiratory disease is present)
2. Avoid standing or sitting with legs dependent for long periods of time
3. Consider the use of Ace bandages or below-knee elastic stockings to prevent venous
   stasis
4. Reduce or removal external venous compression which impedes venous flow
     Avoid pillows behind the knees or Gatch bed which is elevated at the knees
     Avoid leg crossing
     Change positions, move extremities or wiggle fingers and toes every hour
     Avoid garters and tight elastic stockings above the knees
5. Measure baseline circumference of calves and thighs if individual is at risk for deep
   venous thrombosis, or if it is suspected

D. Initiate health teaching as indicated

1. Teach to:
     Avoid long car or plane rides (get up and walk around at least every hour)
     Keep dry skin lubricated (cracked skin eliminates the physical barrier to
       infection)
     Wear warm clothing during cold weather
     Wear cotton or wool socks
     Use gloves or mittens if hands are exposed to cold (including home freezers)
     Avoid dehydration in warm weather
     Give special attention to feet and toes
       Wash feet and dry well daily
       Do not soak feet
       Avoid harsh soaps or chemicals (including iodine) on feet
       Keep nails trimmed and filed smooth
     Inspect feet and legs daily for injuries and pressure points
     Wear clean socks
     Wear shoes that offer support and fit comfortably
     Inspect the inside of shoes daily for rough lining
2. Teach risk factor modification
     Diet
       Avoid foods high in cholesterol
       Modify sodium intake to control hypertension
       Refer to dietitian
     Relaxation techniques to reduce effects of stress
     Smoking cessation (see *Altered Health Maintenance Related to Tobacco Use*)
     Exercise program

3. Teach methods to relieve pain
    Dependent position for ischemic pain
    Elevated extremities for relief of venous aching
    Phantom pain after an amputation may be relieved by massaging or tapping stump or opposite limb
    Use other nursing measures such as relaxation or distraction to assist in pain relief
    If pain is not relieved by above methods, refer to a physician
    Teach symptoms/signs of underlying disease and when to call the physician or health care professional

References/Bibliography

Barnes RW: Managing peripheral vascular disease. J Cardiovasc Med 6(1):33–40, 1981

Bates B: A Guide to Physical Examination. Philadelphia, JB Lippincott, 1980

Coffman JD: Intermittent claudication and rest pain: Physiologic concepts and therapeutic approaches. Prog Cardiovasc Dis 22(1):53–72, 1979

Craven R, Curry T: When the diagnosis is Raynauds. Am J Nurs 81:1097, 1981

Doyle JE: All leg ulcers are not alike: Managing and preventing arterial and venous ulcers. Nursing 13(1):58–62, 1983

Doyle JE: If your legs hurt the reason may be arterial insufficiency. Nursing 4(4):74–79, 1981

Herman JA: Nursing assessment and nursing diagnosis in patients with peripheral vascular disease. Nurs Clin North Am 21(2):219–231, 1986

Holloway NM: Vascular assessment and shock. In Nursing the Critically Ill Adult. Massachusetts, Addison-Wesley, 1979

Miller KA: Assessing peripheral perfusion. Am J Nurs 8(10):1673–1674, 1978

Scandrett S, Becker S: Relaxation training. In Bulechek G, McCloskey JC (eds): Nursing Interventions: Treatments for Nursing Diagnoses. Philadelphia, WB Saunders, 1986

Snow CJ, Carter SA: Is exercise therapy beneficial in intermittent claudication? Vasc Diag Ther 5(1):20–25, 1984

Taggart E: Physical assessment of the patient with arterial disease. Nurs Clin North Am 12(1):109–117, 1977

Ventura MR, Young D, Feldman MJ et al: Effectiveness of health promoting interventions. Nurs Res 33(3):62–167, 1984

West CM: Ischemia. In Carrieri VK, Lindsey AM, West CM (eds): Pathophysiological Phenomena in Nursing: Human Responses to Illness. Philadelphia, WB Saunders, 1986

Unilateral Neglect

Related to **(Specify)**

Definition

Unilateral neglect: The state in which an individual is unable to attend to or "ignores" the hemiplegic side of his body and/or objects, persons, or sounds on the affected side of his environment.

Defining Characteristics

Major (must be present)

Neglect of involved body parts and/or extrapersonal space, and/or
Denial of the existence of the affected limb or side of body

Minor (may be present)

Left homonymous hemianopsia
Difficulty with spatial–perceptual tasks
Hemiplegia (usually left side)

Etiological, Contributing, Risk Factors

Pathophysiological

Neurological disease/damage   Brain injury/trauma
Cerebrovascular accident   Cerebral aneurysms
Cerebral tumors

Focus Assessment Criteria

Subjective Data

The person does not verbalize or perceive a problem, but if asked will give an excuse such as:

"There is someone else in this bed."
"This arm does not belong to me."
"This arm is dead."
The person gives the affected limb a pet name

Objective Data

1. Assess for presence of etiological and contributing factors
   Determine the extent of neurological involvement
   Determine the person's dominance (handedness)
2. Assess for the presence of factors that complicate the neglect syndrome
   Sensory loss of involved body parts
   Apraxia
   Visual field deficit (homonymous hemianopsia)
   Impulsiveness

Short attention span
Lack of insight into extent of disability
Diminished learning skills
Overestimation of abilities
Inability to recognize faces
Concrete thinking (inability to abstract)
Body schema changes
Confusion

3. Assess the effect the neglect has on the ability of the person to safely care for self in the environment

Activities of daily living (ADL)

Bathing, grooming and hygiene

Does the person:

Wash the affected side of his body?
Shave both sides of his face?
Brush all his teeth?
Put dentures in straight?
Comb only part of his hair?
Apply makeup to both sides of face?
Put eyeglasses on straight?

Feeding

Does the person:

Pocket food on the affected side of his mouth?
Eat only half of his food (*e.g.,* eat only food on one side of plate/ tray)?

Dressing

Does the person:

Dress the affected limb(s)?

Mobility/positioning

When sitting in a wheelchair, does the person lean or tilt toward the un- affected side?
Does the affected arm dangle off the lapboard?
Are the head and eyes turned toward the unaffected side?
When propelling the wheelchair or when ambulating, does the person bump or run into objects on affected side?

Safety

Does the person:

Have sensation in the affected limb(s)?
Frequently injure the affected arm or hand (cuts, bumps, bruises)? Does he feel pain when injured? Does he know when he injures himself?
Scan the entire visual field? Will he turn his head to the affected side to compensate?
Respond to stimuli presented from the affected side?
Does the affected arm dangle at the side and get caught in the wheelchair spokes, siderails, doorways, etc.?

Principles and Rationale for Nursing Care

1. Unilateral neglect is also called hemi-inattention, unilateral asomatognosia (uni- lateral spatial agnosia, Anton-Babinski syndrome), anosognosia, and autopagnosia.
2. The most common cause of unilateral neglect is right hemispheric brain damage; specifically, lesions in the right (nondominant) parietal lobe cause this defect much more frequently than lesions on the left.

3. Unilateral neglect is characterized by an unawareness or denial of the affected half of the body, often extending to extrapersonal space.
4. Homonymous hemianopsia (loss of vision on the contralateral side) is usually present with unilateral neglect, but unilateral neglect is different from hemianopsia. These are two separate phenomena, and either can be present without the other. When they are present together, the person has more difficulty compensating for the loss.
5. Anosognosia (ignorance of paralysis) and dressing apraxia may occur in lesions of either hemisphere but have been observed more frequently with lesions of the nondominant hemisphere.
6. The person with a parietal lobe injury will demonstrate problems with body schema, spatial judgment, and sensory interpretation.

Unilateral Neglect
Related to (Specify)

Assessment
See preceding Defining Characteristics.

Outcome Criteria

The person will
- Demonstrate an ability to scan the visual field to compensate for loss of function/sensation in affected limb(s)
- Identify safety hazards in the environment
- Describe the deficit and rationale for treatment

Interventions
1. Assist the person to recognize the perceptual deficit
   - Initially adapt the environment to the deficit
        Position person, call light, bedside stand, television, telephone, and personal items on the unaffected side
        Position person's bed with unaffected side toward the door
        Approach and speak to person from his involved side
        If you must approach person from affected side, announce your presence as soon as you enter the room to avoid startling the person
        Gradually change the person's environment as you teach him to compensate and learn to recognize the forgotten field; move furniture and personal items out of visual field
        For a person in a wheelchair, obtain a lapboard (preferably Plexiglas) and position affected arm on lapboard with fingertips at midline; encourage person to look for arm on board
        For an ambulatory person, obtain an arm sling to prevent the arm from dangling and causing shoulder subluxation

When in bed, elevate affected arm on a pillow to prevent dependent edema

Constantly cue person to his environment

2. Assist the individual with adaptations needed for self care (activities of daily living skills [ADLs])

- Encourage person to wear prescribed corrective lens or hearing aids

    Bathing, dressing and toileting

        Instruct person to attend to affected extremity/side first when performing ADLs

        Instruct person always to look for affected extremity when performing ADLs, to know where it is at all times

        Encourage person to integrate affected extremity during bathing, encourage person to feel extremity by rubbing and massage

        Utilize adaptive equipment as appropriate

        Refer to *Self Care Deficit* for additional interventions

    Feeding

        Instruct person to eat in small amounts; place food on unaffected side of mouth

        Instruct person to use tongue to sweep out "pockets" of food from affected side after every bite

        After meals/medications check oral cavity for pocketed food/medication

        Provide oral care t.i.d. and p.r.n.

        Initially place food in visual field, gradually move food out of field and teach person to scan entire visual field

        Utilize adaptive equipment as appropriate

        Refer to *Feeding Self Care Deficit* for additional interventions

        Refer to *Impaired Swallowing* if person has difficulty in chewing and swallowing food

3. Teach the individual measures to prevent injury

- Retrain person to scan his entire environment

    Turn head past midline to view scene of his affected side

    Have person do activities that require him to turn his head in order to complete them

    Cue person to remind him to scan when ambulating or propelling wheelchair

- Use tactile sensation to reintroduce affected arm/extremity to person

    Have person stroke involved side with uninvolved hand; the person should watch his arm or leg as he strokes it

    Rub different textured materials to stimulate sensations (hot, cold, rough, soft)

- Instruct the person to keep his affected arm and/or leg in view

    Position arm on lapboard (Plexiglas lapboard allows person to view affected leg and thereby helps to integrate the leg into the body schema)

    Use of arm sling if ambulatory

    Instruct person that extra care should be taken around sources of heat or cold, moving machinery or parts to prevent affected arm from becoming injured

4. Initiate health teaching and referrals

- Assess to ensure that both person and family understand the purpose and rationale of all interventions

- Proceed with teaching as needed

    Explain what denial is and its course (see Principles and Rationale for Nursing Care)

Instruct family on how to facilitate relearning techniques (*e.g.,* cueing, scanning visual field)

Teach use of adaptive equipment if appropriate

Maintain a safe environment

References/Bibliography

Adams RD, Victor M: Principles of Neurology. New York, McGraw-Hill, 1981

Anderson MD, Choy E: Parietal lobe syndromes in hemiplegia. Am J Occup Ther 24(1):13–18, 1970

Hopkins HL, Smith HD: Willard and Spackman's Occupational Therapy, 6th ed. Philadelphia, JB Lippincott, 1983

Licht S: Stroke and Its Rehabilitation. Baltimore, Waverly Press, 1975

Taylor JW, Ballenger S: Neurological Dysfunctions and Nursing Interventions. New York, McGraw-Hill, 1980

Trombly CA: Occupational Therapy for Physical Dysfunction, 2nd ed. Baltimore, Williams & Wilkins, 1983

Washburn KB: Physical Medicine and Rehabilitation. Essentials of Primary Care. Garden City, NY, Medical Examination Publishing Co, 1981

Urinary Elimination: Altered Patterns of

Maturational Enuresis*

Related to **(Specify)**

Functional Incontinence

Related to **(Specify)**

Reflex Incontinence

Related to **(Specify)**

* This diagnostic category is not currently on the NANDA list but has been included for clarity and usefulness.

Stress Incontinence

Related to **(Specify)**

Total Incontinence

Related to **(Specify)**

Urge Incontinence

Related to **(Specify)**

Urinary Retention

Related to **(Specify)**

Author's Note: All of these categories pertain to alteration of urine elimination, not urine formulation. Anuria, oliguria, and renal failure should be labeled as collaborative problems as in *Potential Complication: Anuria. Altered Patterns of*

(Continued)

Urinary Elimination represents a broad diagnosis, which is probably too broad for clinical use. It is recommended that a more specific diagnostic category, such as stress incontinence, be used instead. When the etiological or contributing factors have not been identified for incontinence, the diagnosis can temporarily be written *Altered Patterns of Urinary Elimination* related to unknown etiology as manifested by incontinence.

Urinary Elimination: Altered Patterns of

Definition

Altered patterns of urinary elimination: The state in which the individual experiences or is at risk of experiencing urinary elimination dysfunction.

Defining Characteristics

Major (must be present)

Reports or experiences a urinary elimination problem

Urgency	Dribbling
Frequency	Bladder distention
Hesitancy	Incontinence
Nocturia	Large residual urine volumes
Enuresis	

Etiological, Contributing, Risk Factors

Pathophysiological

Congenital urinary tract anomalies

Strictures	Bladder-neck contractures
Hypospadias	Megalocystis (large-capacity
Epispadias	bladder without tone)
Ureterocele	

Disorders of the urinary tract

Infection	Urethritis
Trauma	

Neurogenic disorders or injury

Cord injury/tumor/infection	Diabetic neuropathy
Brain injury/tumor/infection	Alcoholic neuropathy
Cerebrovascular	Tabes dorsalis
Demyelinating diseases	Parkinsonism
Multiple sclerosis	

Prostatic enlargement

Estrogen deficiency

Atrophic vaginitis	Atrophic urethritis

Herpes zoster

Treatment-related

Surgical
Post prostatectomy   Extensive pelvic dissection
Diagnostic instrumentation
General or spinal anesthesia
Drug therapy (iatrogenic)
Antihistamines   Immunosuppressant therapy
Epinephrine   Diuretics
Anticholinergics   Tranquilizers
Sedatives   Muscle relaxants
Post-indwelling catheters

Situational (personal, environmental)

Loss of perineal tissue
Obesity   Childbirth
Aging
Recent substantial weight loss
Irritation to perineal area
Sexual activity   Poor personal hygiene
Pregnancy
Inability to communicate needs
Fecal impaction
Dehydration
Stress or fear
Decreased attention to bladder cues
Depression   Confusion
Intentional suppression (self-induced deconditioning)
Environmental barriers to bathroom
Distant toilets   Bed too high
Poor lighting   Siderails
Unfamiliar surroundings
Impaired mobility

Maturational

Child: Small bladder capacity, lack of motivation
Elderly: Motor and sensory losses, loss of muscle tone, inability to communicate
needs, depression

Focus Assessment Criteria

Subjective Data

1. History of symptoms
Complaints of
Lack of control   Frequency
Dribbling   Pain or discomfort
Hesitancy   Burning
Urgency   Change in voiding pattern
Onset and duration
Description
Frequency
Precipitated by what?
Relieved by what?

Aggravated by what?
Effects on life-style

Social	Sexual
Occupational	Role responsibilities

2. Incontinence (adult)
History of continence
Is degree of continence acceptable?
Age of attainment of continence?
Previous history of enuresis?
History of "weak" bladder?
Family history of incontinence?
Onset and duration (day, night)
History of

Urinary disorders	Prostate problems
Medical problems	Neurological disorders
Kidney or bladder disorders	

Perception of need to void

Present	Absent
Diminished	

Ability to delay urination after urge

Present (how long)?	Absent

Sensations occurring before or during micturition
Difficulty starting stream
Difficulty stopping stream
Painful straining (tenesmus)
Need to force urine out
Lack of sensation to void
Relief after voiding
Complete
Continued desire to void after bladder is emptied

3. Enuresis (child)
Onset and pattern (day, night)
Toilet training history
Family history of bed-wetting
Response of others to child (parents, siblings, peers)

Objective Data

1. Urination stream

Slow	Sprays
Small	Starts and stops
Drops	Slow or hard to start
Dribble	

2. Urine
Color

Yellow	Yellow brown
Amber	Green brown
Straw colored	Dark brown
Red brown	Black

Odor

Faint	Offensive
Ammoniac	Acetonic

Appearance
    Clear   Cloudy
Reaction (normal, 4.6–7.5, or alkaline, greater than 7.5)
Specific gravity
    Dilute (<1.003)
    Concentrated (>1.025)
    Normal (1.003–1.025)
Negative or positive for
    Glucose   Bacteria
    Protein   Red blood cells
    Ketone
3. Voiding and fluid intake patterns (record for 2–4 days to establish a baseline)
    What is daily fluid intake?
    When does incontinence occur?
4. Muscle tone
    Abdomen firm, or soft and pendulous?
    History of recent significant weight loss or gain?
5. Reflexes
    Presence or absence of cauda equina reflexes
        Anal   Bulbocavernosus
6. Bladder
    Distention (palpable)
    Can it be emptied by external stimuli? (Credé's method, gentle suprapubic
        tapping or warm water over the perineum, Valsalva, pulling of pubic hair,
        anal stretch)
    Capacity (at least 300-350 ml)
7. Residual urine
    None   Present in what amount?
8. Assess for presence of
    Constipation   Depression
    Fecal impaction   Mobility disorders
    Dehydration   Sensory disorders
9. Diagnostic studies
    Urinalysis; culture and sensitivity
    Blood (creatinine, urea nitrogen)
    Roentgenograms (intravenous pyelogram, kidney, ureters, bladder), cystometro-
        gram
    Electromyography of the muscles of the external urinary sphincter and muscles
        of the pelvic floor

Principles and Rationale for Nursing Care

Anatomy and Physiology

1. The kidneys produce urine, and the rest of the urinary system serves as a drainage or
   storage system until the urine is excreted.
2. The three components of the lower urinary tract that assist to maintain continence
   are: (Plymat)
   • Detrusor muscle in the bladder wall, which allows bladder expansion to increase
     volume of urine
   • Internal sphincter or proximal urethra which, when contracted, prevents urine
     leakage

- External sphincter, which by voluntary control provides added support during stressed situations (*e.g.,* overdistended bladder)
3. Innervation of the bladder arises from the spinal cord at the sacral levels of 2, 3, and 4. The bladder is under parasympathetic control.
4. Voluntary control over urination is influenced by the cortex, midbrain, and medulla.
5. The female urethra is 3 cm to 5 cm long. The male urethra is approximately 20 cm long.
6. Continence is maintained primarily by the urethra, but the cerebral cortex is the principal area for suppression of the desire to micturate.
7. Capacity of the normal bladder (without experiencing discomfort) is 250 ml to 400 ml.

Urination

1. During urination there is simultaneous relaxation of the external urinary sphincter and contraction of the bladder.
2. The sitting position for the female and the standing position for the male allow for optimal relaxation of the external urinary sphincter and perineal muscles.
3. The desire to void occurs when there is 150 ml to 250 ml of urine in the bladder.
4. Stress, anger, and anxiety can inhibit relaxation of the urinary sphincter.
5. Bladder tissue tone can be lost if the bladder is distended to 1000 ml (atonic bladder) or continuously drained (Foley catheter).
6. Mechanisms to stimulate the voiding reflex or Credé's method may be ineffective if the bladder capacity is less than 200 ml.
7. Alcohol, coffee, and tea have a natural diuretic effect and are bladder irritants.
8. Injury to the spinal cord above sacral 2, 3, 4 produces a spastic or reflex bladder tone.
9. Injury to the spinal cord below sacral 2, 3, 4 produces a flaccid or atonic bladder.
10. Lesions affecting inhibitory centers in the brain or the pathways transmitting inhibitory impulses to the bladder result in an uninhibited bladder.

Enuresis (involuntary voiding during sleep)

1. Enuresis before the age of four may be physiological. Causes include a small bladder, structural disorders of the urinary tract, infection, diabetes (mellitus, insipidus), and nocturnal epilepsy.
2. Enuresis after the age of four may be physiological or maturational. Common contributing factors are the arrival of a new sibling and being a deep sleeper.
3. Enuresis is primarily a maturational problem and usually ceases between the ages of six and eight years. It is more common in boys.
4. There is a high frequency of bed-wetting in children whose parents or other near relatives were bed-wetters.
5. Behavioral problems usually are not the cause of enuresis but may result from lack of understanding or insensitivity to the problem. The child should not be punished or shamed but motivated toward control.

Infection

1. Stasis or pooling of urine contributes to bacterial growth.
2. Bacteria can travel up the ureters to the kidney (ascending infection).
3. Recurrent bladder infections cause fibrotic changes in the bladder wall with resultant decrease in bladder capacity.
4. Urinary stasis, infections, alkaline urine, and decreased urine volume contribute to the formation of urinary tract calculi.

5. Dilute acid urine helps prevent infection and allows for solubility of inorganic materials.

High-risk Elderly

1. Urinary incontinence affects 5% to 15% of elderly people living in the community, and its prevalence increases to about 40% in hospitalized patients and 50% in the institutionalized patients. (Resnick and Yalla, 1985). One of the major problems of incontinence in the elderly is that it may be overlooked and not adequately evaluated by professionals, and as a result, appropriate treatment is denied. Elderly people themselves may not admit to the problem because of attitudes about the inevitability of complications such as incontinence.
2. The incidence of incontinence increases with age, and as age increases the more likely it is that there will be neurologic causes for incontinence.
3. Regardless of the presence or absence of incontinence, the aged genitourinary system is pathophysiologically altered in four ways: bladder capacity is diminished; quantity of residual urine is increased; bladder contractions become uninhibited; and desire to urinate is delayed.
4. Other physiological components of aging that contribute to incontinence are the diminished ability of kidneys to concentrate urine, decreasing muscle tone of the pelvic floor muscles, and the ability to postpone urination.
5. Detrusor instability is the most common cause of incontinence in the elderly; it is frequently combined with functional or iatrogenic causes.
6. Frequent voiding out of habit may contribute to urgency in the elderly because the bladder is rarely fully expanded.
7. The diminished vision, impaired mobility, and decreased energy level that may accompany aging mean that increased time is needed to locate the toilet, which also requires the person to be able to delay urination.

Incontinence

1. Incontinence is transient in as many as 50% of individuals presenting with the problem, and of the remaining group, about two thirds can be cured or markedly improved with treatment (Resnick and Yalla, 1985). There are many effective corrective measures for the management of urinary tract pathology in the elderly, and a positive approach should be taken to minimize the incidence of urinary incontinence.
2. It is important to determine the natural history of the incontinence pattern. A new onset of incontinence is likely to be due to an external precipitating factor outside of the urinary tract (such as medications, acute illness, inaccessible toilets, impaired mobility preventing getting to the toilet on time, etc.) which can often be easily corrected.
3. Incontinence can be either reversible or controllable. Controllable incontinence cannot be cured, but urine removal can be planned.
4. Generally, women are more likely than men to have trouble with bladder control.
5. Obstruction of the bladder neck that progresses to bladder distention and overflow (incontinence) can be caused by fecal impaction and enlarged prostate gland.
6. Persons with diabetes mellitus, which can contribute to increased residual urine, frequency, and urgency, may be less aware of bladder fullness.
7. Dehydration can cause incontinence by eliminating the sensation of a full bladder (the signal to urinate) and also by reducing the person's alertness to the sensation.
8. Social isolation of incontinent persons can be self-imposed because of fear and embarrassment or imposed by others because of odor and esthetics.

9. Depression can prevent the person from recognizing or responding to bladder cues and thus contributes to incontinence.

Intermittent Catheterization

1. Intermittent self-catheterization is the periodic drainage of urine by the individual by the use of a catheter in the bladder.
2. This method maintains the tonicity of the bladder muscle, prevents overdistention, and provides for complete emptying of the bladder.
3. Intermittent catheterization, when performed in a health care facility, should follow aseptic technique because the organisms present in such a facility are more virulent and resistent to drugs than organisms found outside. Persons at home can practice clean technique because of the lack of virulent organisms in the home environment.
4. The initial removal of more than 500 ml of urine from a chronically distended bladder can cause severe hemorrhage, which results when bladder veins, previously compressed by the distended bladder, rapidly dilate and rupture when bladder pressure is abruptly released. (After the initial release of 500 ml of urine, alternate the release of 100 ml of urine with 15-minute catheter clamps).
5. An overdistended bladder reduces blood flow to the bladder wall, making it more susceptible to infection from bacterial growth.
6. The accumulation of more than 500 ml to 700 ml of urine in a bladder should not be permitted.
7. Intermittent catheterization provides for a decrease in morbidity associated with long-term use of indwelling catheters, increased independence, a more positive self-concept, and more normal sexual relations.

Urinary Retention

1. Urinary retention can be caused by three different entities; bladder outlet obstruction, detrusor inadequacy and impaired afferent pathways.
2. Bladder outlet obstruction is commonly caused by impacted stool or an enlarged prostate. The impacted stool or enlarged prostate will compress the urethra so that urine is retained until the bladder distends, causing overflow incontinence.
3. Detrusor inadequacy is characterized by the pressure of uninhibited detrusor contractions sufficient to cause urinary incontinence. One cause of detrusor inadequacy is deconditioned voiding reflexes characterized by anxiety or discomfort associated with voiding. Another cause is central nervous system diseases.
4. Impaired afferent pathways occur when both the sensory and motor branches of the simple reflex arc are damaged. Therefore, there are no sensations to tell the individual the bladder is full or no motor impulses for emptying the bladder. Thus, the individual develops a neurogenic bladder (autonomous).
5. With this type of neurogenic bladder the individual is likely to dribble urine when the pressure in the bladder rises because of the bladder filling beyond its normal capacity or because of coughing, straining, or exercising.
6. Other common names for this type of bladder are lower motor neuron, hypotonic, flaccid, cord, tabetic and atonic bladder.
7. External manual compression and/or abdominal straining are the most effective methods to empty an autonomous bladder.

Reflex Incontinence

1. A lesion above the sacral cord segments (above T12) involving both motor and sensory tracts of the spinal cord will result in a reflex bladder. Other common names for this type of bladder dysfunction are spastic, supraspinal, hypertonic, automatic, and upper motor neuron bladder.

2. A lesion that does not completely transect the spinal cord can produce variable findings.
3. Control from higher cerebral centers is removed in the reflex neurogenic bladder. Therefore, micturition cannot be started or stopped in a voluntary manner.
4. The simple spinal reflex arc takes over the control of micturition.
5. A positive bulbocavernosus reflex suggests that the voiding reflex (spinal reflex arc) is intact.
6. Since the voiding reflex located in the sacral cord segments is spared, micturition can occur automatically after external cutaneous stimulation (manual triggering).
7. Individuals with reflex neurogenic bladders can learn methods for stimulating the reflex arc in order to stimulate bladder emptying.
8. Preferred cutaneous triggering methods are light, rapid suprapubic tapping, light pulling of pubic hairs, massage of the abdomen, and digital rectal stimulation.
9. Avoid the use of Credé's maneuver with a reflex bladder because the urethra may be damaged or vesicoureteral reflux may occur if the external sphincter is contracted.
10. If the opening of the urinary sphincter and the relaxation of the striated muscle surrounding the urinary sphincter are uncoordinated, there is a potential for large residual urine volumes after triggered voiding.
11. Autonomic dysreflexia (dysreflexia) is an abnormal hyperactive reflex activity which occurs only in spinal cord injured individuals with a lesion above T8. Most often, these individuals have an upper motor neuron bladder (reflex incontinence). This is a life-threatening situation in which the blood pressure rises to lethal levels. Autonomic hyperreflexia is most often set off by stimuli resulting from an overstretched bladder or bowel.

Stress Incontinence

1. Urinary continence is maintained by the junction of the bladder and the urethra, by support from the perineal floor, and by the muscle around the urethra.
2. Stress incontinence is the leakage of small amounts of urine when the urethral outlet is unable to control passage of urine in the presence of increased intra-abdominal pressure.
3. In stress incontinence, the pelvic floor muscles (pubococcygeus) and levator ani muscles have been weakened or stretched by childbirth, trauma, menopausal atrophy, or obesity.
4. Stress incontinence is usually made worse by the menopausal decrease in elasticity.
5. A trial of vaginal estrogen cream in the postmenopausal woman who exhibits a pale, atrophic vaginal vault may be helpful in reducing the incidence of incontinence.
6. Kegel exercises will strengthen and tone the muscles of the pelvic floor. They may provide enough augmentation or urethral pressure to prevent mild stress incontinence. They should be taught to all women as a preventive measure.
7. A stress test is used to help diagnose stress incontinence. It involves observation of the urethral meatus of a patient with a full bladder in the standing position while she coughs or strains. Short spurts of urine escaping simultaneously with cough or strain suggest a probable diagnosis of stress incontinence.
8. The patient with pure stress incontinence will have a normal cystometrogram.
9. The degrees of stress incontinence are designated as:
    Grade 1—Loss of urine with sudden increase in abdominal pressure, but never at night.
    Grade 2—Lesser degress of physical stress such as walking, standing erect from a sitting position or sitting up in bed produce incontinence.
    Grade 3—In this stage, there is total incontinence, and urine is lost without any relation to physical activity or to position.

Urge Incontinence

1. Urge incontinence is an involuntary loss of urine associated with a strong desire to void. This is characterized by loss of large volumes of urine and may be triggered by emotional factors, body position changes, or the sight and sound of running water. This type of urge incontinence is commonly called bladder detrusor instability or vesical instability.
2. Detrusor instability is characterized by the presence of uninhibited detrusor contractions sufficient to cause urinary incontinence. Common causes include central nervous system disease, hyperexcitability of the afferent pathways, and deconditioned voiding reflexes.
3. Deconditioning of the voiding reflex can result in incontinence through self-induced or iatrogenic causes. Frequent toileting (more than every 2 hours) causes chronic low-volume voiding, which reduces bladder capacity and increases detrusor tone and bladder wall thickness, which potentiates incontinent episodes.
4. Iatrogenic causes include placing a person on the toilet after the incontinent episode or using uncomfortable equipment to make him continent.
5. A person with an uninhibited neurogenic bladder will have damage to the cerebral cortex affecting the ability to inhibit urination. Sensation of bladder fullness is also limited; this is manifested by urgency. There is little time between the sensation to void and the uninhibited contraction (CVA, Parkinson's disease, brain injury/tumor).
6. Factors that contribute to urgency include acute urinary tract infection, neurological impairments, diuretics, diabetes mellitus, inadequate fluid intake, and habitual frequent voiding.
7. Older persons experience urgency owing to the bladder's limited capacity and their decreased ability to inhibit bladder contractions.
8. Warning time is the amount of time the individual can delay urination after the urge to void is felt.
9. Diminished warning time can cause incontinence if the individual is unable to reach a toilet in time.

Functional Incontinence

1. Functional incontinence is the inability or unwillingness of the person with a normal bladder and sphincter to reach the toilet in sufficient time.
2. Functional incontinence may be caused by conditions affecting the individual's physical and emotional ability to manage the act of urination.
3. Underlying psychological problems can be a functional etiology of incontinence.
4. Environmental barriers such as unfamiliar surroundings, uncomfortable equipment, and/or lack of privacy may aggravate this situation.
5. Approximately 45% of all nursing home residents are incontinent. Of those with bladder incontinence, 82% are mobility limited.

Total Incontinence

1. The person may lose urine without warning; this may be a constant or periodic symptom.
2. The person may or may not be aware of incontinence.
3. Injury to the urethral smooth muscle sphincters may occur during prostatectomy or childbirth.
4. Congenital or acquired neurogenic diseases may lead to dysfunction of the bladder and incontinence.
5. This individual has tried methods to control the bladder and has been unsuccessful for a variety of reasons.

6. Commonly, this type of incontinence is controlled with an indwelling catheter, or, for males, use of an external condom catheter, or use of incontinence garments for females.

Interventions

The following are general interventions for bladder reconditioning or retraining.

A. Assess for causative or contributing factors

See each specific nursing diagnosis

B. Reduce or eliminate contributing factors

Infection or inflammation
Consult with physician

C. Provide for factors that influence micturition

1. Maintain optimal hydration

   Increase fluid intake to 2000–3000 ml per day, unless contraindicated.
   Space fluids every two hours.
   Decrease fluid intake after 7 P.M. and provide only minimal fluids during the night.
   Reduce intake of coffee, tea, dark colas, alcohol, and grapefruit juice because of their diuretic effect.
   Avoid large amounts of tomato and orange juice because they tend to make the urine more alkaline.
   Encourage cranberry juice to acidify urine.

2. Maintain adequate nutrition to ensure bowel elimination at least once every 3 days

   Monitor elimination pattern; check for fecal impaction if indicated.
   Asssess daily dietary intake for daily requirements of roughage, basic four food groups, and adequate fluids.
   See *Altered Nutrition* and *Constipation* for additional interventions.

3. Promote micturition

   Ensure privacy and comfort.
   Use toilet facilities, if possible, instead of bedpans.
   Provide male with opportunity to stand, if possible.
   Assist person on bedpan to flex knees and support back.
   Teach postural evacuation (bend forward while sitting on toilet).
   Ensure safe access to facilities
       Provide person with access to urinal or bedpan.
       Provide person with call light.
       Reduce obstacles to toilet facilities (path that is well lighted and free of obstacles, bed at lowest level).
   Stimulate the cutaneous surface to trigger the voiding reflex
       Have person brush or stroke inner thigh or abdomen.
       Pour warm water over perineum.
       Give glass of water to drink while sitting on the toilet.

4. Promote personal integrity and provide motivation to increase bladder control

   Encourage person to share his feelings about incontinence and determine its effect on his social patterns.
   Convey to him that incontinence can be cured or at least controlled to maintain dignity.
   Expect him to be continent, not incontinent (*e.g.*, encourage street clothes, discourage use of bedpans).

Use protective pads or garments only after conscientious reconditioning efforts have been completely unsuccessful after 6 weeks.

Work to achieve daytime continence before expecting nighttime continence.

Encourage socialization

Encourage and assist person to groom self.

If hospitalized, provide opportunities to eat meals outside bedroom (dayroom, lounge).

If fear or embarrassment is preventing socialization, instruct person to use sanitary pads or briefs temporarily until control is established.

Change clothes as soon as possible when wet to avoid indirectly sanctioning wetness.

Advise the oral use of chlorophyll tablets to deodorize urine and feces.

See *Social Isolation* and *Ineffective Individual Coping Related to Depression* for additional interventions if indicated.

5. Promote skin integrity

Identify individuals at risk of developing pressure ulcers.

Wash area, rinse, and dry well after incontinent episode.

Use a protective ointment if needed (for area burns, use hydrocortisone cream; for fungal irritations, use antifungal ointment).

See *Potential Impaired Skin Integrity* for additional information.

6. Promote personal hygiene

Take showers rather than baths, to prevent bacteria from entering urethra.

Instruct women to cleanse the perineum and urethra from front to back after each bowel movement.

D. **Develop a bladder retraining or reconditioning program to include communication, assessment of voiding pattern, scheduled fluid intake, and scheduled voiding times.**

1. Promote communication among all staff members and among individual, family, and staff

Provide all staff with sufficient knowledge concerning the program planned.

Assess staff's response to program.

2. Assess the person's potential for participation in a bladder retraining program

    Cognition   Willingness to participate

    Desire to change behavior

Assess individual's ability to cooperate.

Provide individual with rationale for plan and acquire his informed consent.

Encourage individual to continue program by providing accurate information concerning reasons for success or failure.

3. Assess voiding pattern (see Fig. II-5)

Monitor and record intake and output

Time and amount of fluid intake

Type of fluid

Amount of incontinence; measure if possible or estimate amount as small, moderate, or large

Amount of void, whether it was voluntary or involuntary

Presence of sensation of need to void

Amount of retention (retention is the amount of urine left in the bladder after an unsuccessful attempt at manual triggering or voiding)

Amount of residual (residual is the amount of urine left in the bladder after either a voluntary or manual triggered voiding; also called a postvoid residual)

	Intake	Output					
Time	Type of Fluids	Incontinence	Void	Manual Trigger	Retention	Residual	Behavior/ Activity
12M							
01							
02							
03							
04							
05							
06							
07							
08							
09							
10							
11							
12N							
1							
2							
3							
4							
5							
6							
7							
8							
9							
10							
11							
Totals							

Fig. II-5   Chart used for the assessment of voiding patterns.

Amount of triggered urine (triggered voiding is urine that is expelled after manual triggering [*e.g.,* tapping, Credé's method])

Identify certain activities which precede voiding (*e.g.,* restlessness, yelling, exercise)

Record in appropriate column

4. Schedule fluid intake and voiding times

Provide for fluid intake of 2000 ml each day unless contraindicated.

Discourage fluids after 7 P.M.

Initially, bladder emptying is done at least every 2 hours and at least twice during the night; goal is between 3 to 6 hours.

If the person is incontinent before scheduled voids, shorten the time between voids.

If the person has a postvoid residual greater than 100 ml to 150 ml, schedule intermittent catheterization.

E. Schedule intermittent catheterization program (ICP)

Monitor intake and output.

Fluid intake should be at least 2000 ml per day.

Use sterile catheterization technique in the hospital, clean technique at home.

Desired catheter volumes are less than 500 ml.

Increase or decrease the interval between catheterization to obtain the desired catheter volumes.

Usual catheterization times are every 4 to 6 hours.

Urine volumes may increase at night; thus, it may be necessary to catheterize more frequently at night.

Encourage the individual to attempt to void before scheduled catheterization time.

Initially obtain postvoid residuals at least every six hours.

Terminate ICP when the bladder is consistently emptied voluntarily or by triggering with less than a 50-ml residual urine after each void.

F. **Teach intermittent catheterization to person and family for long-term management of bladder (see Principles and Rationale for Nursing Care)**

Explain the reasons for the catheterization program.

Explain the relationship of fluid intake and the frequency of catheterization.

Explain the importance of emptying the bladder at the prescribed time regardless of circumstances because of the hazards of an overdistended bladder (*e.g.,* circulation contributes to infection, and stasis of urine contributes to bacterial growth).

G. **Teach prevention of urinary tract infections (UTI)**

Encourage regular complete emptying of the bladder.

Ensure adequate fluid intake.

Keep urine acidic; avoid citrus juices, dark colas, and coffee.

Monitor urine pH.

Teach individual to recognize abnormal changes in urine properties.

    Increase in mucus and sediment

    Blood in urine (hematuria)

    Change in color (from normal straw-colored) or odor

Teach individual to monitor for signs and symptoms of UTI.

    Elevated temperature, chills, and shaking

    Changes in urine properties

    Suprapubic pain

    Painful urination

    Urgency

    Frequent small voids or frequent small incontinences

    Increased spasticity in spinal cord injured individuals

    Increase in urine pH

    Nausea/vomiting

    Lower back and/or flank pain

H. **Teach the individual about his bladder reconditioning program**

Explain rationale and treatments of bladder reconditioning program (see Principles and Rationale for Nursing Care).

Explain the schedule of fluid intake, voiding attempts, manual triggering, and catheterization to control incontinence (see Interventions).

Teach person and family the importance of positive reinforcement and adherence to program for best results.

Refer to community nurses for assistance in bladder reconditioning if indicated.

Maturational Enuresis*

Related to **(Specify)**

Definition

Maturational enuresis: The state in which a child experiences involuntary voiding during sleep which is not pathophysiological in origin.

> **Author's Note:** This diagnostic category represents enuresis that is not caused by pathophysiological or structural deficits (*e.g.*, strictures).

Defining Characteristics

Major (must be present)

Reports or demonstrates episodes of involuntary voiding during sleep

Etiological, Contributing, Risk Factors

Situational (personal, environmental)
    Stressors (school, siblings)
    Inattention to bladder cues
    Unfamiliar surroundings

Maturational

Child
    Small bladder capacity
    Lack of motivation
    Attention-seeking behavior

Principles and Rationale for Nursing Care

See *Altered Patterns of Urinary Elimination*

Maturational Enuresis
Related to (Specify)

Assessment

See Defining Characteristics

* This diagnostic category is not currently on the NANDA list but has been included for clarity or usefulness.

Outcome Criteria
- The child will remain dry during the sleep cycle
- The child or family will be able to state the nature and causes of enuresis

Interventions

A. Assess for contributing factors

Small bladder capacity
Sound sleeper
Response to stress (at school or at home; *e.g.*, new sibling)

B. Promote a positive parent–child relationship

- Explain the nature of enuresis to parents and child
- Explain to parents that disapproval (shaming, punishing) is useless in stopping enuresis but can make child shy, ashamed, and afraid
- Offer reassurance to child that other children wet the bed at night and he is not bad or sinful

C. Reduce contributing factors if possible

1. Small bladder capacity
   - After child drinks fluids, encourage him to postpone voiding to help stretch the bladder
2. Sound sleeper
   - Have child void prior to retiring
   - Restrict fluids at bedtime
   - If child is awakened later (about 11 P.M.) to void, attempt to awaken child fully for positive reinforcement
3. Too busy to sense a full bladder (if daytime wetting occurs)
   - Teach child awareness of sensations that occur when it is time to void
   - Teach child ability to control urination (have him start and stop the stream; have him "hold" the urine during the day, even if for only a short time)
   - Have child keep a record of how he is doing; emphasize dry days or nights (*e.g.*, stars on a calendar)
   - If child wets, have him explain or write down, if he can, why he thinks it happened

D. Initiate health teaching and referrals as indicated

1. For children with enuresis
   - Teach child and parents the facts about enuresis
   - Teach child and family techniques to control the adverse effects of enuresis (*e.g.,*. use of plastic mattress covers, use of child's own sleeping bag (machine washable) when staying overnight away from home)
2. Seek out opportunities to teach the public about enuresis and incontinence (*e.g.*, school and parent organizations, self-help groups)

Functional Incontinence

Related to **(Specify)**

Definition

Functional incontinence: The state in which an individual experiences a difficulty or inability to reach the toilet in time due to environmental barriers, disorientation, and physical limitations.

Defining Characteristics

Major (must be present)

Incontinence before or during an attempt to reach the toilet

Etiological, Contributing, Risk Factors

Pathophysiological

Neurogenic disorders
    Brain injury/tumor/infection
    Cerebrovascular accident
    Demyelinating diseases
    Multiple sclerosis
    Alcoholic neuropathy
    Parkinsonism
Progressive dementia

Treatment-related

Drug therapy (iatrogenic)
    Antihistamines
    Epinephrine
    Anticholinergics
    Sedatives
    Immunosuppressant therapy
    Diuretics
    Tranquilizers
    Muscle relaxants

Situational (personal, environmental)

    Impaired mobility
    Stress or fear
    Decreased attention to bladder cues
        Depression
        Confusion
        Intentional suppression (self-induced deconditioning)

Environmental barriers to bathroom
    Distant toilets
    Poor lighting
    Unfamiliar surroundings
    Bed too high
    Siderails

Maturational

Elderly: Motor and sensory losses, loss of muscle tone, inability to communicate needs, depression

Principles and Rationale for Nursing Care

See *Altered Patterns of Urinary Elimination*

Functional Incontinence
Related to (Specify)

Assessment

See Defining Characteristics

Outcome Criteria

The person will
- Eliminate or reduce incontinent episodes (specify number of hours)
- Remove or minimize environmental barriers from home
- Utilize proper adaptive equipment to assist with voiding, transfers, and dressing
- Describe causative factors for incontinence

Interventions

A. Assess causative or contributing factors

  1. Determine if there is another cause contributing to incontinence (*e.g.*, stress, urge or reflex incontinence, urinary retention, or infection)

  2. Environmental barriers

  Assess obstacles to bathroom

      Obstacles to toilet

          Poor lighting, slippery floor, misplaced furniture and rugs, inadequate footwear, toilet too far, bed too high, siderails up

        Toilet inadequate

          Too small for walkers, wheelchair, seat too low/high, no grab bars

        Inadequate signal system for requesting help

        Lack of privacy

3. Sensory/cognitive deficits
Visual deficits
Blindness, field cuts, poor depth perception
Cognitive deficits
Aging, trauma, stroke, tumor, infection
4. Motor/mobility deficits
Limited upper and/or lower extremity movement/strength (inability to remove clothing)
Barriers to ambulation
Vertigo, fatigue, altered gait, hypertension

B. Reduce or eliminate contributing factors if possible

1. Other causes of incontinence
Establish appropriate bladder reconditioning program (see General Interventions)
2. Environmental barriers
Assess path to bathroom for obstacles, lighting, and distance
Assess adequacy of toilet height and need for grab bars
Assess adequacy of room size
Provide a commode between bathroom and bed
3. Sensory/cognitive deficits
For an individual with diminished vision
Ensure adequate lighting
Encourage person to wear prescribed corrective lens
Provide clear, safe pathway to bathroom
Keep call bell easily accessible
If bedpan or urinal is used, make sure it is within easy reach in the same location at all times
Assess person for safety in bathroom
Assess person's ability to provide self-hygiene
For an individual with cognitive deficits
Offer toileting reminders every two hours, after meals, and before bedtime
Establish appropriate means to communicate need to void
Answer call bell immediately
Encourage wearing ordinary clothes
Provide a normal environment for elimination (use bathroom if possible)
Allow for privacy while maintaining safety
Allow sufficient time for task
Reorient individual to where he is and what task he is doing
Be consistent in your approach to person
Give simple step-by-step instructions, use verbal and nonverbal cues
Give positive reinforcement for success
Assess person for safety in bathroom
Assess need for adaptive devices on clothing to make dressing and undressing easier
Assess person's ability to provide self-hygiene
4. Motor/mobility deficits
For persons with limited hand function
Assess person's ability to remove and replace clothing
Clothing that is loose is easier to manipulate
Provide dressing aids as necessary; Velcro closures in seams for wheelchair

patients, zipper pulls; all garments with fasteners may be adapted with Velcro closures

C. Initiate referral when indicated

Initiate referral to visiting nurse (occupational therapy department) for assessment of bathroom facilities at home

Reflex Incontinence

Related to **(Specify)**

Definition

Reflex incontinence: The state in which the individual experiences an involuntary loss of urine caused by damage to the spinal cord between the cortical and sacral (S1, S2, S3) bladder centers.

Defining Characteristics

Major (must be present)

Uninhibited bladder contractions
Involuntary reflexes producing spontaneous voiding
Partial or complete loss of sensation of bladder fullness or urge to void

Etiological, Contributing, Risk Factors

Pathophysiological
Cord injury/tumor/infection

Principles and Rationale for Nursing Care

See *Altered Patterns of Urinary Elimination*

Reflex Incontinence
Related to (Specify)

Assessment
See Defining Characteristics

Outcome Criteria

The person will
- Report a state of dryness that is personally satisfactory
- Have a residual urine volume of less than 50 ml
- Utilize triggering mechanisms to initiate reflex voiding

Interventions

A. Assess for causative and contributing factors

Spinal cord lesion above T12
Traumatic injury
Infection
Tumor
Syringomyelia
Multiple sclerosis
Brown-Séquard syndrome
Transverse myelitis
Pernicious anemia

B. Explain to person rationale for treatment (see Principles and Rationale for Nursing Care)

C. Develop a bladder retraining or reconditioning program (see General Interventions)

D. Teach techniques to stimulate reflex voiding

Cutaneous triggering mechanisms:
Repeated deep, sharp suprapubic tapping (most effective)
Instruct individual to:
Position self in a half-sitting position
Tapping is aimed directly at bladder wall
Rate is 7 to 8 times per 5 seconds (50 single blows)
Use only one hand
Shift site of stimulation over bladder to find most successful site
Continue stimulation until a good stream starts
Wait approximately 1 minute, repeat stimulation until bladder is empty
One or two series of stimulations without response signifies that nothing more will be expelled
If the above is ineffective perform each of the following for 2 to 3 minutes each. Wait 1 minute between facilitation attempts.
Stroking glans penis
Punching abdomen above inguinal ligaments (lightly)
Stroking inner thigh
Encourage person to void or trigger at least every 3 hours
Indicate on intake and output sheet which mechanism was used to induce voiding.
Persons with abdominal muscle control should use the Valsalva maneuver during triggered voiding.

Teach person that if he increases his fluid intake he also needs to increase the frequency of triggering to prevent overdistention.

Schedule intermittent catheterization program (see General Interventions).

E. Initiate health teaching as indicated

Teach bladder reconditioning program (see General Interventions).

Teach intermittent catheterization (see General Interventions).

Teach prevention of urinary tract infections (see General Interventions).

Teach about autonomic dysreflexia (see Principles and Rationale for Nursing Care).

Instruct person in prevention of dysreflexia:

Establish and maintain a scheduled fluid intake and bladder-emptying routine

Establish and maintain a regulated bowel-emptying program (see *Altered Bowel Elimination*)

Establish and maintain a preventive skin care program (see *Potential Impaired Skin Integrity*)

Instruct person in signs and symptoms of dysreflexia:

Elevated blood pressure, decreasing pulse

Flushing and sweating above the level of the lesion

Cool and clammy below the level of the lesion

Pounding headache

Nasal stuffiness

Anxiety "feeling of impending doom"

Goose pimples

Blurred vision

Instruct person in measures to reduce or eliminate symptoms:

Elevate head

Check blood pressure

Rule out bladder distention; empty bladder by catheter (do not trigger); use lidocaine lubricant for catheter

If condition persists after emptying bladder, check for bowel distention. If stool is present in the rectum, use a Nupercainal suppository to desensitize the area before removing stool.

If condition persists or person has not been able to identify cause, notify physician immediately or seek help in an emergency room

Instruct person to carry an identification card that states signs, symptoms, and management in the event that the person would not be able to direct others

Stress Incontinence

Related to **(Specify)**

Definition

Stress incontinence: The state in which an individual experiences an immediate involuntary loss of urine upon an increase in intra-abdominal pressure.

Defining Characteristics

Major (must be present)

The individual reports
    Loss of urine (usually less than 50 ml) occurring with increased abdominal pressure
        from standing, sneezing, or coughing

Etiological, Contributing, Risk Factors

Pathophysiological
    Congenital urinary tract anomalies
        Strictures
        Hypospadias
        Epispadias
        Ureterocele
        Bladder-neck contractures
        Megalocystis (large-capacity bladder without tone)
    Disorders of the urinary tract
        Infection
        Trauma
        Urethritis
    Estrogen deficiency
        Atrophic vaginitis
        Atrophic urethritis

Situational (personal, environmental)
    Loss of perineal tissue tone
        Obesity
        Aging
        Recent substantial weight loss
        Childbirth
    Irritation to perineal area
        Sexual activity
        Poor personal hygiene
    Pregnancy
    Stress or fear

Maturational
Elderly: loss of muscle tone

Principles and Rationale for Nursing Care
See *Altered Patterns of Urinary Elimination*

Stress Incontinence
Related to (Specify)

Assessment
See Defining Characteristics

Outcome Criteria

The person will
- Report a reduction or elimination of stress incontinence
- Be able to explain the cause of incontinence and rationale for treatment

Interventions

A. Assess for contributing factors

1. Loss of tissue or muscle tone

Childbirth	Cystocele
Obesity	Rectocele
Aging	Prolapsed uterus
Recent weight loss	Atrophic vaginitis or urethritis

2. History of surgery of the bladder and urethra with adhesions to the vaginal wall
3. Increased intra-abdominal pressure

Pregnancy   Obesity

Overdistention between voidings
4. Assess pattern of voiding/incontinence and fluid intake

Promote optimal hydration (see General Intervention)

Assess voiding (see General Intervention)

Instruct person to avoid fluids such as coffee, tea, dark colas, and alcohol, which act as diuretics and irritants

B. Reduce or eliminate causative or contributing factors

1. Loss of tissue and muscle tone

Explain to the person the effect of incompetent floor muscles on continence (see Principles and Rationale for Nursing Care).

Teach person to identify her pelvic floor muscles and strengthen them with exercise (Kegel exercises).

"For posterior pelvic floor muscles, imagine you are trying to stop the passage of stool and tighten your anal muscles without tightening your legs or your abdominal muscles."

"For anterior pelvic floor muscles, imagine you are trying to stop the passage of urine, tighten the muscles (back and front) for four seconds and then release them; repeat ten times, four times a day." (Can be increased to four times an hour if indicated)

Instruct person to stop and start the urine stream several times during voiding.
2. Increased abdominal pressure with pregnancy

Teach to avoid prolonged periods of standing.

Teach the benefit of frequent voidings at least every 2 hours.

Teach Kegel exercises.
3. Increased abdominal pressure with obesity

Instruct person to void every 2 hours.

Avoid prolonged periods of standing.

Explain the relationship of obesity and stress incontinence.

Teach Kegel exercises.

If person desires to lose weight, refer to *Altered Health Maintenance*.

C. Initiate health teaching

For persons who continue to remain incontinent after attempts at bladder reconditioning or muscle retraining:

Promote personal integrity (see General Interventions)

Promote skin integrity (see General Interventions)

Schedule intermittent catheterization program if appropriate (see General Interventions)

Discuss use of incontinence briefs to contain incontinence.

Total Incontinence

Related to **(Specify)**

Definition

Total incontinence: The state in which an individual experiences continuous, unpredictable loss of urine.

Author's Note: This category is used only after the other types of incontinence have been ruled out.

Defining Characteristics

Major (must be present)

Constant flow of urine without distention

Nocturia more than two times during sleep time

Incontinence refractory to other treatments

Minor (may be present)

Unaware of bladder cues to void

Unaware of incontinence

Etiological, Contributing, Risk Factors

Pathophysiological

Congenital urinary tract anomalies

Strictures

Hypospadias

Epispadias

Ureterocele

Megalocystis (large-capacity bladder without tone)

Disorders of the urinary tract

Infection

Trauma

Urethritis

Neurogenic disorders or injury
    Cord injury/tumor/infection
    Brain injury/tumor/infection
    Cerebrovascular accident
    Demyelinating diseases
    Multiple sclerosis
    Diabetic neuropathy
    Alcoholic neuropathy
    Tabes dorsalis

Treatment-related

Surgical
    Post prostatectomy
    Extensive pelvic dissection
General or spinal anesthesia
Post-indwelling catheters

Situational (personal, environmental)

Inability to communicate needs
Dehydration
Stress or fear
Decreased attention to bladder cues
    Depression
    Confusion

Maturational

Elderly: Motor and sensory losses, loss of muscle tone, inability to communicate needs, depression

Principles and Rationale for Nursing Care

See *Altered Patterns of Urinary Elimination*

Total Incontinence
Related to (Specify)

Assessment

See Defining Charateristics

Outcome Criteria

The person will
- Be continent (specify during day, night, 24 hours)
- Be able to identify the cause of incontinence and rationale for treatment

Interventions

A. Assess causative or contributing factors

Physiological
> Congenital abnormalities   Hypospadias/epispadias
> Exstrophy of the bladder

Vesicovaginal fistula
Ectopic urethral orifice
Surgery
Neurogenic diseases
> Brain trauma/tumor/infection   Demyelinating disease
> Cerebrovascular accident   Alzheimer's disease
> Coma

Loss of tissue and muscle tone (grade III stress incontinence)
Psychological
> Disorientation
> Depression

B. Reduce or eliminate causative and contributing factors when possible

Initiate bladder retraining program (see General Intervention)
In persons who are unable to respond to bladder cues
> Establish method to communicate urge to void
> Provide opportunity to void prior to person's usual time for incontinence
> Offer opportunity to void in response to person's usual behavior prior to incontinence (restlessness, screaming)
> Wake person during the night and provide opportunity to void
> If person is unable to void, institute intermittent catheterization (see General Intervention)

Determine if incontinence briefs or external condom catheters are needed

C. If bladder retraining fails, consider use of an indwelling catheter

For males, a catheter no larger than #16 Fr.
For females, up to a #18 Fr. for routine use
Teach care of indwelling catheter
> The person should:
> Maintain 3000 ml fluid intake every day
> Keep urine acidic
> Change catheter at least every 2 weeks or when it does not drain properly
> Tape catheter to prevent pulling:
> > Males—to suprapubic abdominal area
> > Females—to inner aspect of thighs
> Perform thorough cleaning of the meatus, distal catheter, and perineum at least twice a day
> Maintain sterile drainage system at all times in the hospital; at home may use clean system
> Know that the urine collection system should drain by gravity
> Do not lift collection bag above the level of the bladder without pinching off the tubing to prevent backflow
> Connect the catheter to a leg bag drainage system during the day

D. Initiate health teaching

If appropriate, teach intermittent catheterization (see General Intervention)
Instruct person in prevention of urinary tract infection (see General Intervention)
Teach person how to change indwelling catheter
For persons living in the community, initiate a referral to the visiting nurse for
follow-up and/or regular indwelling catheter changes.

Urge Incontinence

Related to **(Specify)**

Definition

Urge incontinence: The state in which an individual experiences an involuntary loss of
urine associated with a strong sudden desire to void.

Defining Characteristics

Major (must be present)

Urgency followed by incontinence

Etiological, Contributing, Risk Factors

See *Altered Patterns of Urinary Elimination*

Pathophysiological

Disorder of the urinary tract
Infection
Trauma
Urethritis
Neurogenic disorders or injury
Brain injury/tumor/infection
Cerebrovascular accident
Demyelinating diseases
Diabetic neuropathy
Alcoholic neuropathy
Parkinsonism

Treatment-related

Diagnostic instrumentation
General or spinal anesthesia
Post-indwelling catheters

Situational (personal, environmental)

Loss of perineal tissue
   Obesity
   Aging
   Recent substantial weight loss
   Childbirth
Irritation to perineal area
   Sexual activity
   Poor personal hygiene
Intentional suppression (self-induced deconditioning)

Maturational

Child: Small bladder capacity

Principles and Rationale for Nursing Care

See *Altered Patterns of Urinary Elimination*

Urge Incontinence
Related to (Specify)

Assessment

See Defining Characteristics

Outcome Criteria

The person will
   • Report an absence or decreased episodes of incontinence (specify)
   • Explain causes of incontinence

Interventions

A. Assess for causative or contributing factors

1. Bladder irritants
   Infection
   Inflammation
   Alcohol, caffeine, or dark cola ingestion
   Concentrated urine
2. Diminished bladder capacity
   Self-induced deconditioning (frequent small voids)
   Post-indwelling catheter
3. Overdistended bladder
   Increased urine production (diabetes mellitus, diuretics)
   Intake of alcohol and/or large quantities of fluids

4. Uninhibited bladder contractions
   Neurologic disorders
   >Cerebrovascular accident
   >Brain tumor/trauma/infection
   >Parkinson's disease
5. Assess pattern of voiding/incontinence and fluid intake
   Maintain optimal hydration (see General Intervention)
   Assess voiding pattern (see General Intervention)

B. Reduce or eliminate causative and contributing factors when possible

1. Bladder irritants
   Infection/inflammation
   >Refer to physician for diagnosis and treatment.
   >Initiate bladder reconditioning program (see General Intervention).
   >Explain the relationship between incontinence and intake of alcohol, caffeine and dark colas. (irritants)
   Explain the risk of insufficient fluid intake and its relation to infection and concentrated urine.
2. Diminished bladder capacity
   Determine amount of time between urge to void and need to void (record how long person can hold off urination).
   For a person with difficulty prolonging waiting time, communicate to personnel the need to respond rapidly to his request for assistance for toileting (note on care plan).
   Teach person to increase waiting time by increasing bladder capacity:
   >Determine volume of each void.
   >Ask person to "hold off" urinating as long as possible.
   >Give positive reinforcement.
   >Discourage frequent voiding that is result of habit, not need.
   >Develop bladder reconditioning program (see General Interventions).
3. Overdistended bladder
   Explain that diuretics are given to help reduce the amount of water in the body; they work by acting on the kidneys to increase the flow of urine.
   Explain that in diabetes mellitus, insulin deficiency causes high levels of blood sugar. The high level of blood sugar pulls fluid from body tissues, causing osmotic diuresis and increased urination (polyuria).
   Explain that because of the increased urine flow, regular voiding is needed to prevent overdistention of the bladder. Explain that overdistention can result in loss of bladder sensation, which increases incontinent episodes (diabetic neuropathy).
   Assess voiding pattern (see General Interventions).
   Check postvoid residual; if greater than 100 ml, include intermittent catheterization in bladder reconditioning program.
   Initiate bladder reconditioning program (see General Interventions).
4. Uninhibited bladder contractions
   Assess voiding pattern (see Interventions)
   Establish method to communicate urge to void (document on care plan).
   Communicate to personnel the need to respond rapidly to a request to void.
   Establish a planned voiding pattern.
   >Provide an opportunity to void upon awakening, after meals, physical exercise, bathing, and drinking coffee or tea, and before going to sleep.

Begin by offering bedpan, commode, or toilet every one-half hour initially, and gradually lengthen the time to at least every 2 hours.

If person has incontinent episode, reduce the time between scheduled voidings.

Document behavior/activity that occurs with void or incontinence (see Assessment of voiding pattern in General Interventions).

Encourage person to try to "hold" urine until set voiding time if possible.

Refer to interventions for additional information on developing a bladder reconditioning program.

C. Initiate health teaching

Instruct person on prevention of urinary tract infections (see General Interventions).

If appropriate, teach bladder reconditioning program (see General Interventions).

If appropriate, teach intermittent catheterization (see General Interventions).

Urinary Retention

Related to **(Specify)**

Definition

Urinary retention: The state in which an individual experiences a chronic inability to void followed by involuntary voiding (overflow incontinence).

> **Author's Note:** This category is not recommended for use with individuals with acute episodes of urinary retention (*e.g.*, fecal impaction, postanesthesia, postdelivery) where catheterization, treatment of the cause, or surgery (prostatic hypertrophy) will cure urinary retention.

Defining Characteristics

Major (must be present)

Bladder distention (not related to acute reversible etiology) or
Bladder distention with small frequent voids or dribbling (overflow incontinence)
100 ml or more residual urine

Minor (may be present)

The individual states that it feels like the bladder is not emptying after voiding

Etiological, Contributing, Risk Factors

Pathophysiological

Congenital urinary tract anomalies
    Strictures

      Ureterocele
      Bladder-neck contractures
      Megalocystis (large-capacity bladder without tone)
   Neurogenic disorders or injury
      Cord injury/tumor/infection
      Brain injury/tumor/infection
      Cerebrovascular accident
      Demyelinating diseases
      Multiple sclerosis
      Diabetic neuropathy
      Alcoholic neuropathy
      Tabes dorsalis
   Prostatic enlargement

Treatment-related

   Surgical
      Post-prostatectomy
      Extensive pelvic dissection
   Diagnostic instrumentation
   General or spinal anesthesia
   Drug therapy (iatrogenic)
      Antihistamines
      Epinephrine
      Anticholinergics
      Theophylline
      Isoproterenol
   Post-indwelling catheters

Situational (personal, environmental)

   Loss of perineal tissue tone
      Obesity
      Aging
      Recent substantial weight loss
      Childbirth
   Irritation to perineal area
      Sexual activity
      Poor personal hygiene
   Pregnancy
   Inability to communicate needs
   Fecal impaction
   Dehydration
   Stress or fear
   Decreased attention to bladder cues
      Depression
      Confusion
      Intentional suppression (self-induced deconditioning)
   Environmental barriers to bathroom
      Distant toilets
      Poor lighting
      Unfamiliar surroundings
      Bed too high
      Siderails

Maturational

Child: Small bladder capacity, lack of motivation

Elderly: Motor and sensory losses, loss of muscle tone, inability to communicate needs, depression

Principles and Rationale for Nursing Care

See *Altered Patterns of Urinary Elimination*

Urinary Retention
Related to (Specify)

Assessment

See Defining Characteristics

Outcome Criteria

The person will
- Empty the bladder using the Credé's and/or Valsalva maneuvers with a residual urine of less than 50 ml if indicated
- Void voluntarily
- Achieve a state of dryness that is personally satisfactory

Interventions

A. Assess for causative or contributing factors

1. Factors that cause impaired afferent pathways
   Cerebrovascular accidents
   Demyelinating diseases
   Spinal cord injury/trauma/infection
   Peripheral nerve damage
      Diabetic neuropathy
      Alcoholic neuropathy
      Pelvic fractures/extensive surgery
2. Loss of bladder tone (detrusor weakness)
   Benign prostatic hypertrophy (postoperative)
   Spinal cord injury/tumor/infection
   Cerebrovascular accident
   Brain injury/tumor/infection
   Medications
      Anticholinergics
      Alpha-adrenergics

3. Conditions contributing to bladder neck obstruction
   Strictures/contracture/spasms
   Edema (postsurgical, postpartum, vaginal or rectal packing)
   Prostatic hypertrophy
   Fecal impaction
   Tumor
   Congenital abnormalities
4. Conditions which inhibit micturition
   Poor fluid intake
   Anxiety

B. Explain to the person the rationale for treatment (see Principles and Rationale for Nursing Care)

C. Develop a bladder retraining or reconditioning program (see General Interventions)

D. Instruct on methods to empty bladder

1. Assist person to a sitting position
   Teach person abdominal strain and Valsalva maneuver
      Instruct person to:
         Lean forward on thighs
         Contract abdominal muscles if possible and strain or "bear down"; hold breath while straining (Valsalva maneuver)
         Hold strain or breath until urine flow stops; wait 1 minute and strain again as long as possible
         Continue until no more urine is expelled
   Teach person Credé's maneuver
      Instruct person to:
         Place hands flat (or place fist) just below umbilical area
         Place one hand on top of the other
         Press firmly down and in toward the pelvic arch
         Repeat six or seven times until no more urine can be expelled
         Wait a few minutes and repeat to ensure complete emptying
   Teach person anal stretch maneuver
      Instruct person to:
         Sit on commode or toilet
         Lean forward on thighs
         Place one gloved hand behind buttocks
         Insert one to two lubricated fingers into the anus to the anal sphincter
         Spread fingers apart; or pull to posterior direction
         Gently stretch the anal sphincter and hold it distended
         Bear down and void
         Take a deep breath and hold it while straining (Valsalva)
         Relax and repeat the procedure until the bladder is empty
2. Instruct individual to try all three techniques or a combination of techniques to determine which is most effective in emptying the bladder.
3. Indicate on the intake and output record which technique was used to induce voiding.
4. Obtain postvoid residuals after attempts at emptying bladder; if residual urine volumes are greater than 100 ml, schedule intermittent catheterization program (see General Interventions).

E. Initiate health teaching

Teach bladder reconditioning program (see General Interventions).

Teach intermittent catheterization (see General Interventions).

Instruct person on prevention of urinary tract infections (see General Interventions).

References/Bibliography

Burgio L, Jones L, Engel B: Studying incontinence in an Urban Nursing Home. J Ger Nurs 14(4):40–45, 1988

Gibbon NOK: Nomenclature of neurogenic bladder. Urology 8(5):423–431, 1976

Jacobs M, Geels W: Signs and Symptoms in Nursing: Interpretation and Management. Philadelphia, JB Lippincott, 1985

Johnson JH: Rehabilitative aspects of neurologic bladder dysfunction. Nurs Clin North Am 15(2):293–307, 1980

Long ML: Incontinence. J Gerontol Nurs 11(1):30–41, 1985

Martin N, Holt N, Hicks D: Comprehensive Rehabilitation Nursing. New York, McGraw-Hill, 1981

McCormick KA, Burgio KL: Incontinence: An update on nursing care measures. J Gerontol Nurs 10(10):16–23, 1984

Niederpruem MS: Autonomic dysreflexia. Rehab Nurs 9(1):29–31, 1984

Opitz JL: Bladder retraining an organized program. Mayo Clin Proc 51(2):367–372, 1976

Pierson CA: Assessment and quantification of urine loss in incontinent women. Nurse Practitioner 9(12):18–30, 1984

Piotrowski MM: Functioning of the normal and neurogenic bladder. Rehabil Nurs Mar–April:13–20, 1980

Plymat K, Turner S: In-home management of urinary incontinence. Home Healthcare Nurse, 6(4):30–34, July/August 1988

Ramphal M: Urinary incontinence among nursing home patients: Issues in research. Geriatr Nurs 8(5):249–254, 1987

Resnick N, Yalla S: Management of urinary incontinence in the elderly. N Engl J Med 5(13):800-805, 1985

Tunink P: Alteration in Urinary Elimination. J Gerontol Nurs 14(4):25–30, April 1988

Voith AM: A conceptual framework for nursing diagnosis: Alteration in urinary elimination. Rehab Nurs 11(1):18–21, 1986

Wahlquist GI, McGuire E, Greene W et al: Intermittent catheterization and urinary tract infection. Rehab Nurs 8(1):18–41, 1983

Walsh P, Gittes R, Perlmutter A et al: Campbell's Urology. Philadelphia, WB Saunders, 1986

Wein AJ, Raezer DM, Benson GS: Management of neurogenic bladder dysfunction in the adult. Urology 8(5):432–443, 1976

Resources for the Consumer

Literature

The HIP Report, Help for Incontinent People,
    Katherine F. Jeter (ed)
    PO Box 544,
    Union, SC 29379

Managing Incontinence: A Guide to Living With Loss of Bladder Control
    Simon Foundation
    Box 835
    Wilmette, IL 60091
    1-800-23SIMON

Violence, Potential for

Related to **(Specify)**

Definition

Potential for violence: A state in which an individual is or may be assaultive toward persons or objects.

> **Author's Note:** This diagnostic category can be made more specific by adding *Potential for Violence directed at others or self-directed. Potential for Self Harm* has been added by the author to describe individuals at risk for self-inflicted injuries, so the descriptor "self-directed" is not needed. Therefore, the content for *Potential for Violence* will focus exclusively on violence directed at others or at objects.

Defining Characteristics

Major (must be present)
Presence of Risk Factors
   See also Etiological Factors

Etiological, Contributing, Risk Factors

Pathophysiological
   Temporal lobe epilepsy
   Progressive central nervous system disorder
   Deterioration (brain tumor)
   Head injuries
   Hormonal imbalance
   Viral encephalopathy
   Mental retardation
   Minimal brain dysfunction
   Toxic response to alcohol or drugs
   Mania

Treatment-related
   Toxic reaction to medication

Situational (personal, environmental)
   History of overt aggressive acts
   Increase in stressors within a short period of time
   Physical immobility
   Suicidal behavior
   Environmental controls
   Perceived threat to self-esteem
   Hallucination
   Argumentative
   Acute agitation

Suspiciousness
Persecutory delusions
Verbal threats of physical assault
Low frustration tolerance
Poor impulse control
Feelings of helplessness
Excessively controlled, inflexible
Fear of the unknown
Response to catastrophic event
Rage reaction
Misperceived messages from others
Antisocial character
Response to dysfunctional family throughout developmental stages
Dysfunctional communication patterns
Drug or alcohol abuse

Maturational

Adolescent: Role identity, peer pressure, separation from family

Focus Assessment Criteria

(Refer also to Focus Assessment Criteria for Ineffective Individual Coping, Ineffective Family Coping, Altered Thought Processes, Anxiety.)

Subjective Data

1. Medical history

   Epilepsy   Alcohol abuse
   Head injury   Drug abuse
   Brain disease   (amphetamines, PCP,
   Hormonal imbalance   marijuana)
   Present medication

2. Psychiatric history

   Previous hospitalizations   Outpatient therapy

3. History of emotional difficulties in individual and/or family

   Alcoholism   Parental brutality
   Cruelty to animals   Pyromania

4. Interaction patterns (note changes)

   Family   Co-workers
   Friends   Others

5. Coping patterns (past and present)
6. Sources of stress in current environment
7. Work/school history

   How does he function under   Employment
      stress?   Stable
   Level of education attained   Frequency of job changes
   Learning disabilities   Periods of unemployment
   Fights in school

8. Legal history

   Arrests and convictions for   Juvenile offenses for violent
      violent crimes   behavior

9. History of violence

Assess recency, severity, and frequency

"What is the most violent thing you have ever done?"

"What is the closest you have ever come to striking someone?"

"In what kinds of situations have you hit someone or destroyed property?"

"When was the last time this happened?"

"How often does this occur?"

"Were you using drugs or alcohol when these episodes occurred?"

10. Present thoughts about violence

Identify possible victim and weapon

"How do you feel after an incident?"

"Are you currently having thoughts about harming someone?"

"Is there anyone in particular you think about harming?" (Identify the victim and the person's access to victim)

"Do you have a specific plan for how you might accomplish this?" (Identify plan, type of weapon, and availability of weapon)

11. Thought content

Helplessness	Fear of loss of control
Suspiciousness or hostility	Persecutory delusions
Perceived intention	Disorientation
(*e.g.*, "He meant to hit me"	
in response to a slight bump)	

Objective Data

1. Body language

Posture (relaxed, rigid)	Hands (relaxed, rigid, clenched)
Facial expression (calm,	
annoyed, tense)	

2. Motor activity

Within normal limits	Pacing
Immobile	Agitation
Increased	

3. Affect

Within normal limits	Flat
Labile	Inappropriate
Controlled	

4. Diagnostic studies

Electrolyte levels	CT scans
Renal function	Blood glucose
EEG	Drug levels (blood, urine, gastric)
Blood gases	Blood alcohol levels

Principles and Rationale for Nursing Care

General

1. A central theme in violent individuals is helplessness. Assaultive behavior is a defense against passivity and helplessness.

2. Aggressive behavior is a defense against anxiety. This coping mechanism is reinforced, since it reduces anxiety by increasing the individual's sense of power and control. (Refer to Principles and Rationale for Nursing Care—*Anxiety* for further

discussion of anger.) Interventions that encourage "acting out of anger" will reinforce assaultiveness, and thus are to be avoided.

3. Fear and anxiety can distort the individual's perception of external stimuli.

4. Violence usually occurs in response to dynamically significant stresses or situations and is not random.

5. When brain dysfunction is a prime or contributing factor in violent behavior, social and environmental variables still need to be evaluated. Organic impairment may interfere with an individual's ability to handle certain stresses. A person's normal behavior can be altered by exposure to or ingestion of toxic chemicals, such as lead and pesticides.

6. Examples of violent behavior in brain dysfunction are biting, scratching, temper outbursts, and mood lability.

7. Alcohol and drug abuse/use impairs judgment and decreases internal controls over behavior.

8. Suspicious, delusional patients may misinterpret the environment or the motives of staff or others.

9. Individuals who had a history of emotional deprivation in childhood are particularly vulnerable to attacks on their self-esteem.

10. Even though the individual may identify the person with whom he is angry, this may not be the real object of his aggression. Individuals often cannot allow themselves to express anger toward a person on whom they are dependent.

11. Staff frequently respond to violent individuals with actual fear or over-reactions. This can lead to punitive sanctions such as heavier medication, seclusion, or attempts to cope by avoidance and withdrawal from the individual.

12. Staff must identify their own reactions to violent individuals so that they can more effectively manage the situation. Trust your intuition that the person is potentially violent.

13. Although individuals may verbalize hostile threats and take a defensive stance, most are fearful of losing control and want assistance in maintaining their control.

Potential for Violence
Related to (Specify)

Assessment
See Defining Characteristics

Outcome Criteria

The person will
- Experience control of behavior with assistance from others
- Have a decreased number of violent responses
- Describe causation and possible preventive measures
- Explain rationale for interventions

Interventions

The nursing interventions for the diagnosis *Potential for Violence* apply to any individual who is potentially violent regardless of etiological or contributing factors.

A. Promote interactions that will increase the individual's sense of trust

1. Acknowledge the individual's feelings (*e.g.,* "You are having a rough time").
    Be genuine and empathetic
    Tell individual that you will help him control his behavior and not let him do anything destructive
    Be direct and frank ("I can see you are angry")
    Be consistent, firm
2. Set limits when individual presents a risk to others. Refer to *Anxiety* for further interventions on limit-setting.
3. Offer the individual choices and options. At times, it is necessary to give in on some demands in order to avoid a power struggle.
4. Encourage individual to express anger and hostility verbally instead of "acting out."
    Encourage walking or exercise as activities that may diffuse aggression
5. Maintain person's personal space.
    Do not touch the individual
    Avoid feelings of physical entrapment of individual or staff
6. Be aware of your own feelings and reactions.
    Do not take verbal abuse personally
    Remain calm, if you are becoming upset, leave the situation in the hands of others, if possible
    Following a threatening situation, ventilate your feelings with other staff

B. Initiate immediate management of high-risk person

1. Allow the acutely agitated individual space that is five times greater than that for an individual who is in control. Do not touch the person unless you have a trusting relationship. Avoid physical entrapment of individual or staff.
2. Convey empathy by acknowledging the individual's feelings. Let him know you will not let him lose control.
3. Do not approach a violent individual alone. Often the presence of three to four staff members will be enough to reassure the individual that you will not let him lose control.
4. Give the individual control by offering him alternatives (*e.g.,* walking, talking)
5. Set limits. Use concise, easily understood statements.
6. When assault is imminent, quick, coordinated action is essential.
7. Approach individual in a calm, self-assured manner so as not to communicate your anxiety or fear.
8. Avoid using force in giving intramuscular injections when possible, since it serves to increase the person's sense of powerlessness. Use only when a clear danger to others or self exists.
9. If the person has a weapon, do not attempt to grab it. Instruct the person to put it down. Attempt to calm the person without risking bodily harm to yourself.

C. Establish an environment that reduces agitation

Decrease noise level
Give short, concise explanations
Control the number of persons present at one time
Provide single or semiprivate room

Allow individual to arrange personal possessions
Be aware that darkness can increase disorientation and enhance suspiciousness
Decrease situations in which the individual is frustrated

D. Assist the individual in maintaining control over his behavior

1. Establish the expectation that he can control his behavior, and continue to reinforce the expectation.
2. Provide positive feedback when person is able to exercise restraint.
3. Reassure individual that the staff will provide control if he cannot ("I am concerned about you, I will get [more staff, medications, etc.] to keep you from doing anything impulsive").
4. Set firm, clear limits when individual presents a danger to self or others. ("Put the chair down").
5. Allow appropriate verbal expressions of anger. Give positive feedback.
6. Set limits on verbal abuse. Do not take insults personally. Support others (clients, staff) who may be targets of abuse.
   Do not give attention to person who is being verbally abusive. Tell the person what you are doing and why.
7. Assist with external controls, as necessary.
   Maintain observation every 15 to 30 minutes
   Remove items that could be used as weapons (glass, sharp objects, etc.)
   Assess ability to tolerate off-unit procedures
   If person is acutely agitated, be cautious with items such as hot coffee

E. Plan for unpredictable violence

Assess person's potential for violence and past history
Ensure availability of staff prior to potential violent behavior (never try to assist person alone when physical restraint is necessary)
Determine who will be in charge of directing personnel to intervene in violent behavior if it occurs
Ensure protection for oneself (door nearby for withdrawal, pillow to protect face)

F. Utilize seclusion and/or restraint, if indicated

1. Remove individual from situation if environment is contributing to aggressive behavior, using the least amount of control needed (*e.g.,* ask others to leave, and take individual to quiet room).
2. Reinforce that you are going to help him control himself.
3. Repeatedly tell the person what is going to happen before external control is begun.
4. Protect individual from injuring self or others through use of restraints or seclusion.*
5. When using seclusion, institutional policy will provide specific guidelines; the following are general
   - Observe individual at least every 15 minutes
   - Search the individual before secluding to remove harmful objects
   - Check seclusion room to see that safety is maintained
   - Offer fluids and food periodically (in nonbreakable containers)
   - When approaching an individual to be secluded, have sufficient staff present
   - Explain concisely what is going to happen ("You will be placed in a room by yourself until you can better control your behavior") and give person a chance to cooperate

* May require a physician's order.

- Assist person in toileting and personal hygiene (assess his ability to be out of seclusion; a urinal or commode may need to be used)
- If person is taken out of seclusion, someone must be present continually
- Maintain verbal interaction during seclusion (provides information necessary to assess person's degree of control)
- When person is allowed out of seclusion, a staff member needs to be in constant attendance to determine whether person can handle additional stimulation

G. Assist individual in developing alternative coping strategies when crisis has passed and learning can occur

1. Explore what precipitates the person's loss of control ("What was happening before you began to feel like hitting her?").
2. Assist the person in recalling the physical symptoms associated with anger.
3. Help person evaluate where in the chain of events change was possible.
   Use role play to practice communication techniques
   Discuss how issues of control interfere with communication
   Help the person recognize negative thinking patterns associated with low self-esteem
4. Practice negotiation skills with significant others and people in authority.
5. Encourage an increase in recreational activities.
6. Use group therapy to decrease sense of aloneness and increase communication skills.
   Instruct or refer for assertiveness training
   Instruct or refer for negotiation skills development

References/Bibliography

APA Task Force: Clinical Aspects of the Violent Individual. Washington, DC, American Psychiatric Association, 1974

Barash D: Defusing the violent patient before he explodes. RN 47(3):35–37, 1984

Grigson J: Beyond patient management: The therapeutic use of seclusion and restraints. Perspect Psychiatr Care 22(4):137–142, 1984

Knowles RD: Dealing with feelings: Managing anger. Am J Nurs 81:2196–2197, 1981

Lion J: Evaluation and Management of the Violent Patient. Springfield, IL, Charles C Thomas, 1972

Misik I: About using restraint. Nursing 11(8):50–55, 1981

Stewart A: Handling the aggressive patient. Perspect Psychiatr Care 18(3):228–232, 1978

Saunders S, Anderson A, Hart C et al (eds): Violent Individuals and Families: A Handbook for Practitioners. Springfield, IL, Charles C Thomas, 1984

Appendixes

Appendix I: Data Base Assessment Guide

This guide directs the nurse to collect data to assess functional heath patterns* of the individual and to determine the presence of actual, potential, or possible nursing diagnoses. Should the person have medical problems, the nurse will also have to assess for data in order to collaborate with the physician in monitoring the problem.

As with any printed assessment tool, the nurse must determine whether to collect or defer certain data. The symbol Δ identifies data that should be collected on hospitalized persons. The collection of data in sections not marked with Δ probably should be deferred with most acutely ill persons or when the information is irrelevant to the particular individual.

As the nurse interviews the person, significant data may surface. The nurse should then ask other questions (focus assessment) to determine the presence of a pattern. Each diagnostic category in Section II has a focus assessment to help the nurse gather more pertinent data in a particular functional area.

For example, the client reports during the initial interview that she has a problem with incontinence. The nurse should ask specific questions utilizing the focus assessment for *Altered Patterns of Urinary Elimination* to determine which incontinence diagnosis is present. After the nurse has identified the factors, the plan of care can be initiated.

Adult Data Base Assessment Format

1. Health perception–health management pattern
   a. Health management
   "How would you usually describe your health?"

Excellent	Fair
Good	Poor

   "How would you describe your health at this time?"
   Review the daily health practices of the individual

Dental care	Exercise regime
Food intake	Leisure activities
Fluid intake	Responsibility in the family

   Use of

Tobacco	Drugs (over-the-counter,
Salt, sugar, fat products	prescribed)
Alcohol	

   Knowledge of safety practices

Fire prevention	Automobile (maintenance, seat
Water safety	belts)
Children	Bicycle
	Poison control

---

* The functional health patterns have been adapted from Gordon M: Nursing Diagnosis: Application and Process. New York, McGraw-Hill, 1982.

Knowledge of disease and preventive behavior
Specific disease (*e.g.*, heart disease, cancer, respiratory disease, childhood diseases, infections, dental disease)
Susceptibility (*e.g.*, presence of risk factors, family history)
"What do you do to keep healthy and to prevent disorders in yourself? In your children?"

Adequate nutrition	Professional examinations
Weight control	(gynecological,
Exercise program	dental)
Self-examinations (breast,	Immunizations
testicular)	

b. Developmental history*
Family history

Maternal grandparents		Paternal grandparents
Mother	Patient	Father
Spouse	Children	Siblings

Assess for achievement of developmental tasks
Young adult:
(Intimacy vs. isolation)
Accepting himself and stabilizing self-concept
Establishing independence from parental home and financial aid
Becoming established in a vocation or profession that provides personal satisfaction, economic independence, and a feeling of making a worthwhile contribution to society
Learning to appraise and express love responsibility through more than sexual contexts
Establishing an intimate bond with another, either through marriage or with a close friend
Establishing and managing a residence/home
Finding a congenial social group
Deciding whether or not to have a family
Formulating a meaningful philosophy of life
Becoming involved as a citizen in the community
Middle age:
(Generativity vs. stagnation)
Developing a sense of unity and abiding intimacy with mate
Helping growing and grown children become happy and responsible adults—relinquishing central position in their life
Taking pride in accomplishments of self and spouse
Finding pleasure in generativity and recognition in work
Balancing work with other roles
Preparing for retirement
Role reversal with parents/parental loss
Achieving mature social and civic responsibility
Developing or maintaining active organizational membership
Accepting and adjusting to changes of middle age (physical)
Socialization with new and old friends
Use of leisure time

* Source: Nursing History Guide. Nursing Dept, Southeastern Missouri University, Cape Girardeau, MO

Older adult:

(Integrity vs. despair)

Deciding how and where to live out remaining years

Continuing supportive, close, and warm relationship with significant others, including a satisfying sexual relationship

Satisfactory living arrangements—safe, comfortable household routine

Supplemental retirement income, if possible

Maintaining maximum level of self-health care

Maintaining interest in people outside of family

Maintaining social, civic, and political responsibility

Pursuing interests

Finding meaning in life after retirement

Facing inevitable illness and death of self and significant others

Formulating a philosophy of life

Finding meaning to life through philosophy/religion

Adjusting to death of spouse or loved one

c. Health perception

Δ Reason for and expectations of hospitalization (and previous hospital experiences)

Δ "Describe your illness"

| Cause | Onset |

Δ "What treatments or practices have been prescribed?"

Diet	Surgery
Weight loss	Cessation of smoking
Medications	Exercises

Δ "Have you been able to follow the prescribed instructions?" If not, "What has prevented you?"

Δ "Have you experienced or do you anticipate a problem with caring for yourself (your children, your home)?"

Mobility problems	Financial concerns
Sensory deficits	Structural barriers (stairs,
(vision, hearing)	narrow doorway)

Δ Are there any problems that could contribute to falls or accidents?

Unfamiliar setting

Decreased sensorium (vertigo, confusion)

Sensory deficits (visual, auditory, tactile)

Motor deficits (gait, tremors, ROM coordination)

Urinary/bowel urgency

2. Δ Nutritional–metabolic pattern

"What is the usual daily food intake (meals, snacks)?"

"What is the usual fluid intake (type, amounts)?"

"How is your appetite?"

| Indigestion | Vomiting |
| Nausea | Sore mouth |

"What are your food restrictions or preferences?"

"Any supplements (vitamins, feedings)?"

"Has your weight changed in the last 6 months?" If yes, "Why?"

"Any problems with ability to eat?"

| Swallow liquids | Chew |
| Swallow solids | Feed self |

Skin

"What is the skin condition?"

Color, temperature, turgor

Lesions (type, description, location)

Edema (type, location)

Pruritus (location)

Are there any factors present that could contribute to pressure ulcer development?

Immobility

Dehydration

Malnourishment

Decreased circulation

Sensory deficits

3. Δ Elimination pattern

Bladder

"Are there any problems or complaints with the usual pattern of urinating?"

Oliguria

Polyuria

Dysuria

Dribbling

Retention

Burning

Incontinence

"Are assistive devices used?"

Intermittent catheterization

Catheter (Foley, external)

Incontinence briefs

Cystostomy

Bowel

"What is the usual time, frequency, color, consistency, pattern?"

"Assistive devices (type, frequency)?"

Ileostomy

Colostomy

Enemas

Cathartics

Laxatives

Suppositories

4. Activity–exercise pattern

"Describe usual daily/weekly activities of daily living"

Occupation

Leisure activities

Exercise pattern (type, frequency)

Δ "Are there any limitations in ability?"

Ambulating (gait, weight-bearing, balance)

Bathing self (shower, tub)

Dressing/grooming (oral hygiene)

Toileting (commode, toilet, bed-pan)

"Are there complaints of dyspnea or fatigue?"

Δ Are there factors present that could interfere with self-care after discharge?

Motor deficits

Cognitive/sensory deficits

Emotional deficits

Environmental barriers

Lack of knowledge

Lack of resources

5. Δ Sleep–rest pattern

"What is the usual sleep pattern?"

Bedtime

Hours slept

Sleep aids (medication, food)

Sleep routine

"Any problems?"

Difficulty falling asleep

Difficulty remaining asleep

Not feeling rested after sleep

6. Δ Cognitive–perceptual pattern
   "Any deficits in sensory perception (hearing, sight, touch)?"
Glasses	Hearing aid
   "Any complaints?"
   Vertigo

Insensitivity to superficial pain	Insensitivity to cold or heat
   "Able to read and write?"

7. Self-perception pattern
   Δ "What are you most concerned about?"
   "What are your present health goals?"
   Δ "How would you describe yourself?"
   "Has being ill made you feel differently about yourself?"
   "To what do you attribute the following?"

Becoming ill	Maintaining health
Getting better	

8. Role–relationship pattern
   Δ Communication
   Any hearing deficits? (hearing aids, lip-reading)
   What language is spoken?
   Is speech clear? Relevant?
   Assess ability to express self and understand others (verbally, in writing, with gestures)
   Relationships
   "Do you live alone?" "If not, with whom?"
   "To whom do you turn for help in time of need?"
   Assess family life (members, educational level, occupations)

Cultural background	Decision-making
Activities (lone or group)	Communication patterns
Roles, discipline	Finances
   "Any complaints?"

Parenting difficulties	Marital difficulties
Difficulties with relatives, (in-laws, parents)	Abuse (physical, verbal, substance)

9. Sexuality–sexual functioning
   "Has there been or do you anticipate a change in your sexual relations because of your condition?"

Fertility	Pregnancy
Libido	Contraceptives
Erections	History
Menstruation	
   Assess knowledge of sexual functioning

10. Coping–stress management pattern
    Δ "How do you make decisions (alone, with assistance, who)?"
    Δ "Has there been a loss in your life in the past year (or changes—moves, job, health)?"
    "What do you like about yourself?"
    "What would you like to change in your life?"
    "What is preventing you?"
    "What do you do when you are tense or under stress (*e.g.*, problem-solve, eat, sleep, take medications, seek help)?"

Δ "What can the nurses do to provide you with more comfort and security during your hospitalization?"

11. Value–belief system

"With what (whom) do you find a source of strength or meaning?"

"Is religion or God important to you?"

"What are your religious practices (type, frequency)?"

"Have your values or moral beliefs been challenged recently? Describe."

Δ "Is there a religious person or practice (diet, book, ritual) that you would desire during hospitalization (institutionalization)?"

12. Δ Physical assessment (objective)

General appearance

Weight and height

Eyes (appearance, drainage)

    Pupils (size, equal, reactive to light)

    Vision (glasses)

Mouth

    Mucous membrane (color, moisture, lesions)

    Teeth (condition, loose, broken, dentures)

Speech

Hearing (hearing aids)

Pulses (radial, apical, peripheral)

    Rate, rhythm, volume

Respirations

    Rate, quality, breath sounds (upper and lower lobes)

Blood pressure

Temperature

Skin (color, temperature, turgor)

    Lesions, edema, excoriations

Bowel sounds

Functional ability (mobility and safety)

    Dominant hand

    Use of right and left hands, arms, legs

    Strength, grasp

    Range of motion

    Gait (stability)

    Use of aids (wheelchair, braces, cane, walker)

    Weight-bearing (full, partial, none)

Mental status

    Orientation (time, place, person, events)

    Memory

    Affect

    Eye contact

Appendix II: Psychiatric Data Base Assessment Guide*

This data base supplements the data base in Appendix I, with additional focus on:
    Cognitive–perceptual pattern
    Role–relationship pattern
    Coping–stress management pattern
Cognitive–perceptual pattern (See No. 6, Appendix I)
    Mental status questionnaire (complete for patient 60 years of age or older) (Kahn)
    Are the following questions answered correctly?

	Yes	No
1. Where are you now?		
2. Where is this place located?		
3. What is today's date? Day of the week?		
4. What month is it?		
5. What year is it?		
6. How old are you?		
7. When is your birthday?		
8. What year were you born?		
9. Who is the president of the U.S.?		
10. Who was president before him?		
11. Spell the word "world" backwards?		

Total the number of questions on the mental status questionnaire answered incorrectly and check below to indicate the degree of cognitive impairment.
_____ 1–2 Absent to mild
_____ 3–5 Mild to moderate
_____ 6–8 Moderate to severe
_____ 8–11 Severe

Orientation   Person: _____ Place: _____ Time: _____

Pain perception/pain tolerance
    How do you manage pain? _____
    What causes you to have pain? _____

* Source: Developed by Leanne Sladewski, Bridget Thiel, Constance Harris, and Julia Voss (Courtesy of Dept of Nursing, Hanna Pavilion, University Hospitals of Cleveland, Cleveland, OH)

Sensory–perceptual alterations	*Yes*	*No*	*Describe*
Delusions Persecutory			
Grandiose			
Religious			
Self-accusatory			
Somatic			
Hallucinations Auditory			
Visual			
Tactile			
Olfactory			
Homicidal ideation Past thoughts			
Past action			
Current thoughts			
Current plan			
Action on plan			
Suicide potential Control over your life			
Feel like giving up			
Feel guilty			
Past thoughts of suicide			
Past suicide attempt			
Current thoughts of suicide			
Plan for suicide			
Recent suicide attempt			
Attempt in the hospital			
Currently at risk			
Nursing suicide precautions			
Family history			

Rationale for nursing suicide precautions _____

_____

_____

Obsessions			
Compulsive behavior			
Ritualistic behavior			
Phobias			

Education: _____

_____

Employment: _____

_____

Assessment
   Speech: _____
   Hearing: _____
   Vision: _____
   Gait: _____
   Psychomotor activity: _____
   Ability to follow directions: _____

Comments: _____
_____
_____
_____
_____
_____

Role–relationship pattern (See No. 8, Appendix I)

Family name	Age	Role	Quality of relationship			Supportive	
			Good	Fair	Poor	Yes	No
Significant others							

Satisfaction with relationships	Very dissatisfied			Very satisfied
Family members	1	2	3	4
Friends	1	2	3	4
Social acquaintances	1	2	3	4
Co-workers	1	2	3	4
Classmates	1	2	3	4
Employer	1	2	3	4
Teachers	1	2	3	4

"How are problems handled in your family?" _____
_____

"How do family members/significant others feel about your problems?" _____
_____
_____

"Who makes decisions in your family?" _____
Family activities: _____
_____

"Do you ever feel lonely?" _____ "When?" _____
"What do you do when you feel lonely?" _____
_____

Describe:
 Speech _____
 Eye contact _____
 Nonverbal behavior _____
 Interactions with family/significant others if observed _____

Coping–stress tolerance pattern (See No. 10, Appendix I)

Recent changes	Yes	No	Comments
School			
Work			
Family unit			
Health			
Finances			
Home			
Own illness			
Other's illness			
Death of significant other			
Marital status			

"What makes you feel tense (or other appropriate term)?" _____

"What do you do when you are feeling tense (or other appropriate term)?" _____

"What helps relieve tension for you?" _____

Comments: _____

References/Bibliography

Kahn RL, Goldfarb M, Pollack M et al: Brief objective measures for the determination of mental status in the aged. Am J Psychiatry 117:326–328, 1960 (Questions 1–10)

Appendix III: Pediatric Data Base Assessment*

I. Identifying Information

Child's initials _____

Birthdate _____   Age _____

Sex _____

Weight _____   Percentile _____

Length or height _____   Percentile _____

Head circumference (if appropriate) _____   Percentile _____

Allergies _____

II. Data Base Assessment*

A. Health perception–health management pattern

1. For all children
   a. How is your child's health in general?
   b. How is your child's health today?
   c. What do you do to keep your child well?
      (1) Nutrition
      (2) Opportunities for exercise and play
      (3) Professional health care
      (4) Immunization status
      (5) Any regular medication? What are they? What is their purpose?
2. For the hospitalized or ill child
   a. Why was your child admitted to the hospital?
      (1) What caused the illness/injury?
      (2) When did the illness begin?
   b. What treatment is your child receiving?
      What is your understanding of the purpose of the treatment?
      How do you think the treatment is working?
   c. Has your child ever been hospitalized before? For what reason? How did that go for you and the child?
   d. What expectations do you have about this hospitalization?
   e. Do you anticipate any problems in caring for your child when he goes home: What are the anticipated problems?
3. For both well and ill children: complete for all children under 24 months of age and when appropriate because of related problems (*e.g.*, developmental disabilities, complications of prematurity, etc.)
   a. Did the mother have prenatal care? How long?
   b. Did the mother take any medications during pregnancy?
   c. Were there any complications during pregnancy?
   d. What were the infant's birth weight and length?

* Developed by Susan Ross, RN, MS, and Linda H. Snow, RN, MS, Assistant Professors, Department of Nursing, American International College, Springfield, MA, March 1985. Used with permission. Adapted from Appendix I, Adult Data Base Assessment Guide.

e. What was the length of gestation?
f. Were there any complications with the infant during the first month of life?

B. Nutritional–metabolic pattern

1. How is the child's appetite?
2. Describe a typical day for your child in terms of what he eats and drinks at meals and snacks.
   a. Breast-fed
       (1) How often?
       (2) How long at each feeding?
       (3) Any difficulties?
       (4) Plans for continuing or weaning
   b. Formula-fed
       (1) Name of formula
       (2) Number of feedings in 24 hours
       (3) Amount of formula at each feeding
       (4) Any difficulties perceived
       (5) Plans for continuing or weaning
   c. Solid foods
       (1) When begun
       (2) Food groups that child eats
       (3) Approximate amounts at each meal
       (4) Describe a typical after-school snack
   d. General
       (1) Are there any food restrictions or special diet due to allergies, intolerances, other health problems, or religious practice?
       (2) What vitamins and/or supplements does the child take?
       (3) How much milk does the child drink in 24 hours?
       (4) Does the child use a bottle or cup?
3. What are the child's special food likes and dislikes?
4. How often does the child go to "fast-food" restaurants? What does he usually order?
5. How much candy, other sweets, processed snack foods, and soda does your child eat/drink?
6. What, if any concerns do you have about your child's appetite, feeding behavior, or diet?

C. Elimination pattern

1. Bowel
   a. How many stools does your child have daily?
   b. What is the color, amount, and consistency?
   c. Is he toilet trained?
   d. Does he ever need laxatives, enemas, or suppositories? How often? How do you decide that one of the above is necessary?
   e. What is the usual colostomy/ileostomy care (if applicable)?
2. Bladder
   a. Does your child have any problems with urination?
       (1) Bed-wetting (enuresis)
       (2) Burning or other dysuria
       (3) Dribbling

(4) Oliguria
(5) Polyuria
(6) Urinary retention
  b. Are any assistive devices used?
      (1) Intermittent catheterization
      (2) Indwelling catheter
      (3) Stoma for urinary drainage—describe routine of care
  c. Is the child toilet trained?
      (1) Daytime
      (2) Nighttime
      (3) Accidents?
3. Skin—Does your child ever have any trouble with his skin (*e.g.*, itching, swelling, rashes, sores, acne, color, or temperature changes)? Describe.

D. Activity–exercise pattern

1. Gross motor abilities
   a. When did your child roll over? Sit unsupported? Walk alone? Climb stairs? Ride tricycle? (etc.) (Obtain information appropriate to child's age and developmental abilities)
   b. What sports/exercise does your child enjoy and participate in?
   c. What, if any, concern do you have about your child's abilities in these areas?
2. Fine motor abilities
   a. Does your baby reach for things? Grasp? Transfer objects from one hand to another? Use his fingers to pick up objects? Feed himself a cracker? Use a spoon?
   b. What hobbies does your child have?
   c. What, if any, concerns do you have about your child's abilities to use his hands?
3. Self-care abilities or activities
   a. How independent is your child in feeding himself? Describe the help he needs, if any.
   b. How much help does your child need with toileting? If assistive devices are used, is child independent or does he need help? Describe. Does child use diapers, a potty chair, or toilet?
   c. How much help does your child need with dressing (buttons, ties, zippers, etc.)?
   d. How much help does your child need with hygiene practices (bathing, brushing teeth, etc.)? Does he prefer a shower or tub?

E. Sleep–rest patterns

1. How many hours does the child sleep each 24 hours?
   a. At night
   b. Naps
2. What is the child's usual sleep routine?
   a. Bedtime
   b. Naptime
   c. Rituals (stories, drink, etc.)
   d. Security object(s)
3. Are there any problems related to sleep?
   a. Nightmares, night terrors
   b. Difficulty falling asleep
   c. Refusal at bedtime
   d. Waking up during night

F. Cognitive–perceptual pattern

1. Does the child have any sensory perception deficits (hearing, smell, sight, touch)? Describe.
2. What grade in school is child?
   a. How does he do in school?
   b. What, if any, problems are perceived by parent, teacher, or child relative to school achievement?

G. Self-perception pattern

1. How has your child's illness made you feel? What are you most concerned about?
2. For school-age and adolescent child: How does your illness (injury) make you feel? What are you most concerned about?
3. For well older school-age child and adolescent: How do you feel about yourself?

H. Role-relationship pattern

1. Communication
   a. Language development
      (1) When did child coo? Babble? Say words? Phrases? Sentences? Use pronouns? (Use questions appropriate to child's age and developmental abilities.)
      (2) Does the child use language appropriate for his age?
      (3) What, if any, concerns do you have about your child's language development or characteristics of speech?
   b. What language is spoken at home?
2. Relationships
   a. Describe family life
      (1) Composition of household (family members, ages)
      (2) Cultural background
      (3) Roles
      (4) Occupations and educational background of adults
      (5) Decision-making patterns
      (6) Communication patterns
      (7) Discipline
      (8) Problems (*e.g.,* finances, family violence, problems with parenting, marital problems)
   b. Peer relationships
      (1) Does your child play with other children? Describe the quality of the child's play (*e.g.,* solitary, parallel, interactive, cooperative, aggressive).
      (2) Does the child have a "best friend" of the same sex? Belong to a "gang"?
      (3) Does your child prefer playmates who are older, younger, same age?
      (4) Does your child have imaginary playmates?
      (5) What concerns, if any, do you have about your child's relationships with others?

I. Sexuality–sexual functioning

1. What interest does your child show in sexuality/sexual function? How do you feel about this? How do you handle your child's curiosity and behavior?
2. For adolescent, assess:
   a. Knowledge of sexual functioning
   b. Sexual activity
   c. Use of contraceptives

    d. History of pregnancy

    e. Feelings about opposite sex

J. Coping–stress management pattern

1. How do you make decisions? (alone? with whom?)
2. Have there been any losses or changes in your life in the past year? In your child's? (*e.g.,* move, death of significant other or pet, loss of parental job)
3. To whom do your turn for support and help when you are feeling stressed?
4. How do you manage child care, housework, and other responsibilities? For the teenager: How do you manage school work, sports and other activities, and work responsibilities?
5. What can the nurses do to help you during this hospitalization?

K. Value-belief system

1. What religious affiliation or preference do you hold?
2. Is there a religious person or practice (diet, book, ritual) that you desire during your child's hospitalization

L. Physical assessment (objective)

1. General appearance
2. Temperature (note whether oral, rectal, or auxiliary)
3. Skin
   a. Color
   b. Temperature
   c. Turgor
   d. Lesions
   e. Edema
   f. Excoriations
4. Head
   a. Size, shape
   b. Fontanelles and cranial sutures
5. Neck
6. Eyes (appearance, drainage)
   a. Pupils (size, equal, reactive to light)
   b. Vision
       (1) Responds to visual stimulus
       (2) Wears glasses
7. Mouth and pharynx
   a. Mucous membranes (color, moisture, lesions)
   b. Teeth (number, primary and/or secondary, condition, orthodontic devices)
   c. Pharynx (redness, exudate, tonsils)
8. Ears (appearance, drainage)
   a. TMs
   b. Responds to auditory stimulus
   c. Uses hearing aids
9. Pulses (radial, apical, peripheral)
   a. Rate
   b. Rhythm
   c. Quality
10. Blood pressure (note if by palpation, Doppler)

11. Respirations
    a. Rate
    b. Quality (include signs of respiratory distress)
    c. Breath sounds
12. Abdomen
    a. Bowel sounds
    b. Scars
    c. Prostheses
13. Genitalia
14. Functional ability (mobility and safety)
    a. Presence/absence of primary reflexes
    b. Gross and fine motor ability
    c. Dominant hand
    d. Mobility and use of four extremities
    e. Strength, grasp
    f. Use of aids (*e.g.,* wheelchair, braces, crutches)
    g. Weight-bearing
15. Mental status
    a. Orientation (time, person, place, events)
    b. Level of consciousness
    c. Pain (presence/absence, location, description)
    d. Affect
    e. Eye contact
    f. Use of language (ability and amount)
    g. Personal–social abilities (*e.g.,* self-care, nonverbal communication)
    h. Growth and development
       (1) Cognitive development
           (a) Objective data
           (b) Stage of development according to Piaget
       (2) Psychosocial development
           (a) Objective data
           (b) State of development according to Erikson

Appendix IV: High-Risk Elderly Assessment Guide*

Guiding Principles in Geriatric Assessment

1. Aging is not a uniform process. Aging intensifies one's individuality, and the accumulation of unique life experiences contributes to increased diversity in the elderly. Progressive uniqueness is an intrinsic part of a person's identity. Because of this diversity, health norms for the elderly are not well established. Alterations in health should be compared with the individual's previous patterns and changes.

2. Aging leads to a generalized slowing down in organ system and cellular processes. This results in a decline of compensatory reserve and functional capacity, leading to increased vulnerability to disease. New illness, even minor illness, can produce debilitating effects in the elderly. For example, problems such as infection and hypotension can produce acute confusion as a significant early symptom.

3. Chronic illness is common in the elderly, and multisystem disorders often complicate the individual's physiologic response. Often, the medical diagnosis alone provides little information about the individual's ability to care for himself and manage his needs. Functional impairment is often an indication of new illness or poorly managed chronic disease.

4. Some aging changes appear universal in the elderly, differing only in the degree to which symptoms are manifested. Sensory decrements, such as presbycusis, presbyopia, and cataracts, and musculoskeletal disorders, such as osteoporosis and arthritis, are a few examples.

5. Symptom or disease presentation in the elderly may be absent, delayed, or different in comparison with that of younger persons. Vague symptoms such as lethargy, confusion, shortness of breath, weakness, fatigue, or absence of an elevated temperature may replace more classic symptomatology. Pain may not be well localized, and instead there may be complaints of "hurting all over." New illness or disease is often signaled by a new loss of function or a decline in function such as immobility or a decline in ADL performance, not wanting to eat, cognitive decline or confusion, sleep disorders, agitation, lethargy, and decreased motivation. Physical disorders often present initially as mental disorders (dementia, depression, acute confusion).

6. Developmental issues related to ego integrity vs. despair emphasize the importance of life review as a developmental imperative in the elderly. Life review is a process of remembering and resolving, in which past griefs or losses are put in their proper perspective and the individual derives a sense of self-worth, self-respect, and acceptance of his strengths as well as his mistakes. Failure to engage in life review may deny the individual the opportunity to achieve ego integrity.

7. Many elderly persons face major life adjustments: the need for long-term care (in-home care or nursing home care), outliving family and friends, and accepting increasing dependency. Filial responsibility, or the role that children play in caring for elders, comes into focus as a major issue.

8. Numerous and concurrent losses characterize older adulthood. Loss of employment, friends, and other social contacts through retirement, illness, death or relocation;

* Developed by Deborah Lekan-Rutledge, RN, MSN, C.

loss of mobility and physical capacity through declining health; and loss of social status, financial stability, and significant relationships such as one's spouse are common in the elderly. There are few positive images of growing older, and society induces fear associated with aging.

9. The following special considerations must be taken into account when assessing the elderly:
   a. Begin at a slow, relaxed pace and gauge the pace to the individual.
   b. Ensure that comfort needs are met before beginning the interview (*e.g.,* using the toilet, pain medicine, body positioning).
   c. Monitor the environment for comfortable temperature, minimal background noise, adequate lighting, adequate space, and privacy.
   d. An awareness of sensory decrements should modify verbal and nonverbal approaches. Position self closely to maximize voice contact, use medium-pitched tone of voice, speak slowly and clearly, do not shout, face the individual to allow lip-reading, and use touch appropriately and liberally to convey interest and concern and to accentuate verbal content. Use sentences that are concise and clearly stated and that contain a simply stated question or comment. Avoid sentences that are lengthy or complex or that contain multiple questions
   e. Assess at more than one encounter and at different times of the day. Individuals have good days and bad days, and in some cases, early mornings may reveal more pain and stiffness, or evening may show greater fatigue.
   f. Validate information obtained from the individual with other sources (spouse, family, friends) to establish accuracy of data collected.

10. Functional assessment is an approach to the elderly which focuses on abilities and strengths related to self-management of health problems rather than on disease pathology and medical diagnosis. Functional assessment includes assessment of physical health (mobility and ADL, continence, feeding, bathing, dressing), cognitive and affective status, social abilities and social support, and other areas of home management such as housekeeping, transportation, and shopping. Changes in functional ability ultimately affect independence and self-care. The actual performance of skills is emphasized rather than relying on self-report, which can be exaggerated or underestimated. Also, functional capacity and actual ability should be determined so that reasonable goals may be established.

11. By living longer, the elderly have demonstrated their adaptability and success at survival. The majority of elderly people are in good health and live independently in the community. Only 5% of elderly persons are in long-term care institutions at any one time, although about 20% may at some point need long-term care services. For many, the burden of managing chronic disease is very small, and only a few changes in health habits are necessary to remain functioning independently.

(Refer to the focus assessments under each diagnostic category for detailed guidelines.)

Nursing Assessment of the High-Risk Elderly

Purpose: To identify patterns of aging that deviate from the individual's norm or from accepted standards for the elderly so that timely and appropriate intervention may occur in the endeavor to prevent unnecessary disability and dependency.

Demographics

Name   D.O.B.   Sex

Demographics give basic information about the era in which the individual grew up and the life experiences he is likely to have had at a certain age (the Great War, the depression, invention of modern products). Chronological age is not a good indicator of health or fitness.

Medical Diagnoses

The number of medical diagnoses may not be a key factor in the degree of disability. In some cases, one diagnosis, such as senile dementia of the Alzheimer's type, can produce a high level of functional impairment, while another composite of several diagnoses that are well compensated for may produce minimal functional impairment. Medical diagnoses give cues to the potential health problems that may exist.

Medications

Both prescription and over-the-counter medications should be determined by having the individual bring the medication bottle and instructions with him to the first encounter. Questioning the individual about what the drug is for, when it is taken, and any side-effects to watch out for gives information about memory, knowledge, compliance, manual dexterity, and social support (how he gets the prescription filled). Polypharmacy and "poly-providers" are common in the elderly.

Date of Last Screening Tests

    Eye examination, glaucoma check:
    Audiometry examination:
    Blood chemistry:
    Hematocrit:
    Hemoccult:
    Gynecological examination (women):
    Urological examination (men):
    Blood pressure:

Determining whether the individual uses health resources is a valuable bit of information about his access to health providers, knowledge and use of community services, health practices, social support, and general health status.

Health Status/Perception

    How would you describe your health?
    Describe the health problems you are having now, and how they are being managed.
    Do you feel your life has had meaning?
    What is your philosophy of life?
    Do you anticipate any future problems?
    If you could change any part of your life, past or present, what would you change?
    Describe a typical day.

Self-perception of health has been shown to be a good indicator of overall health status. The individual's perception of his own health problems may be at variance with the provider's option. Elderly persons tend to rate their health higher than do providers. It is important to assess sensory function early in the encounter so that modifications in interaction style can be made.

    Ask the individual to recount a usual day's activities and a recent day's activities (such as yesterday). Assess activity patterns, eating patterns, out-of-house activities, sleep and rest periods, socialization, interests, and hobbies. Also ask if there are things the individual would like very much to do but cannot. Ask to describe these. Assess for recent changes in each of these areas and ask to describe the reasons for these changes. New health problems often result in changes in normal routines, usually limitations or restrictions. Information about memory and the ability to organize and communicate complex information can be obtained.

The nurse is encouraged to use the Data Base Assessment Guide in Appendix I as a tool for assessing adults according to functional health patterns. Special high-risk problems of the elderly include impaired mobility, falls, fall-related injuries, social isolation, impaired thought processes, incontinence, and losses (of meaning in life, function, significant others). Factors that identify elderly individuals at high risk for each problem are outlined in the section that follows.

High-Risk Profile for Impaired Mobility and Activities of Daily Living

- Advanced age
- Musculoskeletal disorders (joint pain and stiffness, deformity, limited range of motion, contractures, fracture, foot problems, amputation)
- Gait instability and balance disorders, vertigo
- Incontinence
- History of falling
- Pressure sores
- Cognitive impairment or depression
- Sensory deficits (visual, auditory, kinesthetic)
- Medications affecting sensorium: tranquilizers, sedatives, psychotropics, narcotic analgesics, hypnotics, antidepressants; and medications affecting blood pressure
- Easy fatigability related to low cardiac output, hypotension, sleep disorders, disuse atrophy and weakness, nutritional deficiency, hypoxia, anemia, depression

High-Risk Factors for Falls

- History of falls
- Sensory–motor deficits (*e.g.,* vision, hearing, hemianopsia, paresis, aphasia)
- Gait instability
- Improper footwear or foot problems (corns, bunions, calluses)
- Postural hypotension, especially with complaints of dizziness
- Confusion (persistent or acute)
- Incontinence, urinary urgency
- Cardiovascular disease affecting cerebral perfusion and oxygenation: dysrhythmias, syncopal episodes, congestive heart failure, fibrillation
- Neurological disease affecting movement or judgment: cerebrovascular accident with impulsivity; Parkinsonism; moderate Alzheimer's disease; seizure disorder, vertigo
- Orthopedic disorders or devices affecting movement or balance: casts, splints, slings, prostheses, recent surgery, severe arthritis
- Medications affecting blood pressure or level of consciousness: psychotropics, sedatives, analgesics, diuretics, antihypertensives, medication change, more than five drugs
- Agitation, increased anxiety, emotional lability
- Willfulness, uncooperativeness
- Situational factors: new admission, room change, roommate change

High-Risk Factors for Fall-Related Injury

- Debilitating disease conditions: cancer, advanced congestive heart failure and heart disease, multisystem failure, cardiovascular accident, parkinsonism, dementing illnesses
- Osteoporosis
- Advanced age

- Female
- History of falls
- Undernutrition
- History of fracture
- Use of mobility device
- Lives alone
- Relocation
- Cognitive impairment
- Impaired physical mobility (paresis, excessive fatigue, joint pain or deformity)
- Lack of or inadequate transportation
- Vision and hearing deficits that are uncorrected
- Incontinence
- Recent loss of spouse or significant relationship, including pet
- Advanced age
- Lack of at least one close affiliate (confidant)
- Depression
- Language and cultural barriers
- Communication disorders including aphasia
- Personal crisis and grief, anxiety

High-Risk Factors for Pain

- Chronic diseases such as arthritis, cardiovascular disease and angina, osteoporosis with vertebral compression, cancer
- Communication barriers (aphasia, dementing illnesses such as senile dementia, Alzheimer's type [SDAT], language barriers)
- Neurological deficits involving loss of sensation or pain (CVA, herpes zoster)
- Neuropathy (diabetes, peripheral neuropathy)
- Medications which alter sensorium (psychotropics, sedatives, hypnotics, narcotic analgesics, antidepressants)
- Emotional crises involving anxiety, grief, fear
- Disuse atrophy as a result of a greater degree of immobility when capabilities suggest a higher level of mobility
- Pain as a result of therapeutic treatment (iatrogenic), including surgical intervention

Pain assessment should include a pain history, pain coping inventory, and a pain record or diary (initiated at the first encounter). Assessment of pain coping is particularly important because it allows the nursing staff to assist, reinforce, and support the person's coping efforts and to back up his inner resources (Copp).

High-Risk Factors for Nutritional Deficiency

- Anorexia due to medications, grief, depression, illness
- Diuretic therapy which depletes fluid and electrolytes
- Lactose intolerance leading to avoidance of dairy products and as a result, insufficient calcium and vitamin D
- Impaired mental status (related to dementing illnesses, drugs, other diseases) leading to inattention to hunger or selecting insufficient kinds or amounts of foods
- Impaired mobility or manual dexterity (paresis, tremors, weakness, joint pain or deformity)
- Difficulty with chewing or swallowing
- Acute illness or disease which increases metabolic needs
- Urinary incontinence leading to voluntary fluid restriction

- Constipation or diarrhea may reduce appetite
- Food preferences (including cultural food traditions) not available or food preferences not sufficient to meet nutritional needs
- Lactose intolerance
- Small framed or history of undernutrition
- Inadequate income to purchase food
- Lack of transportation to buy food or facility to cook
- New dentures or poor dentition
- Dislike of cooking and eating alone
- Refusal to eat related to death wish or depression

Nutritional assessment may include a 24-hour recall, a 3-day diary, a food preference inventory, calorie count and food intake over a period of time, and other objective measures such as skinfold test, height and weight, and blood chemistries.

High-Risk Factors for Urinary Incontinence

- Female
- Acute illness
- Urinary tract infection
- Prostatic hyperplasia in men
- Constipation and stool impaction
- Neurologic impairment
- Relocation to a new equipment
- Impaired mobility including joint pain, stiffness, paresis, amputation, fracture, limited range of motion
- Impaired manual dexterity
- Impaired cognition, confusion
- Psychological disorders, especially depression
- Iatrogenic factors—medications that cause rapid bladder filling (diuretics), impair sensorium (sedatives, tranquilizers, hypnotics, narcotic analgesics), anticholinergics, calcium-channel-entry blockers, alpha-adrenoreceptor agonists and antagonists

High-Risk Factors for Acute Confusion

- Sensory deficits, especially if uncorrected
- Drugs with central nervous system effects: toxic effects and drug interactions
- Advanced age, especially over 80
- Living alone
- Social isolation
- Relocation
- Hospitalized, institutionalized
- Sensory overload or deprivation
- Postoperative status
- Use of tubes such as nasotracheal tubes, Foley and intravenous catheters
- Restraints
- Physiologic problems which interfere with oxygen transport: hypothermia, hyperthermia, dehydration or excessive hydration, hypoxia, hypotension
- Communication and language barriers
- Undernutrition
- Acute illness
- Anxiety and fear

High-Risk Factors for Hopelessness/Spiritual Distress

- Memory loss and cognitive impairment
- Institutionalization
- Life-threatening illness or disease
- Few or no family members or friends living
- Social isolation
- Psychological conditions, especially depression
- Impaired mobility
- Unresolved conflict or guilt
- Underdeveloped spiritual identity
- Inability to practice religious rituals

References/Bibliography

Brody J, Foley E: Epidemiologic considerations. In Schneider E (ed): The Teaching Nursing Home: A New Approach to Geriatric Research, Education, and Clinical Practice, pp 9–25. New York, Raven Press, 1985

Copp L: Pain coping model and typology. Image 17(3):69–71, 1985

Drugay M: Nutritional evaluation: Who needs it. J Gerontol Nurs 12(4):14–18, 1986

Hogue C: Mobility. In Schneider E (ed): The Teaching Nursing Home: A New Approach to Geriatric Research, Education, and Clinical Care, pp 231–244. New York, Raven Press, 1985

Kwentus J, Harkins S, Lignon N et al: Current concepts of geriatric pain and its treatment. Geriatrics 40(4):48–57, 1985

Pfeiffer E: A short portable mental status questionnaire for the assessment of organic brain deficit in elderly patients. J Am Geriatr Soc 23:433–437, 1975

Resnick N, Yalla S: Management of urinary incontinence in the elderly. N Engl J Med 313(13):800–805, 1985

Wolanin M, Phillips L: Confusion: Prevention and Care. St. Louis, CV Mosby, 1981

Appendix V: Maternal Data Base Assessment Guide

This data base is divided into four sections. Section I directs the initial data collection on admission to the labor and delivery unit. Section II focuses on the collection of specific data during the immediate postdelivery period. Section III, organized under the functional health patterns, focuses on the collection of data on the family unit after the immediate postdelivery period. In Section III, the nurse can choose to defer the collection of certain data that are determined to be inappropriate. Section IV represents a Parental–Infant Interaction Assessment that is initiated during labor and delivery and is completed on the postpartum unit.

I. Intrapartal Assessment

1. Support person present
2. Childbirth preparation classes (type, location)
3. Prenatal history
   - Estimated date of confinement (EDC)
   - Past/present medical problems
     - Hospitalizations
     - Infections
     - Diabetes mellitus
     - Hypertension
4. Contact with communicable disease (gonorrhea, herpes, rubella, measles, hepatitis, mumps, AIDS)
   - Medications taken during pregnancy
   - Gravida, para (abortions, C-sections, miscarriages)
   - Previous labor history (length, medications, problems)
   - Tobacco, alcohol, drug use
5. Labor history
   - When labor became apparent
   - Character and amount of show
   - Membranes (intact, ruptured, color)
   - Contractions (frequency, character)
6. Last food intake (time, type)
7. Last bowel movement
8. Present status
   - Rested
   - Alert
   - Tired
   - Excited
   - Exhausted
   - In control
   - Fearful
   - Out of control
   - Anxious
9. Physical assessment
   - Vital signs
   - Cervix (effacement, dilatation)
   - Contractions (frequency, character)
   - Urine (glucose, acetone)
   - Fetal heart sounds

II. Immediate Postdelivery Assessment

1. Physical assessment
   Vital signs
   Uterine involution (position in cm)
   Lochia (amount, color)
   Perineal area (episiotomy,
     lacerations)
   Breasts
   Bowel sounds
   Bladder (voiding, distention,
     incontinence)
2. Present status (mother, significant other)
   Emotional status (describe)   Discomforts (describe)

III. Postpartum Assessment

Assess each pattern for usual functioning and evaluate its impact on parenting, child care, and lactation as indicated. Proceed with health teaching under each pattern when indicated.

1. Health perception–health maintenance pattern
   "How would you usually describe your health?"
     Excellent   Fair
     Good   Poor
   "How would you describe your health at this time?
   Review the daily health practices of the individual (adults, children)
     Dental care   Exercise regimen
     Food intake   Leisure activities
     Fluid intake   Responsibilities in the family
   Use of
     Tobacco   Drugs (over-the-counter,
     Salt, sugar, fat products   prescribed)
     Alcohol
   Knowledge of safety practices
     Fire prevention   Automobile (maintenance, seat
     Water safety   belts, infant seats)
     Children/infants   Bicycle
                                         Poison control
   Knowledge of disease and preventive behavior
     Specific diseases (e.g., heart disease, cancer, respiratory disease, childhood
       diseases, infections, dental disease)
     Susceptibility (e.g., presence of risk factors, family history)
   "What do you do to keep healthy and to prevent disorders in yourself? In your
     children?"
     Adequate nutrition   Professional examinations
     Weight control   (gynecological,
     Exercise program   dental)
     Self-examinations (breast,   Immunizations
       testicular)
2. Nutritional–metabolic pattern
   "What is the usual daily food intake (meals, snacks)"
   "What is the usual fluid intake (type, amounts)?"
   "How is your appetite?"
     Indigestion   Vomiting
     Nausea   Sore mouth

"What are your food restrictions or preferences?"
"Any supplements (vitamins, feedings)?"
"Has your weight changed prior to pregnancy?" If yes, "Why?"
3. Elimination pattern
   Bladder
   "Are there any problems or complaints with the usual pattern of urinating?"

Oliguria	Retention
Polyuria	Burning
Dysuria	Stress incontinence
Dribbling	

   Bowel
   "What is the usual time, frequency, color, consistency, pattern?"
   "Assistive devices (type, frequency)?"

Enemas	Cathartics
Laxatives	Suppositories

4. Activity–exercise pattern
   "Describe usual daily/weekly activities of daily living."

Occupation	Exercise pattern (type,
Leisure activities	frequency)

   "Will you return to work? When?"
   "Are there factors present that could interfere with activities at home (self-care, home care)?"
   Lack of knowledge
   Lack of resources
5. Sleep–rest pattern
   "What is the usual sleep pattern?"

Bedtime	Sleep aids (medication, food)
Hours slept	Sleep routine

   "Any problems?"

Difficulty falling asleep	Not feeling rested after sleep
Difficulty remaining asleep	

6. Cognitive–perceptual pattern
   "Any deficits in sensory perception (hearing, sight, touch)?"

Glasses	Hearing aid

   "Any complaints?"

Vertigo	Insensitivity to cold or heat
Insensitivity to superficial pain	

   "Able to read and write?"
7. Self-perception pattern
   "What are you most concerned about?"
   "What are your present health goals?"
   "How would you describe yourself?"
   "Has being ill made you feel differently about yourself?"
   "How do you think your life will change with this baby?"
8. Role-relationship pattern
   Relationships
   "To whom do you turn for help in time of need?"
   Assess family life (members, educational level, occupations)

Cultural background	Decision-making
Activities (lone or group)	Communication patterns
Roles	Finances

"Any complaints?"
    Parenting difficulties
    Difficulties with relative
        (in-laws, parents)

Marital difficulties
Abuse (physical, verbal,
    substance

9. Sexuality–reproductive pattern
    Age at menarche
    Contraceptive use (type, years of use)
    Leukorrhea, vaginal itching, postcoital bleeding, pain, or cystitis
    Sexual activities
        "Have you been satisfied with the quality and quantity of your sexual
            activities (your partner)?"
        "Any pain or discomfort with intercourse?"
        "Has there been or do you expect a change in your sexual relations (related to
            pregnancy, child care, breast feeding)?"

10. Coping–stress pattern
    Δ "How do you make decisions (alone, with assistance, with whom)?"
    Δ "Has there been a loss in your life in the past year (or changes—moves, job,
        health)?"
    "What do you like about yourself?"
    "What would you like to change in your life?"
    "What is preventing you?"
    "What do you do when you are tense or under stress (*e.g.*, problem-solve, eat,
        sleep, take medication, seek help)?"

11. Values–belief pattern
    "With what (whom) do you find a source of strength or meaning?"

12. Physical assessment
    General appearance
    Weight and height
    Eyes (appearance, drainage)
        Pupils (size, equal, reactive to light)
        Vision (glasses)
    Mouth
        Mucous membrane (color, moisture, lesions)
        Teeth (condition, loose, broken, dentures)
    Hearing (hearing aids)
    Pulses (radial, apical, peripheral)
        Rate, rhythm, volume
    Respirations
        Rate, quality, breath sounds (upper and lower lobes)
    Blood pressure
    Temperature
    Skin (color, temperature, turgor)
        Lesions, edema, pruritus
    Uterine involution (position in cm)
    Lochia (amount, color)
    Perineal area (episiotomy, lacerations)
    Breasts
    Bowel sounds
    Bladder (voiding, distention, incontinence)

IV. Parental–Infant Interaction Assessment

Place check marks in front of data that are present. Add additional data as indicated.
A. Delivery room assessment
  1. Attempts to see infant as soon as delivered
  2. Response
    Happy   Angry
    Disappointed   Ambivalent
    Apathetic   Sad
  3. Holds and talks to infant
  4. Uses baby's name
  5. Response to partner
    Happy   Angry
    Ignores him   Indifferent
B. Postpartum assessment
  1. Verbal responses of mother
    Verbalizes positive feelings
    Seeks proximity by holding infant closely; touches and hugs
    Smiles and gazes at infant; seeks eye-to-eye contact
    Seeks family resemblance (*i.e.,* "has my eyes," "sleeps like his father")
    Refers to infant by name and sex
    Expresses interest in learning infant care
    Performs nurturing behavior (*i.e.,* feeding, changing)
  2. Requests that baby be taken to nursery
  3. Complains about baby
  4. Does not refer to baby by name
  5. Nonverbal responses of mother*
    Looks, reaches out to baby   Tenses face, arms
    Hugs, kisses baby   Turns head from baby
    Smiles at baby   Unresponsive to partner/nurse
    Positive eye contact with partner Doesn't touch baby
    Holds hand of partner   Doesn't look at baby
    Breast-feeds baby   Pushes baby away
    Sleepy, not drug-induced Cries unhappily
  Comments:

_____

_____

* Source: Neeson JD, May KA: Comprehensive Maternity Nursing, p 646. Philadelphia, JB Lippincott, 1986

Appendix VI: Noninvasive Pain Relief Techniques

Noninvasive pain relief techniques are external measures that influence the person internally.

General Principles

1. Convey to the person that you believe that the pain is present.
2. Explain the relationship of stress and muscle tension to pain.
3. Explain the various methods of relief and allow the person to choose one or two.
4. Attempt to teach the method when pain is absent or mild.
5. Perform the technique with the person to coach him and encourage him to focus on details of the distraction.
6. Encourage the person to practice the technique when the pain is mild.
7. Teach the person to use the technique before feeling pain (if the pain can be anticipated) and to increase the complexity of the distraction as the pain increases in intensity (*e.g.,* increase the volume of music via earphones as discomforts increase during a bone-marrow aspiration).
8. Inform others (staff, family) about the technique and its purpose.
9. Explain that noninvasive pain relief can be utilized with medications and usually increases their effects.

Specific Techniques

- Distraction
- Cutaneous stimulation
- Relaxation

Distraction

Distraction is the deliberate focusing of attention on stimuli other than the pain sensation. The ability to be distracted from pain does not denote that the pain is nonexistent or mild. Even persons with severe pain can choose to be distracted from their pain.

Distraction can be taught to children. (Caution parent not to confuse this therapeutic distraction technique that the child chooses to practice with the surprise distraction of a child prior to painful events. This latter technique serves only to produce feelings of mistrust and fear in children.)

Distraction cannot usually be practiced for very long periods. After the distraction ends, the person may have an increased awareness of the pain and fatigue.

1. Examples of distraction methods
   a. Visual distractions
      - Counting objects (flowers on wallpaper, spots on wall, animals in picture, someone's blinks)
      - Describe objects (pictures, slides)
   b. Auditory distractions (songs, tapes)
   c. Tactile kinesthetic distractions (holding, stroking, rocking, rhythmic breathing)
   d. Guided imagery (see Appendix X)

2. Breathing techniques
   a. Slow rhythmic
      - Have person take slow deep breaths through nose and exhale through mouth
      - Try to slow rate to nine breaths a minute if possible
      - Instruct person to take extra breaths if needed
   b. Heartbeat breathing (McCaffery). Teach person to
      - Take a slow deep breath
      - Count pulse on wrist
      - Inhale as you count two beats
      - Exhale as you count the next three beats
   c. He-who breathing (McCaffery). Instruct person to
      - Take a slow deep breath
      - Inhale and say *he* on inhaling
      - Exhale and say *who* on exhaling
      - Rate can be increased (should not exceed 40 per minute) if pain increases

Cutaneous Stimulation

Cutaneous stimulation is stimulation of the skin's surface. Examples of methods follow.
1. Massage
   Rub with warm lubricant over painful part or over the opposite adjacent part if the actual painful part cannot be massaged (*e.g.,* if a fractured left leg is casted, the person can massage the fracture site on the right leg)
2. Application of cold
   a. The therapeutic effects of cold are (Lehmann et al)
      Reduces small-diameter nerve conduction, which lessens the perception of pain
      Decreases the inflammatory response of tissues
      Decreases blood flow
      Decreases edema
   b. The use of cold is indicated with
      Trauma (first 24–48 hours)
      Fractures
      Insect bites
      Hemorrhage
      Muscle spasms
      Rheumatoid arthritis (if relief is acquired)
      Pruritus
      Headaches
   c. The use of cold is contraindicated
      With Raynaud's disease
      With cold allergy
      48 hours after trauma
   d. Guidelines for use of cold
      - Protect skin from cold burn (*e.g.,* layers of cloth between skin and cold source)
      - Caution its use with persons with limited communication ability or decreased sensorium (infants, sedated persons)
      - Caution its use on areas with impaired sensation (*e.g.,* diabetic's foot)
   e. Examples of cold application methods
      Towel or washcloth soaked in ice water and wrung out
      Ice bags (Zip-loc plastic bag filled with ice water or frozen)

        Reusable gel pak (stored in refrigerator or freezer)

        Massage of painful site with ice

3. Application of heat

  a. The therapeutic uses of heat are

        Slows small-diameter nerve conduction, which lessens the perception of pain

        Increases the inflammatory response of stress

        Increases blood flow

        Increases edema

  b. The use of heat is indicated with

        Trauma (past 48 hours)

        Cystitis

        Hemorrhoids

        Backache

        Arthritis (if relief is attained)

        Bursitis

  c. The use of heat is contraindicated with

        Trauma (first 24–48 hours)

        Edema/hemorrhage

        Vascular insufficiency

        Malignant sites

        Pruritus

  d. Examples of heat application methods

        Towel or washcloth soaked in warm water and wrung out (cover cloth with plastic around area to trap heat longer)

        Heating pads (moist or dry)

        Warm bath or shower

        Sunbathing

        Moist heat pack (commercially available)

4. External analgesic preparations (McCaffery)

        External analgesic preparations—ointments, lotions, liniments—produce a sensation (usually warmth) that may persist for several hours

  a. Guidelines for use

      • Do not use on broken skin

      • Do not apply to mucous membranes (anus, vagina)

      • Always skin-test each product before using

      • Follow directions and use sparingly or painful burning may occur

  b. Examples of external analgesic preparations

        Products with methyl salicylate (oil of wintergreen)

        Products with menthol

Relaxation

Relaxation is a state of relief from skeletal muscle tension that the person achieves through the practice of deliberate techniques

1. The therapeutic effects of relaxation are that it

        Decreases anxiety

        Provides the person with some control over pain

        Decreases skeletal muscle tension

        Serves as a distraction from pain

2. Examples of relaxation techniques

        Biofeedback

Yoga
Meditation
Progressive relaxation exercises (see Appendix X)

References/Bibliography

Benson H: The Relaxation Response. New York, Avon Books, 1976
Breeden SA, Kondo C: Using biofeedback to reduce tension. Am J Nurs 75:2010–2012, 1975
Brown B: Stress and the Art of Biofeedback. New York, Bantam Books, 1977
Donovan M: Relaxation with guided imagery: A useful technique. Cancer Nursing 3(1):27–32, 1980
Flynn PAR: Holistic Health. Maryland, Chap 3. Psychosomatics. Robert J Brady, 1980
Lehmann JF, Warren CG, Scham SM: Therapeutic heat and cold. Clin Orthop 99:207–245, 1974
McCaffery M: Pain relief for the child: Problem areas and selected non-pharmacological methods. Pediatric Nursing 3(4):11–16, 1977
McCaffery M: Technique to help a patient relax. Am J Nurs 77:794–795, 1977
McCaffery M: Nursing Management of the Patient with Pain, 2nd ed, Chapters 7 and 8. Philadelphia, JB Lippincott, 1979
McCoy P: Further proof that touch speaks louder than words. RN 40(11):43–46, 1977
Mennell JM: The therapeutic use of cold. American Osteopathic Journal 74:1146–1158, 1975
Michelsen D: Giving a back rub. Am J Nurs 78:1197–1199, 1978
Petrello JM: Temperature maintenance of hot moist compresses. Am J Nurs 73:1050–1051, 1973
Simonton C, Mathews-Simonton S, Creighton J: Getting Well Again: A Step-by-Step Self-Help Guide to Overcoming Cancer for Patients and Their Families. Los Angeles, JP Tarcher, 1978
Wilson RL: An introduction to yoga. Am J Nurs 76:261–263, 1976

Appendix VII: Guidelines for Problem-Solving and Crisis Intervention

The two basic coping behaviors in response to problems are emotion-focused behaviors and problem-focused behaviors.*

Emotion-Focused Behaviors

1. *Minimization* occurs when the seriousness of a problem is minimized. This may be useful as a way to provide needed time for appraisal, but it may become dysfunctional when it precludes appraisal.
2. *Projection, displacement, and suppression of anger* occur when anger is attributed to or expressed toward a less threatening person or thing, which may reduce the threat enough to allow an individual to deal with it. Distortion of reality and disturbance of relationships may result, which further compound the problem. Suppression of anger may result in stress-related physical symptoms.
3. *Anticipatory preparation* is the mental rehearsal of possible consequences of behavior or outcomes of stressful situations, which provides the opportunity to develop perspective as well as to prepare for the worst. It becomes dysfunctional when the anticipation creates unmanageable stress, as, for example, in anticipatory mourning.
4. *Attribution* is the finding of personal meaning in the problem situation, which may be religious faith or individual belief. Examples are fate, the will of the divine, luck. Attribution may offer consolation but becomes maladaptive when all sense of self-responsibility is lost.

Problem-Focused Behaviors

1. *Goal-setting* is the conscious process of setting time limitations on behaviors, which is useful when goals are attainable and manageable. It may become stress-inducing if unrealistic or short-sighted.
2. *Information-seeking* is the learning about all aspects of a problem, which provides perspective and, in some cases, reinforces self-control.
3. *Mastery* is the learning of new procedures or skills, which facilitates self-esteem and self-control: for example, self-care of colostomies, insulin injection, or catheter care.
4. *Help-seeking* is the reaching out to others for support. Sharing feelings with others provides an emotional release, reassurance, and comfort, as, for example, with Weight Watchers and other self-help and support groups.

Problem-Solving Techniques

1. Identify the problem
    What is wrong?
    What are the causes?
    Refer to pertinent literature, individuals, and organizations for more knowledge about the problem, if indicated
2. Find the cause
    Who or what is responsible for the problem?

* Lazarus RS, Folkman S: Analysis of coping in a middle-age community sample. J Health Soc Behav 21(9):219–239, 1980

How have you contributed to the problem?

Put yourself in the place of each person and consider the problem from his perspective

3. Discover the options

What are your goals?

What do you want to accomplish?

What are the goals of the others involved in the problem?

List all possible options for dealing with the problem (including not doing anything)

4. List advantages and disadvantages for each option

What will happen if you do nothing?

What is the worst thing that could happen with each option?

5. Choose an option and a plan

What preparation do you need before implementing the plan?

How do others fit into the plan?

How will you know if the plan is working or not?

Guidelines for Crisis Intervention

1. Assist the victim to confront reality (*e.g.*, encourage viewing of dead body)
2. Encourage persons involved to display emotions of crying and anger (within limits)
3. Do not encourage the person to focus on all the implications of the crisis at once—*e.g.*, divorce, death—for they may too overwhelming
4. Avoid giving false reassurances such as "It will be all right" or "Don't worry"
5. Clarify fantasies with facts: encourage verbalization to assist with catharsis and to identify misinformation
6. Avoid encouraging person or family to blame others, but allow ventilation of anger (*e.g.*, rape)
7. Encourage person or family to seek help and validate its acceptability (*e.g.*, "A friend of mine found the American Cancer Society very helpful")
8. Assist person or family to identify resources (agencies, people) to help with everyday tasks of living until resolution is attained

Appendix VIII: Guidelines for Preparing Diagnostic Categories*

Components

A. *Name:* This part provides a name for the diagnosis, a concise phrase, term, or label.
B. *Definition:* This part provides a clear, precise definition of the named diagnosis. The definition expresses the essential nature of the diagnosis named and delineates its meaning. The definition should enable one to differentiate this diagnosis from all others.
C. *Defining Characteristics:* This part provides the clinical criteria that validate the presence of the diagnosis. These criteria are observable or reportable cues. For actual nursing diagnoses, defining characteristics are signs and symptoms separated into two sets: major and minor.
   1. Major defining characteristics: Those that appear to be present in 80% or more clients experiencing the diagnosis (research-based).
   2. Minor defining characteristics: Those that appear to be present in 50%–79% of the clients experiencing the diagnosis (research-based).
For potential nursing diagnoses the defining characteristics are risk factors
D. *Substantiating/supportive materials:* This part provides documentation that substantiates the existence, nature, and characteristics of the phenomena of concern. Minimal validation documentation is a narrative review of relevant literature.

Proposed New Nursing Diagnostic Category: Optional Components for Submission

A. *Supplemental information:* The following types of supplemental information may be submitted to further clarify the nursing phenomena identified by the proposed nursing diagnosis.
   1. *Related factors*[†]: In some cases, there may be specific factors that appear to show some type of patterned relationship with the phenomena of concern, named as a nursing diagnosis. Where this situation exists, it may be helpful to name and describe these. Such factors may be described variously as antecedent to, associated with, related to, contributing to, or abetting.
   2. *Sources of variance:* In some cases, unique sources of variance in the experience of the phenomena may be possible. Where this situation exists, it may be helpful to identify these. Such sources of variance may include developmental stage variance, ethnic or cultural variance, levels of risk variance, acuity variance, and multidiagnosis variance.
B. *Supplemental validation:* If it is available, supplemental validation of the nursing diagnosis may be submitted. This may include research abstracts, brief reports of validation projects, or reports of intervention or treatment studies.

---

* Source: North American Nursing Diagnosis Association, St. Louis University School of Nursing, 3525 Caroline Street, St. Louis, MO 63104
† Etiology was deleted as a requirement for submission but can be optional.

Appendix IX: Guidelines for Play Therapy

Play is a natural means of expression for children and is essential to their mental, emotional, and social well-being. The need for play during stress (*e.g.*, developmental, illness, treatments) is essential in order to provide the child with an outlet for emotional release and a sense of mastery over the situation. Play provides parents and professionals with opportunities to assess the mood, words, and actions of a child and identify the child's present perception of the situation.

A. General

1. Professionals and parents utilize play to assist the child to
   Recognize his feelings
   Cope with a new concept
   Identify his fears
   Understand threatening or unknown events
   Clarify distortions received from others (parents, peers)
   Gain a sense of mastery
2. Play can be utilized to diagnose the child's perception of the situation, his perception of caregivers, and his mental responses to events
3. Guidelines for therapeutic play
   Promote spontaneity by reflecting only what the child expresses
   Avoid forcing the child to participate
   Allow sufficient time without interruption
   Identify when it is appropriate to encourage child to share concerns
   Play for the child who cannot play for himself
   Allow child to work freely on his project without direction or adult comment
   Allow child to engage in violent nondestructive acts

B. Types of play

1. Drawing and painting
   • Supplies: Crayons, paint, brushes, paper
      Artwork usually requires little direction
      Older children can be asked to draw what they like or do not like about the hospital
      An old sheet can cover the bed clothes of a child confined to bed
      Ask child to explain picture when it is done
      Clarify misconceptions
2. Dramatic play
   • Supplies: Puppets, dolls, stuffed animals, replicas of hospital equipment, actual hospital equipment, miniature hospital furniture
      Assign roles to the child and to the doll or puppet ("Mary, you are the nurse and the puppet is you")
      Ask child to administer a treatment to the puppet or doll
      Supervise the child when playing with equipment

3. Needle play (dramatic play)
- Supplies: Doll, stuffed animals, clean syringes and needles, alcohol wipes, water vial, Band-Aids, miniature IV sets (tubing, tourniquets, tongue blade for arm board)

>>>Introduce immediately after or in between the child's experiences
>>>Expect reluctance to touch syringe
>>>Demonstrate injection and ask the child to help you push the fluid in
>>>Allow child to give injections on the doll anywhere and however he wants to
>>>Make appropriate sounds of crying and protest to show the child that crying is permitted
>>>Show child how to give the doll love after the injection
>>>Encourage child to talk about why injections are needed
>>>Use group play to encourage participation
>>>Overly aggressive children should be shown acceptance

References/Bibliography

Axline V: Play Therapy. New York, Ballantine Books, 1969

Brooks M: Why play in the hospital? Nurs Clin North Am 5:431–441, 1970

Levinson P, Ousterhout D: Art and play therapy with pediatric burn patients. Journal of Burn Care and Rehabilitation 1(5):42–46, 1980

Oehler J: The frog family books: Color the pictures sad or glad. Matern Child Nurs J 6:281–283, 1981

Petrillo M, Sanger S: Emotional Care of Hospitalized Children, 2nd ed. Philadelphia, JB Lippincott, 1980

Smallwood S: Preparing children for surgery. AORN, 47(1):177–182, 1988

Taylor M, Williams H: Use of therapeutic play in the ambulatory pediatric hematology clinic. Cancer Nursing 3:433–437, 1980

Resources for Parents and Children

Literature

Books That Help Children Deal with a Hospital Experience (Publication number 017-031-00020-1)

When Your Child Goes to the Hospital (Publication number 793-30092)

A Reader's Guide for Parents of Children with Mental, Physical, or Emotional Disabilities. (Publication number [HSA]77-5290). An annotated reference on basic reading, books on teaching and playing at home, books that deal with particular issues, and books written by parents and children.

The foregoing three titles are available from the U.S. Government Printing Office, Washington, DC 20402

Preparing Children and Families for Health Care Encounters. A compilation of articles for parents and professionals on various aspects of preparation. Available from the Association for the Care of Children's Health, 3615 Wisconsin Avenue NW, Washington, DC 20016

Appendix X: Stress Management Techniques

The following techniques can be taught to provide an individual with an opportunity to control his response to stressors and, in turn, increase his ability to manage stress constructively. Suggested readings are listed at the end to provide more specific information.

Progressive Relaxation Technique

Progressive relaxation is a self-taught or instructed exercise that involves learning to constrict and relax muscle groups in a systematic way, beginning with the face and finishing with the feet. This exercise may be combined with breathing exercises that focus on inner body processes. It usually takes 15 to 30 minutes and may be accompanied by a taped instruction that directs the person concerning the sequence of muscles to be relaxed.

1. Wear loose clothing; remove glasses and shoes.
2. Sit or recline in a comfortable position with neck and knees supported; avoid lying completely flat
3. Begin with slow, rhythmic breathing
   a. Close your eyes or stare at a spot and take in a slow deep breath
   b. Exhale the breath slowly
4. Continue rhythmic breathing at a low steady pace and feel the tension leaving your body with each breath
5. Begin progressive relaxation of muscle groups
   a. Breathe in and tense (tighten) your muscles and then relax the muscles as you breathe out
   b. Suggested order for tension-relaxation cycle (with tension technique in parentheses)
      Face, jaw, mouth (squint eyes, wrinkle brow)
      Neck (pull chin to neck)
      Right hand (make a fist)
      Right arm (bend elbow in tightly)
      Left hand (make a fist)
      Left arm (bend elbow in tightly)
      Back, shoulders, chest (shrug shoulders up tightly)
      Abdomen (pull stomach in and bear down on chair)
      Right upper leg (push leg down)
      Right lower leg and foot (point toes toward body)
      Left upper leg (push leg down)
      Left lower leg and foot (point toes toward body)
6. Practice technique slowly
7. End relaxation session when you are ready by counting to three, inhaling deeply, and saying, "I am relaxed"

Self-coaching

Self-coaching is a procedure to decrease anxiety by understanding one's own signs of anxiety (such as increased heart rate or sweaty palms) and then coaching oneself to relax.

For example, "I am upset about this situation but I can control how anxious I get. I will take things one step at a time, and I won't focus on my fear. I'll think about what I must do to finish this task. The situation will not be forever. I can manage until it is over. I'll focus on taking deep breaths."

Thought Stopping

Thought stopping is a self-directed behavioral procedure learned to gain control of self-defeating thoughts. Through repeated systematic practice, a person does the following:
1. Says "Stop" when a self-defeating thought crosses the mind (*e.g.*, "I'm not smart enough" or "I'm not a good nurse")
2. Allows a brief period—15 to 30 seconds—of conscious relaxation (because of an increased focus on negative thoughts, it may seem at first that self-defeating thoughts increase; however, eventually the self-defeating thoughts will decrease)

Assertive Behavior

Assertive behavior is the open, honest, empathetic sharing of your opinions, desires, and feelings. Assertiveness is not a magical acquisition but learned behavioral skill. Assertive persons do not allow others to take advantage of them and thus are not victims. Assertive behavior is not domineering but remains controlled and non-aggressive. An assertive person

Does not hurt others

Does not wait for things to get better

Does not invite victimization

Listens attentively to the desires and feelings of others

Takes the initiative to make relationships better

Remains in control or uses silences as an alternative

Examines all the risks involved before asserting

Examines personal responsibilities in each situation before asserting

Refer to suggested readings for specific techniques or participate in an assertiveness training course led by a competent instructor. Assertive behavior is best learned slowly in several sessions rather than in one lengthy session or workshop.

Guided Imagery

This technique is the purposeful use of one's imagination in a specific way to achieve relaxation and control. The person concentrates on the image and pictures himself involved in the scene. The following is an example of the technique.
1. Discuss with person an image he has experienced that is pleasurable and relaxing to him, such as

Lying on a warm beach

Feeling a cool wave of water

Floating on a raft

Watching the sun set
2. Choose a scene that will involve at least two senses
3. Begin with rhythmic breathing and progressive relaxation
4. Have person travel mentally to the scene
5. Have the person slowly experience the scene; how does it look? sound? smell? feel? taste?
6. Practice the imagery
   a. Suggest tape-recording the imagined experience to assist with the technique

 b. Practice the technique alone to reduce feelings of embarrassment

7. End the imagery technique by counting to three and saying, "I am relaxed" (if the person does not utilize a specific ending, he may become drowsy and fall asleep, which defeats the purpose of the technique)

References/Bibliography

Alberti RE, Emmons L: Your Perfect Right: A Guide to Assertive Behavior, 2nd ed. San Luis Obispo, CA, Impact, 1974

Benson H: The Relaxation Response. New York, Avon Books, 1976

Bloom L, Coburn K, Pearlman J: The New Assertive Woman. New York, Dell, 1976

Chenevert M: Special Techniques in Assertiveness Training for Women in the Health Professions. St. Louis, CV Mosby, 1978

Gridano D, Everly G: Controlling Stress and Tension. Englewood Cliffs, NJ, Prentice-Hall, 1979

Herman S: Becoming Assertive: A Guide for Nurses. New York, D Van Nostrand, 1978

Hill L, Smith N: Self-Care Nursing. Englewood Cliffs, NJ, Prentice-Hall, 1985 (especially Part II, Self-Care Primarily Associated with the Mind)

McCaffery M: Nursing Management of the Patient with Pain, 2nd ed. Philadelphia, JB Lippincott, 1979 (especially Chapter 10, Imagery; Chapter 9, Relaxation)

Appendix XI: Collaborative Problems*

Potential Complication: Gastrointestinal–Hepatic

PC: Paralytic Ileus/Small Bowel Obstruction
PC: Hepatorenal Syndrome
PC: Hyperbilirubinemia
PC: Evisceration
PC: Hepatosplenomegaly
PC: Curling's Ulcer
PC: Ascites
PC: G.I. Bleeding

Potential Complication: Metabolic/Immune

PC: Hypoglycemia
PC: Hyperglycemia
PC: Negative Nitrogen Balance
PC: Electrolyte Imbalances
PC: Thyroid Dysfunction
PC: Hypothermia (severe)
PC: Hyperthermia (severe)
PC: Sepsis
PC: Acidosis/Alkalosis
PC: Diabetes
PC: Anasarca
PC: Hypo/Hyperthyroidism
PC: Allergic Reaction
PC: Donor Tissue Rejection
PC: Adrenal Insufficiency

Potential Complication: Neurologic/Sensory

PC: Increased Intracranial Pressure
PC: Stroke
PC: Seizures
PC: Spinal Cord Compression
PC: Autonomic Dysreflexia
PC: Birth Injuries
PC: Hydrocephalus
PC: Microcephalus
PC: Meningitis
PC: Cranial Nerve Impairment

* The most frequently used collaborative problems are represented on this list.

PC: Paresis/Paresthesia/Paralysis
PC: Peripheral Nerve Impairment
PC: Increased Intraocular Pressure
PC: Corneal Ulceration
PC: Neuropathies

Potential Complication: Cardiovascular

PC: Dysrhythmias
PC: Congestive Heart Failure
PC: Cardiogenic Shock
PC: Thromboemboli/Deep Vein Thrombosis
PC: Hypovolemic Shock
PC: Peripheral Vascular Insufficiency
PC: Hypertension
PC: Congenital Heart Disease
PC: Thrombocytopenia
PC: Polycythemia
PC: Anemia
PC: Compartmental Syndrome
PC: Disseminated Intravascular Coagulation
PC: Endocarditis
PC: Sickling Crisis
PC: Embolism (air, fat)
PC: Spinal Shock
PC: Ischemic Ulcers

Potential Complication: Respiratory

PC: Atelectasis/Pneumonia
PC: Asthma
PC: C.O.P.D
PC: Pulmonary Embolism
PC: Pleural Effusion
PC: Tracheal Necrosis
PC: Ventilator Dependency
PC: Pneumothorax
PC: Laryngeal Edema

Potential Complication: Renal/Urinary

PC: Acute Urinary Retention
PC: Renal Failure
PC: Bladder Perforation

Potential Complication: Reproductive

PC: Fetal Compromise
PC: Uterine Atony
PC: Pregnancy-Induced Hypertension
PC: Eclampsia

PC: Hydramnios
PC: Hypermenorrhea
PC: Polymenorrhea
PC: Syphilis

Potential Complication: Muscular/Skeletal

PC: Stress Fractures
PC: Osteoporosis
PC: Joint Dislocation

Lynda Juall Carpenito

Index

Page numbers in *italics* indicate illustrations; those followed by t indicate tables.